# Beyond
# Food Labels

# Beyond Food Labels

**EATING HEALTHY WITH THE % DAILY VALUES**

## Roberta Schwartz Wennik, M.S., R.D.

A PERIGEE BOOK

A Perigee Book
Published by The Berkley Publishing Group
200 Madison Avenue
New York, NY 10016

Copyright © 1996 by Roberta Schwartz Wennik, M.S., R.D.
Book design by Irving Perkins Associates
Cover design by James R. Harris
Photograph of the author on page 399 by Yuen Lui Studios.

First edition: May 1996

Published simultaneously in Canada.

The Putnam Berkley World Wide Web site address is
http://www.berkley.com

**Library of Congress Cataloging-in-Publication Data**

Wennik, Roberta Schwartz.
    Beyond food labels : eating healthy with percentage daily values /
Roberta Schwartz Wennik. — 1st ed.
        p.    cm.
    "A Perigee book."
    ISBN 0-399-52201-8
    1. Nutrition—Tables.    2. Food—Composition—Tables.    I. Title.
TX551.W44    1996
641—dc20                                                                    95-40407
                                                                                    CIP

Printed in the United States of America

10  9  8  7  6  5  4  3  2  1

*This is for Annette Schwartz, my mother (1918–1993).*
*When I was younger, she told me I should become a writer.*
*I only wish she were here to see her vision come true.*

*And for Ernest Schwartz, my father (1918–1996).*
*He showed me by his actions that nothing is impossible*
*if you believe in it strongly.*

# Acknowledgments

To my dear husband, Larry, who has supported me and been there for me each step of the way. You're a great sounding board, critic, proofreader, and believer.

To my wonderful girls, Debbie and Shari, who tolerated listening to all my nutrition facts to finally find it was worthwhile stuff.

Many, many thanks to my literary agent, Judith Riven, who saw the potential in this book and had the expertise to see it through on its journey. I have appreciated your abilities, your encouragement and the friendship we've developed.

And thank you, Debra Waterhouse, M.P.H., R.D., for telling me about Judith Riven.

Where would a book be without its editor? John Duff is a great person to work with: patient, instructive, supportive, with invaluable input and excellent guidance.

Thanks to my family, friends, and colleagues. Forgive me for not mentioning you all by name; but if I do, this will begin to sound like an awards ceremony.

# Contents

# Healthy Facts

As you wheel your cart down the supermarket aisle, you'll notice more people stopping to read food labels. As a health-conscious consumer, it's the smart thing to do. With so many foods from which to choose, it's the information on the label that can help you make your selection, from the words on the front of the package to the nutrient values listed on the side. This book not only explains what's on the label and how to use it, but provides the % Daily Values (percent daily values) for over 10,000 foods.

You may not be familiar with % Daily Values (% DV) yet, but after reading this book, you will come to appreciate that it is one of the most useful numbers on the new label. With it you can see how a food fits into your nutrient allowance for the day. No longer will you judge foods as "good" or "bad." It's just a matter of balancing your selection of foods to make up a healthful diet. Because a food is, say, high in fat, doesn't mean you have to avoid it. As long as your nutrient account (just as with your bank account) still has some "funds" available, you can spend it as you wish.

## A Brief History

The new food labeling has come a long way since 1906, when Congress passed both the Federal Food and Drugs Act and Federal Meat Inspection Act. Back then, the main concern of Congress was regulating the safety and quality of our food supply. By 1938, there was a move to include more information on the label. All products had to display the name of the food, its net weight, and the name and address of the manufacturer. Certain products also had to list ingredients.

During the 1940s, lawmakers didn't foresee the day scientists would find a link between the foods we eat and chronic diseases. The major concern had been to be sure people were getting enough of certain vitamins and minerals. By the 1950s, evidence pointed to a connection between high blood cholesterol and heart disease. However, the Food and

Drug Administration (FDA) wouldn't allow health claims on the labels. It felt that the cholesterol/heart disease relationship and the effects of fat from food hadn't been firmly proven. It wasn't until 1965 that the FDA finally allowed the statement "Information on fat and cholesterol is provided for individuals who, on the advice of a physician, are modifying their dietary intake of fat and cholesterol."

By the 1970s, the FDA set up a voluntary nutrition labeling program. Only fortified foods or foods that made **nutrient content claims** had to include information about calories, protein, fat, carbohydrate, and eight vitamins and minerals. To provide uniformity, this information had to be arranged on the label in a specific way. Serving size, servings per container, calories, and the major nutrients were listed first, followed by the percentages of the U.S. Recommended Daily Allowances (U.S. RDA) for the required vitamins and minerals.

At the time, a favorite nutrient content claim to entice you to buy a product was "Contains No Cholesterol." That the product was high in fat didn't seem to matter. With the media's help, many Americans were convinced a diet high in cholesterol could lead to high blood cholesterol, and, in turn, heart disease.

Even though a diet high in cholesterol can increase the risk of heart disease, it is total fat and, most especially, saturated fat, that are greater offenders. Since heart disease is the number-one killer in the United States, this book was written to help you keep your intake of these nutrients within healthy limits.

Today, the product must meet strict government standards for fat, cholesterol, and sodium to display statements such as "no cholesterol," "fat free," and "reduced calorie." When you see these claims, they have a uniform meaning.

In the late 1980s, the *Surgeon General's Report on Nutrition and Health* and *Diet and Health: Implications for Reducing Chronic Disease Risk* from the National Research Council of the National Academy of Sciences were published. The information they contained prompted the FDA and the Food Safety and Inspection Service (FSIS) to initiate a new effort toward food labeling reform. The FSIS is part of the U.S. Department of Agriculture (USDA), which governs meat and poultry products. The FDA regulates almost all other food products and ingredients added to food. After much debate in Congress concerning what should and should not be included on food labels, the Nutrition Labeling and Education Act (NLEA) was passed in 1990. NLEA gave the FDA the power to regulate and enact new labeling requirements.

Americans are interested in how nutrition can affect their health. Therefore, regulating **health claims** on the label is paramount on the FDA's agenda. It became an important issue in 1984 when a major cereal manufacturer placed a health message on one of its high-fiber products saying that the fiber in the cereal could reduce the risk of cancer. The FDA decided it was time to set down some rules.

The FDA now allows some claims that explain the relationship between particular nutrients and foods to diseases or health-related conditions. However, that's only after experts in the field have agreed that the scientific evidence resulting from well-designed studies confirms the relationship. An example of a health claim would be "While many factors affect heart disease, diets low in saturated fat and cholesterol may reduce the risk of the disease." No longer do you have to worry that this is sales hype by the food manufacturer to get you to buy the product. The product must be low in fat, cholesterol, and sodium to carry a health claim.

In 1991, the USDA/FSIS announced it would also enact the new labeling, even though neither Congress nor the NLEA required it. Labeling for all products would now be uniform. The government requires most processed meat and poultry foods (such as luncheon meats, hot dogs, chicken franks, ham, corned beef, burritos, and pizza) to have nutrition labeling. On the other hand, raw meats and poultry are presently only subject to voluntary nutrition labeling programs where the grocery store must display or provide a brochure with nutrient information. The FDA and USDA set May 1994 and July 1994, respectively, as the deadlines for manufacturers to change over to the new labeling.

Although restaurants are not required to provide nutrition facts for the dishes they serve, many fast food and convenience restaurants have been very good about giving the consumer that information. However, in most cases, they don't supply % Daily Values. Therefore, you should find the section in the back of the book on fast foods very helpful.

The old expression, "You can't tell a book by its cover," no longer applies to packaged foods. It's what's on the label that may make up your mind whether to purchase it or not. Considering that it is costing the food industry around $2 billion to change over to the new labeling, it's definitely a cover worth reading.

# 1. Reduce the Fat and Cholesterol: Just a Fad or Good Advice?

Being told to reduce the amount of fat and cholesterol you eat is good advice. It's one way you can decrease your risk of heart disease, cancer, diabetes, hypertension, and obesity.

You do need some fat in your diet, though. Fat helps transport the fat-soluble vitamins (A, D, E, and K) throughout your body. Fat acts as insulation against the cold, as well as serving as a shock absorber around your organs. It is an efficient form of storing energy, which your body calls upon at times of prolonged energy use. However, the average American eats far more fat than he or she needs, especially saturated fat, which contributes to high blood cholesterol.

As for dietary cholesterol, you could give up eating it entirely and your body would do fine. Your body is able to make all the cholesterol it needs. Cholesterol is a fatlike substance produced by the body that becomes part of cell membranes, hormones (such as estrogen, progesterone, and testosterone), and bile acids that help digest dietary fat. When you eat too much cholesterol, your body tries to compensate by making less.

Because fat and cholesterol are not water soluble, they are packaged in a way that allows them to travel around in the watery environment of the bloodstream. The liver encloses them in bundles called LDL cholesterol (low-density lipoprotein) and HDL cholesterol (high-density lipoprotein). You might have heard LDL cholesterol referred to as the "bad" cholesterol and HDL cholesterol as the "good" kind.

LDL cholesterol has its negative reputation because, as it travels around the bloodstream dropping off some of its fat and cholesterol content to the cells, it also may leave some in the bloodstream. There it can make its way into the walls of the arteries and possibly cause problems.

Cholesterol and fat can cause injury to the artery walls—something like a sore. The body's defense is to form a scab, such as you get when you cut yourself. In time, enough scarring or plaque can cause narrowing of the arteries, and, in turn, promote heart disease, hypertension, and a possible stroke.

Even after the LDL packets have dropped off some of their load, whether to the cells or the artery walls, they normally have some left. With whatever fat and cholesterol they still contain, the LDL packets travel back to the liver where the liver reabsorbs about 70% to 80% of them. Unfortunately, if the LDL packets are rich in saturated fat (because you have eaten a diet high in saturated fat), the liver closes its doors. The packets have to continue traveling around, dropping off more of their fat and cholesterol into the bloodstream as they do. The liver makes matters worse by continuing to make more LDL cholesterol.

HDL cholesterol, the "good" cholesterol, travels around the bloodstream trying to pick up the excess fat and cholesterol left behind by the LDL cholesterol, but HDL's holding capacity is limited. The more HDL cholesterol you have, the more efficient the cleanup. That's why it's worth having your blood tested for total cholesterol, LDL cholesterol, and HDL cholesterol. Look for a total cholesterol of less than 200 mg/dL (milligrams per deciliter), an LDL of less than 130 mg/dL, and an HDL of greater than 35 mg/dL. You can increase your HDL count with exercise and a low-fat diet.

One mistake many people make is thinking that foods contain LDL and HDL cholesterol. They do not. Cholesterol in food comes in just one kind: cholesterol. It's when it gets into your body that the liver packages it into LDL and HDL cholesterol bundles, which contain the cholesterol and fat you eat, along with that made by the liver.

The American Heart Association recommends you eat less than 30% of total calories from total fat, less than 10% of total calories from saturated fat, and less than 300 milligrams of cholesterol per day. By using this book and % Daily Values, you should be able to select foods that keep you within these guidelines.

# 2. The Food Label

Serving Size ①

List of Nutrients ③

Vitamins & Minerals ⑤

Calories Per Gram ⑦

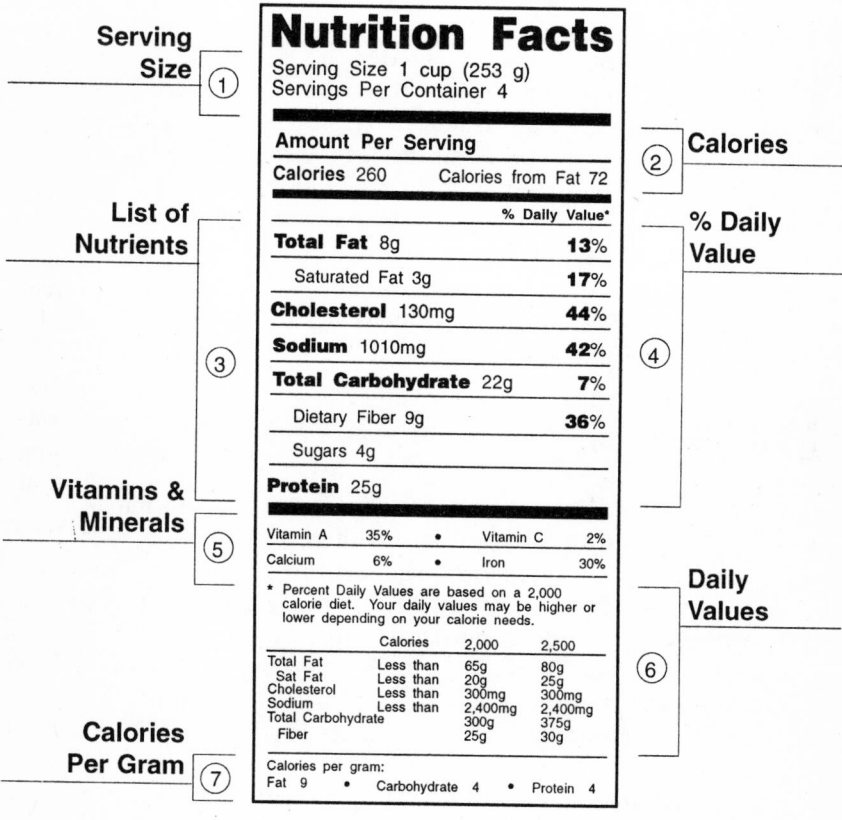

Calories ②

% Daily Value ④

Daily Values ⑥

## Nutrition Facts

Serving Size 1 cup (253 g)
Servings Per Container 4

**Amount Per Serving**

Calories 260          Calories from Fat 72

% Daily Value*

**Total Fat** 8g — **13%**

Saturated Fat 3g — **17%**

**Cholesterol** 130mg — **44%**

**Sodium** 1010mg — **42%**

**Total Carbohydrate** 22g — **7%**

Dietary Fiber 9g — **36%**

Sugars 4g

**Protein** 25g

Vitamin A 35%   •   Vitamin C 2%

Calcium 6%   •   Iron 30%

\* Percent Daily Values are based on a 2,000 calorie diet. Your daily values may be higher or lower depending on your calorie needs.

| | Calories | 2,000 | 2,500 |
|---|---|---|---|
| Total Fat | Less than | 65g | 80g |
| Sat Fat | Less than | 20g | 25g |
| Cholesterol | Less than | 300mg | 300mg |
| Sodium | Less than | 2,400mg | 2,400mg |
| Total Carbohydrate | | 300g | 375g |
| Fiber | | 25g | 30g |

Calories per gram:
Fat 9   •   Carbohydrate 4   •   Protein 4

Food Label for Chili

Most foods are displayed on the supermarket shelves so you can see the front of their packages. On the front you'll find the name of the product and the brand name (which could either be the manufacturer's name and/or the name of the product line). There will possibly be a short description of the contents and the weight. As you hold the package in your hand, turn it clockwise. You should now be looking at the nutrition information panel. It should say **"Nutrition Facts"** at the top and look like the example above.

The nutrients listed on the label are there because of their impact on such diseases as heart disease, high blood pressure, stroke, obesity, diabetes, osteoporosis, and some forms of cancer. These nutrients include: total fat, saturated fat, cholesterol, sodium, total carbohydrate, dietary fiber, sugars, protein, vitamins A and C, calcium, and iron. The label no longer must display the B vitamins since most people get a sufficient amount in their diets.

Some diseases may be related to an excess of certain nutrients, such as fat and cholesterol; others may be due to a deficiency of a nutrient in the diet, such as dietary fiber or calcium. That's why the recommended amounts for the nutrients listed on the bottom of the label (section 6, as shown on the illustration) for either a 2,000-calorie and 2,500-calorie diet are stated as maximums or minimums. The maximums for total fat, saturated fat, cholesterol, and sodium are not set as goals to achieve, but values not to exceed. The less you eat of these nutrients, the better. The minimums, set for carbohydrate and dietary fiber, are another story. Since most Americans don't eat enough dietary fiber, you may need to work on picking foods that are high in fiber.

## The New Format

The FDA conducted many studies to determine what format was the most useful and easiest to read. The result is the Nutrition Facts label you see on packaged foods today. The label is divided into numerous sections. **Serving Size** appears at the top (section ①), given in both metric weight and household measures (cups, tablespoons, slices, etc.).

Section ② provides **Total Calories Per Serving** and **Calories from Fat**. Some people feel there should have been one more number included in this section: percentage fat in the food. The FDA chose not to for a good reason.

The government recommends eating no more than 30% of **total** daily calories from fat. We're not talking here about individual foods, but the total intake for the day. However, many people mistakenly think that if any food contains more than 30% fat, it's off limits.

What if the new labels had included "% Calories From Fat"? These same people would look at the label on margarine or vegetable oil, for example, find they are 100% fat, and immediately put the products back on the shelf. With that kind of thinking, many foods, which could be part of a healthy diet, are avoided. That is why, instead, the FDA developed the concept of % Daily Values (% DV), which you can see in section ④. **(Just remember, it's the amount of fat eaten during an entire day that counts, not what is in one serving of a food.)**

% DVs help people learn to balance higher-fat foods with lower-fat ones. The numbers in section ④ will serve as your guide. They show you how much of your day's allowance for a nutrient you use up when eating the food. From that you can figure what you have left for the day. A quick example might help. A teaspoon of oil has a % DV of 8%. After eating the oil, you still have 92% of your daily fat allowance left to spend.

Just looking at the way the label displays % DVs tells you how important they are. They are set off in a column and presented in bold type. % DV will probably, in time and with use, be the standard to which people turn. It's so easy and tells you so much.

In a moment, we'll go into more detail about % DVs and how you can put those numbers to work for you. For now, just appreciate that the current government recommendations, known as **Daily Values** (found in section⑥), serve as the basis for the % DVs.

Section③ includes the list of **nutrients** with their gram or milligram values. The layout and bold letters help to bring attention to specific nutrient headings (total fat, cholesterol, sodium, total carbohydrate, and protein). Grams and milligrams are intentionally less conspicuous than % DVs to get readers of labels to rely more on % DVs than counting grams and milligrams.

Below sections ③ and ④ is the section with the **vitamins** and **minerals** (vitamins A and C, iron, and calcium)—the ones that are most often deficient in the diet. Cereal products tend to list the B vitamins, along with phosphorus, magnesium, zinc, and copper. While not required, the manufacturers provide this information since cereals are good sources of these nutrients. Vitamins and minerals, as with the other major nutrients, also have Daily Values (DVs). Their DVs are not listed on the label, but are shown as percentages. Looking at the label on page 7, you can see that a serving of chili provides you with 30% of the DV for iron. At this level, chili is a high source of iron. You're getting about a third of your day's iron needs in just one serving.

The sections so far mentioned provide product-specific information. The bottom sections, ⑥ and ⑦, on the other hand, give general information for interpreting the label values. This information, when included, will be the same no matter what the product. The footnote regarding calories per gram of fat, carbohydrate, and protein is there so you can convert the grams of these nutrients into calories, if you want. (If your calculations don't work out to the same answer as on the label, but are close, it's probably due to mathematical rounding.)

## Format Variations

In most cases, you will see the complete Nutrition Facts label on the foods you buy. However, you may see a shortened or simplified version depending upon what the food contains or the package size. The complete label, such as the one on page 7, includes the fourteen mandatory nutrients. If the package is too small to hold any of the information, the food manufacturer must provide its address or phone number so you can contact them if you want.

Some products may contain insignificant amounts of many of these nutrients (insignificant meaning zero or less than 1 gram). When this is true for at least half of the fourteen mandatory nutrients, the label must still display the five core nutrients (calories, total fat, sodium, total carbohydrate, and protein). If food manufacturers omit some nutrients, they may add the footnote, "Not a significant source of ——" listing those particular nutrients.

Another variation of the format appears on products that require additional preparation before eating. The FDA encourages food manufacturers to include the nutrient information for the product as it is in the package and also after preparation. For example, you may see two columns on a cake mix: the first column is for the mix in the box; the second column is for the cake prepared as instructed on the box.

The label for baby foods (for children under two years old) will not carry information about calories from fat or saturated fat, nor values for saturated fat, polyunsaturated fat, monounsaturated fat, and cholesterol. The exception to this is infant formula. Many people wrongly assume that, because they, as adults, are limiting their amount of fat, infants should also have their fat intake restricted. At this stage, adequate amounts of fat are necessary for growth and development. Not until a child has reached two years old, should fat be limited in the same proportions as an adult.

The labels on toddler foods (children under four) list % DVs for protein, vitamins, and minerals since the government has assigned DVs to these nutrients. Because total fat, saturated fat, cholesterol, sodium, total carbohydrate, and dietary fiber have no DVs set, the labels can't list % DVs for those nutrients.

## The Exemptions

Some foods are exempt from labeling. You won't find it on:

1. Foods served for immediate consumption (e.g., hospital cafeterias, airplanes)
2. Foods prepared on site and ready to eat, but not for immediate consumption (e.g., bakery, deli, candy store)

3. Foods shipped in bulk form
4. Foods sold by vendors (e.g., vending machines, mall cookie counters, sidewalk vendors)
5. Foods served in a restaurant (Voluntary labeling is permitted. If a restaurant makes any nutrient content claims or health claims, they must adhere to government standards.)
6. Foods that contain insignificant amounts of the nutrients (e.g., plain coffee, tea, some spices)
7. Foods produced by small businesses (based on number of employees and food sales)
8. Medical foods (e.g., foods to meet nutritional needs of patients with certain diseases)
9. Infant formulas

You also won't find labeling on raw foods. However, the FDA and USDA have asked supermarkets to voluntarily post Nutrition Facts for many raw foods. This applies to the most commonly eaten fruits, vegetables, and fish (twenty in each category), and the forty-five best-selling cuts of meat (red meats and poultry). Previously frozen meats are affected similarly. The supermarket must display this information in a visible place on a poster or in a brochure.

# 3. % Daily Value—A Piece of the Pie

% Daily Values are an important new addition to food labels. They represent a new approach to nutrition information where you don't judge a food by its specific grams or milligrams of a nutrient. The FDA, along with many health professionals, believe % DV will help people appreciate that no individual food is good or bad nutritionally. Rather, % DV is a way of looking at a food's nutrient contribution to the overall diet.

## Daily Values

To understand % DV, you first must know about **Daily Values**. Daily Values (DVs) are the currently accepted nutrition recommendations set by the government. They are based on eating 2,000 calories a day, a level referred to as the reference diet.

The DVs, which appear at the bottom of the label, are calculated as follows:

### CALCULATING DAILY VALUES

| Nutrient | Calculated As* | DV for 2,000 Calories |
|---|---|---|
| Total Fat | 30% of total calories | 65 g |
| Saturated Fat | 10% of total calories | 20 g |
| Total Carbohydrate | 60% of total calories | 300 g |
| Fiber | 11.5 g per 1,000 calories | 25 g |
| Cholesterol | — | 300 mg |
| Sodium | — | 2,400 mg |

g = gram    mg = milligram

* Some numbers may be rounded off for nutrition labeling.
• The DVs for cholesterol and sodium stay the same, 300 mg and 2,400 mg respectively, no matter the number of calories you need.
• Protein, while not included on the bottom of the label nor required to have % DV listed, is calculated as 10% of total calories. For 2,000 calories, the DV for protein is 50 g.

The FDA had to make a major decision (for labeling purposes) about what calorie level to select for the reference diet. It chose 2,000 calories because that level provides a midway point between the caloric needs of two groups. The first group with caloric needs less than 2,000 calories includes dieters, women, sedentary men, and older people. On the other hand, many men, athletes, and more active people fall into the second group whose needs are greater.

Originally, the FDA wanted to set the level at 2,300 calories. However, many health professionals argued against it, stating it was too high a level for too many Americans. As a compromise, the FDA set the reference diet at 2,000 calories, but also required that the DVs for 2,500 calories be listed for those people with greater caloric needs.

Your needs may be more or less. Refer to the charts "How Many Calories Do You Need?" on page 35 to determine your calorie level and then use the following table to find your DVs.

### DAILY VALUES FOR DIFFERENT CALORIE LEVELS

(Based on the recommendations in the "Calculating Daily Values" Table on page 12)

| CALORIES | Total Fat (g) | Sat. Fat (g) | Total Cholesterol (g) | Fiber (g) | Protein (g) |
|---|---|---|---|---|---|
| 1,200 | 40 | 16 | 180 | 20 * | 46 ** |
| 1,400 | 47 | 16 | 210 | 20 * | 46 ** |
| 1,600 | 53 | 17 | 240 | 20 | 46 ** |
| 1,800 | 60 | 20 | 270 | 21 | 46 ** |
| 2,000 (Reference Diet) | 65 | 21 | 300 | 25 | 50 |
| 2,200 | 73 | 24 | 330 | 25 | 55 |
| 2,500 | 80 | 25 | 375 | 30 | 65 |
| 2,800 | 93 | 31 | 420 | 32 | 70 |
| 3,200 | 107 | 36 | 480 | 37 | 80 |
| 3,500 | 117 | 39 | 525 | 40 | 88 |

\* 20 g is the minimum amount of fiber recommended for all calorie levels below 2,000. Source: *National Cancer Institute*.

\*\* 46 g is the minimum amount of protein recommended for all calorie levels below 1,800. Source: *Recommended Dietary Allowances*, 1989.

Vitamins A and C, calcium, and iron also have DVs. However, on the label they are only expressed as % DVs based on the following Daily Values.

**DAILY VALUES FOR VITAMINS AND MINERALS**

| | |
|---|---|
| Vitamin A | 5,000 IU |
| Vitamin C | 60 mg |
| Calcium | 1,000 mg |
| Iron | 18 mg |

## % Daily Value

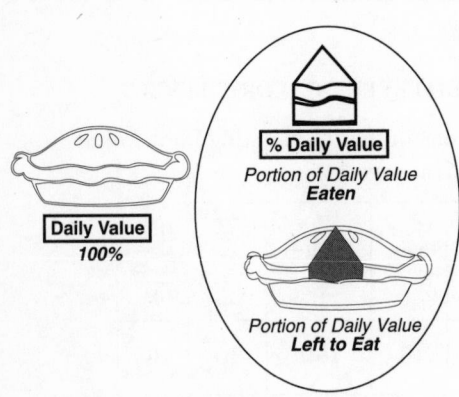

There is an easy way to understand Daily Value and % Daily Value. Picture the DV **for each nutrient** as a whole pie. The pie represents the total amount (or DV) you can eat of a particular nutrient for the day. % DV is like having a slice of that pie. Each time you eat a food, you take out another slice of the pie equal to the % DV listed on the label for that nutrient. Eating enough slices to add up to 100% of a particular nutrient means you've eaten your whole pie or all of your DV for that nutrient.

You may wonder how the food manufacturers come up with the % DVs. It's just a matter of arithmetic.

First, divide the grams or milligrams of a nutrient by the DV for that nutrient. (You'll find the grams listed right after the name of the nutrient in section ③ of the label. The DV is at the bottom of the label in section ⑥.)

Then, multiply the results by 100, rounding your answer to a whole number.

For example, the label on page 7 shows that the chili has 8 g Total Fat. The DV for Total Fat is 65 g for the 2,000-calorie reference diet. Therefore,

$$(8 \text{ g} \div 65 \text{ g}) \times 100 = 13\% \text{ DV.}$$

**NOTE:** % Daily Value is *not* the percentage of the nutrient in the food. It is the portion of your day's allowance used up when eating the food.

Grams and milligrams, while quantitative, can be misleading. If the label states that a food contains 6 grams of saturated fat, what is your first impression? "Oh, I can have that. Six grams of fat isn't much." As it turns out, six grams of saturated fat is equal to 30% DV. It uses up 30% of your daily allowance for saturated fat.

On the other hand, you may look at the grams or milligrams of a nutrient, think the number sounds large and, therefore, avoid the food. Had you looked at the % DV first, you would have had a better idea of how the food would fit into your daily intake of the nutrient. For example, if you're being careful about the amount of sodium you eat each day, you might think that 150 milligrams sounds like too much in one food. Yet, the % DV for 150 milligrams of sodium is only 6%.

### Rules of Thumb

% DV gives you an idea whether a food contains a lot or a little of each nutrient. The **5% & 20%** Rules will also help.

When reading the label for % DV, create a picture in your mind of how much of the whole DV pie you're eating. It's also a great way to compare different food products.

### The 5% Rule

When you're looking for a food that is a **low source** of a nutrient, look for a % DV that is less than or equal to 5%. You would apply this rule when you are trying to limit the amount of fat, cholesterol, or sodium you eat. The **5% Rule** comes in handy when you've had foods high in these nutrients and you need to balance them with some low sources.

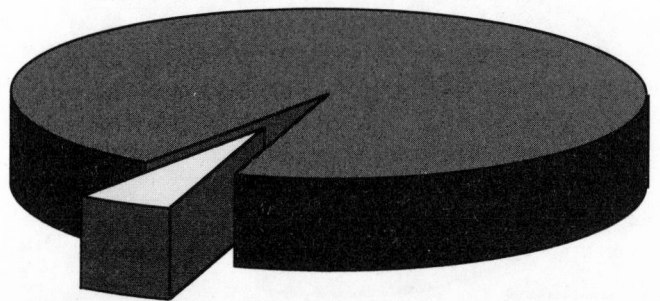

**Less than or equal to 5%**

### *The 20% Rule*

A food is considered a **high source** of a nutrient when its % DV is greater than 20%. Let's say you need to increase the amount of fiber in your diet. Looking back at the sample label on page 7, you can see that the chili has a 36% DV for dietary fiber, certainly a high source of the nutrient. A food with a % DV for fat of more than 20% is a high-fat food. You can use the **20% Rule** as a guide to increase your intake of some nutrients, such as fiber, or decrease others, such as fat, sodium, or cholesterol.

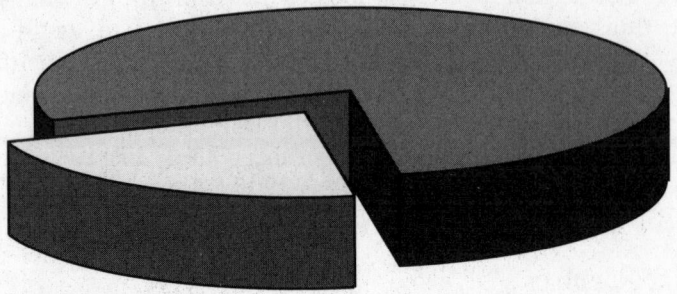

**Greater than 20%**

### *The 25% Rule*

Another rule of thumb is the **25% Rule**. After you've made the food selections for your meal, add up separately the % DVs **for each nutrient**. If the totals for each nutrient equal less than 25% per meal, you probably will be able to stay within your DV allowance for the day. This rule takes into account that you may have a couple of snacks during the day.

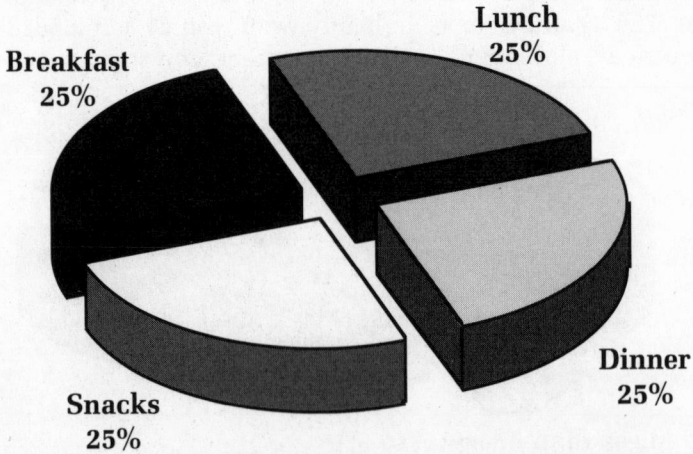

**Lunch 25%**

**Breakfast 25%**

**Dinner 25%**

**Snacks 25%**

## Planning Your Day's Meals with % Daily Values

Up to this point, we've basically been talking about % DVs of individual foods, showing their sole effect on the whole pie. While it is a useful approach for selecting individual foods or comparing different foods, you need to start thinking about your complete diet. You won't always be serving just one "slice of pie" at a time. Depending upon what you eat at a meal, you could end up taking out several slices for each nutrient pie. You'll quickly see whether you're going over your limit for certain nutrients, such as fat, sodium, and cholesterol, or not getting enough of others, such as fiber, vitamins A and C, calcium, and iron. Let's go through an example to show you how it works.

Imagine you started out your day with a breakfast of orange juice, hot oatmeal with brown sugar, a slice of whole wheat toast with margarine, and milk. You can find the % DVs for these foods either on their package labels or in this book. Since this is a book on fat and cholesterol, those are the nutrients we'll focus on for this example.

Looking at the following table and using the rules of thumb, you can see that after breakfast the total % DVs for each nutrient works with the **25% Rule**. (Make sure you don't add the % DVs for the different nutrients together.) Most of the foods are low in fat or fairly low in fat with their % DVs being close to the **5% Rule**. The last line of the table shows you how much of the % DVs you have left for the remainder of the day.

| Foods | % Daily Values | | |
| --- | --- | --- | --- |
| | **Total Fat** | **Saturated Fat** | **Cholesterol** |
| **Breakfast** | | | |
| 4 oz orange juice | 1% | 0% | 0% |
| 1 cup hot oatmeal | 4% | 2% | 0% |
| 1 tsp brown sugar | 0% | 0% | 0% |
| 1 slice whole wheat toast | 1% | 0% | 0% |
| 1 tsp margarine | 6% | 3% | 0% |
| 1 cup low-fat milk (1%) | 4% | 8% | 3% |
| Approx. 360 calories | | | |
| **Totals** | 16% | 13% | 3% |
| **% DV Remaining** | 100%−16% = **84%** | 100%−13% = **87%** | 100%−3% = **97%** |

Fortunately, with your low-fat breakfast, you still have a good portion of your nutrient allowance or % DVs remaining to spend during the rest of the day. Notice how the hot oatmeal, whole wheat toast, and low-fat milk all satisfy the 5% Rule for total fat. They're equal to or less than 5% DV. The other foods are not far off.

For lunch, you join your friends at the corner deli. As you can see in the following table, while the selections you made at the deli blew the 5% Rule for each food and the 25% Rule for the meal, you didn't go over your day's allowance for the nutrients. You even have plenty of % DV available for dinner.

| Foods | % Daily Values | | |
| --- | --- | --- | --- |
| | Total Fat | Saturated Fat | Cholesterol |
| **Lunch** | | | |
| Ham and cheese sandwich | 24% | 32% | 19% |
| Tossed green salad with 2 tbsp red wine vinaigrette | 11% | 5% | 0% |
| Potato chips (20) | 12% | 10% | 0% |
| Banana | 1% | 0% | 0% |
| Approx. 760 calories | | | |
| **Totals** | 48% | 47% | 19% |
| **% DV Remaining** | 84%−48% = **36%** | 87%−47% = **40%** | 97%−19% = **78%** |

In the afternoon, you decide to have a package of animal crackers for a snack. They're not very high in calories or fat (110 calories, 3% DV total fat, 2% DV saturated fat, and 0% DV cholesterol).

| **% DV Remaining** | 36%−3% = **33%** | 40%−2% = **38%** | 78%−0% = **78%** |
| --- | --- | --- | --- |

Knowing how much % DV you have remaining, you can plan your dinner accordingly.

| Foods | % Daily Values | | |
| --- | --- | --- | --- |
| | Total Fat | Saturated Fat | Cholesterol |
| **Dinner** | | | |
| 3 oz turkey roll (light meat) | 9% | 9% | 12% |
| 2 tbsp gravy | 6% | 3% | 2% |
| 1 medium baked potato | 0% | 0% | 0% |
| 2 tbsp sour cream | 9% | 18% | 7% |
| 1 cup steamed vegetables | 0% | 0% | 0% |
| 1/2 cup applesauce | 0% | 0% | 0% |
| Approx. 460 calories | | | |
| **Totals** | 24% | 30% | 21% |
| **% DV Remaining** | 33%−24% = **9%** | 40%−30% = **10%** | 78%−21% = **57%** |

The turkey breast was a good choice since its % DV is quite low. You can even splurge on some gravy for your turkey and sour cream on your potato, if you'd like. And with that, you still have calories and % DV left to spend. Not only that, the foods you ate provided you with a healthy, balanced diet, both from the standpoint of % DVs and by selecting foods from each of the food groups (grains and breads, vegetables, fruits, milk and dairy, meat and dried beans).

As it turns out, you can even have a dish of frozen yogurt in the evening and still not go over your % DVs for 2,000 calories a day.

While your meals this day met the nutrition recommendations, you will find that some days will work out better than others. What's important is how your meals average out over several days.

Most people would jump to the conclusion that having such foods as a ham and cheese sandwich, potato chips, or sour cream is really "being bad." Yet, as you can see, it really came down to balancing a variety of foods to come up with a healthy day's intake. If you use this approach each day, no food need be off limits (unless your physician has told you otherwise).

You get to choose how you want to spend your fat allowance. Always keep in mind, though, that low-fat or fat-free foods are not calorie-free. Therefore, while you may be keeping within your DV allowance for fat, you could be ending up with too many calories.

# 4. Answers to Frequently Asked Questions

**Q. What do some of the other terms on the Nutrition Facts label mean?**

**A. —**

- **Cholesterol** is a fatlike substance that can only be found in foods of animal origin (meat, poultry, fish, eggs, and dairy products).

- **Dietary Fiber** includes both soluble and insoluble fibers. Food manufacturers only have to give a value for the total dietary fiber. *Soluble fiber*, found in such foods as oats, barley, legumes (dried beans), fruits, and vegetables, is useful in slowing the emptying of your stomach. This can give you a fuller feeling longer. Soluble fiber also helps to lower blood cholesterol by binding bile and dietary cholesterol so they can't be absorbed into the bloodstream. Foods such as bran, whole grains, fruits, and vegetables contain *insoluble fiber*. It helps to increase fecal bulk and decrease the transit time of fecal material, reducing the risk of constipation, diverticulitis, and colon cancer.

- **Protein** grams must appear on the label, but a % DV doesn't have to be declared. The DV for protein is 50 grams, based on 10% of a 2,000-calorie reference diet. Food manufacturers only have to provide % DV if they make a nutrient content claim regarding protein. Since most Americans get plenty of protein and there are no chronic diseases associated with the nutrient, the FDA doesn't require the % DV for protein to be listed.

- **Saturated Fat** is one of three types of fat that make up total fat (the others being monounsaturated and polyunsaturated). There is a higher risk of heart disease when there is too much saturated fat in the diet. Whereas monounsaturated and polyunsaturated fats are normally liquid at room temperature, saturated fat is solid.

Foods of animal origin such as meat, butter, whole milk, and whole milk products are high in saturated fat. A good source of mono-unsaturated and polyunsaturated fats is vegetable oil. However, palm kernel oil and coconut oil are the exception, both being high in saturated fat.

- **Serving Size** is listed in household measures, such as cups and tea-spoons, as well as slices and pieces. Food manufacturers must also give the metric measure (grams or milliliters) of a serving. More consistent serving sizes for similar food products make comparing foods easier. Based on national food consumption surveys, serving sizes are now more realistic, reflecting what the average American eats.

The government set *reference amounts* for over 100 categories of food based on what most people eat at a time for a particular food. The purpose of reference amounts is (1) to determine serving sizes listed on the label and (2) establish the criteria for nutrient content claims and health claims. It's no longer up to the manufacturer to determine the serving size (to make the nutrient numbers look good).

You may notice that there is some variation among serving sizes of similar foods. This is especially evident with foods that come in discrete units or single-serving containers. Looking at the category of cookies, the reference amount is 30 grams. The serving size is the number of cookies that comes closest to the 30 gram weight. If one cookie weighs 14 grams, then the label would say that a serving was two cookies (28 g).

A cookie weighing, for example, 48 grams, would be considered a one-cookie serving size. While the 48 grams is greater than the reference amount of 30 grams, the government allows for variations on unit sizes. The manufacturer has up to a 200% leeway. That means, if a single cookie weighs up to 60 grams, it is still considered one serving. This approach is valid for many different foods, such as bread, crackers, and muffins, due to differences in thickness of a slice or the size or weight of one piece.

This 200% leeway prevents the manufacturer from listing serving sizes in fractions. In the past, you might have seen on the label fractions of slices or pieces as a serving size. Now, a serving size has to be a whole number that is closest to the reference amount, and it should be close enough to allow you to compare nutrient information.

Because of the 200% leeway, manufacturers can decide whether a product that doesn't come in discrete units should provide one serving or two. A can of soup that contains 15 ounces (420 grams), provides us with a good example. The reference amount for soup is 245 grams per serving.

| *At two servings in a can:* | 420 g ÷ 2 = 210 g of soup per serving (close enough to the 245 gram reference amount). |
|---|---|
| *At one serving in a can:* | 420 g, still within the 200% allowed by law (245 × 2 = 490 grams). |

Of course, it's up to you how much you want to eat. Just be aware of what you're comparing by looking at the serving sizes and why the serving sizes don't always agree.

One of the more helpful additions to the label is the actual number of crackers, chips, and cookies in a serving. Of course, it's best to count them out into a bowl and put the package away. No point in tempting fate!

- **Sugars** refer to both naturally occurring (such as lactose in milk and fructose in fruits) and added sugars. Some dairy and fruit products may appear high in sugars even though they contain no added sugars. One way to tell if that's the case is to refer to the list of ingredients. Besides the obvious word *sugar*, look for the words *sucrose, fructose, honey, corn syrup, dextrin, dextrose,* and *fruit juice concentrate,* to name a few.

  If you want to know how much sugar has been added, you'll need to compare an unsweetened version of the food to one that has been sweetened. For example, compare 1 cup of plain, fat-free, unsweetened yogurt containing 16 grams of "Sugars" to 1 cup of strawberry fat-free yogurt with 36 grams of "Sugars." While some of the 20-gram difference comes from the strawberries, most of it is from added sugar. By the way, that 20 grams is equal to 5 teaspoons of sugar. (Divide grams of sugar by 4, since there are 4 grams of sugar in 1 teaspoon.)

  You won't find % DV for sugars because there is no DV set for sugars. There is no scientific evidence associating sugar with any chronic diseases. The major health problems related to sugar are its ability to cause dental caries (cavities) and, when eaten in excess, obesity.

- **Total Carbohydrate** includes both simple and complex carbohydrates. Two types of carbohydrates are specifically listed: Dietary Fiber, which is a complex carbohydrate, and Sugars, which are simple carbohydrates. When adding the grams of Dietary Fiber and Sugars together, the sum doesn't always equal the grams of Total Carbohydrate. That's because there are still more complex carbohydrates (such as starches) that don't have to be accounted for specifically on the label but are included in the Total Carbohydrate count. Besides listing Dietary Fiber and Sugars, you may also see "Other Carbohydrate," as well as "Soluble Fiber" and "Insoluble Fiber."

  Grams of "Sugar Alcohols" will be listed when foods, such as sugar-free candies and gums, carry "sugar-free" or "low-sugar" claims. Sorbitol, xylitol, and mannitol are a few of the sugar alcohols.

- **Total Fat** includes saturated fat, polyunsaturated fat, and monounsaturated fat. Food manufacturers must list total fat and saturated fat, along with their grams and % DVs. It's up to them if they want to include values for the polyunsaturated and monounsaturated fats in the food.

Total fat also consists of glycerol (a building block of fat) and trans-fatty acids. Some trans-fatty acids occur naturally in some of our food. However, most are the product of *hydrogenation*, a process that makes polyunsaturated fats, such as corn oil, more saturated and more solid at room temperature. Most margarines are made using this process. If you were to add the grams of saturated fat, along with monounsaturated and polyunsaturated fats, the result might not equal the grams of total fat. That's because total fat doesn't have to include grams of glycerol and trans-fatty acids.

With many scientific studies showing that trans-fatty acids raise blood cholesterol the same way as saturated fats, many people would like to see trans-fatty acids listed separately on the label. For now, though, the FDA hasn't approved the request. Fortunately, trans-fatty acids make up only a minor part of the fat content of most foods. Look at the list of ingredients for the words "hydrogenated" or "partially hydrogenated" to see if a food contains trans-fatty acids through processing. However, it doesn't mean that the food is bad for you.

**Q. How can I make use of the information on the Nutrition Facts label?**

**A. —**

### Comparing Food Products

You can compare different brands or varieties of food products by looking at the % Daily Value for the various nutrients. You will be able to tell three things from the % DVs:

1. Which product has more or less of certain nutrients
2. Which product, using the **5% & 20% Rules** (page 15), is a high or low source of certain nutrients
3. Which foods can fit into the **25% Rule** (page 16) for a meal

For example, you might be interested in comparing the fat content of different brands of spaghetti sauce. Let's say the total fat for Brand A is 25% DV and Brand B is 18% DV.

1. Brand B obviously has less total fat (since its % DV is smaller).
2. Using the **5% & 20% Rules**, Brand A, with 25% DV, falls into the greater than 20% DV category, making it a high source of fat.

3. Brand B works into the **25% Rule** for a meal better than Brand A. At least you would still have 7% DVs remaining of total fat to apply to the rest of your meal.

You can use % DVs to compare a particular food with its low-fat or fat-free version to see how much you save by eating the low-fat or fat-free version (for instance, low-fat cream cheese instead of regular cream cheese). While there's no reason you can't eat the regular version, it's just a matter of how you want to spend your DV or nutrient allowance.

### Knowing Exactly What's in the Food

Since 1938, certain products such as dairy foods, mayonnaise, ketchup, jelly, and orange juice didn't have to include a list of ingredients. They were made according to the FDA's official recipe. These foods were said to have a "standard of identity." Over the years, the FDA has standardized more than 300 products. That's not to say that food manufacturers, in all cases, avoided including a list of ingredients. However, with the new labeling, no matter whether a product fits the standard or not, *ingredients must be shown and appear in descending order of weight, from most to least.*

The labeling of ingredients is much more detailed and informative now. Before the 1990 Nutrition Labeling and Education Act, additives were listed collectively under the general terms *flavorings*, *colorings*, and *spices*. For people with allergies to these additives or religious or cultural beliefs against eating them, there was no way to know just what they were getting. Things have changed.

- **Caseinate:** Buying products that call themselves nondairy doesn't necessarily mean they don't contain some milk derivative. People with allergies to dairy products may be misled by the label saying nondairy, when the product contains caseinate. Caseinate is a milk protein used to whiten coffee creamers or texturize products. Therefore, checking the list of ingredients becomes very important for casein-sensitive individuals.

- **Colors:** Food, Drug and Cosmetic (FD&C) colors will have to be listed specifically, referred to by name (such as FD&C Blue No.1), except on butter, cheese, and ice cream. Colors derived from such foods as paprika and beet juice can be identified simply as artificial colors.

- **Hydrolyzed Protein:** The words *hydrolyzed protein* used to be allowed in the list of ingredients, though people never knew what the protein was that had been hydrolyzed. (Hydrolysis is a process using an acid or enzyme to break down proteins into their amino acid building blocks.) These proteins are very useful ingredients for leavening, thickening, and enhancing flavor, to name a few functions. However, as with other additives, people with allergies or religious or cultural reasons for avoiding certain proteins didn't know what proteins were used. No longer will that be the case. The source of the protein must be identified (for instance, hydrolyzed soy protein). The label will also have to specifically state that the food "contains glutamate" (MSG).

- **Ice Cream Products:** It used to be that if the frozen dessert product did not contain a certain amount of fat, it had to be called "ice milk" or "frozen dairy dessert." Now, terms such as *no-fat ice cream* (less than 0.5% fat), *low-fat ice cream* (0.5% to 3% fat), *reduced-fat ice cream* (3% to 7% fat), and *regular ice cream* (10% or more fat) will be allowed. Manufacturers will no longer use the term "ice milk."

- **Juices:** With the new labeling, you'll finally know what you're getting when you purchase vegetable or fruit juices, whether carbonated or not, made from concentrate, or containing no juice at all. The container cannot display luscious-looking fruits and vegetables, implying something that the product is not. Right up front on the label will be the words "Contains ____ % ____ juice." The first blank states the actual percentage of juice and the second blank gives the name of the fruit or vegetable (e.g., Contains *50% apple* juice). No longer will you buy a fruit juice, such as peach juice, only to find that you bought apple juice with a little peach juice for flavoring.

    The name of the beverage will give you a general idea of how much juice is included. **"Juice"** is the word you should look for when you want 100% fruit juice (e.g., *Apple Juice*). A "juice **beverage**," "juice **drink**" or "juice **cocktail**" does not contain 100% juice. The part that isn't juice is probably water and added sugar. A **"flavored"** juice means you're getting very little of that named juice. However, in most cases, a percentage will be given so you'll know whether the juice has much nutritional value. A juice **blend** must list on the front label those juices, from most to least, that make up the blend or percentages present must be declared.

### Calculating the % Fat in the Food

For years people have been told that they must keep their intake of fat down to 30% of total calories. Many misinterpreted this to mean that no food should contain more than 30% of calories from fat. Since some foods can be as much as 100% fat, considering a food's contribution to one's daily allowance for fat is more useful than calculating the percentage calories from fat.

% DV allows you to indulge in some of your favorite higher-fat foods and not have to feel guilty. However, for those of you who can't seem to break the "% Calories from Fat" habit, do the following calculations: Divide Calories from Fat by Calories and then multiply by 100.

As an example, taking the label information found on page 7, we know that the Calories from Fat are 72 and Total Calories are 260.

Therefore, the percentage of fat in the chili equals 28% (as compared to 13% DV).

### Calculating the Grams of Fat

This is a book on % Daily Values. As you look through the food list, you will not see grams of total fat and saturated fat listed, nor milligrams of cholesterol. As mentioned earlier, % DV is a much more useful number since it gives you a better picture of how much of your day's allowance for a nutrient is used up when you eat a particular food. However, for those of you who need to know the grams and milligrams of fat and cholesterol, there is a way to use the % DVs listed in the second part of this book to calculate those values.

**For Total Fat:** Multiply the % DV for total fat by 65 grams (Daily Value for 2,000 calories). The answer you get is the grams of total fat.

**For Saturated Fat:** Multiply the % DV for saturated fat by 20 grams (Daily Value for 2,000 calories). The answer you get is the grams of saturated fat.

**For Cholesterol:** Multiply the % DV for cholesterol by 300 milligrams (Daily Value). The answer you get is the milligrams of cholesterol.

**Q. Can I believe the claims on the label?**

**A. —**

Yes. No longer will you have to worry that the claims on the label are put there by the manufacturer so you'll be enticed to buy the product. **Nutrient content claims** and **health claims** can help you choose foods for a healthy diet.

**Q. What do some of the Nutrient Content Claims mean?**

**A. —**

There are three types of nutrient content claims, all of which tell you about the amount of a nutrient in the food:

1. *Absolute claims* state the level or range of a nutrient (e.g., "fat free")
2. *Relative* or *comparative claims* compare the amount of nutrient in one food with the amount in another similar food (e.g., "reduced cholesterol")
3. *Implied claims* describe the food in a way suggesting that a nutrient is absent or present in certain amounts (e.g., "high in oat bran")

- **Cholesterol-Free Food** is a good example of some of the subtleties in terms to watch for on the label. By including the word "food," the claim means that the food is naturally free of cholesterol. **Cholesterol-Free**, on the other hand, means that the cholesterol has been removed from a food that naturally contained cholesterol. This same approach to labeling applies to such nutrients as sodium, fat, etc.

- **Free** means there is none or only a trace amount of the particular nutrient in the food. For example, a product that is "fat free" has less than 0.5 grams of fat. While you can feel "free" to eat these foods, keep in mind that they aren't calorie free.

- **Fresh** refers to a food that is unprocessed, raw, has never been frozen or heated, and contains no preservatives. In the case of milk, since people understand that in almost all cases, milk has been pasteurized, it may display the term fresh.

- **Fresh frozen** and **frozen fresh** mean that the food was quickly frozen while it was still fresh.

- **Good** source and **High** source of a nutrient mentioned on the label alert you to a particular level of the nutrient in the food. "Good" provides between 10% and 19% of the DV for that nutrient. A product that is "high" in a particular nutrient must provide 20% or more of the DV for that nutrient. For example, when a container of orange juice states it is "high in vitamin C," it means you are getting at least 12 milligrams of vitamin C (DV for vitamin C is 60 milligrams; therefore, 20% of 60 milligrams = 12 milligrams).

- **Healthy** is another term that manufacturers love to put on their products because of what it conveys in the consumer's mind. To use the term, whether as a claim or as a brand name, the food must meet certain criteria. It must be low in fat (no more than 3 grams), low in saturated fat (no more than 1 gram), and cholesterol to be no more than 60 milligrams. Foods must contain at least 10% of the DV of either vitamin A, vitamin C, iron, calcium, protein, or fiber. Raw meat and poultry products can be called "healthy" if they meet the definition for "extra lean" (less than 5 grams of fat, 2 grams of saturated fat, and 95 milligrams of cholesterol per serving). Over a specified period of time, food manufacturers will have to reduce the sodium levels for individual foods down to 360 milligrams and down to 480 milligrams for meal-type products.

- **Lean** or **extra lean** are terms that are presently being used to describe the amount of fat in raw meat, as well as the level of fat in processed foods. The most familiar example is ground beef (e.g., extra lean ground beef has less than 10% fat). Using these terms for both raw meat and processed foods is confusing to some consumers. They can't be sure that the term is referring to the level of fat in the meat or a nutrient content claim (see the table on Fat on page 29 for details). Therefore, the USDA is in the process of formulating new rulings on how to refer to the different levels of fat in raw meats. There has been discussion of stating the level of fat as "_____% lean /_____% fat."

- **Less** can refer to a food that has been reformulated or not. In either case, it must contain 25% less of that nutrient compared to another food. It's a way to advertise that the particular food is a better choice. A mayonnaise product label could say, "Less calories than regular mayonnaise." In the case of pretzels, which are naturally low in fat, the label might state, "Less fat than potato chips."

- **Light** or **lite** caused much confusion before the new labeling took effect. These terms can now mean two things. They can apply to the amount of calories, fat, or sodium in a serving (see the tables on pages 29, 30, and 31 for details). The terms can also be used when describing the texture or color of a food. To do so, the food manufacturer must actually state what is light, such as "light brown sugar" or "light and fluffy."

- **Low** tells you that if you frequently eat food labeled as such for certain nutrients, you will probably not go over your daily allowance for those nutrients. Let's say the label states, "Low Sodium." That means the food must contain less than or equal to 140 milligrams of sodium. Since you're allowed 2,400 milligrams of sodium a day, you could have many servings of low-sodium foods without going over the daily allowance.

- **Natural** is one of those terms for which the FDA still hasn't established a final ruling. Look further than the word "natural" to see what the nutrient information and ingredients tell you.

- **Reduced** is another phrase you will see frequently. It means that the manufacturer has reformulated the food product so it has less of certain nutrients than the regular or reference product. However, the food may still contain large amounts of certain nutrients. The major point here is that the food contains at least 25% less of that nutrient. For example, 1 tablespoon of the regular mayonnaise contains 100 calories. Therefore, the reduced-calorie version must contain 75 or fewer calories.

- **See side / back panel for nutrition information** is displayed on the front of the package when a product has made a nutrient content claim. To make such a claim, the product must adhere to set levels for fat, saturated fat, cholesterol, and sodium per serving. If the product can't live up to being low in all these nutrients, then you'll see, **"See side / back panel for information about _____ and other nutrients."** (The nutrients that aren't low enough are written in the blank. For example, if a cheese says "Fat Free," but is high in sodium, it will say "See side panel for information about sodium and other nutrients.")

The following tables provide the specific amounts for each nutrient that qualifies a food product to use certain descriptors on the label. The criteria for nutrient levels may differ for meal-type products (entrées, main dish products, and dinners).

| FAT | |
|---|---|
| **Claim** | **Definition (per reference amount)** |
| Free | Less than 0.5 g |
| Low | 3 g or less |
| Light or Lite | Product has 1/3 fewer calories *or* 50% less fat per reference amount |
| Reduced | At least 25% less fat than comparison food |
| _____ % fat free | If product meets low-fat requirements (3 g or less); the percentage is based on the amount of fat, by weight, per 100 grams of food. For example:<br><br>Serving size: 100 g<br>Total Fat: 5 g<br>5 g ÷ 100 g = 5% fat<br>Therefore, food is 95% fat free<br>(100%−5% = 95%) |
| Lean | For meat, poultry, and seafood products; main dish, meal, and meal-type products<br><br>Per reference amount, labeled serving and/or 100 grams<br>Total Fat: Less than 10 g<br>Saturated Fat: Less than 4 g<br>Cholesterol: Less than 95 mg |
| Extra Lean | For meat, poultry, and seafood products; main dish, meal, and meal-type products<br><br>Per reference amount, labeled serving and/or 100 grams<br>Total Fat: Less than 5 g<br>Saturated Fat: Less than 2 g<br>Cholesterol: Less than 95 mg |

Note: "Low fat" or "Fat free" may still be high in calories.

## SATURATED FAT

| Claim | Definition (per reference amount) |
|---|---|
| Free | Less than 0.5 g |
| Low | 1 g or less *and* no more than 15% of calories from saturated fat |
| Reduced | At least 25% less saturated fat than comparison food |

## CHOLESTEROL

| Claim | Definition (per reference amount) |
|---|---|
| Free | Less than 2 mg *and* 2 g or less saturated fat |
| Low | 20 mg or less *and* 2 g or less saturated fat |
| Reduced | At least 25% less cholesterol *and* 2 g or less saturated fat than comparison food |

Cholesterol and fat are not the same thing. Cholesterol claims are allowed only if food contains 2 g or less of **saturated fat** per reference amount. "Low Cholesterol" also means "Low Saturated Fat" but not necessarily "Low Total Fat."

## CALORIES

| Claim | Definition (per reference amount) |
|---|---|
| Free | Less than 5 calories |
| Low | 40 calories or less |
| Light or Lite | Product has 1/3 fewer calories *or* 50% less fat per reference amount; if more than half the calories are from fat, fat content must be reduced by 50% or more |
| Reduced | At least 25% fewer calories than comparison food |

| SODIUM | |
|---|---|
| **Claim** | **Definition**<br>**(per reference amount)** |
| Free | Less than 5 mg |
| Very low | 35 mg or less |
| Low | 140 mg or less |
| Light in sodium | Product has 50% less sodium per reference amount; only foods that have more than 40 calories or 3 g of fat per serving can use these terms |
| Lightly salted | Product has added 50% *less* sodium than is normally added to food; label must state "not a low-sodium food" if the food contains more than 140 mg sodium |
| Reduced | At least 25% less sodium than comparison food |
| Unsalted, Without Added Salt, or No Salt Added | Permitted if<br>1. No salt added during processing<br>2. The product it resembles and substitutes for is normally made with salt<br>3. Label must say "not a sodium-free food" if it doesn't meet the requirement as such |

Salt is not the same thing as sodium. Salt refers to sodium chloride, which is 40% sodium. One teaspoon of salt is about 2,300 mg of sodium.

| SUGARS | |
|---|---|
| **Claim** | **Definition**<br>**(per reference amount)** |
| Free | Less than 5 g |
| Reduced | At least 25% less sugar than comparison food |
| No Added Sugar, Without Added Sugar, No Sugar Added | Permitted if<br>1. No sugars added during processing or packing, including ingredients that contain sugars (e.g., jam, fruit juices, dried fruit)<br>2. The product this food is a substitute for normally contains added sugars |

| | OTHER TERMS |
|---|---|
| **Claim** | **Definition (per reference amount)** |
| High, Rich In, Excellent Source Of | Contains 20% or more of the *Daily Value* for the nutrient |
| Good Source Of, Contains, Provides | Contains 10%–19% of the *Daily Value* for the nutrient |
| More, Fortified, Enriched, Added | Contains 10% or more of the *Daily Value* for the nutrient |

Certain Nutrient Content Claims can be labeled with other words.

| **Claim** | **Also Labeled As** |
|---|---|
| Free | No, free of, zero, without, trivial source of, negligible source of, dietarily insignificant source of |
| Low | Low in, contains small amount of, few, low source, little |
| Reduced | Reduced in, less, lower, lower in, fewer |

## Q. Can I believe the health claims on the labels?

**A. —**

More and more scientific studies are revealing a relationship between what we eat and particular diseases or health-related conditions. Having a health claim on a food label can alert you to those foods that may help fight coronary heart disease, cancer, hypertension, and osteoporosis.

Label information becomes extremely important when you realize the consequences of too much or not enough of certain nutrients. Too much dietary fat, especially saturated fat, and dietary cholesterol may increase the blood cholesterol levels in some adults. In turn, their risk of heart disease increases. A high-fat diet also increases the risk for cancer and obesity. Diets high in sodium may promote or aggravate high blood pressure in some adults. High blood pressure is a risk factor for a heart attack or stroke. Increasing your intake of dietary fiber found in fruits, vegetables, and grain products may reduce the risk of some cancers.

It's reassuring to know that now when food manufacturers put a health claim on the label, the food meets certain requirements for fat, cholesterol, sodium, and fiber. Only health claims approved by the FDA are allowed. As you will see, the requirements for including a health claim are quite strict. The result will probably be that few foods will qualify for health claims. While diet can help reduce the risk of certain diseases, you must consider your overall lifestyle (e.g., exercise and smoking), as well.

An example of a health claim would be:

*Development of cancer depends on many factors. Eating a diet low in fat and high in grain products, fruits, and vegetables that contain dietary fiber may reduce your risk for some types of cancer.*

Any food that makes a health claim must have *no more* than the following nutrient levels. In many cases, the nutrient levels may have to be much lower, depending upon the health claim.

|  | Food Product * | Main Dish Product ** | Meat Product ** |
|---|---|---|---|
| **Total Fat** | 13 g | 19.5 g | 26 g |
| **Saturated Fat** | 4 g | 6 g | 8 g |
| **Cholesterol** | 60 mg | 90 mg | 120 mg |
| **Sodium** | 480 mg | 720 mg | 960 mg |

\* Per reference amount, per label serving size, and per 50 g when reference amount is 30 g or less *or* 2 tablespoons or less

\*\* Per labeled serving

For a food to carry a health claim, it must also contain at least 10% of the DV of one or more of the following nutrients: protein, dietary fiber, vitamin A, vitamin C, calcium, or iron.

Lastly, each of the seven health claims has its own specific nutrient requirements as outlined in the table that follows.

| If the Label Talks About: | You Can Be Sure a Serving of the Food Is: |
|---|---|
| *Coronary heart disease and:*<br>Dietary saturated fat and cholesterol | Low fat, low saturated fat, and low cholesterol |
| | Fish and game meats must be extra lean |
| Fruits, vegetables, and grain products that contain fiber, particularly soluble fiber | Low fat, low saturated fat, and low cholesterol |
| | At least 0.6 g of soluble fiber per reference amount (without fortification) |
| *Osteoporosis and:*<br>Calcium | High in calcium (at least 200 mg), which is easily absorbed into the body |
| | Food contains no more phosphorus than calcium<br>*(continued)* |

| If the Label Talks About: | You Can Be Sure a Serving of the Food Is: |
|---|---|
| *Hypertension and:* | |
| Sodium | Low sodium |
| *Cancer and:* | |
| Dietary fat | Low fat |
| | Fish and game meats must be extra lean |
| Fiber-containing grain products, fruits, and vegetables | Low fat |
| | Good source of dietary fiber (without fortification) |
| Fruits and vegetables | Good source (without fortification) of at least one of the following: vitamin A, vitamin C, or dietary fiber |

See Nutrient Content tables on pages 29 to 32 for specific nutrient levels for the above nutrient content claims.

## Q. What's in a name?

**A. —**

The government made a major move forward when they set up the NLEA rules for labeling. No longer are deceptive nutrient or health claims allowed. The one area that has not yet been tackled, though, is deceptive ingredient claims.

While many of the names manufacturers devise for their products are quite clever, realize that statements on the front of the package may or may not tell you exactly what you're getting inside. Many foods have labels that tout "Made with _____," whether it be real fruit, real vegetables, etc. You'll need to look a little farther than the front of the package to be sure just how much of the "made with" you're getting. Oftentimes, if a package has a "made with" statement on it, it means "made with just a little bit." Looking at the % Daily Values for vitamins and minerals, as well as the list of ingredients, may give you a better idea.

Pictures on the front of the package can also be misleading. Seeing a package covered with pictures of fruits or vegetables or whatever may lead you to believe that the food is loaded with these ingredients, when, in fact, it may not be.

Watch out for foods that say they are sweetened with concentrated fruit juices. In many cases, the juice has been clarified to such an extent that the vitamin content is lost, leaving you with just sugar. Many foods use apple juice as a sweetener, which is virtually void of vitamins. While these foods aren't bad for you, don't be misled into thinking that they are healthier.

If a package says "Gravy with Beef" as compared to "Beef with Gravy," there is a clear message here. A dish called Gravy with Beef is just that—a lot of gravy with a little bit of beef added. At least the manufacturer was honest with the name. The amount of protein in the dish would give you a good clue as to just how much meat you're getting. For those who are curious, one ounce of meat has about 7 grams of protein.

## Q. How do I use the % Daily Value Converter Card?

**A. —**

The % DV provided on the labels are based on a 2,000 calorie reference diet. However, you may eat more or less calories. You can use the **% Daily Value Converter Card** (found on the inside back cover) to adjust the % DV listed on the label to your calorie needs. Unless you already know how many calories you should be eating, the following information can help you to determine that number.

First, **what is your activity level?** Look over the following activities to see which one applies to you most of the time.

❑ **Light Activity:** sit-down job or one that requires standing for long periods of time; no regular physical activity; weekend exerciser
❑ **Moderate Activity:** participate in regular recreation or fitness activities such as brisk walking, jogging, swimming, or cycling at least three times per week for 30 to 50 minutes each session
❑ **Heavy Activity:** experience vigorous physical activity for 60 minutes or more at least four days per week

Next, check the following table to see what your approximate daily calorie intake should be. Make sure that you're looking in the correct table. There's one for women and another for men.

### HOW MANY CALORIES DO YOU NEED?

| WOMEN Age | Light | Activity Level Moderate | Heavy |
|---|---|---|---|
| If Dieting: 1,200 to 1,500 | | | |
| 19–24 | 1,800 | 2,200 | 2,600 |
| 24–50 | 1,800 | 2,200 | 2,600 |
| 50+ | 1,700 | 2,000 | 2,400 |

| MEN Age | Light | Activity Level Moderate | Heavy |
|---|---|---|---|
| If Dieting: 1,500 to 1,800 | | | |
| 19–24 | 2,300 | 3,000 | 3,700 |
| 24–50 | 2,300 | 3,000 | 3,800 |
| 50+ | 2,000 | 2,600 | 3,200 |

Derived from *Recommended Dietary Allowances,* 10th edition. National Research Council, 1989.

Now, follow the simple steps given on the front of the card. You will simply be looking in the first column of the card for the % DV listed on the label and then look across that row to your calorie level. The number you see there is your *adjusted % DV*.

All the discussion so far about % DVs (the 5% & 20% Rules, the 25% Rule, etc.) still applies. The only difference is that instead of using the % DV listed on the label, you use the adjusted % DV.

# 5. How to Use the Food Listings

By now you should have a better idea about the new food labeling. You've seen how you can use the % Daily Value information on the label to select foods that will keep you within your daily allowance (Daily Value) for the various nutrients.

The next part of this book provides you with the % Daily Values for total fat, saturated fat, and cholesterol of over 10,000 foods, both generic and brand names. You can use this information to compare and select foods for a healthy day's intake.

## Types of Foods Included in the List

You will find foods listed in two ways: generically and by brand names. When you see a generic listing, it may be because: (1) the food has not been processed in any way, such as fresh fruits and vegetables, cuts of meat, poultry, and fish or (2) the food can be purchased at the deli counter, salad bar, in bulk, etc. where you won't find any labeling. The typical market is organized in such a way that most generic-type foods are stocked along the walls and perimeter of the store. Next time you're in your market, check out where you find the produce, meat, and fish departments, dairy goods, bakery, deli, and salad bar. That's where most of the generically listed foods in this book will be found.

If you don't have a particular brand name in mind for a food, look in the generic listing. As you probably have already noticed, there is a listing of the food categories in the table of contents to make it easier to find the food you want. If you can't find it in the generic listing, then go through the brand named foods to find something similar. At least that way you'll have a general idea of the % Daily Value of the type of food you want to eat.

Unless most of your shopping is from the dairy, produce, and meat counters, you'll quickly realize how many processed and packaged foods you do purchase. This book includes many of the popular brands by the major food manufacturers.

You may find that some of the % Daily Values listed in this book differ slightly from those found on the label. This can be due to (1) rounding of numbers, (2) changes in serving sizes used by the food manufacturer, or (3) improvements in products by manufacturers (after this book was published) resulting in different nutrient declarations. Therefore, when you're in the supermarket, check the actual label for the most current information.

In some cases, the values may reflect the product before preparation. If the values are for a prepared product, the food listing will say "prep as dir" (prepared as directed).

Some foods listed in this book may not be in your supermarket. This could be due to one of several reasons. First, the product may not be distributed in your region of the country. Second, your market may have chosen not to carry it. Lastly, with food manufacturers constantly changing their product line, adding and deleting different foods, the food may no longer be available.

On the other hand, you may find products in your store that are not included in this book. With so many products manufactured, it would be impossible to include them all. Also, there were manufacturers who didn't want to have their products included because they are constantly changing their product line.

## The Way the Products Are Listed

This book lists foods in a way similar to how supermarkets stock their shelves. For example, there's a bread aisle in the supermarket, and there is a section in this book called "Bread and Bread Products." Looking at the shelves of bread in the market, you'll see sliced bread, rolls, pita, etc. Those different types of bread serve as subcategories in this book. The same approach holds true for the other sections of the market.

In this way, when you're in a particular area of the store, you can pull this book out and compare various products within a particular category. Refer to the table of contents for not only the major categories, but the subcategories. You'll also find the major categories stated at the top of each page and the sub-categories at the bottom. Finding a particular product should be quite simple.

At the beginning of each new section, whether it be a major category or subcategory, the **generic foods** are listed alphabetically. These are then followed by the **brand name foods**, also listed alphabetically.

There are several rules of thumb for locating brand name foods in this book. The way you look them up will be very similar to how you would ask a clerk in the supermarket where to find a product. Think about how you refer to the food. In most cases, you would ask for a certain brand and then possibly the variety of that brand. For example, if you want to know where to find the cracker, Wheat Thins Low Sodium, by Nabisco, you'd probably ask for Wheat Thins, not the manufacturer, Nabisco. Once you're in the right part of the cracker aisle and find the family of Wheat Thin crackers, you then would look for the low-sodium variety. The same would hold true for many other products.

Manufacturers spend millions of dollars establishing name recognition for their products. Just as cattle are branded with a distinguishing mark, food products are likewise branded. This could be the manufacturer's name, when a unique name hasn't been created for the product or product line (for example, BEN & JERRY'S Chocolate Ice Cream).

On the other hand, foods might be distinguished by their type or product line name. This name, which may or may not be a registered name, is given to a group of foods that are similar due to packaging or food content. An example would be Kraft's STOVE TOP Stuffing Mixes.

In most cases, the brand names will be in UPPERCASE letters. As mentioned above, the brand name can either be the name for a line of products or the manufacturer's name. Following the brand name may be the variety or description of the food, which appears in lowercase letters (for example, STOVE TOP Stuffing Mix). A product that has both a brand name and sub–brand name will have the sub–brand name in *italics* (for example, SEVEN SEAS *Viva* Salad Dressing). If the brand name is different from the manufacturer's name, the manufacturer is shown in SMALL CAPS (for example, SEVEN SEAS *Viva*—KRAFT).

A quick summary—

| UPPERCASE | = | Brand name or manufacturer's name |
| Lowercase | = | Variety or description |
| *Italics* | = | Sub–brand name |
| SMALL CAPS | = | Manufacturer |

### Symbols Used in the Food List

As you go through the food list, you will notice certain symbols to the left of the name of the food. They are a guide to give you an idea whether the food falls into the **5% Low Source Rule** (see page 15), the **20% High Source Rule** (see page 16) or somewhere in between. The symbols serve as a quick reference that is extremely useful when you've had some high-fat and/or high-cholesterol foods. If that's the case, to stay within your Daily Value allowances for the day, you will need to look for foods that are low in fat and cholesterol. The symbols will help you do that.

★ Foods with this symbol have less than or equal to 5% DV for **all** three nutrients: total fat, saturated fat, and cholesterol (5% Low Source Rule).

❖ Foods with this symbol have **at least one** of the three nutrients greater than 5% DV but less than or equal to 20% DV.

☒ Foods with this symbol have **at least one** of the three nutrients greater than 20% DV (20% High Source Rule).

The symbols are not meant to imply that one food is better than another or that some foods are bad and others are good. Always keep your total daily intake in mind. If you eat a food with the ☒ symbol, it just means that to keep from going over your daily allowance for fat or cholesterol, you should then select foods with the other two symbols.

There is another way of enjoying the high-fat foods, yet cutting their % DVs in half at the same time. Simply eat half a serving. Whatever the % DV is on the label, you can divide that by two.

While these symbols represent the levels of total fat, saturated fat, and cholesterol, they do not consider the amount of calories, milligrams of sodium, etc. in the food. It's up to you to read the label to make sure that, if you're watching your sodium or calorie intake, you don't go overboard just because the food is low in fat. Remember that low fat doesn't necessarily mean low calories.

Sadly, obesity in America is on the rise. It could partially be due to consumers believing that as long as they're eating low-fat or fat-free foods, they can have as many servings of them as they want. (Other factors are lack of exercise and leading a sedentary lifestyle.) Therefore, when you're looking through the food list, take note of the number of calories per serving. The same **5% and 20% Rules** (based on 2,000 calories) work here, too.

| 5% Rule | = | A food with 100 calories or less |
| 20% Rule | = | A food with 400 calories or more |

Also, when adding up your calories for each meal, try to keep the total below 25% of the number of calories you should have for the day.

| 25% Rule | = | A meal with 500 calories |

### Abbreviations Used in the Food List

Take note whether the % DVs given in the food list are for a prepared product or just the mix. After the name of the food, it might say "prep as dir," which is the abbreviation for "prepared as directed." That means the values given are for the finished product. In some cases, the manufacturer only lists the values for the mix, leaving it up to the consumer to decide whether to choose a low-fat method of preparation. If the % DVs are just for the mix, you must look up the values for the ingredients you add to make the final product.

| | | | | | |
|---|---|---|---|---|---|
| ~ | = | approximately/about | oz | = | ounce |
| " | = | inch | pc(s) | = | piece(s) |
| < | = | less than | pkg | = | package |
| avg | = | average | pkt | = | packet |
| blk(s) | = | block(s) | prep as dir | = | prepared as directed |
| choc | = | chocolate | serv | = | serving |
| diam | = | diameter | slc(s) | = | slice(s) |
| env | = | envelope | tbsp | = | tablespoon |
| fl oz | = | fluid ounce | tsp | = | teaspoon |
| g | = | gram | w/ | = | with |
| lb | = | pound | w/o | = | without |

## Measurement Equivalents

| VOLUME | | | WEIGHT | | |
|---|---|---|---|---|---|
| 1 teaspoon | = | 1/3 tablespoon | 1 ounce | = | 28.4 grams |
| | | 1/6 fluid ounce | 3 1/2 ounces | = | 100 grams |
| 1 tablespoon | = | 3 teaspoons | 4 ounces | = | 1/4 pound |
| | | 1/2 fluid ounce | 8 ounces | = | 1/2 pound |
| 2 tablespoons | = | 1/8 cup | 16 ounces | = | 1 pound |
| | | 1 fluid ounce | | | |
| 4 tablespoons | = | 1/4 cup | | | |
| | | 2 fluid ounces | | | |
| 16 tablespoons | = | 1 cup | | | |
| | | 8 fluid ounces | | | |
| | | 1/2 pint | | | |
| | | 1/4 quart | | | |
| 2 pints | = | 1 quart | | | |
| | | 32 fluid ounces | | | |
| 1 quart | = | 4 cups | | | |
| | | 32 fluid ounces | | | |
| 4 quarts | = | 1 gallon | | | |
| 1 liter | = | 33.3 fluid ounces | | | |
| | | 1.06 quarts | | | |

# 6. Food Section

<table>
<tr><td></td><td></td><td></td><td colspan="3" align="center">% DAILY VALUE</td></tr>
<tr><td>FOOD</td><td>Serving Size</td><td>Calories</td><td>Tot Fat</td><td>Sat Fat</td><td>Chol</td></tr>
</table>

## Baked Goods

<u>COFFEE CAKES, DANISH, AND SWEET ROLLS</u>

**Generic Foods**

| FOOD | Serving Size | Calories | Tot Fat | Sat Fat | Chol |
|---|---|---|---|---|---|
| ❖ Cinnamon Crumb Coffee Cake | 1 slc (~2 oz) | 210 | 15% | 10% | 9% |
| ❖ Cinnamon Roll | 1 roll (~2 oz) | 200 | 13% | 6% | 0% |
| ❖ Danish Pastry | 1 pc (~2 oz) | 210 | 18% | 19% | 0% |
| ❖ Sweet Roll | 1 roll (~2 oz) | 190 | 12% | 10% | 9% |

**Brand Name Foods**

| FOOD | Serving Size | Calories | Tot Fat | Sat Fat | Chol |
|---|---|---|---|---|---|
| ENTENMANN'S Fat Free Cholesterol Free Coffee Cakes—KRAFT | | | | | |
| ★ Apple Buns | 1 bun | 150 | 0% | 0% | 0% |
| ★ Blueberry Cheese Buns | 1 bun | 140 | 0% | 0% | 0% |
| ★ Cinnamon Raisin Buns | 1 bun | 160 | 0% | 0% | 0% |
| ★ Pineapple Cheese Buns | 1 bun | 140 | 0% | 0% | 0% |
| ★ Raspberry Cheese Buns | 1 bun | 160 | 0% | 0% | 0% |
| AUNT FANNY'S Honey Buns—PET | | | | | |
| ✇ Applesauce filled | 1 bun | 330 | 26% | 20% | 0% |
| ✇ Banana Creme | 1 bun | 350 | 28% | 20% | 0% |
| ✇ Chocolate Creme filled | 1 bun | 350 | 28% | 20% | 0% |
| ✇ Iced Honey Bun | 1 bun | 350 | 28% | 20% | 0% |
| ✇ Large Honey Bun | 1 bun | 500 | 45% | 35% | 0% |
| ✇ Raspberry filled | 1 bun | 350 | 26% | 25% | 0% |
| ✇ Regular Honey Bun | 1 bun | 360 | 31% | 25% | 0% |
| ✇ Vanilla Creme filled | 1 bun | 350 | 28% | 20% | 0% |
| ❖ AUNT JEMIMA Coffee Cake, Easy Mix—QUAKER | 1/3 cup | 170 | 8% | 5% | 0% |

| FOOD | Serving Size | Calories | Tot Fat | Sat Fat | Chol |
|---|---|---|---|---|---|
| **BREAKFAST ON-THE-GO!—** | | | | | |
| WEIGHT WATCHERS | | | | | |
| ★ Cinnamon Streusel Coffee Cake | 1 cake | 190 | 5% | 5% | 0% |
| ❖ Glazed Cinnamon Rolls | 1 roll | 200 | 8% | 8% | 2% |
| Ⓐ ENTENMANN'S Cinnamon Buns—KRAFT | 1 bun | 220 | 15% | 28% | 19% |
| ENTENMANN'S Coffee Cakes—KRAFT | | | | | |
| ❖ Cheese Coffee Cake | 1/9 cake | 190 | 13% | 17% | 10% |
| ❖ Cheese Filled Crumb Coffee Cake | 1/8 cake | 210 | 15% | 19% | 13% |
| Ⓐ Cinnamon Filbert Ring | 1/6 danish | 270 | 26% | 15% | 10% |
| ❖ Crumb Coffee Cake | 1/10 cake | 250 | 19% | 15% | 6% |
| Ⓐ Pecan Danish Ring | 1/8 danish | 230 | 22% | 15% | 8% |
| ❖ Raspberry Danish Twist | 1/8 danish | 220 | 18% | 16% | 6% |
| Ⓐ Walnut Danish Ring | 1/8 danish | 230 | 22% | 15% | 8% |
| ENTENMANN'S Fat Free Cholesterol Free Coffee Cakes—KRAFT | | | | | |
| ★ Apricot Danish Twist | 1/8 danish | 150 | 0% | 0% | 0% |
| ★ Cinnamon Apple Coffee Cake | 1/9 cake | 130 | 0% | 0% | 0% |
| ★ Cinnamon Apple Twist | 1/8 danish | 150 | 0% | 0% | 0% |
| ★ Lemon Twist | 1/8 danish | 130 | 0% | 0% | 0% |
| ★ Raspberry Twist | 1/8 danish | 140 | 0% | 0% | 0% |
| LITTLE DEBBIE Individual Snacks—MCKEE | | | | | |
| ❖ Coffee Cake | 1 pkg (60 g) | 230 | 11% | 6% | 3% |
| Ⓐ Honey Bun | 1 pkg (85 g) | 380 | 36% | 31% | 0% |
| ❖ *Pecan Spinwheels* Coffee Cakes | 1 pkg (57 g) | 220 | 14% | 5% | 0% |
| ❖ MORTON Honey Buns | 1 bun | 250 | 15% | 13% | 0% |
| PEPPERIDGE FARM Danish— CAMPBELL'S | | | | | |
| ❖ Apple | 1 danish | 210 | 14% | 13% | 5% |
| ❖ Cheese | 1 danish | 230 | 17% | 18% | 18% |
| ❖ Raspberry | 1 danish | 210 | 14% | 13% | 5% |
| Ⓐ PEPPERIDGE FARM Apple Fruit Squares—CAMPBELL'S | 1 danish | 210 | 15% | 23% | 0% |
| ❖ PEPPERIDGE FARM Cinnamon Roll—CAMPBELL'S | 1 roll | 250 | 18% | 13% | 5% |
| PILLSBURY Sweet Rolls | | | | | |
| ❖ Apple Cinnamon Roll w/Icing | 1 roll | 140 | 8% | 8% | 0% |
| ❖ Caramel Roll | 1 roll | 170 | 11% | 8% | 0% |
| ❖ Cinnamon Raisin Roll w/Icing | 1 roll | 180 | 11% | 8% | 0% |
| ❖ Cinnamon Roll w/Icing | 1 roll | 140 | 8% | 8% | 0% |
| ❖ Orange Roll w/Icing | 1 roll | 170 | 11% | 8% | 0% |
| Ⓐ SARA LEE Cinnamon Roll, All Butter w/Icing | 1 roll | 300 | 22% | 40% | 12% |
| SARA LEE Coffee Cake | | | | | |

★ Foods with this symbol have less than or equal to 5% *Daily Value* for <u>all</u> three nutrients (5% Rule).

❖ Foods with this symbol have <u>at least one</u> of the three nutrients greater than 5% *Daily Value* but less than or equal to 20% *Daily Value.*

Ⓐ Foods with this symbol have <u>at least one</u> of the three nutrients greater than 20% *Daily Value* (20% Rule).

| FOOD | Serving Size | Calories | Tot Fat | Sat Fat | Chol |
|------|------|------|------|------|------|
| ✦ Butter Streusel | 1/6 cake | 220 | 18% | 30% | 12% |
| ❖ Crumb | 1/8 cake | 220 | 14% | 8% | 5% |
| ✦ Pecan | 1/6 cake | 220 | 18% | 30% | 13% |
| ❖ SUN MAID Cinnamon Rolls— | | | | | |
|    CAMPBELL TAGGART | 1 roll | 180 | 10% | 12% | 2% |

## MUFFINS AND PAN BREADS

### Generic Foods

| | | | | | |
|------|------|------|------|------|------|
| ❖ Banana Bread | 1 slc | 200 | 10% | 8% | 9% |
| ❖ Blueberry Muffin | 1 muffin | 160 | 7% | 4% | 4% |
| ❖ Corn Muffin | 1 muffin | 170 | 9% | 7% | 9% |
| ❖ Cornbread | 1 pc | 180 | 8% | 7% | 11% |
| ❖ Oat Bran Muffin | 1 muffin | 150 | 6% | 3% | 0% |
| ❖ Pumpkin Bread | 1 slc | 200 | 12% | 6% | 9% |
| ❖ Wheat Bran Muffin | 1 muffin | 160 | 11% | 6% | 6% |

### Brand Name Foods

| | | | | | |
|------|------|------|------|------|------|
| ARROWHEAD MILLS | | | | | |
| ★ Cornbread Mix | 1/4 cup mix | 120 | 2% | 0% | 0% |
| ★ Wheat Bran Muffin Mix | 1/3 cup mix | 150 | 3% | 0% | 0% |
| AUNT FANNY'S Muffins—PET | | | | | |
| ❖ Almond Poppy Seed | 2 muffins | 310 | 20% | 10% | 5% |
| ❖ Apple Bran | 2 muffins | 290 | 17% | 10% | 5% |
| ✦ Banana Nut | 2 muffins | 320 | 22% | 10% | 5% |
| ❖ Blueberry | 2 muffins | 290 | 17% | 10% | 5% |
| AUNT JEMIMA Corn Bread | | | | | |
| Mix—QUAKER | | | | | |
| ★ Buttermilk | 3 tbsp | 80 | 0% | 0% | 0% |
| ❖ Easy Mix | 1/3 cup | 150 | 6% | 5% | 0% |
| ★ White | 3 tbsp | 80 | 0% | 0% | 0% |
| ★ Yellow | 3 tbsp | 80 | 0% | 0% | 0% |
| ★ B & M Brown Bread: Plain or | | | | | |
| Raisin—PET | 1/2" slice | 130 | 1% | 0% | 0% |
| ❖ BALLARD Corn Bread | | | | | |
| (prep as dir)—PILLSBURY | 1/16 pan | 130 | 4% | 5% | 8% |
| BETTY CROCKER Muffin Mixes | | | | | |
| (prep as dir)—GENERAL MILLS | | | | | |
| ★ Apple Cinnamon | 1 muffin | 140 | 6% | 4% | 6% |
| ❖ Banana Nut | 1 muffin | 150 | 8% | 5% | 6% |
| ❖ Cinnamon Streusel | 1 muffin | 170 | 11% | 7% | 6% |
| ❖ Lemon Poppyseed | 1 muffin | 190 | 11% | 6% | 6% |
| ❖ Light Blueberry | 1 muffin | 130 | 1% | 0% | 6% |
| ❖ Twice the Blueberry | 1 muffin | 140 | 6% | 4% | 6% |
| ❖ Wild Blueberry | 1 muffin | 170 | 8% | 5% | 6% |

| FOOD | Serving Size | Calories | Tot Fat | Sat Fat | Chol |
|---|---|---|---|---|---|
| BREAKFAST ON-THE-GO! Muffins—WEIGHT WATCHERS | | | | | |
| ❖ Banana Nut | 1 muffin | 190 | 8% | 8% | 2% |
| ❖ Blueberry | 1 muffin | 250 | 8% | 5% | 15% |
| ❖ Chocolate Chocolate Chip | 1 muffin | 200 | 6% | 8% | 2% |
| ❖ Harvest Honey Bran | 1 muffin | 220 | 6% | 5% | 0% |
| DUNCAN HINES Muffin Mix (prep as dir)—PROCTER & GAMBLE | | | | | |
| ❖ Bakery Style Blueberry | 1 muffin | 190 | 8% | 7% | 5% |
| ❖ Bakery Style Cinnamon Swirl | 1 muffin | 200 | 10% | 7% | 6% |
| ❖ Blueberry | 1 muffin | 110 | 5% | 3% | 6% |
| ENTENMANN'S Blueberry Muffins—KRAFT | | | | | |
| ❖ Regular | 1 muffin | 160 | 10% | 7% | 13% |
| ★ Fat Free Cholesterol Free | 1 muffin | 120 | 0% | 0% | 0% |
| ❖ FLAKO Corn Muffin Mix—QUAKER | 1/3 cup | 160 | 6% | 5% | 0% |
| ★ FRIEND'S Brown Bread: Plain or Raisin—PET | 1/2" slice | 130 | 1% | 0% | 0% |
| GOLD MEDAL Muffin Mixes (prep as dir)—GENERAL MILLS | | | | | |
| ❖ Apple Cinnamon | 1 muffin | 170 | 11% | 9% | 12% |
| ❖ Banana Nut | 1 muffin | 170 | 12% | 9% | 12% |
| ❖ Blueberry | 1 muffin | 160 | 10% | 7% | 12% |
| ❖ Caramel Nut | 1 muffin | 170 | 10% | 8% | 12% |
| ❖ Corn Muffin | 1 muffin | 170 | 9% | 7% | 12% |
| ❖ KRUSTEAZ Honey Cornbread Mix (prep as dir) (2" square)—CONTINENTAL MILLS | 1 pc | 120 | 5% | 5% | 7% |
| KRUSTEAZ Muffin Mix (prep as dir)—CONTINENTAL MILLS | | | | | |
| ❖ Almond Poppyseed | 1 muffin | 180 | 8% | 8% | 10% |
| ❖ Apple Cinnamon | 1 muffin | 160 | 6% | 10% | 1% |
| ★ Apple Cinnamon, Fat Free | 1 muffin | 130 | 0% | 0% | 0% |
| ❖ Blueberry | 1 muffin | 180 | 9% | 13% | 12% |
| ★ Blueberry, Fat Free | 1 muffin | 130 | 0% | 0% | 0% |
| ❖ Blueberry Bran | 1 muffin | 190 | 9% | 13% | 10% |
| ❖ Honey Bran | 1 muffin | 160 | 7% | 5% | 8% |
| ❖ Lemon Poppyseed | 1 muffin | 180 | 8% | 10% | 10% |
| ❖ Oat Bran | 1 muffin | 190 | 8% | 5% | 0% |
| PEPPERIDGE FARM *Wholesome Choice* Muffins—CAMPBELL'S | | | | | |
| ★ Apple Oatmeal | 1 muffin | 160 | 5% | 3% | 0% |
| ★ Blueberry | 1 muffin | 140 | 4% | 0% | 0% |
| ★ Bran w/Raisins | 1 muffin | 150 | 4% | 3% | 0% |

★ Foods with this symbol have less than or equal to 5% *Daily Value* for <u>all</u> three nutrients (5% Rule).
❖ Foods with this symbol have <u>at least one</u> of the three nutrients greater than 5% *Daily Value* but less than or equal to 20% *Daily Value*.
Ⓐ Foods with this symbol have <u>at least one</u> of the three nutrients greater than 20% *Daily Value* (20% Rule).

| FOOD | Serving Size | Calories | Tot Fat | Sat Fat | Chol |
|---|---|---|---|---|---|
| ★ Corn | 1 muffin | 150 | 5% | 0% | 0% |
| ❖ PILLSBURY Gingerbread Mix (prep as dir) | 1/8 pan | 220 | 8% | 8% | 0% |
| QUICK BREAD Mix (prep as dir)—PILLSBURY | | | | | |
| ❖ Apple Cinnamon | 1/12 loaf | 180 | 9% | 5% | 7% |
| ❖ Banana | 1/12 loaf | 170 | 9% | 5% | 12% |
| ❖ Blueberry | 1/12 loaf | 180 | 9% | 5% | 7% |
| ❖ Carrot | 1/16 loaf | 140 | 8% | 5% | 8% |
| ❖ Cranberry | 1/12 loaf | 160 | 6% | 5% | 7% |
| ❖ Date | 1/12 loaf | 180 | 6% | 5% | 7% |
| ❖ Nut | 1/12 loaf | 170 | 9% | 5% | 7% |
| ❖ Pumpkin | 1/12 loaf | 170 | 9% | 5% | 12% |
| ROBIN HOOD Muffin Mixes (prep as dir)—GENERAL MILLS | | | | | |
| ❖ Apple Cinnamon | 1 muffin | 170 | 11% | 9% | 12% |
| ❖ Banana Nut | 1 muffin | 170 | 12% | 9% | 12% |
| ❖ Blueberry | 1 muffin | 160 | 10% | 7% | 12% |
| ❖ Caramel Nut | 1 muffin | 170 | 10% | 8% | 12% |
| ❖ Corn Muffin | 1 muffin | 170 | 9% | 7% | 12% |
| SARA LEE Breakfast Quick Breads | | | | | |
| ❖ Apple Cinnamon | 1/8 loaf | 190 | 12% | 8% | 8% |
| ❖ Banana | 1/8 loaf | 180 | 9% | 8% | 8% |
| ❖ Blueberry | 1/8 loaf | 200 | 14% | 8% | 7% |
| ❖ Oatmeal Raisin | 1/8 loaf | 210 | 12% | 8% | 8% |
| SARA LEE Muffins | | | | | |
| ⊛ Hearty Corn | 1 muffin | 260 | 22% | 15% | 8% |
| ❖ Hearty Fruit Blueberry | 1 muffin | 220 | 17% | 10% | 5% |
| ★ THOMAS' Date-Nut Loaf—CPC | 1 oz | 80 | 3% | 0% | 1% |

# Beverages and Beverage Mixes

## ALCOHOLIC BEVERAGES AND MIXERS

**Generic Foods**

| | | | | | |
|---|---|---|---|---|---|
| ★ Ale | 12 fl oz | 150 | 0% | 0% | 0% |
| ★ Light | 12 fl oz | 100 | 0% | 0% | 0% |
| ★ Malt | 12 fl oz | 150 | 0% | 0% | 0% |
| ★ Regular | 12 fl oz | 160 | 0% | 0% | 0% |
| ★ Gin | 1 1/2 fl oz | 110 | 0% | 0% | 0% |
| ★ Rum | 1 1/2 fl oz | 100 | 0% | 0% | 0% |
| ★ Vodka | 1 1/2 fl oz | 100 | 0% | 0% | 0% |
| ★ Whiskey | 1 1/2 fl oz | 110 | 0% | 0% | 0% |
| ★ Anisette | 1 1/2 fl oz | 100 | 0% | 0% | 0% |
| ★ Apricot Brandy | 1 1/2 fl oz | 100 | 0% | 0% | 0% |

| FOOD | Serving Size | Calories | Tot Fat | Sat Fat | Chol |
|------|--------------|----------|---------|---------|------|
| ★ Brandy | 1 1/2 fl oz | 110 | 0% | 0% | 0% |
| ★ Crème de Menthe | 1 1/2 fl oz | 190 | 0% | 0% | 0% |
| ★ Curacao | 1 1/2 fl oz | 80 | 0% | 0% | 0% |
| ★ Kahlua | 1 1/2 fl oz | 180 | 0% | 0% | 0% |
| ★ Dessert | 3 1/2 fl oz | 160 | 0% | 0% | 0% |
| ★ Madeira | 3 1/2 fl oz | 110 | 0% | 0% | 0% |
| ★ Sauterne | 3 1/2 fl oz | 80 | 0% | 0% | 0% |
| ★ Sherry | 3 1/2 fl oz | 80 | 0% | 0% | 0% |
| ★ Table Wine, Red | 3 1/2 fl oz | 70 | 0% | 0% | 0% |
| ★ Table Wine, Rosé | 3 1/2 fl oz | 70 | 0% | 0% | 0% |
| ★ Table Wine, White | 3 1/2 fl oz | 70 | 0% | 0% | 0% |
| ★ Vermouth | 3 1/2 fl oz | 110 | 0% | 0% | 0% |
| ★ Wine Cooler | 8 fl oz | 120 | 0% | 0% | 0% |

**Brand Name Foods**

CANADA DRY Mixers—
CADBURY BEVERAGES

| | | | | | |
|------|--------------|----------|---------|---------|------|
| ★ Collins Mixer | 8 fl oz | 100 | 0% | 0% | 0% |
| ★ Sour Mixer | 8 fl oz | 90 | 0% | 0% | 0% |
| ★ Tonic Water | 8 fl oz | 100 | 0% | 0% | 0% |
| ❖ COCA CASA Cream of Coconut Drink Mix—CADBURY BEVERAGES | 3 tbsp | 170 | 5% | 15% | 0% |
| ★ HOLLAND HOUSE Cooking Wines: All types—CADBURY BEVERAGES | 2 tbsp | 35 | 0% | 0% | 0% |

HOLLAND HOUSE Drink Mixes
—CADBURY BEVERAGES

| | | | | | |
|------|--------------|----------|---------|---------|------|
| ★ Daiquiri | 3.5 fl oz | 150 | 0% | 0% | 0% |
| ★ Manhattan | 2 fl oz | 60 | 0% | 0% | 0% |
| ★ Margarita | 3.5 fl oz | 150 | 0% | 0% | 0% |
| ★ Old Fashioned | 2 fl oz | 80 | 0% | 0% | 0% |
| ★ Pina Colada | 4.5 fl oz | 180 | 0% | 0% | 0% |
| ★ Strawberry Daiquiri | 3.5 fl oz | 150 | 0% | 0% | 0% |
| ★ Sweet & Sour | 4 fl oz | 100 | 0% | 0% | 0% |
| ★ Tom Collins | 3 fl oz | 160 | 0% | 0% | 0% |
| ★ Whiskey Sour | 3.5 fl oz | 150 | 0% | 0% | 0% |

MR. & MRS. "T" Drink Mixes—
CADBURY BEVERAGES

| | | | | | |
|------|--------------|----------|---------|---------|------|
| ★ Bloody Mary | 8 fl oz | 40 | 0% | 0% | 0% |
| ★ Grenadine | 2 tbsp | 80 | 0% | 0% | 0% |
| ★ Mai Tai | 4.5 fl oz | 140 | 0% | 0% | 0% |
| ★ Margarita | 4 fl oz | 130 | 0% | 0% | 0% |
| ★ Pina Colada | 4.5 fl oz | 180 | 0% | 0% | 0% |
| ★ Strawberry Daiquiri | 3.5 fl oz | 150 | 0% | 0% | 0% |

---

★  Foods with this symbol have less than or equal to 5% *Daily Value* for <u>all</u> three nutrients (5% Rule).

❖  Foods with this symbol have <u>at least one</u> of the three nutrients greater than 5% *Daily Value* but less than or equal to 20% *Daily Value*.

Ⓐ  Foods with this symbol have <u>at least one</u> of the three nutrients greater than 20% *Daily Value* (20% Rule).

| FOOD | Serving Size | Calories | Tot Fat | Sat Fat | Chol |
|---|---|---|---|---|---|
| ★ Sweet & Sour | 4 fl oz | 100 | 0% | 0% | 0% |
| ★ Whiskey Sour | 4 fl oz | 100 | 0% | 0% | 0% |
| ROSE'S—CADBURY BEVERAGES | | | | | |
| ★ Grenadine | 2 tbsp | 90 | 0% | 0% | 0% |
| ★ Sweet & Sour Mix (ready-to-use) | 4 fl oz | 100 | 0% | 0% | 0% |
| ★ Sweetened Lime Juice | 1 tsp | 10 | 0% | 0% | 0% |
| BACARDI Frozen Tropical Fruit Mixers—COCA-COLA | | | | | |
| ★ Banana Daiquiri (11% lime juice) | 2 fl oz | 150 | 0% | 0% | 0% |
| ★ Margarita (17% lime juice) | 2 fl oz | 100 | 0% | 0% | 0% |
| Ⓐ Pina Colada | 2 fl oz | 190 | 9% | 25% | 0% |
| ★ Rum Runner (13% fruit juice) | 2 fl oz | 140 | 0% | 0% | 0% |
| ★ Strawberry Daiquiri (10% fruit juice) | 2 fl oz | 140 | 0% | 0% | 0% |
| ★ SCHWEPPES Collins Mixer— CADBURY BEVERAGES | 8 fl oz | 100 | 0% | 0% | 0% |

## CARBONATED BEVERAGES

**Generic Foods**

| FOOD | Serving Size | Calories | Tot Fat | Sat Fat | Chol |
|---|---|---|---|---|---|
| ★ Club Soda | 8 fl oz | 0 | 0% | 0% | 0% |
| ★ Cola | 8 fl oz | 100 | 0% | 0% | 0% |
| ★ Cola, Diet | 8 fl oz | 2 | 0% | 0% | 0% |
| ★ Cream Soda | 8 fl oz | 130 | 0% | 0% | 0% |
| ★ Ginger Ale | 8 fl oz | 80 | 0% | 0% | 0% |
| ★ Mineral Water | 8 fl oz | 0 | 0% | 0% | 0% |
| ★ NonCola, Diet | 8 fl oz | 0 | 0% | 0% | 0% |
| ★ Root Beer | 8 fl oz | 100 | 0% | 0% | 0% |
| ★ Tonic/Quinine Water | 8 fl oz | 85 | 0% | 0% | 0% |

**Brand Name Foods**

| FOOD | Serving Size | Calories | Tot Fat | Sat Fat | Chol |
|---|---|---|---|---|---|
| A & W Cream Soda— CADBURY BEVERAGES | | | | | |
| ★ Diet | 8 fl oz | 0 | 0% | 0% | 0% |
| ★ Regular | 8 fl oz | 110 | 0% | 0% | 0% |
| A & W Root Beer—CADBURY BEVERAGES | | | | | |
| ★ Diet | 8 fl oz | 0 | 0% | 0% | 0% |
| ★ Regular | 8 fl oz | 110 | 0% | 0% | 0% |
| ALL SPORT—PEPSI | 12 fl oz | | | | |
| ★ Fruit Punch | 12 fl oz | 80 | 0% | 0% | 0% |
| ★ Grape | 12 fl oz | 80 | 0% | 0% | 0% |
| ★ Lemon Lime | 12 fl oz | 70 | 0% | 0% | 0% |
| ★ Orange | 12 fl oz | 70 | 0% | 0% | 0% |
| ★ CANADA DRY Diet Sodas: All flavors—CADBURY BEVERAGES | 8 fl oz | 0 | 0% | 0% | 0% |

| FOOD | Serving Size | Calories | Tot Fat | Sat Fat | Chol |
|------|------|------|------|------|------|
| **CANADA DRY Sodas—** | | | | | |
| CADBURY BEVERAGES | | | | | |
| ★ Barrelhead Root Beer | 8 fl oz | 110 | 0% | 0% | 0% |
| ★ Birch Beer | 8 fl oz | 110 | 0% | 0% | 0% |
| ★ Black Cherry Wishniak | 8 fl oz | 130 | 0% | 0% | 0% |
| ★ Cactus Cooler | 8 fl oz | 110 | 0% | 0% | 0% |
| ★ California Strawberry | 8 fl oz | 110 | 0% | 0% | 0% |
| ★ Cherry Ginger Ale | 8 fl oz | 100 | 0% | 0% | 0% |
| ★ Concord Grape | 8 fl oz | 120 | 0% | 0% | 0% |
| ★ Cranberry Ginger Ale | 8 fl oz | 90 | 0% | 0% | 0% |
| ★ Ginger Ale | 8 fl oz | 90 | 0% | 0% | 0% |
| ★ Golden Ginger Ale | 8 fl oz | 100 | 0% | 0% | 0% |
| ★ Half and Half | 8 fl oz | 110 | 0% | 0% | 0% |
| ★ Hi-Spot | 8 fl oz | 110 | 0% | 0% | 0% |
| ★ Island Lime | 8 fl oz | 140 | 0% | 0% | 0% |
| ★ Jamaica Cola | 8 fl oz | 110 | 0% | 0% | 0% |
| ★ Lemon Ginger Ale | 8 fl oz | 90 | 0% | 0% | 0% |
| ★ Lemon Sour | 8 fl oz | 110 | 0% | 0% | 0% |
| ★ Peach Soda | 8 fl oz | 120 | 0% | 0% | 0% |
| ★ Pine Pineapple | 8 fl oz | 110 | 0% | 0% | 0% |
| ★ Sunripe Orange | 8 fl oz | 140 | 0% | 0% | 0% |
| ★ Tahitian Treat | 8 fl oz | 150 | 0% | 0% | 0% |
| ★ Vanilla Cream Soda | 8 fl oz | 120 | 0% | 0% | 0% |
| ★ Wild Cherry | 8 fl oz | 110 | 0% | 0% | 0% |
| ★ **CANADA DRY Sparkling** | | | | | |
| **Water: All flavors—**CADBURY | | | | | |
| BEVERAGES | 8 fl oz | 0 | 0% | 0% | 0% |
| **COCA-COLA: All varieties** | | | | | |
| ★ Diet | 8 fl oz | 1 | 0% | 0% | 0% |
| ★ Regular | 8 fl oz | 97 | 0% | 0% | 0% |
| **COTT Diet Sodas—**CADBURY | | | | | |
| BEVERAGES | | | | | |
| ★ Ginger Ale | 8 fl oz | 5 | 0% | 0% | 0% |
| ★ Tonic | 8 fl oz | 5 | 0% | 0% | 0% |
| **COTT Sodas—**CADBURY BEVERAGES | | | | | |
| ★ Cola | 8 fl oz | 110 | 0% | 0% | 0% |
| ★ Cream Soda | 8 fl oz | 120 | 0% | 0% | 0% |
| ★ Ginger Ale | 8 fl oz | 90 | 0% | 0% | 0% |
| ★ Grape | 8 fl oz | 130 | 0% | 0% | 0% |
| ★ Half & Half | 8 fl oz | 120 | 0% | 0% | 0% |
| ★ Lemon Up | 8 fl oz | 110 | 0% | 0% | 0% |
| ★ Mint Ginger Ale | 8 fl oz | 110 | 0% | 0% | 0% |
| ★ Orange | 8 fl oz | 140 | 0% | 0% | 0% |
| ★ Pineapple | 8 fl oz | 130 | 0% | 0% | 0% |
| ★ Punch | 8 fl oz | 130 | 0% | 0% | 0% |

★ Foods with this symbol have less than or equal to 5% *Daily Value* for all three nutrients (5% Rule).

❖ Foods with this symbol have at least one of the three nutrients greater than 5% *Daily Value* but less than or equal to 20% *Daily Value*.

Ⓐ Foods with this symbol have at least one of the three nutrients greater than 20% *Daily Value* (20% Rule).

| FOOD | Serving Size | Calories | Tot Fat | Sat Fat | Chol |
|------|------|------|------|------|------|
| ★ Red Cherry | 8 fl oz | 130 | 0% | 0% | 0% |
| ★ Root Beer | 8 fl oz | 110 | 0% | 0% | 0% |
| ★ Tonic | 8 fl oz | 100 | 0% | 0% | 0% |
| CRUSH Orange Soda— CADBURY BEVERAGES | | | | | |
| ★ Diet | 8 fl oz | 20 | 0% | 0% | 0% |
| ★ Regular | 8 fl oz | 140 | 0% | 0% | 0% |
| ★ Cherry | 8 fl oz | 140 | 0% | 0% | 0% |
| CRUSH Sodas—CADBURY BEVERAGES | | | | | |
| ★ Grape | 8 fl oz | 140 | 0% | 0% | 0% |
| ★ Peach | 8 fl oz | 140 | 0% | 0% | 0% |
| ★ Pineapple | 8 fl oz | 140 | 0% | 0% | 0% |
| ★ Strawberry | 8 fl oz | 130 | 0% | 0% | 0% |
| ★ Tropical Fruit Punch (5% juice) | 10 fl oz | 180 | 0% | 0% | 0% |
| ★ Tropical Punch | 8 fl oz | 210 | 0% | 0% | 0% |
| ★ CRYSTAL—PEPSI | 12 fl oz | 150 | 0% | 0% | 0% |
| FANTA Sodas—COCA-COLA | | | | | |
| ★ Ginger Ale | 8 fl oz | 90 | 0% | 0% | 0% |
| ★ Grape | 8 fl oz | 120 | 0% | 0% | 0% |
| ★ Orange | 8 fl oz | 120 | 0% | 0% | 0% |
| ★ Root Beer | 8 fl oz | 110 | 0% | 0% | 0% |
| ★ FRESCA—COCA-COLA | 8 fl oz | 3 | 0% | 0% | 0% |
| HIRES Cream Soda— CADBURY BEVERAGES | | | | | |
| ★ Diet | 8 fl oz | 0 | 0% | 0% | 0% |
| ★ Regular | 8 fl oz | 130 | 0% | 0% | 0% |
| HIRES Root Beer—CADBURY BEVERAGES | | | | | |
| ★ Diet | 8 fl oz | 0 | 0% | 0% | 0% |
| ★ Regular | 8 fl oz | 130 | 0% | 0% | 0% |
| MOUNTAIN DEW: All varieties— PEPSI | | | | | |
| ★ Diet | 12 fl oz | 0 | 0% | 0% | 0% |
| ★ Regular | 12 fl oz | 170 | 0% | 0% | 0% |
| MR. PIBB—COCA-COLA | | | | | |
| ★ Diet | 8 fl oz | 1 | 0% | 0% | 0% |
| ★ Regular | 8 fl oz | 97 | 0% | 0% | 0% |
| MUG Cream Soda—PEPSI | | | | | |
| ★ Diet | 12 fl oz | 5 | 0% | 0% | 0% |
| ★ Regular | 12 fl oz | 170 | 0% | 0% | 0% |
| MUG Root Beer—PEPSI | | | | | |
| ★ Diet | 12 fl oz | 0 | 0% | 0% | 0% |
| ★ Regular | 12 fl oz | 160 | 0% | 0% | 0% |
| PEPSI: All varieties | | | | | |
| ★ Diet | 12 fl oz | 0 | 0% | 0% | 0% |
| ★ Regular | 12 fl oz | 150 | 0% | 0% | 0% |
| SCHWEPPES Diet Sodas— CADBURY BEVERAGES | | | | | |
| ★ Dry Grape Ginger Ale | 8 fl oz | 2 | 0% | 0% | 0% |

| FOOD | Serving Size | Calories | Tot Fat | Sat Fat | Chol |
|---|---|---|---|---|---|
| ★   Ginger Ale | 8 fl oz | 0 | 0% | 0% | 0% |
| ★   Raspberry Ginger Ale | 8 fl oz | 0 | 0% | 0% | 0% |
| ★ SCHWEPPES Seltzer Water: All | | | | | |
|      flavors—CADBURY BEVERAGES | 8 fl oz | 0 | 0% | 0% | 0% |
| SCHWEPPES Sodas—CADBURY | | | | | |
| BEVERAGES | | | | | |
| ★   Bitter Lemon | 8 fl oz | 110 | 0% | 0% | 0% |
| ★   Citrus Tonic | 8 fl oz | 90 | 0% | 0% | 0% |
| ★   Cranberry Tonic | 8 fl oz | 90 | 0% | 0% | 0% |
| ★   Dry Grape Ginger Ale | 8 fl oz | 100 | 0% | 0% | 0% |
| ★   Ginger Ale | 8 fl oz | 90 | 0% | 0% | 0% |
| ★   Ginger Beer | 8 fl oz | 100 | 0% | 0% | 0% |
| ★   Grape | 8 fl oz | 130 | 0% | 0% | 0% |
| ★   Grapefruit | 8 fl oz | 110 | 0% | 0% | 0% |
| ★   Iced Tea | 8 fl oz | 90 | 0% | 0% | 0% |
| ★   Lemon Sour | 8 fl oz | 110 | 0% | 0% | 0% |
| ★   Lemon-Lime | 8 fl oz | 100 | 0% | 0% | 0% |
| ★   Raspberry Ginger Ale | 8 fl oz | 100 | 0% | 0% | 0% |
| ★   Raspberry Tonic | 8 fl oz | 90 | 0% | 0% | 0% |
| ★   Tonic Water | 8 fl oz | 90 | 0% | 0% | 0% |
| SLICE—PEPSI | | | | | |
| ★   Cherry Spice | 12 fl oz | 150 | 0% | 0% | 0% |
| ★   Cola | 12 fl oz | 160 | 0% | 0% | 0% |
| ★   Diet: All flavors | 12 fl oz | 0 | 0% | 0% | 0% |
| ★   Dr. Slice | 12 fl oz | 140 | 0% | 0% | 0% |
| ★   Fruit Punch | 12 fl oz | 190 | 0% | 0% | 0% |
| ★   Grape | 12 fl oz | 190 | 0% | 0% | 0% |
| ★   Lemon Lime | 12 fl oz | 150 | 0% | 0% | 0% |
| ★   Mandarin Orange | 12 fl oz | 190 | 0% | 0% | 0% |
| ★   Pineapple | 12 fl oz | 190 | 0% | 0% | 0% |
| ★   Red | 12 fl oz | 190 | 0% | 0% | 0% |
| ★   Strawberry | 12 fl oz | 170 | 0% | 0% | 0% |
| SPRITE—COCA-COLA | | | | | |
| ★   Diet | 8 fl oz | 3 | 0% | 0% | 0% |
| ★   Regular | 8 fl oz | 100 | 0% | 0% | 0% |
| SUNDROP Sodas—CADBURY | | | | | |
| BEVERAGES | | | | | |
| ★   Diet | 8 fl oz | 5 | 0% | 0% | 0% |
| ★   Regular | 8 fl oz | 140 | 0% | 0% | 0% |
| SUNKIST Sodas—CADBURY BEVERAGES | | | | | |
| ★   Cherry | 8 fl oz | 140 | 0% | 0% | 0% |
| ★   Citrus | 8 fl oz | 100 | 0% | 0% | 0% |
| ★   Citrus, Diet | 8 fl oz | 0 | 0% | 0% | 0% |
| ★   Fruit Punch | 8 fl oz | 130 | 0% | 0% | 0% |

★ Foods with this symbol have less than or equal to 5% *Daily Value* for all three nutrients (5% Rule).

❖ Foods with this symbol have at least one of the three nutrients greater than 5% *Daily Value* but less than or equal to 20% *Daily Value*.

Ⓐ Foods with this symbol have at least one of the three nutrients greater than 20% *Daily Value* (20% Rule).

| FOOD | Serving Size | Calories | Tot Fat | Sat Fat | Chol |
|------|------|------|------|------|------|
| ★ Grape | 8 fl oz | 140 | 0% | 0% | 0% |
| ★ Lemonade | 8 fl oz | 120 | 0% | 0% | 0% |
| ★ Orange | 8 fl oz | 140 | 0% | 0% | 0% |
| ★ Orange, Diet | 8 fl oz | 5 | 0% | 0% | 0% |
| ★ Peach | 8 fl oz | 120 | 0% | 0% | 0% |
| ★ Pineapple | 8 fl oz | 140 | 0% | 0% | 0% |
| ★ Sparkling Lemonade, Diet | 8 fl oz | 0 | 0% | 0% | 0% |
| ★ Strawberry | 8 fl oz | 140 | 0% | 0% | 0% |
| ★ TAB—COCA-COLA | 8 fl oz | 1 | 0% | 0% | 0% |

## COCOA AND COCOA MIXES

**Generic Foods**

| FOOD | Serving Size | Calories | Tot Fat | Sat Fat | Chol |
|------|------|------|------|------|------|
| ★ Carob Powder | 2 tbsp | 50 | 1% | 0% | 0% |
| ★ Cocoa Mix | 2 tbsp | 100 | 2% | 3% | 0% |
| ★ Cocoa Mix, Aspartame sweetened (prep w/water) | 8 fl oz | 60 | 1% | 2% | 1% |

**Brand Name Foods**

| FOOD | Serving Size | Calories | Tot Fat | Sat Fat | Chol |
|------|------|------|------|------|------|
| ❖ ALPINE COCOA: All flavors—CONTINENTAL MILLS | 1 pouch | 160 | 9% | 8% | 0% |
| ★ ALPINE COCOA Light: All flavors—CONTINENTAL MILLS | 1 pouch | 60 | 2% | 3% | 0% |
| ★ FEATHERWEIGHT Hot Cocoa Mix | 1 pouch | 40 | 2% | 5% | 0% |
| GHIRARDELLI Cocoas | | | | | |
| ⊛ Sweet Ground Chocolate & Cocoa | 2 1/2 tbsp | 80 | 19% | 36% | 3% |
| ★ Unsweetened | 1 tbsp | 20 | 2% | 4% | 0% |
| GHIRARDELLI Hot Chocolates | | | | | |
| ★ Double Chocolate | 2 1/2 tbsp | 80 | 2% | 5% | 0% |
| ★ Hazelnut | 2 1/2 tbsp | 80 | 2% | 4% | 0% |
| ★ Mocha | 2 1/2 tbsp | 80 | 3% | 4% | 0% |
| HERSHEY's Bake Shoppe | | | | | |
| ★ Cocoa | 1 tbsp | 20 | 1% | 0% | 0% |
| ★ European Style Cocoa | 1 tbsp | 20 | 1% | 0% | 0% |
| HERSHEY's Hot Cocoa Collection | | | | | |
| ★ Chocolate Almond | 1 pkt | 150 | 5% | 3% | 0% |
| ★ Chocolate Mint | 1 pkt | 150 | 5% | 3% | 0% |
| ★ Chocolate Raspberry | 1 pkt | 150 | 5% | 3% | 0% |
| ★ Dutch Chocolate | 1 pkt | 150 | 5% | 3% | 0% |
| ★ Irish Cream | 1 pkt | 150 | 5% | 3% | 0% |
| ★ NESTLÉ Cocoa, unsweetened | 1 tbsp | 15 | 1% | 0% | 0% |
| SWISS MISS Hot Cocoa Mix—HUNT WESSON | | | | | |
| ❖ Cocoa and Cream | 1 pkt | 150 | 8% | 15% | 2% |
| ★ Diet | 1 pkt | 20 | 0% | 1% | 0% |
| ★ Fat Free | 1 pkt | 50 | 0% | 0% | 1% |
| ★ Lite | 1 pkt | 70 | 1% | 1% | 0% |

| FOOD | Serving Size | Calories | Tot Fat | Sat Fat | Chol |
|---|---|---|---|---|---|
| ★ Marshmallow Lovers | 1 pkt | 140 | 5% | 5% | 1% |
| ★ Milk Chocolate | 1 pkt | 110 | 2% | 1% | 0% |
| ★ Mini-Marshmallow | 1 pkt | 110 | 2% | 2% | 0% |
| ★ Rich Chocolate | 1 pkt | 110 | 2% | 2% | 0% |
| ★ Sugar Free | 1/4 cup | 70 | 0% | 0% | 0% |
| ★ Sugar Free Mini-Marshmallow | 1 pkt | 50 | 1% | 1% | 0% |
| ★ Sugar Free Rich | 1 pkt | 50 | 0% | 1% | 0% |
| ★ Sugar-Free Milk Chocolate | 1 pkt | 50 | 0% | 0% | 0% |
| ★ White Chocolate | 1 pkt | 110 | 2% | 2% | 0% |
| SWISS MISS Premiere Hot Cocoa—HUNT WESSON | | | | | |
| ★ Almond Mocha | 1 pkt | 140 | 4% | 4% | 0% |
| ★ Chocolate English Toffee | 1 pkt | 140 | 4% | 3% | 0% |
| ★ Chocolate Raspberry Truffle | 1 pkt | 140 | 4% | 4% | 0% |
| ★ Suisse Chocolate Truffle | 1 pkt | 140 | 4% | 4% | 0% |

## COFFEE AND TEA

### Generic Foods

| FOOD | Serving Size | Calories | Tot Fat | Sat Fat | Chol |
|---|---|---|---|---|---|
| ★ Coffee, brewed: Regular or Decaffeinated | 8 fl oz | 5 | 0% | 0% | 0% |
| ★ Coffee, instant: Regular or Decaffeinated (prep w/water) | 8 fl oz | 5 | 0% | 0% | 0% |
| ★ Tea, brewed: Regular or Herbal | 8 fl oz | 2 | 0% | 0% | 0% |
| ★ Tea, instant (prep w/water) | 8 fl oz | 2 | 0% | 0% | 0% |

### Brand Name Foods

| FOOD | Serving Size | Calories | Tot Fat | Sat Fat | Chol |
|---|---|---|---|---|---|
| GENERAL FOODS *International Coffees* (prep as dir)—KRAFT | | | | | |
| ★ Cafe Amaretto | 8 fl oz | 60 | 5% | 3% | 0% |
| ★ Cafe Francais | 8 fl oz | 60 | 5% | 4% | 0% |
| ★ Cafe Vienna | 8 fl oz | 70 | 4% | 3% | 0% |
| ★ French Vanilla Cafe | 8 fl oz | 60 | 4% | 3% | 0% |
| ★ Hazelnut Belgian Cafe | 8 fl oz | 70 | 3% | 3% | 0% |
| ★ Italian Cappuccino | 8 fl oz | 50 | 3% | 3% | 0% |
| ★ Kahlua Cafe | 8 fl oz | 60 | 3% | 3% | 0% |
| ★ Orange Cappuccino | 8 fl oz | 70 | 3% | 3% | 0% |
| ★ Suisse Mocha: Regular or Decaf | 8 fl oz | 60 | 4% | 3% | 0% |
| ★ Viennese Chocolate Cafe | 8 fl oz | 60 | 3% | 4% | 0% |
| GENERAL FOODS *International Coffees*, Sugar Free Low Calorie (prep as dir)—KRAFT | | | | | |
| ★ Cafe Vienna | 8 fl oz | 30 | 2% | 3% | 0% |

★ Foods with this symbol have less than or equal to 5% *Daily Value* for all three nutrients (5% Rule).
❖ Foods with this symbol have at least one of the three nutrients greater than 5% *Daily Value* but less than or equal to 20% *Daily Value*.
⊘ Foods with this symbol have at least one of the three nutrients greater than 20% *Daily Value* (20% Rule).

| FOOD | Serving Size | Calories | Tot Fat | Sat Fat | Chol |
|------|------|------|------|------|------|
| ★ French Vanilla Cafe | 8 fl oz | 35 | 3% | 3% | 0% |
| ★ Orange Cappuccino | 8 fl oz | 30 | 2% | 3% | 0% |
| ★ Suisse Mocha: Regular or Decaf | 8 fl oz | 30 | 3% | 3% | 0% |
| MAXWELL HOUSE *Cappio* Iced Cappuccino—KRAFT | | | | | |
| ❖ Coffee | 8 fl oz | 130 | 4% | 8% | 2% |
| ❖ Mocha | 8 fl oz | 140 | 4% | 8% | 2% |
| ❖ Vanilla | 8 fl oz | 140 | 3% | 7% | 2% |
| MAXWELL HOUSE Cappuccino (prep as dir)—KRAFT | | | | | |
| ★ Cinnamon | 8 fl oz | 90 | 2% | 0% | 0% |
| ★ Coffee | 8 fl oz | 90 | 1% | 0% | 0% |
| ❖ Mocha: Regular or Decaf | 8 fl oz | 100 | 4% | 6% | 0% |
| ★ Vanilla: Regular or Decaf | 8 fl oz | 90 | 2% | 0% | 0% |
| POSTUM (prep as dir)—KRAFT | | | | | |
| ★ Coffee Flavor Instant Hot Beverage | 8 fl oz | 10 | 0% | 0% | 0% |
| ★ Instant Hot Beverage | 8 fl oz | 10 | 0% | 0% | 0% |

### FLAVORED MILK BEVERAGES

**Generic Foods**

| FOOD | Serving Size | Calories | Tot Fat | Sat Fat | Chol |
|------|------|------|------|------|------|
| Chocolate Milk | | | | | |
| ❖ 1% milk fat | 8 fl oz | 160 | 4% | 8% | 2% |
| ❖ 2% milk fat | 8 fl oz | 180 | 8% | 16% | 6% |
| ⊛ Whole milk | 8 fl oz | 210 | 13% | 26% | 10% |

**Brand Name Foods**

| FOOD | Serving Size | Calories | Tot Fat | Sat Fat | Chol |
|------|------|------|------|------|------|
| HERSHEY's Milk Drinks | | | | | |
| ❖ 2% Chocolate Milk | 8 fl oz | 90 | 8% | 15% | 5% |
| ★ Banana Split Drink | 8 fl oz | 160 | 4% | 0% | 1% |
| ★ Chocolate Caramel Flavored Drink | 8 fl oz | 160 | 4% | 0% | 1% |
| ★ Chocolate Cherry Flavored Drink | 8 fl oz | 160 | 4% | 0% | 1% |
| ★ Chocolate Marshmallow Drink | 8 fl oz | 160 | 4% | 0% | 1% |
| ★ HERSHEY's Chocolate Milk Mix | 2 tbsp mix | 60 | 0% | 0% | 0% |
| ❖ HERSHEY's Shake Drink Box | 8 fl oz | 230 | 7% | 13% | 7% |
| KRAFT Instant Malted (prep as dir) | | | | | |
| ❖ Chocolate | 1 cup | 200 | 9% | 15% | 7% |
| ❖ Natural | 1 cup | 210 | 11% | 20% | 8% |
| QUIK—NESTLÉ | | | | | |
| ★ Chocolate Flavor Drink Mix | 2 tbsp mix | 90 | 1% | 1% | 0% |
| ★ Strawberry Flavor Drink Mix | 2 tbsp mix | 90 | 0% | 0% | 0% |
| ★ Sugar-Free Chocolate Flavor Drink Mix | 2 tbsp mix | 40 | 1% | 2% | 0% |
| OVALTINE—SANDOZ | | | | | |
| ★ Classic Original Malt Flavor | 4 tbsp mix | 80 | 0% | 0% | 0% |

| FOOD | Serving Size | Calories | Tot Fat | Sat Fat | Chol |
|------|--------------|----------|---------|---------|------|
| ★ Classic Tradition Chocolate Malt Flavor | 4 tbsp mix | 80 | 0% | 0% | 0% |
| ★ Rich Chocolate | 4 tbsp mix | 80 | 0% | 0% | 0% |

## FRUIT-FLAVORED BEVERAGES

### Brand Name Foods

| FOOD | Serving Size | Calories | Tot Fat | Sat Fat | Chol |
|------|--------------|----------|---------|---------|------|
| ALPINE Spiced Cider Drink Mix —CONTINENTAL MILLS | | | | | |
| ★ Regular | 1 packet | 80 | 0% | 0% | 0% |
| ★ Sugar Free | 1 packet | 15 | 0% | 0% | 0% |
| ★ BETTY CROCKER *Squeezit*: All flavors—GENERAL MILLS | 1 bottle | 110 | 0% | 0% | 0% |
| ★ BETTY CROCKER *Squeezit 100*: All flavors—GENERAL MILLS | 1 bottle | 100 | 0% | 0% | 0% |
| BRIGHT & EARLY Beverage— COCA-COLA | | | | | |
| ★ Apple Beverage (1% juice) | 8 fl oz | 120 | 0% | 0% | 0% |
| ★ Fruit Punch (0% juice) | 8 fl oz | 130 | 0% | 0% | 0% |
| ★ Grape (0% juice) | 8 fl oz | 140 | 0% | 0% | 0% |
| ★ Lemonade (1% juice) | 8 fl oz | 120 | 0% | 0% | 0% |
| ★ Orange Beverage (1% juice) | 8 fl oz | 120 | 0% | 0% | 0% |
| ★ CAPRI SUN: All flavors—KRAFT | 6.75 fl oz | 100 | 0% | 0% | 0% |
| COUNTRY TIME—KRAFT | | | | | |
| ★ Sugar Sweetened Drink Mix: All flavors (prep as dir) | 8 fl oz | 70 | 0% | 0% | 0% |
| ★ Sugar Free Low Calorie Drink Mix: All flavors (prep as dir) | 8 fl oz | 5 | 0% | 0% | 0% |
| ★ CRYSTAL LIGHT Low Calorie Soft Drink Mix: All flavors (prep as dir)—KRAFT | 8 fl oz | 5 | 0% | 0% | 0% |
| KOOL-AID—KRAFT | | | | | |
| ★ Sugar Free Low Calorie Soft Drink Mix: All flavors (prep as dir) | 8 fl oz | 5 | 0% | 0% | 0% |
| ★ Sugar Sweetened Soft Drink Mix: All flavors (prep as dir) | 8 fl oz | 70 | 0% | 0% | 0% |
| ★ Unsweetened Soft Drink Mix: All flavors (prep as dir) | 8 fl oz | 100 | 0% | 0% | 0% |
| ★ KOOL-AID *Bursts* Soft Drink: All flavors—KRAFT | 6.75 fl oz | 100 | 0% | 0% | 0% |

★ Foods with this symbol have less than or equal to 5% *Daily Value* for <u>all</u> three nutrients (5% Rule).
❖ Foods with this symbol have <u>at least one</u> of the three nutrients greater than 5% *Daily Value* but less than or equal to 20% *Daily Value*.
Ⓢ Foods with this symbol have <u>at least one</u> of the three nutrients greater than 20% *Daily Value* (20% Rule).

| FOOD | Serving Size | Calories | Tot Fat | Sat Fat | Chol |
|------|-------------|----------|---------|---------|------|
| NATURAL BREWS (0% juice)— | | | | | |
| SMUCKER'S | | | | | |
| ★ Cafe Mocha | 8 fl oz | 150 | 0% | 0% | 0% |
| ★ Cherry Amaretto | 8 fl oz | 160 | 0% | 0% | 0% |
| ★ Draft Rootbeer | 8 fl oz | 180 | 0% | 0% | 0% |
| ★ Ginseng Cola | 8 fl oz | 170 | 0% | 0% | 0% |
| ★ Orange Creme | 8 fl oz | 160 | 0% | 0% | 0% |
| ★ Outrageous Gingerale | 8 fl oz | 170 | 0% | 0% | 0% |
| ★ Spiced Apple | 8 fl oz | 170 | 0% | 0% | 0% |
| ★ Vanilla Creme | 8 fl oz | 170 | 0% | 0% | 0% |
| ★ POWERADE: All flavors— | | | | | |
| COCA-COLA | 8 fl oz | 70 | 0% | 0% | 0% |
| ★ SWISS MISS Spiced Apple | | | | | |
| Cider Mix—HUNT WESSON | 1/4 cup | 80 | 0% | 0% | 0% |
| TANG Drink Mix—KRAFT | | | | | |
| ★ Mango flavored (prep as dir) | 8 fl oz | 100 | 0% | 0% | 0% |
| ★ Orange flavored (prep as dir) | 8 fl oz | 100 | 0% | 0% | 0% |
| ★ Orange flavored, Sugar Free Low Calorie Drink Mix (prep as dir) | 8 fl oz | 5 | 0% | 0% | 0% |

## FRUIT JUICES: COCKTAILS, DRINKS, AND JUICES

**Generic Foods**

| FOOD | Serving Size | Calories | Tot Fat | Sat Fat | Chol |
|------|-------------|----------|---------|---------|------|
| ★ Apple Cider | 8 fl oz | 120 | 0% | 0% | 0% |
| ★ Apple Juice | 8 fl oz | 120 | 0% | 0% | 0% |
| ★ Apricot Nectar | 8 fl oz | 140 | 0% | 0% | 0% |
| ★ Cranberry Juice | 8 fl oz | 150 | 0% | 0% | 0% |
| ★ Grape Juice | 8 fl oz | 140 | 0% | 0% | 0% |
| ★ Grapefruit Juice | 8 fl oz | 100 | 0% | 0% | 0% |
| ★ Lemon Juice | 1 tsp | 1 | 0% | 0% | 0% |
| ★ Lemonade | 8 fl oz | 110 | 0% | 0% | 0% |
| ★ Lemonade Powder (prep w/water) | 8 fl oz | 110 | 0% | 0% | 0% |
| ★ Lime Juice | 1 tsp | 1 | 0% | 0% | 0% |
| ★ Orange Juice | 8 fl oz | 110 | 0% | 0% | 0% |
| ★ Papaya Nectar | 8 fl oz | 140 | 0% | 0% | 0% |
| ★ Passion Fruit Juice | 8 fl oz | 130 | 0% | 0% | 0% |
| ★ Peach Nectar | 8 fl oz | 130 | 0% | 0% | 0% |
| ★ Pear Nectar | 8 fl oz | 150 | 0% | 0% | 0% |
| ★ Pineapple Juice | 8 fl oz | 130 | 0% | 0% | 0% |
| ★ Prune Juice | 8 fl oz | 180 | 0% | 0% | 0% |

**Brand Name Foods**

| FOOD | Serving Size | Calories | Tot Fat | Sat Fat | Chol |
|------|-------------|----------|---------|---------|------|
| DEL MONTE 100% Fruit Juices | | | | | |
| ★ Pineapple | 8 fl oz | 110 | 0% | 0% | 0% |
| ★ Prune | 8 fl oz | 170 | 0% | 0% | 0% |

| FOOD | Serving Size | Calories | Tot Fat | Sat Fat | Chol |
|------|------|------|------|------|------|
| DOLE 100% Fruit Juice Blends (prep from concentrate) | | | | | |
| ★ Country Raspberry | 8 fl oz | 140 | 0% | 0% | 0% |
| ★ Mandarin Tangerine | 8 fl oz | 140 | 0% | 0% | 0% |
| ★ Mountain Cherry | 8 fl oz | 120 | 0% | 0% | 0% |
| ★ Orchard Peach | 8 fl oz | 140 | 0% | 0% | 0% |
| ★ Tropical Fruit | 8 fl oz | 140 | 0% | 0% | 0% |
| DOLE 100% Fruit Juices (prep from concentrate) | | | | | |
| ★ Pine-Grapefruit | 8 fl oz | 130 | 0% | 0% | 0% |
| ★ Pine-Orange | 8 fl oz | 120 | 0% | 0% | 0% |
| ★ Pine-Orange-Banana | 8 fl oz | 130 | 0% | 0% | 0% |
| ★ Pine-Orange-Berry | 8 fl oz | 130 | 0% | 0% | 0% |
| ★ Pine-Orange-Guava | 8 fl oz | 120 | 0% | 0% | 0% |
| ★ Pine-Orange-Strawberry | 8 fl oz | 130 | 0% | 0% | 0% |
| ★ Pine-Passion-Banana | 8 fl oz | 120 | 0% | 0% | 0% |
| ★ Pineapple | 8 fl oz | 130 | 0% | 0% | 0% |
| DOLE Fruit Juice Drink (prep from concentrate) | | | | | |
| ★ Apple Berry Burst (15% juice) | 8 fl oz | 120 | 0% | 0% | 0% |
| ★ Fruit Fiesta (15% juice) | 8 fl oz | 140 | 0% | 0% | 0% |
| ★ Lanai Breeze (20% juice) | 8 fl oz | 120 | 0% | 0% | 0% |
| ★ Pacific Pink Grapefruit (35% juice) | 8 fl oz | 140 | 0% | 0% | 0% |
| ★ Raspberry Lemon Splash (15% juice) | 8 fl oz | 120 | 0% | 0% | 0% |
| ★ Tropical Breeze (20% juice) | 8 fl oz | 120 | 0% | 0% | 0% |
| FARMERS MARKET—SMUCKER'S | | | | | |
| ★ Boysenberry (31% juice) | 8 fl oz | 120 | 0% | 0% | 0% |
| ★ Cherry (33% juice) | 8 fl oz | 120 | 0% | 0% | 0% |
| ★ Cranberry (30% juice) | 8 fl oz | 120 | 0% | 0% | 0% |
| ★ Papaya (43% juice) | 8 fl oz | 130 | 0% | 0% | 0% |
| ★ Peach (46% juice) | 8 fl oz | 120 | 0% | 0% | 0% |
| ★ Pineapple Coconut (43% juice) | 8 fl oz | 120 | 0% | 0% | 0% |
| ★ Raspberry (30% juice) | 8 fl oz | 120 | 0% | 0% | 0% |
| ★ Strawberry (32% juice) | 8 fl oz | 120 | 0% | 0% | 0% |
| ★ Tropical Orange (30% juice) | 8 fl oz | 120 | 0% | 0% | 0% |
| ★ Tropical Punch (30% juice) | 8 fl oz | 120 | 0% | 0% | 0% |
| FIVE ALIVE—COCA-COLA | | | | | |
| ★ Berry Citrus (41% juice) | 8 fl oz | 120 | 0% | 0% | 0% |
| ★ Citrus (41% juice) | 8 fl oz | 120 | 0% | 0% | 0% |
| ★ Tropical Citrus (43% juice) | 8 fl oz | 120 | 0% | 0% | 0% |
| HEINKE'S—SMUCKER'S | | | | | |
| ★ Apple Boysenberry (100% juice) | 8 fl oz | 120 | 0% | 0% | 0% |

★ Foods with this symbol have less than or equal to 5% *Daily Value* for <u>all</u> three nutrients (5% Rule).
❖ Foods with this symbol have <u>at least one</u> of the three nutrients greater than 5% *Daily Value* but less than or equal to 20% *Daily Value*.
Ⓐ Foods with this symbol have <u>at least one</u> of the three nutrients greater than 20% *Daily Value* (20% Rule).

| FOOD | Serving Size | Calories | Tot Fat | Sat Fat | Chol |
|---|---|---|---|---|---|
| ★ Apple Raspberry (100% juice) | 8 fl oz | 120 | 0% | 0% | 0% |
| ★ Berry Patch (100% juice) | 8 fl oz | 120 | 0% | 0% | 0% |
| ★ Black Cherry (100% juice) | 8 fl oz | 180 | 0% | 0% | 0% |
| ★ Boysenberry Cider (100% juice) | 8 fl oz | 120 | 0% | 0% | 0% |
| ★ California Punch (80% juice) | 8 fl oz | 110 | 0% | 0% | 0% |
| ★ Cherry Cider (88% juice) | 8 fl oz | 115 | 0% | 0% | 0% |
| ★ Cranberry 100% (100% juice) | 8 fl oz | 60 | 0% | 0% | 0% |
| ★ Cranberry Lemonade (81% juice) | 8 fl oz | 120 | 0% | 0% | 0% |
| ★ Cranberry Nectar (100% juice) | 8 fl oz | 120 | 0% | 0% | 0% |
| ★ Gravenstein Apple (100% juice) | 8 fl oz | 120 | 0% | 0% | 0% |
| ★ Hibiscus Cranberry (80% juice) | 8 fl oz | 120 | 0% | 0% | 0% |
| ★ Macchu Pichu Punch (100% juice) | 8 fl oz | 120 | 0% | 0% | 0% |
| ★ Mountain Raspberry (100% juice) | 8 fl oz | 120 | 0% | 0% | 0% |
| ★ Natural Apple (100% juice) | 8 fl oz | 120 | 0% | 0% | 0% |
| ★ Old Fashioned Lemon (74% juice) | 8 fl oz | 120 | 0% | 0% | 0% |
| ★ Organic Apple (100% juice) | 8 fl oz | 120 | 0% | 0% | 0% |
| ★ Organic Pear (100% juice) | 8 fl oz | 120 | 0% | 0% | 0% |
| ★ Paradise Punch (63% juice) | 8 fl oz | 110 | 0% | 0% | 0% |
| ★ Passionfruit Mango (77% juice) | 8 fl oz | 130 | 0% | 0% | 0% |
| HI-C Beverage (10% juice)— | | | | | |
| COCA-COLA | | | | | |
| ★ Boppin' Berry | 8 fl oz | 130 | 0% | 0% | 0% |
| ★ Cherry | 8 fl oz | 130 | 0% | 0% | 0% |
| ★ Double Fruit Cooler | 8 fl oz | 130 | 0% | 0% | 0% |
| ★ Exto Cooler | 8 fl oz | 130 | 0% | 0% | 0% |
| ★ Fruit Punch | 8 fl oz | 130 | 0% | 0% | 0% |
| ★ Hula Punch | 8 fl oz | 120 | 0% | 0% | 0% |
| R.W. KNUDSEN Apple Blends | | | | | |
| (100% juice)—SMUCKER'S | | | | | |
| ★ Apple Apricot | 8 fl oz | 120 | 0% | 0% | 0% |
| ★ Apple Banana | 8 fl oz | 120 | 0% | 0% | 0% |
| ★ Apple Boysenberry | 8 fl oz | 120 | 0% | 0% | 0% |
| ★ Apple Cranberry | 8 fl oz | 120 | 0% | 0% | 0% |
| ★ Apple Peach | 8 fl oz | 120 | 0% | 0% | 0% |
| ★ Apple Raspberry | 8 fl oz | 120 | 0% | 0% | 0% |
| ★ Apple Strawberry | 8 fl oz | 120 | 0% | 0% | 0% |
| ★ Cherry Cider | 8 fl oz | 130 | 0% | 0% | 0% |
| ★ Cider & Spice | 8 fl oz | 120 | 0% | 0% | 0% |
| R.W. KNUDSEN Citrus Juices— | | | | | |
| SMUCKER'S | | | | | |
| ★ Cherry Lemonade (84% juice) | 8 fl oz | 120 | 0% | 0% | 0% |
| ★ Cranberry Lemonade (93% juice) | 8 fl oz | 120 | 0% | 0% | 0% |
| ★ Grapefruit Juice (100% juice) | 8 fl oz | 100 | 0% | 0% | 0% |
| ★ Natural Breakfast Juice | | | | | |
| (100% juice) | 8 fl oz | 110 | 0% | 0% | 0% |
| ★ Natural Lemonade (84% juice) | 8 fl oz | 120 | 0% | 0% | 0% |
| ★ Orange Juice (100% juice) | 8 fl oz | 100 | 0% | 0% | 0% |
| ★ Pink Grapefruit Juice (100% juice) | 8 fl oz | 100 | 0% | 0% | 0% |
| ★ Rio Red Grapefruit (100% juice) | 8 fl oz | 140 | 0% | 0% | 0% |

| FOOD | Serving Size | Calories | Tot Fat | Sat Fat | Chol |
|---|---|---|---|---|---|
| **R.W. KNUDSEN Exotic Blends—** SMUCKER'S | | | | | |
| ★ Apricot Nectar (100% juice) | 8 fl oz | 120 | 0% | 0% | 0% |
| ★ Black Cherry Juice (100% juice) | 8 fl oz | 130 | 0% | 0% | 0% |
| ★ Cranberry Juice (100% juice) | 8 fl oz | 70 | 0% | 0% | 0% |
| ★ Cranberry Nectar (100% juice) | 8 fl oz | 150 | 0% | 0% | 0% |
| ★ Cranberry-Raspberry (95% juice) | 8 fl oz | 140 | 0% | 0% | 0% |
| ★ Hibiscus Cranberry (75% juice) | 8 fl oz | 120 | 0% | 0% | 0% |
| ★ Lemon Ginger Echinecea (60% juice) | 8 fl oz | 100 | 0% | 0% | 0% |
| ★ Lime Cactus Cooler (80% juice) | 8 fl oz | 120 | 0% | 0% | 0% |
| ★ Peach Nectar (100% juice) | 8 fl oz | 120 | 0% | 0% | 0% |
| ★ Raspberry Peach (100% juice) | 8 fl oz | 120 | 0% | 0% | 0% |
| ★ Razzleberry (83% juice) | 8 fl oz | 130 | 0% | 0% | 0% |
| ★ Strawberry Banana (96% juice) | 8 fl oz | 120 | 0% | 0% | 0% |
| ★ Strawberry Banana Cactus (77% juice) | 8 fl oz | 120 | 0% | 0% | 0% |
| ★ Strawberry Nectar (100% juice) | 8 fl oz | 120 | 0% | 0% | 0% |
| ★ Watermelon Cooler (76% juice) | 8 fl oz | 120 | 0% | 0% | 0% |
| ★ Yankee Cranberry (100% juice) | 8 fl oz | 120 | 0% | 0% | 0% |
| **R.W. KNUDSEN Fortified Blends** —SMUCKER'S | | | | | |
| ★ Morning Blend (100% juice) | 8 fl oz | 120 | 0% | 0% | 0% |
| ★ Vita Juice (100% juice) | 8 fl oz | 120 | 0% | 0% | 0% |
| **R.W. KNUDSEN Fruit Juices** (100% juice)—SMUCKER'S | | | | | |
| ★ Black Cherry | 8 fl oz | 180 | 0% | 0% | 0% |
| ★ Clear Apple | 8 fl oz | 110 | 0% | 0% | 0% |
| ★ Concord Grape | 8 fl oz | 160 | 0% | 0% | 0% |
| ★ Grape | 8 fl oz | 150 | 0% | 0% | 0% |
| ★ Just Cranberry | 8 fl oz | 60 | 0% | 0% | 0% |
| ★ Natural Apple | 8 fl oz | 120 | 0% | 0% | 0% |
| ★ Organic Apple | 8 fl oz | 120 | 0% | 0% | 0% |
| ★ Organic Concord Grape | 8 fl oz | 160 | 0% | 0% | 0% |
| ★ Organic Grapefruit | 8 fl oz | 100 | 0% | 0% | 0% |
| ★ Organic Gravenstein Apple | 8 fl oz | 120 | 0% | 0% | 0% |
| ★ Organic Pear | 8 fl oz | 120 | 0% | 0% | 0% |
| ★ Organic Prune | 8 fl oz | 170 | 0% | 0% | 0% |
| ★ Organic Tomato | 8 fl oz | 60 | 0% | 0% | 0% |
| ★ Pomegranate | 8 fl oz | 150 | 0% | 0% | 0% |
| **R.W. KNUDSEN Sparkling Fruit** *TeaZers*—SMUCKER'S | | | | | |
| ★ Blackberry Bramble (45% juice) | 12 fl oz | 110 | 0% | 0% | 0% |
| ★ Cherry Spice (44% juice) | 12 fl oz | 110 | 0% | 0% | 0% |

★ Foods with this symbol have less than or equal to 5% *Daily Value* for <u>all</u> three nutrients (5% Rule).

❖ Foods with this symbol have <u>at least one</u> of the three nutrients greater than 5% *Daily Value* but less than or equal to 20% *Daily Value.*

Ⓐ Foods with this symbol have <u>at least one</u> of the three nutrients greater than 20% *Daily Value* (20% Rule).

| FOOD | Serving Size | Calories | Tot Fat | Sat Fat | Chol |
|---|---|---|---|---|---|
| ★ Ginger Peach (49% juice) | 12 fl oz | 110 | 0% | 0% | 0% |
| ★ Hibiscus Blossom (46% juice) | 12 fl oz | 110 | 0% | 0% | 0% |
| ★ Mango Vanilla (48% juice) | 12 fl oz | 110 | 0% | 0% | 0% |
| ★ Raspberry Rose (46% juice) | 12 fl oz | 110 | 0% | 0% | 0% |
| R.W. KNUDSEN Herbal Tea Coolers—SMUCKER'S | | | | | |
| ★ Hibiscus Cooler (61% juice) | 8 fl oz | 90 | 0% | 0% | 0% |
| ★ Lemon Tea Cooler (57% juice) | 8 fl oz | 90 | 0% | 0% | 0% |
| ★ Mango Tea Cooler (61% juice) | 8 fl oz | 90 | 0% | 0% | 0% |
| ★ Orange Tea Cooler (60% juice) | 8 fl oz | 90 | 0% | 0% | 0% |
| ★ Raspberry Tea Cooler (59% juice) | 8 fl oz | 90 | 0% | 0% | 0% |
| R.W. KNUDSEN Juice (from frozen concentrate)—SMUCKER'S | | | | | |
| ★ Cherry Cider (88% juice) | 8 fl oz | 130 | 0% | 0% | 0% |
| ★ Cranberry Nectar (100% juice) | 8 fl oz | 150 | 0% | 0% | 0% |
| ★ Natural Breakfast Juice (100% juice) | 8 fl oz | 110 | 0% | 0% | 0% |
| ★ Natural Lemonade (84% juice) | 8 fl oz | 120 | 0% | 0% | 0% |
| ★ Organic Grape Juice Blend (100% juice) | 8 fl oz | 150 | 0% | 0% | 0% |
| ★ Organic Lemonade (100% juice) | 8 fl oz | 120 | 0% | 0% | 0% |
| ★ Organic Natural Apple Juice (100% juice) | 8 fl oz | 120 | 0% | 0% | 0% |
| ★ Organic Orange (100% juice) | 8 fl oz | 100 | 0% | 0% | 0% |
| ★ Raspberry Nectar (83% juice) | 8 fl oz | 120 | 0% | 0% | 0% |
| ★ Tropical Punch (77% juice) | 8 fl oz | 120 | 0% | 0% | 0% |
| R.W. KNUDSEN Fruit Juice Floats—SMUCKER'S | | | | | |
| ★ Orange Float (82% juice) | 8 fl oz | 140 | 0% | 0% | 0% |
| ★ Raspberry Float (83% juice) | 8 fl oz | 140 | 0% | 0% | 0% |
| ★ Strawberry Float (84% juice) | 8 fl oz | 140 | 0% | 0% | 0% |
| R.W. KNUDSEN Sparkling Fruit Juice Spritzers—SMUCKER'S | | | | | |
| ★ Black Cherry (89% juice) | 12 fl oz | 170 | 0% | 0% | 0% |
| ★ Boysenberry (73% juice) | 12 fl oz | 160 | 0% | 0% | 0% |
| ★ Cherry Cola (70% juice) | 12 fl oz | 170 | 0% | 0% | 0% |
| ★ Cranberry (78% juice) | 12 fl oz | 190 | 0% | 0% | 0% |
| ★ Ginger Ale (65% juice) | 12 fl oz | 160 | 0% | 0% | 0% |
| ★ Grape (71% juice) | 12 fl oz | 170 | 0% | 0% | 0% |
| ★ Jamaican Lemonade (75% juice) | 12 fl oz | 170 | 0% | 0% | 0% |
| ★ Kiwi Lime (73% juice) | 12 fl oz | 160 | 0% | 0% | 0% |
| ★ Lemon Lime (71% juice) | 12 fl oz | 170 | 0% | 0% | 0% |
| ★ Mandarin Lime (72% juice) | 12 fl oz | 170 | 0% | 0% | 0% |
| ★ Mango Fandango (78% juice) | 12 fl oz | 190 | 0% | 0% | 0% |
| ★ Orange Passionfruit (71% juice) | 12 fl oz | 160 | 0% | 0% | 0% |
| ★ Organic Apple (100% juice) | 12 fl oz | 160 | 0% | 0% | 0% |
| ★ Peach (96% juice) | 12 fl oz | 160 | 0% | 0% | 0% |
| ★ Red Raspberry (71% juice) | 12 fl oz | 170 | 0% | 0% | 0% |

| FOOD | Serving Size | Calories | Tot Fat | Sat Fat | Chol |
|---|---|---|---|---|---|
| ★ Strawberry (80% juice) | 12 fl oz | 170 | 0% | 0% | 0% |
| ★ Tangerine (73% juice) | 12 fl oz | 170 | 0% | 0% | 0% |
| ★ Vanilla Creme (67% juice) | 12 fl oz | 160 | 0% | 0% | 0% |
| R.W. KNUDSEN Sports Beverage— SMUCKER'S | | | | | |
| ★ Lemon Recharge (50% juice) | 8 fl oz | 70 | 0% | 0% | 0% |
| ★ Orange Recharge (47% juice) | 8 fl oz | 70 | 0% | 0% | 0% |
| ★ Organic Lemon Recharge (50% juice) | 8 fl oz | 70 | 0% | 0% | 0% |
| ★ Tropical Recharge (47% juice) | 8 fl oz | 70 | 0% | 0% | 0% |
| R.W. KNUDSEN Tropical Blends —SMUCKER'S | | | | | |
| ❖ Coconut Nectar (66% juice) | 8 fl oz | 140 | 8% | 0% | 0% |
| ★ Mango Peach (90% juice) | 8 fl oz | 120 | 0% | 0% | 0% |
| ★ Orange Mango (81% juice) | 8 fl oz | 120 | 0% | 0% | 0% |
| ★ Papaya Nectar (100% juice) | 8 fl oz | 130 | 0% | 0% | 0% |
| ★ Pineapple Coconut (83% juice) | 8 fl oz | 130 | 0% | 0% | 0% |
| ★ Rain Forest Punch (76% juice) | 8 fl oz | 120 | 0% | 0% | 0% |
| ★ Raspberry Hibiscus (61% juice) | 8 fl oz | 90 | 0% | 0% | 0% |
| ★ Strawberry Guava (80% juice) | 8 fl oz | 110 | 0% | 0% | 0% |
| ★ Strawberry Kiwi (81% juice) | 8 fl oz | 120 | 0% | 0% | 0% |
| ★ Tropical Punch (77% juice) | 8 fl oz | 120 | 0% | 0% | 0% |
| MAUNA LA'I—OCEAN SPRAY | | | | | |
| ★ *Island Guava* | 8 fl oz | 130 | 0% | 0% | 0% |
| ★ *Mango, Mango* | 8 fl oz | 130 | 0% | 0% | 0% |
| ★ *Paradise Passion* | 8 fl oz | 13 | 0% | 0% | 0% |
| MINUTE MAID *Fruitopia*— COCA-COLA | | | | | |
| ★ Citrus Consciousness (10% juice) | 8 fl oz | 120 | 0% | 0% | 0% |
| ★ Cranberry Lemonade Meditation (16% juice) | 8 fl oz | 110 | 0% | 0% | 0% |
| ★ Fruit Integration (10% juice) | 8 fl oz | 120 | 0% | 0% | 0% |
| ★ Grape Beyond (10% juice) | 8 fl oz | 130 | 0% | 0% | 0% |
| ★ Lemonade Love (13% juice) | 8 fl oz | 110 | 0% | 0% | 0% |
| ★ Pink Lemonade Euphoria (13% juice) | 8 fl oz | 120 | 0% | 0% | 0% |
| ★ Raspberry Psychic Lemonade (11% juice) | 8 fl oz | 120 | 0% | 0% | 0% |
| ★ Strawberry Passion Awareness (10% juice) | 8 fl oz | 120 | 0% | 0% | 0% |
| MINUTE MAID 100% Fruit Juices—COCA-COLA | | | | | |
| ★ Apple | 8 fl oz | 110 | 0% | 0% | 0% |

★ Foods with this symbol have less than or equal to 5% *Daily Value* for <u>all</u> three nutrients (5% Rule).

❖ Foods with this symbol have <u>at least one</u> of the three nutrients greater than 5% *Daily Value* but less than or equal to 20% *Daily Value*.

Ⓐ Foods with this symbol have <u>at least one</u> of the three nutrients greater than 20% *Daily Value* (20% Rule).

| FOOD | Serving Size | Calories | Tot Fat | Sat Fat | Chol |
|------|------|------|------|------|------|
| ★ Grapefruit | 8 fl oz | 100 | 0% | 0% | 0% |
| ★ Orange: All varieties | 8 fl oz | 110 | 0% | 0% | 0% |
| ★ Pineapple | 8 fl oz | 130 | 0% | 0% | 0% |
| ★ Pineapple/Orange | 8 fl oz | 120 | 0% | 0% | 0% |
| MINUTE MAID Juice Cocktails —COCA-COLA | | | | | |
| ★ Cranberry Apple (15% juice) | 8 fl oz | 170 | 0% | 0% | 0% |
| ★ Pink Grapefruit (50% juice) | 8 fl oz | 110 | 0% | 0% | 0% |
| MINUTE MAID Lemonade— COCA-COLA | | | | | |
| ★ Cranberry Lemonade (16% juice) | 8 fl oz | 110 | 0% | 0% | 0% |
| ★ Lemonade (13% juice) | 8 fl oz | 110 | 0% | 0% | 0% |
| ★ Pink Lemonade (16% juice) | 8 fl oz | 110 | 0% | 0% | 0% |
| ★ Raspberry Lemonade (14% juice) | 8 fl oz | 120 | 0% | 0% | 0% |
| MINUTE MAID Naturals— COCA-COLA | | | | | |
| ★ Apple Cranberry Medley (15% juice) | 8 fl oz | 170 | 0% | 0% | 0% |
| ★ Apple Juice (100% juice) | 8 fl oz | 110 | 0% | 0% | 0% |
| ★ Concord Medley (13% juice) | 8 fl oz | 130 | 0% | 0% | 0% |
| ★ Cranberry Lemonade (16% juice) | 8 fl oz | 110 | 0% | 0% | 0% |
| ★ Fruit Medley (10% juice) | 8 fl oz | 120 | 0% | 0% | 0% |
| ★ Lemonade (13% juice) | 8 fl oz | 110 | 0% | 0% | 0% |
| ★ Orange Grape Blend (100% juice) | 8 fl oz | 120 | 0% | 0% | 0% |
| ★ Raspberry Lemonade (14% juice) | 8 fl oz | 120 | 0% | 0% | 0% |
| ★ Tropical Medley (10% juice) | 8 fl oz | 120 | 0% | 0% | 0% |
| MINUTE MAID Punches— COCA-COLA | | | | | |
| ★ Berry (10% juice) | 8 fl oz | 130 | 0% | 0% | 0% |
| ★ Citrus (14% juice) | 8 fl oz | 120 | 0% | 0% | 0% |
| ★ Concord (10% juice) | 8 fl oz | 130 | 0% | 0% | 0% |
| ★ Fruit (10% juice) | 8 fl oz | 120 | 0% | 0% | 0% |
| ★ Grape (13% juice) | 8 fl oz | 130 | 0% | 0% | 0% |
| ★ Orange (15% juice) | 8 fl oz | 130 | 0% | 0% | 0% |
| ★ Tropical (10% juice) | 8 fl oz | 130 | 0% | 0% | 0% |
| MOTT'S 100% Fruit Juice (prep from concentrate)—CADBURY BEVERAGES | | | | | |
| ★ Apple Juice | 8 fl oz | 120 | 0% | 0% | 0% |
| ★ Grapefruit | 10 fl oz | 120 | 0% | 0% | 0% |
| ★ Orange Juice | 10 fl oz | 130 | 0% | 0% | 0% |
| MOTT'S Fruit Basket Juice (prep from concentrate)—CADBURY BEVERAGES | | | | | |
| ★ Apple | 8 fl oz | 120 | 0% | 0% | 0% |
| ★ Apple Raspberry | 8 fl oz | 130 | 0% | 0% | 0% |
| ★ Grape | 8 fl oz | 130 | 0% | 0% | 0% |
| ★ Peach | 8 fl oz | 130 | 0% | 0% | 0% |

| FOOD | Serving Size | Calories | Tot Fat | Sat Fat | Chol |
|------|--------------|----------|---------|---------|------|
| ★ Tropical Blend | 8 fl oz | 120 | 0% | 0% | 0% |
| MOTT'S Fruit Juice Blends (prep from concentrate)—CADBURY BEVERAGES | | | | | |
| ★ Apple Cranberry (25% juice) | 10 fl oz | 180 | 0% | 0% | 0% |
| ★ Apple Raspberry (25% juice) | 10 fl oz | 140 | 0% | 0% | 0% |
| ★ Fruit Punch (25% juice) | 10 fl oz | 170 | 0% | 0% | 0% |
| ★ Grape Apple (25% juice) | 10 fl oz | 170 | 0% | 0% | 0% |
| MOTT'S Juice Drinks (prep from concentrate)—CADBURY BEVERAGES | | | | | |
| ★ Fruit Punch (25% juice) | 10 fl oz | 170 | 0% | 0% | 0% |
| ★ Grape (17% juice) | 10 fl oz | 170 | 0% | 0% | 0% |
| ★ Lemonade (15% juice) | 10 fl oz | 160 | 0% | 0% | 0% |
| ★ Pineapple Orange (10% juice) | 10 fl oz | 170 | 0% | 0% | 0% |
| ★ NEWMAN'S OWN Roadside Virgin Lemonade | 8 fl oz | 110 | 0% | 0% | 0% |
| OCEAN SPRAY Juices | | | | | |
| ★ 100% Grapefruit Juice | 8 fl oz | 100 | 0% | 0% | 0% |
| ★ Apple Juice | 8 fl oz | 110 | 0% | 0% | 0% |
| ★ *Cran•Blueberry* | 8 fl oz | 160 | 0% | 0% | 0% |
| ★ *Cran•Cherry* | 8 fl oz | 160 | 0% | 0% | 0% |
| ★ *Cran•Grape* | 8 fl oz | 170 | 0% | 0% | 0% |
| ★ *Cran•Raspberry* | 8 fl oz | 140 | 0% | 0% | 0% |
| ★ *Cran•Raspberry*, Reduced Calorie | 8 fl oz | 50 | 0% | 0% | 0% |
| ★ *Cran•Strawberry* | 8 fl oz | 140 | 0% | 0% | 0% |
| ★ *Cranapple* | 8 fl oz | 160 | 0% | 0% | 0% |
| ★ *Cranapple*, Reduced Calorie | 8 fl oz | 50 | 0% | 0% | 0% |
| ★ Cranberry Juice Cocktail | 8 fl oz | 140 | 0% | 0% | 0% |
| ★ Cranberry Juice Cocktail, Reduced Calorie | 8 fl oz | 50 | 0% | 0% | 0% |
| ★ *Cranicot* | 8 fl oz | 160 | 0% | 0% | 0% |
| ★ *Crantastic* Fruit Punch | 8 fl oz | 150 | 0% | 0% | 0% |
| ★ Fruit Punch | 8 fl oz | 130 | 0% | 0% | 0% |
| ★ Orange Juice | 8 fl oz | 120 | 0% | 0% | 0% |
| ★ Pink Grapefruit Juice Cocktail | 8 fl oz | 110 | 0% | 0% | 0% |
| ★ Ruby Red & Tangerine Grapefruit Juice Drink | 8 fl oz | 130 | 0% | 0% | 0% |
| ★ Ruby Red Grapefruit Juice Drink | 8 fl oz | 130 | 0% | 0% | 0% |
| OCEAN SPRAY Lemonade | | | | | |
| ★ Plain | 8 fl oz | 110 | 0% | 0% | 0% |
| ★ w/Cranberry Juice | 8 fl oz | 110 | 0% | 0% | 0% |
| ★ w/Raspberry Juice | 8 fl oz | 110 | 0% | 0% | 0% |
| ★ OCEAN SPRAY *Lightstyle* Low Calorie Cocktails and Drinks: All flavors | 8 fl oz | 40 | 0% | 0% | 0% |

★  Foods with this symbol have less than or equal to 5% *Daily Value* for <u>all</u> three nutrients (5% Rule).

❖  Foods with this symbol have <u>at least one</u> of the three nutrients greater than 5% *Daily Value* but less than or equal to 20% *Daily Value*.

Ⓐ  Foods with this symbol have <u>at least one</u> of the three nutrients greater than 20% *Daily Value* (20% Rule).

| FOOD | Serving Size | Calories | Tot Fat | Sat Fat | Chol |
|------|------|------|------|------|------|
| OCEAN SPRAY *Refreshers* | | | | | |
| ★ Citrus Cranberry Juice Drink | 8 fl oz | 140 | 0% | 0% | 0% |
| ★ Citrus Peach Juice Drink | 8 fl oz | 120 | 0% | 0% | 0% |
| ★ Orange Cranberry Juice Drink | 8 fl oz | 130 | 0% | 0% | 0% |
| ★ REALEMON Juice from Concentrate | 1 tsp | 0 | 0% | 0% | 0% |
| SANTA CRUZ Natural Organic Juice/Blends—SMUCKER'S | | | | | |
| ★ Apple (100% juice) | 8 fl oz | 120 | 0% | 0% | 0% |
| ★ Apricot Nectar (100% juice) | 8 fl oz | 120 | 0% | 0% | 0% |
| ★ Berry Nectar (79% juice) | 8 fl oz | 110 | 0% | 0% | 0% |
| ★ Cherry Nectar (80% juice) | 8 fl oz | 110 | 0% | 0% | 0% |
| ★ Cran-Guava Nectar (80% juice) | 8 fl oz | 110 | 0% | 0% | 0% |
| ★ Cranberry Lemon (82% juice) | 8 fl oz | 120 | 0% | 0% | 0% |
| ★ Cranberry Nectar (77% juice) | 8 fl oz | 110 | 0% | 0% | 0% |
| ★ Gingerale (67% juice) | 8 fl oz | 150 | 0% | 0% | 0% |
| ★ Hawaiian Ginger (75% juice) | 8 fl oz | 110 | 0% | 0% | 0% |
| ★ Lemonade (80% juice) | 8 fl oz | 120 | 0% | 0% | 0% |
| ★ Papaya Nectar (82% juice) | 8 fl oz | 110 | 0% | 0% | 0% |
| ★ Pear Nectar (85% juice) | 8 fl oz | 120 | 0% | 0% | 0% |
| ★ Raspberry Lemon (69% juice) | 8 fl oz | 120 | 0% | 0% | 0% |
| ★ Raspberry Nectar (84% juice) | 8 fl oz | 100 | 0% | 0% | 0% |
| ★ Sparkling Guava (71% juice) | 8 fl oz | 150 | 0% | 0% | 0% |
| ★ Sparkling Lemon Lime (72% juice) | 8 fl oz | 150 | 0% | 0% | 0% |
| ★ Sparkling Lemonade (62% juice) | 8 fl oz | 150 | 0% | 0% | 0% |
| ★ Sparkling Orange Mango (66% juice) | 8 fl oz | 150 | 0% | 0% | 0% |
| ★ Sparkling Raspberry Lemon (63% juice) | 8 fl oz | 150 | 0% | 0% | 0% |
| ★ Strawberry Guava (76% juice) | 8 fl oz | 100 | 0% | 0% | 0% |
| ★ Strawberry Lemonade (72% juice) | 8 fl oz | 120 | 0% | 0% | 0% |

## VEGETABLE JUICES

**Generic Foods**

| FOOD | Serving Size | Calories | Tot Fat | Sat Fat | Chol |
|------|------|------|------|------|------|
| ★ Carrot Juice (canned) | 8 fl oz | 100 | 1% | 0% | 0% |
| ★ Tomato Juice | 8 fl oz | 42 | 0% | 0% | 0% |
| ★ Vegetable Juice Cocktail | 8 fl oz | 50 | 0% | 0% | 0% |

**Brand Name Foods**

| FOOD | Serving Size | Calories | Tot Fat | Sat Fat | Chol |
|------|------|------|------|------|------|
| ★ CAMPBELL'S Tomato Juice | 8 fl oz | 50 | 0% | 0% | 0% |
| ★ DEL MONTE Tomato Juice | 8 fl oz | 50 | 0% | 0% | 0% |
| ★ HAIN Carrot Juice | 1 can (12 oz) | 120 | 2% | 0% | 0% |
| ★ HOLLYWOOD Carrot Juice—HAIN | 1 can (12 oz) | 120 | 2% | 0% | 0% |
| ★ HUNT'S Tomato Juice | 8 fl oz | 50 | 0% | 0% | 0% |

| FOOD | Serving Size | Calories | Tot Fat | Sat Fat | Chol |
|---|---|---|---|---|---|
| ★ HUNT'S Tomato Juice: Regular or No Salt Added—HUNT WESSON | 8 fl oz | 35 | 1% | 0% | 0% |
| ★ KNUDSEN Tomato Juice— SMUCKER'S | 8 fl oz | 60 | 0% | 0% | 0% |
| KNUDSEN Vegetable Blends— SMUCKER'S | | | | | |
| ★ Very Veggie Original Juice | 8 fl oz | 50 | 2% | 0% | 0% |
| ★ Organic Very Veggie | 8 fl oz | 50 | 2% | 0% | 0% |
| ★ Tomato Garlic | 8 fl oz | 60 | 0% | 0% | 0% |
| ★ Very Veggie Low Sodium | 8 fl oz | 50 | 2% | 0% | 0% |
| ★ Very Veggie Original | 8 fl oz | 50 | 2% | 0% | 0% |
| ★ Very Veggie Spicy | 8 fl oz | 50 | 2% | 0% | 0% |
| MOTT'S—CADBURY BEVERAGES | | | | | |
| ★ *Beefamato* | 8 fl oz | 80 | 0% | 0% | 0% |
| ★ *Clamato* | 8 fl oz | 100 | 0% | 0% | 0% |
| ★ *Clamato* Caesar | 8 fl oz | 100 | 0% | 0% | 0% |
| ★ Vegetable Juice from Concentrate | 10 fl oz | 60 | 0% | 0% | 0% |
| ODWALLA | | | | | |
| ★ Carrot Juice (fresh) | 8 fl oz | 70 | 0% | 0% | 0% |
| ★ Vegetable Cocktail (fresh) | 8 fl oz | 70 | 0% | 0% | 0% |
| ★ SNAP-E-TOM Tomato & Chile Cocktail—DEL MONTE | 8 fl oz | 50 | 0% | 0% | 0% |
| V-8 Juice—CAMPBELL'S | | | | | |
| ★ 100% Vegetable Juice | 8 fl oz | 50 | 0% | 0% | 0% |
| ★ Lightly Tangy 100% Vegetable Juice: Regular or Low sodium | 8 fl oz | 60 | 0% | 0% | 0% |
| ★ Picante Vegetable Juice | 8 fl oz | 50 | 0% | 0% | 0% |
| ★ Spicy Hot 100% Vegetable Juice | 8 fl oz | 50 | 0% | 0% | 0% |

*OTHER BEVERAGES*

**Generic Foods**

| | | | | | |
|---|---|---|---|---|---|
| ⊛ Coconut Cream | 2 tbsp | 100 | 17% | 48% | 0% |
| ⊛ Coconut Milk | 2 tbsp | 70 | 11% | 33% | 0% |
| ⊛ Eggnog | 4 fl oz | 335 | 24% | 9% | 31% |
| ★ Sugar Cane Juice | 4 fl oz | 80 | 0% | 0% | 0% |

**Brand Name Foods**

| | | | | | |
|---|---|---|---|---|---|
| ★ GORTON'S Surf Clam Juice— GENERAL MILLS | 1 can | 0 | 0% | 0% | 0% |
| ❖ STONYFIELD FARM Lowfat Egg Nog | 4 fl oz | 110 | 5% | 8% | 14% |

★ Foods with this symbol have less than or equal to 5% *Daily Value* for all three nutrients (5% Rule).
❖ Foods with this symbol have at least one of the three nutrients greater than 5% *Daily Value* but less than or equal to 20% *Daily Value*.
⊛ Foods with this symbol have at least one of the three nutrients greater than 20% *Daily Value* (20% Rule).

| FOOD | Serving Size | Calories | Tot Fat | Sat Fat | Chol |
|------|------|------|------|------|------|

# Breads and Bread Products

## BAGELS

### Generic Foods

| FOOD | Serving Size | Calories | Tot Fat | Sat Fat | Chol |
|------|------|------|------|------|------|
| ★ All Bagels except Egg (3 1/2" diam.) | 1 bagel | 190 | 2% | 1% | 0% |
| ❖ Egg (3 1/2" diam.) | 1 bagel | 200 | 2% | 1% | 6% |

### Brand Name Foods

| FOOD | Serving Size | Calories | Tot Fat | Sat Fat | Chol |
|------|------|------|------|------|------|
| LENDER'S Bagels—KRAFT | | | | | |
| ★ Egg | 1 bagel | 230 | 4% | 3% | 5% |
| ★ Onion | 1 bagel | 220 | 3% | 0% | 0% |
| ★ Plain | 1 bagel | 210 | 2% | 0% | 0% |
| ★ Raisin | 1 bagel | 240 | 5% | 0% | 0% |
| SARA LEE Bagels | | | | | |
| ★ Cinnamon Raisin | 1 bagel | 220 | 2% | 0% | 0% |
| ❖ Egg | 1 bagel | 220 | 2% | 0% | 8% |
| ★ Oat Bran | 1 bagel | 220 | 2% | 0% | 0% |
| ★ Onion | 1 bagel | 210 | 0% | 0% | 0% |
| ★ Plain | 1 bagel | 210 | 1% | 0% | 0% |
| ★ Poppy Seed | 1 bagel | 220 | 2% | 0% | 0% |
| ★ Sesame Seed | 1 bagel | 220 | 2% | 0% | 0% |
| THOMAS' Bagels—CPC | | | | | |
| ★ Cinnamon Raisin | 1 bagel | 170 | 2% | 0% | 0% |
| ❖ Egg | 1 bagel | 170 | 3% | 0% | 10% |
| ★ Multi-Grain | 1 bagel | 150 | 2% | 0% | 0% |
| ★ Onion | 1 bagel | 160 | 3% | 0% | 0% |
| ★ Plain | 1 bagel | 170 | 3% | 0% | 0% |

## BISCUITS

### Generic Foods

| FOOD | Serving Size | Calories | Tot Fat | Sat Fat | Chol |
|------|------|------|------|------|------|
| ⊛ Baking Powder Biscuits | 2 biscuits | 210 | 16% | 23% | 1% |
| ❖ Buttermilk Biscuits | 1 biscuit | 210 | 15% | 13% | 1% |

### Brand Name Foods

| FOOD | Serving Size | Calories | Tot Fat | Sat Fat | Chol |
|------|------|------|------|------|------|
| 1869 BRAND Biscuits—PILLSBURY | | | | | |
| ❖ Baking Powder | 1 biscuit | 100 | 8% | 8% | 0% |
| ❖ Buttermilk | 1 biscuit | 100 | 8% | 8% | 0% |
| ❖ ARNOLD Old Fashioned Biscuits—CPC | 2 biscuits | 130 | 8% | 5% | 0% |
| ★ ARROWHEAD MILLS Biscuit Mix | 1/4 cup mix | 120 | 2% | 0% | 0% |
| BALLARD Extra Lights Oven Ready Biscuits—PILLSBURY | | | | | |
| ★ Buttermilk | 3 biscuits | 150 | 3% | 0% | 0% |

| FOOD | Serving Size | Calories | Tot Fat | Sat Fat | Chol |
|---|---|---|---|---|---|
| ★ Regular | 3 biscuits | 150 | 3% | 0% | 0% |
| BIG COUNTRY Biscuits—PILLSBURY | | | | | |
| ❖ Butter *Tastin'* | 1 biscuit | 100 | 6% | 5% | 0% |
| ❖ Buttermilk | 1 biscuit | 100 | 6% | 5% | 0% |
| ❖ Southern Style | 1 biscuit | 100 | 6% | 5% | 0% |
| ★ GOLDEN DIPT Hush Puppy: | | | | | |
| All varieties—MCCORMICK | ~ 1/4 cup mix | 150 | 0% | 0% | 0% |
| GRANDS! Biscuits—PILLSBURY | | | | | |
| ❖ Butter | 1 biscuit | 200 | 15% | 13% | 0% |
| ❖ Buttermilk | 1 biscuit | 200 | 15% | 15% | 0% |
| ❖ Cinnamon Raisin | 1 biscuit | 200 | 12% | 10% | 0% |
| ❖ Flaky | 1 biscuit | 190 | 14% | 10% | 0% |
| ❖ HomeStyle | 1 biscuit | 190 | 14% | 13% | 0% |
| ❖ Southern Style | 1 biscuit | 200 | 15% | 13% | 0% |
| HUNGRY JACK Biscuits—PILLSBURY | | | | | |
| ❖ Butter *Tastin'* Flaky | 2 biscuits | 170 | 11% | 8% | 0% |
| ❖ Flaky | 2 biscuits | 170 | 11% | 8% | 0% |
| ❖ Flaky Buttermilk | 2 biscuits | 170 | 11% | 8% | 0% |
| ❖ Fluffy | 2 biscuits | 180 | 12% | 10% | 0% |
| ❖ Honey *Tastin'* Flaky | 2 biscuits | 180 | 11% | 8% | 0% |
| ❖ Southern Style Flaky | 2 biscuits | 170 | 11% | 8% | 0% |
| ❖ KRUSTEAZ Cinnamon Raisin Biscuit Mix (3" diam.)— | | | | | |
| CONTINENTAL MILLS | 1 biscuit | 290 | 17% | 15% | 0% |
| PILLSBURY Biscuits | | | | | |
| ★ Butter | 3 biscuits | 150 | 4% | 0% | 0% |
| ★ Buttermilk | 3 biscuits | 150 | 4% | 0% | 0% |
| ★ Country | 3 biscuits | 150 | 4% | 0% | 0% |
| ❖ Tender Layer Buttermilk | 3 biscuits | 160 | 7% | 5% | 0% |
| ROMAN MEAL Biscuits— CAMPBELL TAGGART | | | | | |
| ★ Plain | 1 biscuit | 90 | 3% | 0% | 0% |
| ❖ White | 1 biscuit | 130 | 7% | 0% | 0% |
| ★ SUN MAID Raisin Biscuits— CAMPBELL TAGGART | 1 biscuit | 120 | 3% | 2% | 0% |

## BREADS: MIXES

**Brand Name Foods**

| | | | | | |
|---|---|---|---|---|---|
| ★ ENER-G Eight Grain Bread Mix | 1 slc | 200 | 4% | 3% | 0% |
| KRUSTEAZ Bread Mix— CONTINENTAL MILLS | | | | | |
| ★ Cinnamon Raisin | 1/12 loaf | 180 | 4% | 0% | 0% |
| ★ Country White | 1/10 loaf | 150 | 3% | 0% | 0% |

★ Foods with this symbol have less than or equal to 5% *Daily Value* for <u>all</u> three nutrients (5% Rule).
❖ Foods with this symbol have <u>at least one</u> of the three nutrients greater than 5% *Daily Value* but less than or equal to 20% *Daily Value.*
Ⓐ Foods with this symbol have <u>at least one</u> of the three nutrients greater than 20% *Daily Value* (20% Rule).

| FOOD | Serving Size | Calories | Tot Fat | Sat Fat | Chol |
|---|---|---|---|---|---|
| ★ Cracked Wheat | 1/10 loaf | 150 | 3% | 0% | 0% |
| ★ Dill Rye | 1/10 loaf | 150 | 3% | 0% | 0% |
| ★ Honey Wheat Berry | 1/10 loaf | 150 | 3% | 0% | 0% |
| ★ Italian Herb | 1/10 loaf | 150 | 3% | 0% | 0% |
| ★ Sourdough | 1/10 loaf | 150 | 3% | 0% | 0% |
| PILLSBURY *Bread Machine* Mix (prep as dir) | | | | | |
| ★ Cracked Wheat | 1/12 loaf | 130 | 3% | 0% | 0% |
| ★ Crusty White | 1/12 loaf | 130 | 3% | 0% | 0% |

### BREADS: PACKAGED

**Generic Foods**

| FOOD | Serving Size | Calories | Tot Fat | Sat Fat | Chol |
|---|---|---|---|---|---|
| ❖ Egg Bread | 1 slc | 120 | 4% | 3% | 7% |
| ★ French Bread | 2 slcs | 140 | 2% | 2% | 0% |
| ❖ Indian Fry Bread | 1 pc | 300 | 13% | 9% | 0% |
| ★ Irish Soda Bread | 1 slc | 170 | 5% | 3% | 4% |
| ★ Mixed Grain Bread | 1 slc | 70 | 2% | 1% | 0% |
| ★ Oat Bran Bread | 1 slc | 70 | 2% | 1% | 0% |
| ★ Pumpernickel Bread | 1 slc | 80 | 2% | 1% | 0% |
| ★ Raisin Bread | 1 slc | 70 | 2% | 1% | 0% |
| ★ Rye Bread | 1 slc | 80 | 2% | 1% | 0% |
| ★ Sourdough Bread | 2 slcs | 140 | 2% | 2% | 0% |
| ★ Vienna Bread | 2 slcs | 140 | 2% | 2% | 0% |
| ★ Wheat Bran Bread | 1 slc | 90 | 2% | 1% | 0% |
| ★ Wheat Bread | 1 slc | 130 | 3% | 2% | 0% |
| ★ White Bread | 2 slcs | 120 | 3% | 2% | 0% |
| ★ Whole Wheat Bread | 2 slcs | 120 | 3% | 1% | 0% |

**Brand Name Foods**

| FOOD | Serving Size | Calories | Tot Fat | Sat Fat | Chol |
|---|---|---|---|---|---|
| ARNOLD Breads—CPC | | | | | |
| ★ Cranberry | 1 slc | 70 | 2% | 0% | 0% |
| ★ Deli Rye | 1 slc | 80 | 1% | 0% | 0% |
| ★ Honey Wheat Berry | 1 slc | 70 | 2% | 0% | 0% |
| ★ Onion Rye | 1 slc | 80 | 2% | 0% | 0% |
| ★ Pumpernickel | 1 slc | 90 | 2% | 0% | 0% |
| ★ Raisin & Cinnamon | 1 slc | 70 | 2% | 0% | 0% |
| ★ Real Jewish Dijon Rye | 1 slc | 80 | 2% | 0% | 0% |
| ★ Rye w/Seeds | 1 slc | 90 | 2% | 0% | 0% |
| ★ *Savoni's* Italian | 1 slc | 60 | 1% | 0% | 0% |
| ★ Soft Rye Seeded | 1 slc | 80 | 2% | 0% | 0% |
| ★ Sourdough | 1 slc | 110 | 2% | 0% | 0% |
| ★ Stoneground 100% Whole Wheat | 1 slc | 60 | 2% | 0% | 0% |
| ★ Sunmaid Raisin Bread | 1 slc | 70 | 2% | 0% | 0% |
| ★ Texas Toast | 1 slc | 150 | 5% | 3% | 0% |
| ARNOLD *Brick Oven*—CPC | 2 slcs | 110 | 5% | 2% | 0% |
| ★ Wheat | 2 slcs | 110 | 5% | 2% | 0% |

| FOOD | Serving Size | Calories | Tot Fat | Sat Fat | Chol |
|---|---|---|---|---|---|
| ★ White | 2 slcs | 120 | 4% | 0% | 0% |
| ARNOLD Country—CPC | 1 slc | 100 | 2% | 0% | 0% |
| ★ Buttermilk | 1 slc | 100 | 2% | 0% | 0% |
| ★ Potato | 1 slc | 100 | 3% | 0% | 0% |
| ★ Soft Rye | 1 slc | 70 | 2% | 0% | 0% |
| ARNOLD'S *Levy's*—CPC | 1 slc | 80 | 1% | 0% | 0% |
| ★ Jewish Rye | 1 slc | 70 | 1% | 0% | 0% |
| ★ Pumpernickel | 1 slc | 80 | 1% | 0% | 0% |
| ARNOLD'S *Sunny Valley*—CPC | 2 slcs | 100 | 2% | 0% | 0% |
| ★ Enriched Wheat | 2 slcs | 100 | 2% | 0% | 0% |
| ★ Enriched White | 2 slcs | 100 | 2% | 0% | 0% |
| ARNOLD/BROWNBERRY | | | | | |
| *Bakery Light*—CPC | 2 slcs | 80 | 2% | 0% | 0% |
| ★ Country Bran | 2 slcs | 80 | 2% | 0% | 0% |
| ★ Golden Wheat | 2 slcs | 80 | 1% | 0% | 0% |
| ★ Italian | 2 slcs | 80 | 2% | 0% | 0% |
| ★ Oatmeal | 2 slcs | 80 | 2% | 0% | 0% |
| ★ Premium White | 2 slcs | 80 | 1% | 0% | 0% |
| ★ Soft Rye | 2 slcs | 80 | 2% | 0% | 0% |
| ★ Sourdough | 2 slcs | 80 | 1% | 0% | 0% |
| ARNOLD/BROWNBERRY | | | | | |
| *Bran'Nola*—CPC | 1 slc | 90 | 4% | 2% | 0% |
| ★ 7-Grain White | 1 slc | 90 | 3% | 0% | 0% |
| ★ Country Oat | 1 slc | 90 | 4% | 2% | 0% |
| ★ Dark Wheat | 1 slc | 90 | 3% | 0% | 0% |
| ★ Hearty Wheat | 1 slc | 90 | 5% | 2% | 0% |
| ★ Original | 1 slc | 90 | 3% | 0% | 0% |
| ARNOLD/BROWNBERRY | | | | | |
| *Francisco*—CPC | 2 slcs | 110 | 2% | 0% | 0% |
| ★ Italian Sliced | 2 slcs | 110 | 2% | 0% | 0% |
| ★ Sourdough | 1 slc | 90 | 2% | 0% | 0% |
| BROWNBERRY Breads—CPC | | | | | |
| ★ Apple Honey Wheat | 1 slc | 60 | 2% | 0% | 0% |
| ★ *Bran'Nola* Nutty Grain | 1 slc | 90 | 4% | 0% | 0% |
| ★ Orange Raisin | 1 slc | 70 | 1% | 0% | 0% |
| ★ Raisin Cinnamon | 1 slc | 70 | 2% | 0% | 0% |
| ★ Raisin Walnut | 1 slc | 80 | 4% | 0% | 0% |
| ★ Soft Oatmeal | 1 slc | 70 | 2% | 0% | 0% |
| ★ Soft Wheat | 1 slc | 80 | 3% | 0% | 0% |
| ★ Soft White | 1 slc | 80 | 2% | 0% | 0% |
| BROWNBERRY Hearth—CPC | 1 slc | 90 | 2% | 0% | 0% |
| ★ Grain | 1 slc | 90 | 2% | 0% | 0% |
| ★ Rye | 1 slc | 90 | 2% | 0% | 0% |
| ★ Wheat | 1 slc | 90 | 2% | 0% | 0% |
| BROWNBERRY Natural—CPC | 2 slcs | 100 | 2% | 0% | 0% |

★ Foods with this symbol have less than or equal to 5% *Daily Value* for all three nutrients (5% Rule).

❖ Foods with this symbol have at least one of the three nutrients greater than 5% *Daily Value* but less than or equal to 20% *Daily Value.*

Ⓐ Foods with this symbol have at least one of the three nutrients greater than 20% *Daily Value* (20% Rule).

| FOOD | Serving Size | Calories | Tot Fat | Sat Fat | Chol |
|---|---|---|---|---|---|
| ★ 12 Grain | 2 slcs | 110 | 4% | 0% | 0% |
| ★ Caraway Rye | 1 slc | 70 | 2% | 0% | 0% |
| ★ Dill Rye | 1 slc | 70 | 2% | 0% | 0% |
| ★ *Health Nut* | 1 slc | 70 | 2% | 0% | 0% |
| ★ Oatmeal | 1 slc | 70 | 2% | 0% | 0% |
| ★ Pumpernickel | 1 slc | 70 | 1% | 0% | 0% |
| ★ Unseeded Thin Slice Rye | 2 slcs | 100 | 2% | 0% | 0% |
| ★ Wheat | 1 slc | 80 | 2% | 0% | 0% |
| ★ White | 2 slcs | 120 | 2% | 0% | 0% |
| ★ Whole Bran | 1 slc | 60 | 2% | 0% | 0% |
| **ENER-G FOODS Gluten Free Bread** | | | | | |
| ❖ Brown Rice | 1 slc | 120 | 7% | 2% | 0% |
| ❖ Egg | 1 slc | 180 | 10% | 3% | 2% |
| ❖ Papa's Loaf | 1 slc | 140 | 9% | 2% | 0% |
| ❖ Potato Loaf | 1 slc | 170 | 9% | 3% | 0% |
| ★ Raisin Loaf | 1 slc | 150 | 3% | 0% | 0% |
| ★ Raisin-Egg Loaf | 1 slc | 120 | 4% | 2% | 0% |
| ❖ Tapioca Loaf | 1 slc | 140 | 9% | 2% | 0% |
| ❖ White Rice Loaf | 1 slc | 120 | 8% | 2% | 0% |
| **PEPPERIDGE FARM Bread— CAMPBELL'S** | | | | | |
| ★ Apple Walnut | 1 slc | 80 | 3% | 3% | 0% |
| ★ Cinnamon | 1 slc | 80 | 4% | 3% | 0% |
| ★ Dark Pumpernickel | 1 slc | 80 | 2% | 3% | 0% |
| ★ Golden Swirl (Vermont Maple) | 1 slc | 90 | 4% | 5% | 0% |
| ★ Hearty Country White | 1 slc | 90 | 1% | 0% | 0% |
| ★ Hearty Crunchy Oat | 1 slc | 100 | 3% | 0% | 0% |
| ★ Hearty Honey Wheatberry | 1 slc | 100 | 2% | 0% | 0% |
| ★ Hearty Russet Potato | 1 slc | 90 | 2% | 3% | 1% |
| ★ Hearty Sesame Wheat | 1 slc | 100 | 2% | 0% | 0% |
| ★ Hearty White | 1 slc | 90 | 2% | 0% | 0% |
| ★ Jewish Seeded Rye | 1 slc | 80 | 2% | 3% | 0% |
| ★ Light Style Oatmeal | 3 slcs | 140 | 2% | 0% | 0% |
| ★ Light Style Seven Grain | 3 slcs | 140 | 2% | 0% | 0% |
| ★ Light Style Sourdough | 3 slcs | 130 | 2% | 0% | 0% |
| ★ Light Style Vienna | 3 slcs | 130 | 2% | 3% | 0% |
| ★ Light Style Wheat | 3 slcs | 130 | 2% | 3% | 0% |
| ★ Onion Rye | 1 slc | 80 | 2% | 3% | 0% |
| ★ Raisin w/Cinnamon | 1 slc | 80 | 2% | 0% | 0% |
| ★ Sandwich White | 2 slcs | 130 | 4% | 3% | 0% |
| ★ Texas Toast | 1 slc | 110 | 3% | 3% | 0% |
| ★ Thin Sliced Dijon Rye | 2 slcs | 100 | 2% | 3% | 0% |
| ★ Thin Sliced White | 1 slc | 80 | 2% | 0% | 0% |
| ★ Thin Sliced Whole Wheat | 1 slc | 60 | 2% | 0% | 0% |
| ★ Very Thin Sliced Wheat | 3 slcs | 110 | 3% | 3% | 0% |
| ★ Very Thin Sliced White | 3 slcs | 110 | 2% | 0% | 0% |
| ★ Vienna Thick Sliced | 1 slc | 70 | 2% | 0% | 0% |

| FOOD | Serving Size | Calories | Tot Fat | Sat Fat | Chol |
|---|---|---|---|---|---|
| PEPPERIDGE FARM Garlic Bread & Rolls—CAMPBELL'S | | | | | |
| ❖ Garlic Bread | 1/6 loaf | 160 | 15% | 15% | 10% |
| ❖ Garlic Parmesan Bread | 1/6 loaf | 160 | 11% | 10% | 3% |
| ❖ Monterey Jack w/Jalapeno Cheese Bread | 1/6 loaf | 200 | 15% | 20% | 13% |
| Ⓐ Mozzarella Garlic Bread | 1/6 loaf | 200 | 15% | 25% | 13% |
| ❖ Sourdough Garlic Bread | 1/6 loaf | 180 | 14% | 13% | 3% |
| Ⓐ Two Cheddar Cheese Bread | 1/6 loaf | 210 | 17% | 25% | 17% |
| PILLSBURY Dinner Rolls & Breads | | | | | |
| ★ French Loaf | 1/5 loaf | 150 | 2% | 0% | 0% |
| ★ *Pipin' Hot* Loaf | 1/6 loaf | 110 | 1% | 0% | 0% |

## BREADSTICKS

**Generic Foods**

| | | | | | |
|---|---|---|---|---|---|
| ★ Breadsticks | 3 sticks | 75 | 3% | 1% | 0% |

**Brand Name Foods**

| | | | | | |
|---|---|---|---|---|---|
| PEPPERIDGE FARM Breadsticks— CAMPBELL'S | | | | | |
| ★ Brown & Serve | 1 stick | 150 | 2% | 3% | 0% |
| ★ Cheddar Cheese Thin | 7 sticks | 70 | 4% | 5% | 2% |
| ★ Onion Thin | 7 sticks | 70 | 3% | 0% | 0% |
| ★ Sesame Thin | 7 sticks | 60 | 2% | 0% | 0% |
| ★ PILLSBURY Dinner Rolls & Breads: Breadsticks | 1 stick | 110 | 4% | 3% | 0% |
| STELLA D'ORO Breadsticks | | | | | |
| ★ Garlic | 1 stick | 40 | 2% | 0% | 0% |
| ★ Plain | 1 stick | 40 | 2% | 0% | 0% |
| ★ Sesame | 1 stick | 50 | 4% | 0% | 0% |
| ★ Wheat | 1 stick | 40 | 2% | 0% | 0% |
| STELLA D'ORO Fat Free Breadsticks | | | | | |
| ★ Garlic Grissini-Style | 3 sticks | 60 | 0% | 0% | 0% |
| ★ Original Grissini-Style | 3 sticks | 60 | 0% | 0% | 0% |
| ★ Traditional Original | 2 sticks | 70 | 0% | 0% | 0% |

## ENGLISH MUFFINS

**Generic Foods**

| | | | | | |
|---|---|---|---|---|---|
| ★ English Muffins: All flavors | 1 muffin | 130 | 2% | 1% | 0% |

★ Foods with this symbol have less than or equal to 5% *Daily Value* for <u>all</u> three nutrients (5% Rule).
❖ Foods with this symbol have <u>at least one</u> of the three nutrients greater than 5% *Daily Value* but less than or equal to 20% *Daily Value*.
Ⓐ Foods with this symbol have <u>at least one</u> of the three nutrients greater than 20% *Daily Value* (20% Rule).

| FOOD | Serving Size | Calories | Tot Fat | Sat Fat | Chol |
|------|------|------|------|------|------|
| **Brand Name Foods** | | | | | |
| ARNOLD English Muffins—CPC | | | | | |
| ★ *Bran'Nola* | 1 muffin | 130 | 2% | 0% | 0% |
| ★ Extra Crisp | 1 muffin | 120 | 2% | 0% | 0% |
| ★ Raisin | 1 muffin | 150 | 2% | 0% | 0% |
| ★ Sourdough | 1 muffin | 120 | 2% | 0% | 0% |
| PEPPERIDGE FARM English Muffins—CAMPBELL'S | | | | | |
| ★ Cinnamon Raisin | 1 muffin | 140 | 2% | 0% | 0% |
| ★ Plain | 1 muffin | 130 | 2% | 0% | 0% |
| ★ Seven Grain | 1 muffin | 130 | 2% | 0% | 0% |
| ★ Sourdough | 1 muffin | 130 | 2% | 0% | 0% |
| ROMAN MEAL English Muffins—CAMPBELL TAGGART | | | | | |
| ★ Honey Nut | 1 muffin | 160 | 4% | 0% | 0% |
| ★ Plain | 1 muffin | 140 | 1% | 0% | 0% |
| ★ SUN MAID Raisin English Muffins—CAMPBELL TAGGART | 1 muffin | 160 | 1% | 0% | 0% |
| THOMAS' English Muffins—CPC | | | | | |
| ★ Honey Wheat | 1 muffin | 110 | 2% | 0% | 0% |
| ★ Oat Bran | 1 muffin | 120 | 2% | 2% | 0% |
| ★ Plain | 1 muffin | 120 | 2% | 0% | 0% |
| ★ Raisin | 1 muffin | 140 | 2% | 0% | 0% |
| ★ Sourdough | 1 muffin | 120 | 2% | 0% | 0% |
| THOMAS' English Muffins, Sandwich Size—CPC | | | | | |
| ★ Onion | 1 muffin | 180 | 2% | 0% | 0% |
| ★ Plain | 1 muffin | 190 | 3% | 0% | 0% |
| ★ Sourdough | 1 muffin | 200 | 3% | 0% | 0% |
| ★ Wheat | 1 muffin | 180 | 2% | 0% | 0% |

PITA BREAD

| FOOD | Serving Size | Calories | Tot Fat | Sat Fat | Chol |
|------|------|------|------|------|------|
| **Generic Foods** | | | | | |
| ★ White Pita | 1 pita | 170 | 1% | 0% | 0% |
| ★ Whole Wheat Pita | 1 pita | 170 | 3% | 1% | 0% |
| **Brand Name Foods** | | | | | |
| THOMAS' *Sahara* Pita—CPC | | | | | |
| ★ 100% Whole Wheat | 1 pita | 60 | 1% | 0% | 0% |
| ★ Oat Bran | 1 pita | 130 | 2% | 0% | 0% |
| ★ Onion | 1 pita | 140 | 1% | 0% | 0% |
| ★ Original Style | 1 pita | 70 | 0% | 0% | 0% |
| ★ Sourdough | 1 pita | 150 | 1% | 0% | 0% |

| FOOD | Serving Size | Calories | Tot Fat | Sat Fat | Chol |
|------|--------------|----------|---------|---------|------|

## Pizza Crusts

**Brand Name Foods**

BOBOLI—KRAFT

| | | | | | |
|------|--------------|----------|---------|---------|------|
| ★ Pizza Shell (16 oz) | 1/8 shell | 160 | 5% | 5% | 1% |
| ★ Pizza Shell (8 oz) | 1/2 shell | 160 | 5% | 5% | 1% |
| ❖ Pizza Shell Thin Crust | 1/5 shell | 150 | 5% | 6% | 2% |
| ★ CHEF BOYARDEE Quick & Easy Pizza Crust Mix—AMERICAN | | | | | |
|    HOME FOODS | 1/4 pkg | 150 | 2% | 0% | 0% |
| ★ ENER-G Gluten Free Pizza Shell (6") | 1/5 crust | 60 | 4% | 1% | 0% |
| ★ PILLSBURY Dinner Rolls & Breads: | | | | | |
|    Pizza Crust | 1/4 crust | 180 | 4% | 3% | 0% |
| ★ ROBIN HOOD Pizza Crust— | | | | | |
|    GENERAL MILLS | 1/4 crust | 160 | 3% | 0% | 0% |

## Rolls: Dinner

**Generic Foods**

| | | | | | |
|------|--------------|----------|---------|---------|------|
| ❖ Crescent Roll | 2 rolls | 190 | 12% | 10% | 0% |
| ★ Dinner Roll | 2 rolls | 160 | 5% | 3% | 0% |
| ★ French Roll | 1 roll | 110 | 2% | 2% | 0% |
| ★ Hard Roll | 1 roll | 170 | 4% | 2% | 0% |
| ⓐ Popover (55 g) | 1 popover | 120 | 7% | 7% | 23% |

**Brand Name Foods**

| | | | | | |
|------|--------------|----------|---------|---------|------|
| ARNOLD *Francisco* Rolls—CPC | 1 roll | 80 | 2% | 0% | 0% |
| ★ Brown N' Serve Sourdough | 1 roll | 80 | 2% | 0% | 0% |
| ★ French (6") | 1 roll | 170 | 4% | 0% | 0% |
| ★ French Mini | 1 roll | 110 | 2% | 0% | 0% |
| ARNOLD Rolls—CPC | | | | | |
| ★ *Bran'Nola* Dinner | 1 roll | 70 | 2% | 0% | 0% |
| ★ Potato | 1 roll | 150 | 3% | 0% | 0% |
| ★ Potato Sesame | 1 roll | 150 | 4% | 3% | 0% |
| ★ *Savoni's* 8" Italian | 1 roll | 280 | 5% | 2% | 0% |
| ★ Sesame | 1 roll | 170 | 4% | 0% | 0% |
| ★ Wheat Dinner | 1 roll | 100 | 3% | 0% | 0% |
| ★ White Dinner | 1 roll | 90 | 2% | 0% | 0% |
| ★ PEPPERIDGE FARM *Deli* *Classic* Rolls: Hearty Potato Dinner—CAMPBELL'S | 1 roll | 80 | 4% | 3% | 0% |

---

★   Foods with this symbol have less than or equal to 5% *Daily Value* for <u>all</u> three nutrients (5% Rule).

❖   Foods with this symbol have <u>at least one</u> of the three nutrients greater than 5% *Daily Value* but less than or equal to 20% *Daily Value*.

ⓐ   Foods with this symbol have <u>at least one</u> of the three nutrients greater than 20% *Daily Value* (20% Rule).

| FOOD | Serving Size | Calories | Tot Fat | Sat Fat | Chol |
|---|---|---|---|---|---|
| PEPPERIDGE FARM *European Bake Shoppe* Brown & Serve Rolls—CAMPBELL'S | | | | | |
| ★ Brown & Serve Club | 1 roll | 120 | 2% | 0% | 0% |
| ★ Brown & Serve French | 1 roll | 240 | 4% | 3% | 0% |
| ★ Brown & Serve Hearth | 3 rolls | 150 | 3% | 0% | 0% |
| PEPPERIDGE FARM *European Bake Shoppe* French Rolls— CAMPBELL'S | | | | | |
| ★ French Style | 1 roll | 100 | 2% | 0% | 0% |
| ★ Seven Grain French | 1 roll | 80 | 3% | 0% | 0% |
| ★ Sourdough French Style | 1 roll | 100 | 2% | 0% | 0% |
| PEPPERIDGE FARM Garlic Bread & Rolls—CAMPBELL'S | | | | | |
| ❖ Garlic & Cheese Biscuits | 1 biscuit | 170 | 9% | 13% | 3% |
| ❖ Garlic & Cheese Rolls | 1 roll | 130 | 8% | 8% | 5% |
| PEPPERIDGE FARM Rolls— CAMPBELL'S | | | | | |
| ★ Country Style Classic Dinner | 3 rolls | 150 | 5% | 5% | 0% |
| ❖ Finger Poppy Seeds | 3 rolls | 150 | 7% | 8% | 2% |
| ❖ Finger Sesame Seeds | 3 rolls | 150 | 7% | 8% | 2% |
| ❖ Heat & Serve Butter Crescent | 1 roll | 110 | 8% | 15% | 5% |
| ❖ Heat & Serve Golden Twist | 1 roll | 110 | 6% | 8% | 1% |
| ❖ Petite Croissants | 1 roll | 130 | 12% | 18% | 7% |
| PILLSBURY Dinner Rolls & Breads | | | | | |
| ❖ Butterflake | 1 roll | 130 | 8% | 5% | 0% |
| ❖ Cheese Crescents | 2 rolls | 210 | 18% | 15% | 1% |
| ❖ Cornbread Twists | 1 roll | 130 | 9% | 8% | 0% |
| ❖ Crescents | 2 rolls | 200 | 17% | 13% | 0% |
| ★ PILLSBURY Hot Roll Mix (prep as dir) | 1 roll | 130 | 5% | 3% | 5% |
| ❖ SARA LEE Petite Croissant | 2 croissants | 230 | 17% | 20% | 2% |

### ROLLS: HAMBURGER AND HOT DOG BUNS

**Generic Foods**

| | | | | | |
|---|---|---|---|---|---|
| ★ Hamburger Roll (mixed grain) | 1 roll | 110 | 4% | 3% | 0% |
| ★ Hot Dog Roll (mixed grain) | 1 roll | 110 | 4% | 3% | 0% |

**Brand Name Foods**

| | | | | | |
|---|---|---|---|---|---|
| ARNOLD Buns—CPC | | | | | |
| ★ *Bran'Nola* Hot Dog | 1 bun | 110 | 2% | 0% | 0% |
| ★ Hamburger | 1 bun | 140 | 4% | 3% | 0% |
| ★ Hot Dog | 1 bun | 100 | 3% | 0% | 0% |
| ★ New England Style Hot Dog | 1 bun | 110 | 3% | 0% | 0% |
| ★ Potato Hot Dog | 1 bun | 120 | 3% | 0% | 0% |

| FOOD | Serving Size | Calories | Tot Fat | Sat Fat | Chol |
|---|---|---|---|---|---|
| ★ Wheat Hamburger | 1 bun | 130 | 3% | 0% | 0% |
| BROWNBERRY Buns—CPC | | | | | |
| ★ Sliced Hot Dog . | 1 bun | 110 | 3% | 0% | 0% |
| ★ Wheat Hot Dog | 1 bun | 110 | 3% | 0% | 0% |
| ENER-G FOODS Gluten Free Rolls | | | | | |
| ❖ Hamburger Bun, White Rice | 1 bun | 270 | 18% | 4% | 0% |
| ❖ Hamburger Bun, Brown Rice | 1 bun | 260 | 14% | 4% | 0% |
| ❖ Hamburger Bun, Tapioca | 1 bun | 300 | 20% | 4% | 0% |
| ❖ Hot Dog Bun, Tapioca | 1 bun | 290 | 16% | 5% | 0% |
| ❖ Hot Dog Bun, White Rice | 1 bun | 270 | 18% | 4% | 0% |
| PEPPERIDGE FARM Rolls— | | | | | |
| CAMPBELL'S | | | | | |
| ❖ Dijon Frankfurter | 1 roll | 140 | 5% | 8% | 0% |
| ★ Frankfurter | 1 roll | 140 | 4% | 5% | 0% |
| ★ Hamburger | 1 roll | 130 | 4% | 5% | 0% |

## ROLLS: SANDWICH

### Generic Foods

| | | | | | |
|---|---|---|---|---|---|
| ★ Kaiser Roll | 1 roll | 170 | 4% | 2% | 0% |
| ❖ Submarine/Hoagie Roll | 1 roll | 400 | 6% | 5% | 0% |

### Brand Name Foods

| | | | | | |
|---|---|---|---|---|---|
| ★ ARNOLD *Francisco* Kaiser Roll—CPC | 1 roll | 170 | 3% | 0% | 0% |
| ARNOLD'S *Levy Old Country* Rolls—CPC | | | | | |
| ★ Kaiser | 1 roll | 170 | 3% | 0% | 0% |
| ★ Onion | 1 roll | 160 | 5% | 3% | 2% |
| ★ Sub | 1 roll | 140 | 2% | 0% | 0% |
| ARNOLD Buns—CPC | | | | | |
| ★ *Bran'Nola* | 1 bun | 130 | 2% | 0% | 0% |
| ★ Kaiser Sandwich w/Sesame | 1 bun | 140 | 5% | 3% | 0% |
| ★ Kaiser | 1 roll | 160 | 3% | 0% | 0% |
| ★ Onion | 1 roll | 160 | 3% | 0% | 0% |
| ★ Soft Sandwich | 1 roll | 120 | 4% | 3% | 0% |
| ★ Soft Sandwich Sesame | 1 roll | 140 | 5% | 2% | 0% |
| ★ Steak | 1 roll | 170 | 4% | 0% | 0% |
| ★ Sub | 1 roll | 170 | 4% | 0% | 0% |
| BROWNBERRY Buns—CPC | | | | | |
| ★ Wheat Sandwich | 1 bun | 130 | 3% | 0% | 0% |
| ★ White Sandwich | 1 bun | 140 | 4% | 3% | 0% |
| BROWNBERRY Rolls—CPC | | | | | |
| ★ Hearth Kaiser | 1 roll | 150 | 4% | 0% | 0% |

★ Foods with this symbol have less than or equal to 5% *Daily Value* for <u>all</u> three nutrients (5% Rule).
❖ Foods with this symbol have <u>at least one</u> of the three nutrients greater than 5% *Daily Value* but less than or equal to 20% *Daily Value*.
Ⓐ Foods with this symbol have <u>at least one</u> of the three nutrients greater than 20% *Daily Value* (20% Rule).

| FOOD | Serving Size | Calories | Tot Fat | Sat Fat | Chol |
|---|---|---|---|---|---|
| ★ Natural White Sandwich Seed | 1 roll | 140 | 5% | 3% | 0% |
| ★ Potato Sandwich | 1 roll | 150 | 4% | 0% | 0% |
| ❖ PEPPERIDGE FARM *Deli Classic* | | | | | |
| Soft Hoagie Roll—CAMPBELL'S | 1 roll | 200 | 7% | 13% | 0% |
| PEPPERIDGE FARM Rolls— | | | | | |
| CAMPBELL'S | | | | | |
| ❖ Hoagie | 1 roll | 200 | 7% | 13% | 0% |
| ❖ Multigrain Hoagie Sandwich | 1 roll | 200 | 7% | 13% | 0% |
| ★ Multigrain Sandwich Bun | 1 bun | 150 | 4% | 3% | 0% |
| ★ Onion Sandwich Bun w/ | | | | | |
| Poppy Seeds | 1 bun | 140 | 4% | 5% | 0% |
| ❖ Potato Sandwich Bun | 1 bun | 160 | 6% | 3% | 0% |
| ❖ Sourdough Sandwich Bun | 1 bun | 170 | 5% | 8% | 0% |

## STUFFING

**Generic Foods**

| | | | | | |
|---|---|---|---|---|---|
| ⓐ Bread Stuffing | 1 cup | 390 | 26% | 17% | 0% |
| ⓐ Cornbread Stuffing | 1 cup | 360 | 27% | 18% | 0% |

**Brand Name Foods**

| | | | | | |
|---|---|---|---|---|---|
| ARNOLD/BROWNBERRY | | | | | |
| Stuffing—CPC | | | | | |
| ❖ Cornbread | 2 cups | 250 | 6% | 5% | 0% |
| ★ Herb Seasoned | 2 cups | 240 | 5% | 2% | 0% |
| ★ Sage & Onion | 2 cups | 240 | 5% | 2% | 0% |
| ★ Seasoned | 2 cups | 250 | 5% | 2% | 0% |
| ★ Unseasoned | 2 cups | 250 | 5% | 2% | 0% |
| ★ CROUTETTES Stuffing Mix— | | | | | |
| KELLOGG'S | 1 cup mix | 120 | 0% | 0% | 0% |
| PEPPERIDGE FARM *Distinctive* | | | | | |
| Stuffing—CAMPBELL'S | | | | | |
| ★ Apple & Raisin | 1/2 cup | 140 | 2% | 0% | 0% |
| ★ Classic Chicken | 1/2 cup | 130 | 2% | 0% | 0% |
| ❖ Country Garden & Herb | 1/2 cup | 150 | 8% | 5% | 0% |
| ★ Harvest Vegetable & Almond | 1/2 cup | 140 | 5% | 0% | 0% |
| ❖ Honey Pecan Cornbread | 1/2 cup | 140 | 8% | 3% | 0% |
| ❖ Wild Rice & Mushroom | 1/2 cup | 170 | 9% | 8% | 0% |
| PEPPERIDGE FARM Stuffing— | | | | | |
| CAMPBELL'S | | | | | |
| ★ Corn Bread | 3/4 cup | 170 | 3% | 0% | 0% |
| ★ Country Style | 3/4 cup | 140 | 2% | 0% | 0% |
| ★ Cube | 3/4 cup | 140 | 2% | 0% | 0% |

| FOOD | Serving Size | Calories | Tot Fat | Sat Fat | Chol |
|---|---|---|---|---|---|
| ★ Herb Seasoned | 3/4 cup | 170 | 2% | 0% | 0% |
| ★ Sage & Onion Stuffing for Turkey | 1/2 cup | 150 | 2% | 0% | 0% |
| STOVE TOP Stuffing Mix (prep as dir)—KRAFT | | | | | |
| ❖ Chicken Flavor | 1/2 cup | 170 | 13% | 8% | 0% |
| ❖ Cornbread | 1/2 cup | 170 | 13% | 8% | 0% |
| ❖ For Beef | 1/2 cup | 180 | 13% | 8% | 0% |
| ❖ For Pork | 1/2 cup | 170 | 13% | 8% | 0% |
| ❖ For Turkey | 1/2 cup | 170 | 13% | 8% | 0% |
| ❖ Long Grain & Wild Rice | 1/2 cup | 180 | 13% | 8% | 0% |
| ❖ Mushroom & Onion | 1/2 cup | 180 | 14% | 8% | 0% |
| ❖ San Francisco Style | 1/2 cup | 170 | 13% | 8% | 0% |
| ❖ Savory Herbs | 1/2 cup | 170 | 13% | 8% | 0% |

## TACOS AND TORTILLAS

**Generic Foods**

| FOOD | Serving Size | Calories | Tot Fat | Sat Fat | Chol |
|---|---|---|---|---|---|
| ❖ Taco Shell (baked) | 2 tacos | 120 | 9% | 4% | 0% |
| ★ Tortilla, Corn | 2 tortillas | 110 | 2% | 1% | 0% |
| ★ Tortilla, Flour | 1 tortilla | 160 | 5% | 4% | 0% |

**Brand Name Foods**

| FOOD | Serving Size | Calories | Tot Fat | Sat Fat | Chol |
|---|---|---|---|---|---|
| ❖ GEBHARDT Taco Shells— HUNT WESSON | 3 shells | 160 | 13% | 12% | 0% |
| ❖ LAWRY'S Taco Shells—LIPTON | 2 shells | 120 | 9% | 8% | 0% |
| OLD EL PASO Shells—PET | | | | | |
| ❖ Mini | 7 shells | 160 | 15% | 8% | 0% |
| ❖ Regular | 3 shells | 170 | 15% | 9% | 0% |
| ❖ Super | 2 shells | 190 | 18% | 10% | 0% |
| ❖ Tostaco | 1 shell | 130 | 10% | 6% | 0% |
| ❖ Tostada | 3 shells | 160 | 15% | 10% | 0% |
| ❖ White Corn | 3 shells | 170 | 15% | 9% | 0% |
| OLD EL PASO Tortillas—PET | | | | | |
| ★ Flour Tortilla | 1 tortilla | 150 | 4% | 3% | 0% |
| ★ Soft Taco Tortillas | 2 tortillas | 180 | 5% | 4% | 0% |
| ❖ PANCHO VILLA Taco Shells—PET | 3 shells | 190 | 17% | 11% | 0% |
| ROSARITA Shells—HUNT WESSON | | | | | |
| ❖ Taco | 3 shells | 160 | 13% | 12% | 0% |
| ❖ Tostada | 2 shells | 130 | 7% | 5% | 12% |
| TYSON *Mexican Original* Tortillas | | | | | |
| ❖ Burrito Style Flour | 1 tortilla | 170 | 6% | 5% | 0% |
| ★ Enchilada Style Corn | 3 tortillas | 130 | 2% | 0% | 0% |
| ❖ Fajita Style Flour | 2 tortillas | 180 | 7% | 5% | 0% |

★ Foods with this symbol have less than or equal to 5% *Daily Value* for <u>all</u> three nutrients (5% Rule).
❖ Foods with this symbol have <u>at least one</u> of the three nutrients greater than 5% *Daily Value* but less than or equal to 20% *Daily Value*.
Ⓐ Foods with this symbol have <u>at least one</u> of the three nutrients greater than 20% *Daily Value* (20% Rule).

| FOOD | Serving Size | Calories | Tot Fat | Sat Fat | Chol |
|---|---|---|---|---|---|
| ★ Soft Taco Style Flour | 1 tortilla | 120 | 5% | 3% | 0% |
| ★ Whole Wheat Flour | 1 tortilla | 120 | 5% | 5% | 0% |

# Breakfast Dishes and Breakfast Sandwiches

### BREAKFAST SANDWICHES

**Brand Name Foods**

BREAKFAST ON-THE-GO!—
WEIGHT WATCHERS

| | | | | | |
|---|---|---|---|---|---|
| ❖ Classic Omelet Sandwich | 1 sandwich | 220 | 8% | 5% | 0% |
| ❖ English Muffin Sandwich | 1 sandwich | 220 | 11% | 10% | 7% |
| ❖ Garden Omelet Sandwich | 1 sandwich | 220 | 9% | 10% | 5% |
| ❖ Ham & Cheese Bagel Sandwich | 1 sandwich | 200 | 8% | 10% | 5% |
| ❖ Sausage Biscuit | 1 biscuit | 230 | 17% | 18% | 8% |

QUICK MEAL Breakfast Sandwiches—HORMEL FOODS

| | | | | | |
|---|---|---|---|---|---|
| ⊛ Canadian Bacon/Egg/Cheese Muffin | 1 sandwich | 260 | 14% | 25% | 37% |
| ⊛ Sausage Biscuit | 1 sandwich | 360 | 34% | 30% | 15% |
| ⊛ Sausage/Cheese Biscuit | 1 sandwich | 410 | 40% | 50% | 22% |
| ⊛ Sausage/Egg Biscuit | 1 sandwich | 390 | 37% | 40% | 40% |
| ⊛ Sausage/Egg/Cheese Muffin | 1 sandwich | 390 | 35% | 50% | 43% |
| ⊛ Steak Biscuit | 1 sandwich | 320 | 22% | 20% | 17% |

SWANSON *Great Starts* Breakfast—CAMPBELL'S

| | | | | | |
|---|---|---|---|---|---|
| ⊛ Bacon Burrito & Scrambled Eggs | 1 pkg | 250 | 17% | 20% | 30% |
| ❖ Original Burrito w/ Scrambled Eggs | 1 pkg | 200 | 12% | 15% | 20% |
| ⊛ Sandwich Egg w/Cheese | 1 pkg | 360 | 29% | 40% | 57% |
| ⊛ Sausage Burrito | 1 pkg | 240 | 19% | 20% | 30% |
| ⊛ Sausage, Egg & Cheese on a Biscuit | 1 pkg | 490 | 46% | 60% | 48% |

### CEREAL AND GRANOLA BARS: CEREAL BARS

**Brand Name Foods**

CARNATION Breakfast Bars—
NESTLÉ

| | | | | | |
|---|---|---|---|---|---|
| ❖ Chewy Chocolate Chip | 1 bar | 150 | 9% | 12% | 0% |
| ❖ Chewy Peanut Butter Chocolate Chip | 1 bar | 150 | 8% | 10% | 0% |
| ❖ Chocolate Chunk Granola | 1 bar | 140 | 8% | 9% | 0% |
| ❖ Honey & Oats Granola | 1 bar | 130 | 6% | 6% | 0% |

| FOOD | Serving Size | Calories | Tot Fat | Sat Fat | Chol |
|------|------|------|------|------|------|
| HEALTH VALLEY Fat Free Breakfast Bars | | | | | |
| ★ Apple | 1 bar | 110 | 0% | 0% | 0% |
| ★ Apricot | 1 bar | 110 | 0% | 0% | 0% |
| ★ Blueberry | 1 bar | 110 | 0% | 0% | 0% |
| ★ Cherry | 1 bar | 110 | 0% | 0% | 0% |
| ★ Chocolate | 1 bar | 110 | 0% | 0% | 0% |
| ★ Strawberry | 1 bar | 110 | 0% | 0% | 0% |
| HEALTH VALLEY Fat Free Crisp Rice Bars | | | | | |
| ★ Orange Date | 1 bar | 110 | 0% | 0% | 0% |
| ★ Raisin Apple | 1 bar | 110 | 0% | 0% | 0% |
| ★ Tropical Fruit | 1 bar | 110 | 0% | 0% | 0% |
| HEALTH VALLEY Fat Free Healthy Tarts | | | | | |
| ★ Baked Apple Cinnamon | 1 tart | 150 | 0% | 0% | 0% |
| ★ California Strawberry | 1 tart | 150 | 0% | 0% | 0% |
| ★ Chocolate Fudge | 1 tart | 150 | 0% | 0% | 0% |
| ★ Cranberry Apple | 1 tart | 150 | 0% | 0% | 0% |
| ★ Mountain Blueberry | 1 tart | 150 | 0% | 0% | 0% |
| ★ Red Raspberry | 1 tart | 150 | 0% | 0% | 0% |
| ★ Sweet Red Cherry | 1 tart | 150 | 0% | 0% | 0% |
| KELLOGG'S Cereal Bars | | | | | |
| ❖ *Rice Krispies* Chocolate Chip Cereal Bars | 1 bar | 120 | 6% | 8% | 0% |
| ★ *Rice Krispies Treats* Squares | 1 bar | 90 | 3% | 0% | 0% |
| KUDOS Whole Grain Bars (Chocolate Covered, 1 oz)— M&M/MARS | | | | | |
| ❖ Chocolate Chip | 1 bar | 120 | 8% | 14% | 1% |
| ❖ Milk and Cookies | 1 bar | 130 | 8% | 12% | 1% |
| ❖ Nutty Fudge | 1 bar | 130 | 8% | 12% | 1% |
| ❖ Peanut Butter | 1 bar | 130 | 8% | 13% | 1% |
| KUDOS Whole Grain Bars (Plain, 0.7 oz)—M&M/MARS | | | | | |
| ❖ Chocolate Chunk | 1 bar | 90 | 5% | 6% | 0% |
| ★ Low Fat Blueberry | 1 bar | 90 | 2% | 0% | 0% |
| ★ Low Fat Strawberry | 1 bar | 80 | 2% | 0% | 0% |
| NATURE'S CHOICE Fat Free Fruit Filled Cereal Bars— BARBARA'S BAKERY | | | | | |
| ★ Apple | 1 bar | 110 | 0% | 0% | 0% |
| ★ Blueberry | 1 bar | 110 | 0% | 0% | 0% |
| ★ Raspberry | 1 bar | 110 | 0% | 0% | 0% |

★ Foods with this symbol have less than or equal to 5% *Daily Value* for <u>all</u> three nutrients (5% Rule).

❖ Foods with this symbol have <u>at least one</u> of the three nutrients greater than 5% *Daily Value* but less than or equal to 20% *Daily Value*.

Ⓐ Foods with this symbol have <u>at least one</u> of the three nutrients greater than 20% *Daily Value* (20% Rule).

| FOOD | Serving Size | Calories | Tot Fat | Sat Fat | Chol |
|------|--------------|----------|---------|---------|------|
| ★ Strawberry | 1 bar | 110 | 0% | 0% | 0% |
| NUTRI-GRAIN Cereal Bars— KELLOGG'S | | | | | |
| ★ Apple Cinnamon | 1 bar | 140 | 5% | 3% | 0% |
| ★ Blueberry | 1 bar | 140 | 5% | 3% | 0% |
| ★ Peach | 1 bar | 140 | 5% | 3% | 0% |
| ★ Raspberry | 1 bar | 140 | 5% | 3% | 0% |
| ★ Strawberry | 1 bar | 140 | 5% | 3% | 0% |

## CEREAL AND GRANOLA BARS: GRANOLA BARS

**Brand Name Foods**

| FOOD | Serving Size | Calories | Tot Fat | Sat Fat | Chol |
|------|--------------|----------|---------|---------|------|
| BARBARA'S BAKERY Granola Bars | | | | | |
| ☻ Cinnamon & Oats | 1 bar | 260 | 23% | 20% | 0% |
| ☻ Coconut Almond | 1 bar | 290 | 31% | 40% | 0% |
| ☻ Peanut Butter | 1 bar | 260 | 23% | 20% | 0% |
| BETTY CROCKER Low Fat Granola *Bites*—GENERAL MILLS | | | | | |
| ★ Apple Cinnamon | 1 pouch | 120 | 3% | 0% | 0% |
| ★ Chocolate Chip | 1 pouch | 120 | 3% | 2% | 0% |
| ★ Oats & Honey | 1 pouch | 120 | 3% | 0% | 0% |
| HEALTH VALLEY Fat Free Granola Bars | | | | | |
| ★ Blueberry | 1 bar | 140 | 0% | 0% | 0% |
| ★ Chocolate Chip | 1 bar | 140 | 0% | 0% | 0% |
| ★ Date Almond | 1 bar | 140 | 0% | 0% | 0% |
| ★ Raisin | 1 bar | 140 | 0% | 0% | 0% |
| ★ Raspberry | 1 bar | 140 | 0% | 0% | 0% |
| ★ Strawberry | 1 bar | 140 | 0% | 0% | 0% |
| KELLOGG'S Granola Bar, Low Fat | | | | | |
| ★ Crunchy Almond & Brown Sugar | 1 bar | 80 | 2% | 0% | 0% |
| ★ Crunchy Apple Spice | 1 bar | 80 | 2% | 0% | 0% |
| ★ Crunchy Cinnamon Raisin | 1 bar | 80 | 2% | 0% | 0% |
| NATURE VALLEY Granola Bars —GENERAL MILLS | | | | | |
| ❖ Chocolate Chip | 2 bars | 220 | 13% | 9% | 0% |
| ❖ Cinnamon | 2 bars | 210 | 12% | 5% | 0% |
| ❖ Cinnamon Graham | 2 bars | 170 | 9% | 4% | 0% |
| ❖ Oat Bran | 2 bars | 210 | 12% | 5% | 0% |
| ❖ Oats 'n Honey | 2 bars | 210 | 12% | 5% | 0% |
| ❖ Peanut Butter | 2 bars | 220 | 15% | 6% | 0% |
| NATURE VALLEY Low Fat Chewy Granola Bars—GENERAL MILLS | | | | | |
| ★ Apple Brown Sugar | 1 bar | 110 | 3% | 0% | 0% |
| ★ Chocolate Chip | 1 bar | 110 | 3% | 3% | 0% |

| FOOD | Serving Size | Calories | Tot Fat | Sat Fat | Chol |
|---|---|---|---|---|---|
| ★ Honey Nut | 1 bar | 110 | 3% | 0% | 0% |
| ★ Oatmeal Raisin | 1 bar | 110 | 3% | 0% | 0% |
| ★ Orchard Blend | 1 bar | 110 | 3% | 0% | 0% |
| ★ Triple Berry | 1 bar | 110 | 3% | 0% | 0% |
| NATURE'S CHOICE Fat Free Granola Bars—BARBARA'S BAKERY | | | | | |
| ★ Apple Apricot | 1 bar | 90 | 0% | 0% | 0% |
| ★ Apple Blueberry | 1 bar | 90 | 0% | 0% | 0% |
| ★ Apple Raspberry | 1 bar | 90 | 0% | 0% | 0% |
| ★ Multigrain | 1 bar | 90 | 0% | 0% | 0% |
| NATURE'S CHOICE Granola Bars —BARBARA'S BAKERY | | | | | |
| ★ Carob Chip | 1 bar | 80 | 3% | 0% | 0% |
| ★ Cinnamon-Raisin | 1 bar | 80 | 3% | 0% | 0% |
| ★ Oats 'N Honey | 1 bar | 80 | 3% | 0% | 0% |
| ★ Peanut Butter | 1 bar | 80 | 5% | 0% | 0% |
| NATURE'S CHOICE Grrr-Nola Treats—BARBARA'S BAKERY | | | | | |
| ★ Chocolate Chip | 1 bar | 80 | 3% | 0% | 0% |
| ★ Cinnamon Toast | 1 bar | 80 | 3% | 0% | 0% |
| ★ Peanut & Jelly | 1 bar | 80 | 5% | 0% | 0% |
| ★ Tutti-Frutti | 1 bar | 80 | 3% | 0% | 0% |
| QUAKER Chewy Granola Bars | | | | | |
| ❖ Chewy Nutty Trail Mix | 1 bar | 120 | 8% | 5% | 0% |
| ❖ Chocolate Chip | 1 bar | 120 | 5% | 8% | 0% |
| ★ Granola Bar Caramel Apple | 1 bar | 120 | 5% | 5% | 0% |
| ★ Low Fat Apple Berry | 1 bar | 110 | 3% | 3% | 0% |
| ★ Low Fat Chocolate Chunk | 1 bar | 110 | 3% | 3% | 0% |
| ❖ Peanut Butter | 1 bar | 120 | 6% | 5% | 0% |
| ❖ Peanut Butter & Chocolate Chip | 1 bar | 120 | 7% | 8% | 0% |
| ❖ S'Mores | 1 bar | 120 | 5% | 8% | 0% |

## EGGS

**Brand Name Foods**

| FOOD | Serving Size | Calories | Tot Fat | Sat Fat | Chol |
|---|---|---|---|---|---|
| ❖ BREAKFAST-ON-THE-GO! Handy Ham & Cheese Omelet— WEIGHT WATCHERS | 1 omelet | 230 | 9% | 15% | 12% |
| SWANSON Great Starts Breakfast—CAMPBELL'S | | | | | |
| ⊛ Budget Scrambled Eggs | 1 pkg | 200 | 18% | 40% | 63% |
| ⊛ Eggs & Silver Dollar Pancakes | 1 pkg | 250 | 22% | 30% | 97% |

★ Foods with this symbol have less than or equal to 5% *Daily Value* for all three nutrients (5% Rule).

❖ Foods with this symbol have at least one of the three nutrients greater than 5% *Daily Value* but less than or equal to 20% *Daily Value*.

⊛ Foods with this symbol have at least one of the three nutrients greater than 20% *Daily Value* (20% Rule).

| FOOD | Serving Size | Calories | Tot Fat | Sat Fat | Chol |
|------|------|------|------|------|------|
| ✧ Eggs, Bacon & Cheese On a Muffin | 1 pkg | 290 | 23% | 30% | 32% |
| ✧ Scrambled Eggs & Bacon | 1 pkg | 290 | 29% | 45% | 80% |
| ✧ Scrambled Eggs & Sausage | 1 pkg | 360 | 40% | 50% | 93% |

## FRENCH TOAST

**Brand Name Foods**

| | | | | | |
|------|------|------|------|------|------|
| DOWNYFLAKE French Toast—PET | | | | | |
| ❖ Cinnamon Swirl | 2 pcs | 270 | 9% | 8% | 13% |
| ❖ Regular | 2 pcs | 260 | 10% | 6% | 17% |
| KRUSTEAZ French Toast— CONTINENTAL MILLS | | | | | |
| ✧ Cinnamon Swirl | 2 slcs | 230 | 8% | 5% | 32% |
| ✧ Classic Style | 2 slcs | 230 | 8% | 5% | 32% |
| ❖ Sourdough | 1 slc | 140 | 3% | 3% | 7% |
| SWANSON *Great Starts* Breakfast— CAMPBELL'S | | | | | |
| ✧ Cinnamon Swirl French Toast | 1 pkg | 440 | 43% | 60% | 50% |
| ✧ French Toast w/Sausage | 1 pkg | 410 | 40% | 45% | 37% |

## INSTANT BREAKFAST DRINKS

**Brand Name Foods**

| | | | | | |
|------|------|------|------|------|------|
| CARNATION Instant Breakfast Mix (prep w/skim milk)—NESTLÉ | | | | | |
| ★ Cafe Mocha | 9 fl oz | 220 | 1% | 2% | 2% |
| ★ Classic Chocolate Malt | 9 fl oz | 220 | 3% | 5% | 2% |
| ★ Creamy Milk Chocolate | 9 fl oz | 220 | 2% | 4% | 2% |
| ★ French Vanilla | 9 fl oz | 220 | 1% | 2% | 2% |
| ★ Strawberry Creme | 9 fl oz | 220 | 1% | 2% | 2% |
| CARNATION Instant Breakfast (10 fl oz can)—NESTLÉ | | | | | |
| ★ Cafe Mocha | 1 can | 220 | 4% | 3% | 2% |
| ★ Creamy Milk Chocolate | 1 can | 220 | 4% | 5% | 2% |
| ★ French Vanilla | 1 can | 220 | 5% | 2% | 1% |
| ★ Strawberry Creme | 1 can | 220 | 5% | 3% | 2% |
| CARNATION Instant Breakfast, No Sugar Added—NESTLÉ | | | | | |
| ★ Classic Chocolate Malt | 9 fl oz | 160 | 3% | 4% | 2% |
| ★ Creamy Milk Chocolate | 9 fl oz | 160 | 2% | 4% | 2% |
| ★ French Vanilla | 9 fl oz | 150 | 1% | 2% | 2% |
| ★ Strawberry Creme | 9 fl oz | 150 | 1% | 2% | 2% |
| ★ PILLSBURY Instant Breakfast: Chocolate (prep w/8 oz skim milk)—PILLSBURY | 1 env | 220 | 2% | 4% | 3% |

| FOOD | Serving Size | Calories | Tot Fat | Sat Fat | Chol |
|------|------|------|------|------|------|

## PANCAKES: FROZEN OR REFRIGERATED

**Brand Name Foods**

ACT II Pancakes (4.41 oz)—
GOLDEN VALLEY

| FOOD | Serving Size | Calories | Tot Fat | Sat Fat | Chol |
|------|------|------|------|------|------|
| ⊛ Apple Cinnamon | 1 pkg | 370 | 23% | 15% | 2% |
| ⊛ Blueberry Topped | 1 pkg | 370 | 23% | 15% | 2% |
| ⊛ Maple Topped | 1 pkg | 370 | 23% | 15% | 2% |
| ❖ DOWNYFLAKE Pancakes—PET | 3 pancakes | 270 | 11% | 9% | 2% |

HUNGRY JACK Microwave
Pancakes—PILLSBURY

| FOOD | Serving Size | Calories | Tot Fat | Sat Fat | Chol |
|------|------|------|------|------|------|
| ★ Blueberry | 3 pancakes | 230 | 5% | 3% | 3% |
| ❖ Buttermilk | 3 pancakes | 240 | 6% | 5% | 3% |
| ❖ Buttermilk Mini's | 11 pancakes | 230 | 6% | 5% | 3% |
| ❖ Original* | 3 pancakes | 240 | 6% | 5% | 3% |

KRUSTEAZ Pancakes—
CONTINENTAL MILLS

| FOOD | Serving Size | Calories | Tot Fat | Sat Fat | Chol |
|------|------|------|------|------|------|
| ❖ Blueberry | 3 pancakes | 260 | 8% | 8% | 5% |
| ❖ Buttermilk | 3 pancakes | 270 | 8% | 8% | 3% |
| ★ Mini | 6 pancakes | 120 | 4% | 3% | 1% |

SWANSON *Great Starts*
Breakfast—CAMPBELL'S

| FOOD | Serving Size | Calories | Tot Fat | Sat Fat | Chol |
|------|------|------|------|------|------|
| ⊛ *Budget*, 6 Silver Dollar Pancakes | 1 pkg | 340 | 28% | 45% | 23% |
| ⊛ Pancakes w/Bacon | 1 pkg | 400 | 31% | 35% | 33% |
| ⊛ Pancakes w/Sausage | 1 pkg | 490 | 38% | 55% | 30% |

## PANCAKES: MIXES

**Brand Name Foods**

ARROWHEAD MILLS
Pancake Mixes

| FOOD | Serving Size | Calories | Tot Fat | Sat Fat | Chol |
|------|------|------|------|------|------|
| ★ Blue Corn | 1/3 cup mix | 160 | 2% | 0% | 0% |
| ★ Buckwheat | 1/3 cup mix | 140 | 2% | 0% | 0% |
| ★ Buttermilk | 1/4 cup mix | 120 | 1% | 0% | 1% |
| ★ Multigrain | 1/4 cup mix | 120 | 1% | 0% | 0% |
| ★ Oat Bran | 1/3 cup mix | 140 | 2% | 0% | 0% |
| ★ Whole Grain | 1/4 cup mix | 120 | 1% | 0% | 0% |
| ★ Wild Rice | 1/3 cup mix | 140 | 2% | 0% | 0% |

AUNT JEMIMA—QUAKER

| FOOD | Serving Size | Calories | Tot Fat | Sat Fat | Chol |
|------|------|------|------|------|------|
| ★ Buckwheat | 1/4 cup mix | 120 | 2% | 0% | 0% |
| ★ Buttermilk Complete | 1/3 cup mix | 190 | 3% | 3% | 3% |

★ Foods with this symbol have less than or equal to 5% *Daily Value* for <u>all</u> three nutrients (5% Rule).
❖ Foods with this symbol have <u>at least one</u> of the three nutrients greater than 5% *Daily Value* but less than or equal to 20% *Daily Value*.
⊛ Foods with this symbol have <u>at least one</u> of the three nutrients greater than 20% *Daily Value* (20% Rule).

| FOOD | Serving Size | Calories | Tot Fat | Sat Fat | Chol |
|------|------|------|------|------|------|
| ★ Buttermilk Complete, Reduced Calorie | 1/3 cup mix | 140 | 2% | 3% | 5% |
| ★ Complete | 1/3 cup mix | 190 | 3% | 3% | 5% |
| ★ Whole Wheat | 1/4 cup mix | 130 | 1% | 0% | 0% |
| BETTY CROCKER Pancake Mixes (prep as dir)—GENERAL MILLS | | | | | |
| ★ Complete Buttermilk | 3 pancakes | 200 | 4% | 3% | 4% |
| ★ Complete Original | 3 pancakes | 210 | 4% | 4% | 3% |
| BISQUICK *Shake 'N Pour* Pancake & Waffle Mixes (prep as dir)— GENERAL MILLS | | | | | |
| ❖ Blueberry | 3 pancakes | 220 | 7% | 6% | 0% |
| ★ Buttermilk | 3 pancakes | 200 | 5% | 4% | 0% |
| ❖ Original | 3 pancakes | 210 | 6% | 4% | 0% |
| ★ FEATHERWEIGHT Pancake Mix | 5 tbsp | 160 | 3% | 0% | 0% |
| HUNGRY JACK Pancake Mix (prep as dir)—PILLSBURY | | | | | |
| ④ Buttermilk | 1/3 cup mix | 290 | 20% | 15% | 23% |
| ★ Buttermilk Complete | 1/3 cup mix | 160 | 2% | 0% | 1% |
| ④ *Extra Lights* | 1/3 cup mix | 240 | 12% | 10% | 23% |
| ★ *Extra Lights* Complete | 1/3 cup mix | 150 | 3% | 3% | 0% |
| ④ Original | 1/3 cup mix | 290 | 20% | 13% | 23% |
| KRUSTEAZ Pancake Mix (prep as dir)—CONTINENTAL MILLS | | | | | |
| ❖ Buckwheat (4") | 3 pancakes | 280 | 6% | 5% | 3% |
| ★ Buttermilk (4") | 3 pancakes | 200 | 5% | 3% | 3% |
| ④ Crepe (4") | 3 pancakes | 100 | 5% | 5% | 30% |
| ★ Harvest Apple Spice (4") | 2 pancakes | 210 | 5% | 0% | 0% |
| ★ Imitation Blueberry (4") | 3 pancakes | 210 | 5% | 5% | 3% |
| ★ Lite Oatbran (4") | 3 pancakes | 140 | 2% | 0% | 0% |
| ④ Old Fashioned (4") | 3 pancakes | 230 | 14% | 10% | 50% |
| ★ Whole Wheat & Honey (4") | 3 pancakes | 230 | 2% | 0% | 3% |
| ④ ROBIN HOOD Buttermilk Pancake Mix—GENERAL MILLS | 3 pancakes | 220 | 10% | 10% | 21% |

## TOASTER PASTRIES

**Brand Name Foods**

| FOOD | Serving Size | Calories | Tot Fat | Sat Fat | Chol |
|------|------|------|------|------|------|
| POP-TARTS—KELLOGG'S | | | | | |
| ❖ Apple Cinnamon | 1 pastry | 210 | 8% | 5% | 0% |
| ❖ Blueberry | 1 pastry | 210 | 11% | 5% | 0% |
| ❖ Brown Sugar Cinnamon | 1 pastry | 220 | 14% | 5% | 0% |
| ❖ Cherry | 1 pastry | 200 | 8% | 5% | 0% |
| ❖ Frosted Blueberry | 1 pastry | 200 | 8% | 5% | 0% |
| ❖ Frosted Brown Sugar Cinnamon | 1 pastry | 210 | 11% | 5% | 0% |
| ❖ Frosted Cherry | 1 pastry | 200 | 8% | 5% | 0% |
| ❖ Frosted Chocolate Fudge | 1 pastry | 200 | 8% | 5% | 0% |
| ❖ Frosted Chocolate Vanilla Creme | 1 pastry | 200 | 8% | 5% | 0% |

| FOOD | Serving Size | Calories | Tot Fat | Sat Fat | Chol |
|------|-------------|----------|---------|---------|------|
| ❖ Frosted Grape | 1 pastry | 200 | 8% | 5% | 0% |
| ❖ Frosted Raspberry | 1 pastry | 210 | 9% | 5% | 0% |
| ❖ Frosted S'Mores | 1 pastry | 200 | 8% | 3% | 0% |
| ❖ Frosted Strawberry | 1 pastry | 200 | 8% | 8% | 0% |
| ❖ Milk Chocolate Graham | 1 pastry | 210 | 9% | 5% | 0% |
| ❖ Strawberry | 1 pastry | 200 | 8% | 8% | 0% |
| ★ POP-TARTS, Low Fat: All flavors—KELLOGG'S | 1 pastry | 190 | 5% | 3% | 0% |
| POP-TARTS, *Minis* Bite Size Pastry Snack—KELLOGG'S | | | | | |
| ❖ Frosted Chocolate | 1 pouch | 170 | 6% | 5% | 0% |
| ❖ Frosted Grape | 1 pouch | 170 | 6% | 5% | 0% |
| ❖ Frosted Strawberry | 1 pouch | 170 | 6% | 5% | 0% |
| THOMAS' *Toast-R-Cakes*—CPC | | | | | |
| ❖ Banana Nut | 1 cake | 110 | 8% | 2% | 1% |
| ★ Blueberry | 1 cake | 100 | 5% | 2% | 1% |
| ★ Cinnamon Apple | 1 cake | 100 | 5% | 2% | 1% |
| ❖ Corn | 1 cake | 110 | 6% | 2% | 1% |
| ★ Raisin Bran | 1 cake | 90 | 5% | 0% | 1% |
| TOASTER STRUDEL Pastries—PILLSBURY | | | | | |
| ❖ Apple | 1 pastry | 180 | 11% | 8% | 2% |
| ❖ Blueberry | 1 pastry | 180 | 11% | 8% | 2% |
| ❖ Cherry | 1 pastry | 180 | 11% | 8% | 2% |
| ❖ Cinnamon | 1 pastry | 190 | 12% | 8% | 2% |
| ❖ Cream Cheese | 1 pastry | 190 | 15% | 18% | 5% |
| ❖ Cream Cheese & Blueberry/ Strawberry | 1 pastry | 190 | 14% | 15% | 3% |
| ❖ French Toast Style | 1 pastry | 190 | 11% | 8% | 2% |
| ❖ Raspberry | 1 pastry | 180 | 11% | 8% | 2% |
| ❖ Strawberry | 1 pastry | 180 | 11% | 8% | 2% |
| Frosted TOASTETTES—NABISCO | | | | | |
| ❖ Blueberry | 1 tart | 190 | 8% | 7% | 0% |
| ❖ Brown Sugar Cinnamon | 1 tart | 190 | 8% | 7% | 0% |
| ❖ Cherry | 1 tart | 190 | 8% | 7% | 0% |
| ❖ Fudge | 1 tart | 190 | 8% | 7% | 0% |
| ❖ Strawberry | 1 tart | 190 | 8% | 7% | 0% |

## WAFFLES: FROZEN

**Brand Name Foods**

DOWNYFLAKE Waffles—PET

| | Serving Size | Calories | Tot Fat | Sat Fat | Chol |
|------|-------------|----------|---------|---------|------|
| ★ Apple/Cinnamon | 2 waffles | 180 | 3% | 3% | 0% |
| ❖ Blueberry | 2 waffles | 180 | 6% | 5% | 0% |

---

★ Foods with this symbol have less than or equal to 5% *Daily Value* for <u>all</u> three nutrients (5% Rule).

❖ Foods with this symbol have <u>at least one</u> of the three nutrients greater than 5% *Daily Value* but less than or equal to 20% *Daily Value*.

Ⓐ Foods with this symbol have <u>at least one</u> of the three nutrients greater than 20% *Daily Value* (20% Rule).

---

| FOOD | Serving Size | Calories | Tot Fat | Sat Fat | Chol |
|---|---|---|---|---|---|
| ❖ Butter & Syrup | 2 waffles | 150 | 6% | 4% | 0% |
| ❖ Buttermilk | 2 waffles | 160 | 6% | 5% | 1% |
| ★ Crisp & Healthy | 2 waffles | 170 | 3% | 3% | 0% |
| ❖ Homestyle | 4 waffles | 230 | 8% | 7% | 0% |
| ❖ Homestyle Jumbo | 2 waffles | 170 | 6% | 5% | 0% |
| ❖ Hot 'n Buttery | 2 waffles | 180 | 9% | 6% | 1% |
| ★ Plain | 2 waffles | 170 | 3% | 3% | 0% |
| EGGO Waffles—KELLOGG'S | | | | | |
| ❖ Apple Cinnamon | 2 waffles | 220 | 12% | 8% | 7% |
| ❖ Blueberry | 2 waffles | 220 | 12% | 8% | 7% |
| ❖ Blueberry Minis | 3 sets of 4 waffles | 240 | 12% | 8% | 8% |
| ❖ Buttermilk | 2 waffles | 220 | 12% | 8% | 8% |
| ❖ Cinnamon Toast Minis | 3 sets of 4 waffles | 280 | 14% | 10% | 8% |
| ❖ Common Sense Oat Bran | 2 waffles | 200 | 11% | 8% | 0% |
| ❖ Common Sense Oat Bran with Fruit & Nut | 2 waffles | 220 | 12% | 8% | 0% |
| ❖ Homestyle | 2 waffles | 220 | 12% | 8% | 8% |
| ❖ Homestyle Minis | 3 sets of 4 waffles | 240 | 12% | 8% | 8% |
| ❖ Nut & Honey | 2 waffles | 240 | 15% | 10% | 8% |
| ❖ Nutri-Grain | 2 waffles | 190 | 9% | 5% | 0% |
| ❖ Nutri-Grain Multi-Bran | 2 waffles | 80 | 9% | 5% | 0% |
| ❖ Nutri-Grain Raisin & Bran | 2 waffles | 210 | 9% | 5% | 0% |
| ★ Special K | 2 waffles | 140 | 0% | 0% | 0% |
| ❖ Strawberry | 2 waffles | 220 | 12% | 8% | 7% |
| KRUSTEAZ Waffles—CONTINENTAL MILLS | | | | | |
| ❖ Blueberry | 2 waffles | 230 | 12% | 5% | 7% |
| ❖ Buttermilk | 2 waffles | 220 | 12% | 5% | 7% |
| ❖ Homestyle | 2 waffles | 220 | 12% | 5% | 7% |

## WAFFLES: MIXES

**Brand Name Foods**

| ☮ KRUSTEAZ Belgian Waffle Mix (prep as dir)—CONTINENTAL MILLS | 1,7" round | 440 | 29% | 18% | 37% |

See also Pancakes: Mixes, page 82

| FOOD | Serving Size | Calories | Tot Fat | Sat Fat | Chol |
|------|--------------|----------|---------|---------|------|

# Candy and Confections
## CHOCOLATE CANDY

### Generic Foods

| FOOD | Serving Size | Calories | Tot Fat | Sat Fat | Chol |
|------|--------------|----------|---------|---------|------|
| ⊛ Chocolate Coated Peanuts | 1.4 oz | 230 | 26% | 28% | 0% |
| ❖ Chocolate Covered Fondant | 1.4 oz | 150 | 6% | 11% | 0% |
| ❖ Chocolate Covered Raisins | 40 pcs | 160 | 10% | 15% | 0% |
| ★ Fondant | 1.4 oz | 150 | 2% | 1% | 0% |
| Fudge | | | | | |
| ❖ Chocolate | 1.4 oz | 160 | 7% | 8% | 0% |
| ❖ Chocolate w/Marshmallows | 1.4 oz | 170 | 10% | 20% | 3% |
| ❖ Chocolate w/Marshmallows & Nuts | 1.4 oz | 180 | 12% | 19% | 3% |
| ★ Peanut Butter | 1.4 oz | 150 | 4% | 3% | 1% |
| ❖ w/Nuts | 1.4 oz | 160 | 6% | 4% | 1% |
| ⊛ Milk Chocolate | 1.4 oz | 200 | 20% | 39% | 0% |
| ⊛ Milk Chocolate Peanuts | 1/4 cup | 190 | 19% | 27% | 1% |
| ⊛ Milk Chocolate Raisins | 1/4 cup | 190 | 11% | 21% | 0% |
| ⊛ Milk Chocolate w/Almonds | 1.4 oz | 210 | 22% | 29% | 22% |
| ⊛ Milk Chocolate w/Peanuts | 1.4 oz | 220 | 23% | 33% | 0% |
| ⊛ Milk Chocolate w/Rice Cereal Bar | 1 bar | 200 | 17% | 33% | 3% |
| ⊛ Turtles | 1 pc | 210 | 18% | 23% | 3% |

### Brand Name Foods

| FOOD | Serving Size | Calories | Tot Fat | Sat Fat | Chol |
|------|--------------|----------|---------|---------|------|
| ⊛ 100 GRAND—NESTLÉ | 1.5 oz bar | 200 | 12% | 25% | 3% |
| ⊛ 3 MUSKETEERS Bar—M&M/MARS | 2.1 oz bar | 260 | 13% | 22% | 1% |
| ⊛ 5TH AVENUE—HERSHEY FOODS | 2 oz bar | 280 | 18% | 25% | 1% |
| ⊛ BABY RUTH—NESTLÉ | 1 bar | 280 | 19% | 36% | 0% |
| ⊛ BARNONE—HERSHEY FOODS | 1.65 oz bar | 250 | 23% | 45% | 2% |
| BRACH'S Chocolate | | | | | |
| ⊛ Chocolate Covered Raisins | 34 pcs | 170 | 10% | 23% | 1% |
| ⊛ Clusters | 3 pcs | 230 | 23% | 33% | 1% |
| ⊛ Double Dippers | 15 pcs | 220 | 21% | 32% | 2% |
| ⊛ Malts | 15 pcs | 190 | 14% | 24% | 3% |
| ❖ Mint Patties | 3 pcs | 140 | 5% | 10% | 0% |
| ⊛ Nonpareils | 17 pcs | 200 | 14% | 29% | 2% |
| ⊛ BUNCHA CRUNCH—NESTLÉ | 2.1 oz bag | 200 | 15% | 24% | 2% |
| ⊛ BUTTERFINGER—NESTLÉ | 1.4 oz bar | 280 | 17% | 31% | 0% |
| ⊛ BUTTERFINGER BB's—NESTLÉ | 1.5 oz bag | 220 | 14% | 31% | 0% |
| CADBURY'S Chocolate Bars— HERSHEY FOODS | | | | | |
| ⊛ *Dairy Milk* | 9 blks | 220 | 18% | 40% | 3% |
| ⊛ *Fruit & Nut* | 9 blks | 210 | 17% | 30% | 2% |

★ Foods with this symbol have less than or equal to 5% *Daily Value* for all three nutrients (5% Rule).
❖ Foods with this symbol have at least one of the three nutrients greater than 5% *Daily Value* but less than or equal to 20% *Daily Value*.
⊛ Foods with this symbol have at least one of the three nutrients greater than 20% *Daily Value* (20% Rule).

| FOOD | Serving Size | Calories | Tot Fat | Sat Fat | Chol |
|---|---|---|---|---|---|
| ⊛ *Krisp* | 9 blks | 200 | 15% | 35% | 3% |
| ⊛ *Mint* | 5 blks | 190 | 12% | 25% | 1% |
| ⊛ *Roast Almond* | 9 blks | 220 | 20% | 35% | 3% |
| CADBURY Eggs—HERSHEY FOODS | | | | | |
| ❖ *Creme Egg* | 1 pc | 180 | 9% | 20% | 2% |
| ⊛ *Mini Eggs* | 12 pcs | 200 | 14% | 30% | 3% |
| ⊛ CARAMELLO—HERSHEY FOODS | 1.6 oz bar | 220 | 15% | 30% | 3% |
| CELLA'S—TOOTSIE ROLL | | | | | |
| ❖ Dark Chocolate | 2 pcs | 110 | 7% | 14% | 0% |
| ❖ Milk Chocolate | 2 pcs | 110 | 7% | 13% | 0% |
| ⊛ CHARLESTON CHEW, Chocolatey | | | | | |
| —TOOTSIE ROLL | 1 bar | 230 | 9% | 27% | 0% |
| ⊛ CHUNKY BAR—NESTLÉ | 1.4 oz bar | 200 | 17% | 29% | 1% |
| ⊛ CRUNCH—NESTLÉ | 1.55 oz bar | 230 | 18% | 34% | 2% |
| DOVE—M&M/MARS | | | | | |
| ⊛ Dark Chocolate | 1.3 oz bar | 200 | 19% | 36% | 1% |
| ⊛ Milk Chocolate | 1.3 oz bar | 200 | 18% | 36% | 2% |
| ESTEE | | | | | |
| ⊛ Chocolate Raisins | 1/4 cup | 180 | 9% | 25% | 1% |
| ❖ Chocolate Vanilla Caramels | 5 candies | 150 | 8% | 5% | 0% |
| ⊛ Dark Chocolate Bar | 7 squares | 200 | 22% | 40% | 3% |
| ⊛ Milk Chocolate Bar | 7 squares | 230 | 26% | 50% | 7% |
| ⊛ Milk Chocolate Bar w/Almonds | 7 squares | 230 | 26% | 45% | 7% |
| ⊛ Milk Chocolate Crisp Rice Bar | 1 bar | 370 | 40% | 75% | 10% |
| ⊛ Milk Chocolate Bar w/ Fruits & Nuts | 7 squares | 220 | 25% | 45% | 7% |
| ⊛ Mint Chocolate Bar | 7 squares | 200 | 22% | 40% | 3% |
| FEATHERWEIGHT Milk Chocolate Bar | | | | | |
| ⊛ Plain | 7 squares | 230 | 26% | 50% | 7% |
| ⊛ w/Almonds | 7 squares | 230 | 26% | 45% | 7% |
| ⊛ w/Crisp Rice | 1 bar | 370 | 40% | 75% | 10% |
| GHIRARDELLI Chocolates | | | | | |
| ⊛ Almond Clusters (4 oz pkg) | 3 clusters | 210 | 24% | 22% | 1% |
| ⊛ Cookies & Cream | 2.5 oz bar | 370 | 33% | 61% | 2% |
| ⊛ Dark Chocolate (3 oz bar) | 4 sections | 210 | 22% | 43% | 0% |
| ⊛ Dark Chocolate w/Almonds (3 oz bar) | 4 sections | 220 | 24% | 36% | 0% |
| ⊛ Dark Chocolate w/Raspberries (3 oz bar) | 4 sections | 210 | 21% | 41% | 0% |
| ⊛ Double Chocolate Mocha | 2.5 oz bar | 350 | 30% | 55% | 4% |
| ⊛ Milk Chocolate (3 oz bar) | 4 sections | 220 | 21% | 41% | 3% |
| ⊛ Milk Chocolate Crisp | 2.5 oz bar | 360 | 31% | 61% | 4% |
| ⊛ Milk Chocolate w/Almonds (3 oz bar) | 4 sections | 230 | 24% | 35% | 2% |
| ⊛ Milk Chocolate w/Macadamias | 2.5 oz bar | 380 | 40% | 65% | 4% |
| ⊛ Milk Chocolate w/Pecans (3 oz bar) | 4 sections | 230 | 25% | 35% | 2% |
| ⊛ Milk Chocolate w/Toffee (3 oz bar) | 4 sections | 220 | 20% | 39% | 4% |

| FOOD | Serving Size | Calories | Tot Fat | Sat Fat | Chol |
|------|------|------|------|------|------|
| ⊛ Milk Chocolate Wafers (5 oz pkg) | 11 pcs | 210 | 19% | 36% | 3% |
| ⊛ Mint Chocolate (3 oz bar) | 4 sections | 220 | 24% | 41% | 1% |
| ⊛ Mint Chocolate Wafers (5 oz pkg) | 11 pcs | 220 | 21% | 41% | 1% |
| ⊛ Non-Pareils (5 oz pkg) | 10 pcs | 190 | 14% | 28% | 0% |
| ⊛ Peanut Clusters (4 oz pkg) | 3 pcs | 210 | 23% | 25% | 1% |
| ⊛ White Confection w/Raspberries (3 oz bar) | 4 sections | 230 | 22% | 43% | 2% |
| ⊛ White Mocha w/Biscotti | 2.5 oz bar | 380 | 34% | 63% | 3% |
| ⊛ GOOBERS—NESTLÉ | 1.38 oz bag | 210 | 20% | 25% | 1% |
| HERSHEY Eggs | | | | | |
| ❖ Marshmallow | 0.95 oz | 110 | 5% | 8% | 1% |
| ⊛ Solid Milk Chocolate | 7 pcs | 210 | 18% | 35% | 3% |
| HERSHEY's *Golden Collection* | | | | | |
| ⊛ Almond Bar | 2.8 oz bar | 450 | 46% | 65% | 3% |
| ⊛ Golden Cashew | 2.8 oz bar | 390 | 38% | 65% | 3% |
| ⊛ Golden Macadamia Nut | 2.8 oz bar | 420 | 45% | 65% | 5% |
| ⊛ Golden Pecan | 2.8 oz bar | 400 | 42% | 65% | 5% |
| ⊛ *Solitaires* Chocolate Covered Almonds | 13 pcs | 230 | 23% | 30% | 2% |
| HERSHEY's *Hugs* Chocolates | | | | | |
| ⊛ Chocolate | 8 pcs | 210 | 18% | 30% | 3% |
| ⊛ w/Almonds | 9 pcs | 230 | 20% | 30% | 3% |
| HERSHEY's *Kisses* Chocolates | | | | | |
| ⊛ Milk Chocolate | 8 pcs | 210 | 18% | 40% | 3% |
| ⊛ w/Almonds | 8 pcs | 210 | 20% | 36% | 2% |
| HERSHEY's *Nuggets* Milk Chocolate | | | | | |
| ❖ Almond | 4 pcs | 210 | 20% | 20% | 2% |
| ⊛ Cookies 'n Mint | 4 pcs | 200 | 15% | 25% | 2% |
| ⊛ Milk Chocolate | 4 pcs | 210 | 19% | 40% | 3% |
| HERSHEY's Chocolate Bars | | | | | |
| ⊛ Cookies 'n Mint | 1.5 oz bar | 230 | 18% | 30% | 3% |
| ⊛ Milk Chocolate | 1.55 oz bar | 230 | 20% | 45% | 3% |
| ⊛ Special Dark | 1.45 oz bar | 230 | 20% | 40% | 0% |
| ⊛ w/Almonds | 1.45 oz bar | 230 | 22% | 35% | 2% |
| ❖ JUNIOR MINTS—TOOTSIE ROLL | 1.6 oz box | 190 | 6% | 12% | 0% |
| ⊛ KIT KAT—HERSHEY FOODS | 1.5 oz bar | 220 | 18% | 40% | 2% |
| ⊛ KRACKEL Chocolate Bar— HERSHEY FOODS | 1.45 oz bar | 220 | 18% | 35% | 3% |
| ❖ KRAFT Fudgies | 5 pcs | 180 | 8% | 13% | 0% |
| M&Ms Chocolate Candies | | | | | |
| ❖ Almond | 1.3 oz bag | 200 | 17% | 17% | 1% |
| ⊛ Mint | 1.7 oz bag | 230 | 15% | 30% | 3% |
| ⊛ Peanut | 1.7 oz bag | 250 | 20% | 25% | 2% |
| ⊛ Peanut Butter | 1.6 oz bag | 240 | 20% | 42% | 1% |

★ Foods with this symbol have less than or equal to 5% *Daily Value* for <u>all</u> three nutrients (5% Rule).
❖ Foods with this symbol have <u>at least one</u> of the three nutrients greater than 5% *Daily Value* but less than or equal to 20% *Daily Value*.
⊛ Foods with this symbol have <u>at least one</u> of the three nutrients greater than 20% *Daily Value* (20% Rule).

| FOOD | Serving Size | Calories | Tot Fat | Sat Fat | Chol |
|------|---|---|---|---|---|
| ⓐ   Plain | 1.7 oz bag | 230 | 15% | 30% | 3% |
| ⓐ  MARS Almond Bar—M&M/MARS | 1.8 oz bar | 240 | 19% | 21% | 2% |
| ⓐ  MILK CHOCOLATE Bar—NESTLÉ | 1.45 oz bar | 220 | 20% | 37% | 3% |
|    MILKY WAY Bar—M&M/MARS | | | | | |
| ⓐ   Bar | 2.1 oz bar | 280 | 17% | 27% | 2% |
| ⓐ   Dark Bar | 1.8 oz bar | 220 | 13% | 22% | 2% |
| ⓐ  MR. GOODBAR Chocolate Bar— | | | | | |
|    HERSHEY FOODS | 1.75 oz bar | 280 | 28% | 35% | 2% |
| ⓐ  NUTRAGEOUS—HERSHEY FOODS | 1.6 oz bar | 240 | 22% | 23% | 1% |
| ❖  OH HENRY!—NESTLÉ | 1.8 oz bar | 230 | 14% | 20% | 1% |
|    PEARSON *Nips*—NESTLÉ | | | | | |
| ❖   Chocolate Mint | 2 pcs | 60 | 2% | 7% | 0% |
| ❖   Chocolate Parfait | 2 pcs | 60 | 3% | 9% | 0% |
|    PETER PAUL—HERSHEY FOODS | | | | | |
| ⓐ   *Almond Joy* | 1.76 oz bar | 240 | 20% | 45% | 0% |
| ⓐ   *Mounds* | 1.9 oz bar | 250 | 30% | 55% | 0% |
| ⓐ  RAISINETS—NESTLÉ | 1.58 oz bag | 200 | 12% | 22% | 1% |
|    REESE'S—HERSHEY FOODS | | | | | |
| ⓐ   Crunchy Peanut Butter Cups | 1.4 oz (2 cups) | 220 | 22% | 25% | 1% |
| ⓐ   Peanut Butter Cups | 1.6 oz (2 cups) | 240 | 22% | 30% | 1% |
| ⓐ   *Pieces* | 50 pcs | 190 | 12% | 35% | 0% |
| ⓐ  ROLO Caramels—HERSHEY FOODS | 7 pcs | 210 | 15% | 35% | 2% |
| ⓐ  SKOR English Toffee—HERSHEY FOODS | 1.4 oz | 220 | 20% | 45% | 7% |
|    SNICKERS—M&M/MARS | | | | | |
| ⓐ   Bar | 2.1 oz bar | 280 | 21% | 26% | 3% |
| ⓐ   Munch Bar | 1.4 oz bar | 230 | 23% | 18% | 3% |
| ⓐ   Peanut Butter Bar | 2 oz bar | 310 | 31% | 35% | 2% |
| ⓐ  SNO CAPS—NESTLÉ | 2.3 oz box | 300 | 19% | 38% | 0% |
|    SYMPHONY Chocolate Bar— | | | | | |
|    HERSHEY FOODS | | | | | |
| ⓐ   Creamy Milk Chocolate | 1.5 oz bar | 230 | 22% | 45% | 3% |
| ⓐ   w/Almonds & Toffee Chips | 1.5 oz bar | 240 | 23% | 40% | 3% |
| ★  TOOTSIE ROLL Midgees | 6 pcs | 160 | 4% | 3% | 0% |
| ❖  TURTLES—NESTLÉ | 2 pcs | 160 | 14% | 15% | 1% |
| ⓐ  TWIX Caramel Cookie Bars | | | | | |
|    (2 oz pkg)—M&M/MARS | 2 cookies | 280 | 21% | 26% | 1% |
| ⓐ  WHATCHAMACALLIT— | | | | | |
|    HERSHEY FOODS | 1.7 oz bar | 250 | 20% | 50% | 2% |
| ❖  YORK Peppermint Pattie— | | | | | |
|    HERSHEY FOODS | 1.5 oz pattie | 170 | 6% | 13% | 0% |

## MARSHMALLOWS

**Brand Name Foods**

| | | | | | |
|------|---|---|---|---|---|
|    FUNMALLOWS Marshmallows— | | | | | |
|    KRAFT | | | | | |
| ★  Miniatures | 1/2 cup | 100 | 0% | 0% | 0% |
| ★  Regular | 4 pcs | 110 | 0% | 0% | 0% |

| FOOD | Serving Size | Calories | Tot Fat | Sat Fat | Chol |
|------|--------------|----------|---------|---------|------|
| KRAFT *Jet-Puffed* Marshmallows | | | | | |
| ★ Miniatures | 1/2 cup | 100 | 0% | 0% | 0% |
| ⊛ Regular | 5 pcs | 110 | 0% | 0% | 0% |

## *OTHER* CANDY

### Generic Foods

| FOOD | Serving Size | Calories | Tot Fat | Sat Fat | Chol |
|------|--------------|----------|---------|---------|------|
| ⊛ Candied Coconut | 1.4 oz | 170 | 11% | 22% | 0% |
| ★ Candied Grapefruit Peel | 1/4 cup | 130 | 0% | 0% | 0% |
| ★ Candied Lemon Peel | 1/4 cup | 170 | 0% | 0% | 0% |
| ★ Candied Orange Peel | 1/4 cup | 130 | 0% | 0% | 0% |
| ★ Candied Pears | 1/4 cup | 140 | 0% | 0% | 0% |
| ★ Candied Pineapple | 1/4 cup | 150 | 0% | 0% | 0% |
| ❖ Caramels: Plain or Chocolate | 1.4 oz | 160 | 7% | 11% | 0% |
| ★ Divinity | 1.4 oz | 140 | 0% | 0% | 0% |
| ★ Gum Drops | 1.4 oz | 140 | 0% | 0% | 0% |
| ★ Hard Candy | 1.4 oz | 160 | 0% | 0% | 0% |
| ★ Jelly Beans | 5 pcs | 30 | 0% | 0% | 0% |
| ★ Lollipop | 1 pc | 110 | 0% | 0% | 0% |
| ⊛ Peanut Bar | 1 bar | 240 | 23% | 10% | 0% |
| ❖ Peanut Brittle | 1.4 oz | 170 | 10% | 13% | 0% |
| ⊛ Peanut Butter Cup | 2 pcs | 180 | 16% | 28% | 2% |
| ❖ Praline | 1 pc | 180 | 15% | 4% | 0% |
| ★ Taffy | 3 pcs | 170 | 2% | 5% | 1% |
| ⊛ Toffee | 3 pcs | 200 | 18% | 37% | 13% |

### Brand Name Foods

| FOOD | Serving Size | Calories | Tot Fat | Sat Fat | Chol |
|------|--------------|----------|---------|---------|------|
| AMAZIN' FRUIT—HERSHEY FOODS | | | | | |
| ★ Gummy Bears | 17 pcs | 130 | 0% | 0% | 0% |
| ★ Super Fruits | 11 pcs | 140 | 0% | 0% | 0% |
| BRACH'S | | | | | |
| ★ Butterscotch Disks | 3 pcs | 70 | 0% | 0% | 0% |
| ★ Candy Corn | 26 pcs | 140 | 0% | 0% | 0% |
| ★ Cinnamon Disks | 3 pcs | 70 | 0% | 0% | 0% |
| ★ Cinnamon Imperials | 52 pcs | 60 | 0% | 0% | 0% |
| ★ Circus Peanuts | 6 pcs | 160 | 0% | 0% | 0% |
| ★ Coffee Candy | 3 pcs | 70 | 3% | 0% | 0% |
| ★ Dessert Mints | 37 pcs | 160 | 0% | 0% | 0% |
| ❖ French Burnt Peanuts | 28 pcs | 190 | 14% | 5% | 0% |
| ★ Jelly Beans | 14 pcs | 140 | 0% | 0% | 0% |
| ★ Kentucky Mints | 17 pcs | 150 | 1% | 0% | 0% |
| ★ Lemon Drops | 4 pcs | 70 | 0% | 0% | 0% |
| ❖ Maple Nut Goodies | 7 pcs | 190 | 13% | 5% | 0% |

★ Foods with this symbol have less than or equal to 5% *Daily Value* for <u>all</u> three nutrients (5% Rule).

❖ Foods with this symbol have <u>at least one</u> of the three nutrients greater than 5% *Daily Value* but less than or equal to 20% *Daily Value*.

⊛ Foods with this symbol have <u>at least one</u> of the three nutrients greater than 20% *Daily Value* (20% Rule).

| FOOD | Serving Size | Calories | Tot Fat | Sat Fat | Chol |
|---|---|---|---|---|---|
| ❖ Milk Maid Caramels | 4 pcs | 150 | 6% | 5% | 0% |
| ★ Orange Slices | 2 pcs | 130 | 0% | 0% | 0% |
| ❖ Royals Chewy Toffee | 5 pcs | 150 | 6% | 4% | 0% |
| ★ Sour Balls | 3 pcs | 70 | 0% | 0% | 0% |
| ★ Sparkles | 3 pcs | 70 | 0% | 0% | 0% |
| ★ Spearmint Leaves | 5 pcs | 130 | 0% | 0% | 0% |
| ★ Spice Drops | 12 pcs | 130 | 0% | 0% | 0% |
| Ⓐ Sprinkles | 17 pcs | 200 | 14% | 29% | 3% |
| ★ Star Brites | 3 pcs | 60 | 0% | 0% | 0% |
| Ⓐ Stars | 10 pcs | 200 | 17% | 38% | 6% |
| ★ Wild 'n Fruity Gummy Bears | 15 pcs | 130 | 0% | 0% | 0% |
| Ⓐ CHARLESTON CHEW, Vanilla—TOOTSIE ROLL | 1 bar | 230 | 11% | 32% | 0% |
| ★ CHARMS Blow Pops—TOOTSIE ROLL | 1 pop | 50 | 0% | 0% | 0% |
| ★ CROWS—TOOTSIE ROLL | 12 pcs | 150 | 0% | 0% | 0% |
| ★ DOTS—TOOTSIE ROLL | 12 pcs | 150 | 0% | 0% | 0% |
| ESTEE | | | | | |
| ★ Assorted Fruit Gum Drops | 23 pcs | 140 | 0% | 0% | 0% |
| ★ Assorted Fruit Gummy Bears | 16 pcs | 140 | 0% | 0% | 0% |
| ★ Assorted Hard Candy | 2–5 pcs | 60 | 0% | 0% | 0% |
| ❖ Candy Coated Peanuts | 1/4 cup | 200 | 14% | 20% | 1% |
| ★ Licorice Gum Drops | 23 pcs | 140 | 0% | 0% | 0% |
| ❖ Peanut Brittle | 1 1/2 oz | 210 | 14% | 10% | 3% |
| Ⓐ Peanut Butter Cups | 5 pcs | 200 | 18% | 35% | 1% |
| FEATHERWEIGHT | | | | | |
| ❖ Chewy Caramels | 5 pcs | 150 | 8% | 5% | 0% |
| ★ Hard Candy: All flavors | 2–5 pcs | 50–60 | 0% | 0% | 0% |
| KRAFT | | | | | |
| ★ Butter Mints | 7 pcs | 60 | 0% | 0% | 0% |
| ★ Caramels | 5 pcs | 170 | 5% | 5% | 2% |
| ★ Party Mints | 7 pcs | 60 | 0% | 0% | 0% |
| ❖ Peanut Brittle | 5 pcs | 170 | 8% | 5% | 0% |
| ★ LIFESAVERS: All flavors | 4 pcs | 60 | 0% | 0% | 0% |
| ★ Gummi Savers: All flavors | 11 pcs | 130 | 0% | 0% | 0% |
| ★ Holes: All flavors | 20 pcs | 20 | 0% | 0% | 0% |
| ★ Sugar Free Mints: All flavors | 1 mint | 10 | 0% | 0% | 0% |
| NIBS—HERSHEY FOODS | | | | | |
| ★ Cherry | 22 pcs | 140 | 2% | 0% | 0% |
| ★ Licorice | 22 pcs | 140 | 2% | 0% | 0% |
| ★ NOW AND LATER: All flavors —PLANTERS LIFESAVERS | 1 pc | 18 | 0% | 0% | 0% |
| ★ Giant: All flavors | 1 pc | 44 | 1% | 0% | 0% |
| ★ Mighty Bite: All flavors | 1 pc | 44 | 1% | 0% | 0% |
| PEARSON Nips—NESTLÉ | | | | | |
| ❖ Butter Rum | 2 pcs | 60 | 2% | 6% | 0% |
| ❖ Caramel | 2 pcs | 60 | 2% | 7% | 0% |
| ★ Coffee | 2 pcs | 60 | 2% | 5% | 0% |
| ❖ Licorice | 2 pcs | 60 | 2% | 6% | 0% |
| ❖ Peanut Butter | 2 pcs | 60 | 3% | 9% | 0% |

| FOOD | Serving Size | Calories | Tot Fat | Sat Fat | Chol |
|------|--------------|----------|---------|---------|------|
| ★ SKITTLES Bite Size Candies: | | | | | |
|    All flavors—M&M/MARS | 2.2 oz bag | 250 | 4% | 3% | 0% |
| ❖ STARBURST Fruit Chews | | | | | |
|    (2.1 oz pkg): All flavors— | | | | | |
|    M&M/MARS | 1 stick | 240 | 7% | 5% | 0% |
| ❖ SUGAR BABIES—TOOTSIE ROLL | 1 pouch | 190 | 3% | 9% | 0% |
| ❖ SUGAR DADDY—TOOTSIE ROLL | 1.7 oz pop | 200 | 4% | 11% | 1% |
| TOOTSIE ROLL | | | | | |
| ★   Blow Pops | 1 pop | 80 | 0% | 0% | 0% |
| ★   Pops | 1 pop | 60 | 0% | 0% | 0% |
| TWIZZLERS—HERSHEY FOODS | | | | | |
| ★   Chocolate | 5 pcs | 140 | 2% | 3% | 0% |
| ★   Licorice | 4 pcs | 140 | 1% | 0% | 0% |
| ★   *Pull n' Peel:* All flavors | 1.5 oz | 130 | 2% | 0% | 0% |
| ★   Strawberry | 1. 75 oz | 170 | 1% | 0% | 0% |

# Cereals

## COOKED CEREALS

*Note:* Values are for cooked cereal, unless otherwise noted.

**Generic Foods**

| FOOD | Serving Size | Calories | Tot Fat | Sat Fat | Chol |
|------|--------------|----------|---------|---------|------|
| ★ Corn Grits (uncooked) | 1/4 cup | 150 | 1% | 0% | 0% |
| ★ Corn Grits, White | 1 cup | 150 | 1% | 0% | 0% |
| ★ Corn Grits, Yellow | 1 cup | 150 | 1% | 0% | 0% |
| ★ Farina, Enriched | 1 cup | 120 | 0% | 0% | 0% |
| Bran: | | | | | |
| ★   Corn Bran (uncooked) | 2 tbsp | 20 | 0% | 0% | 0% |
| ★   Oat Bran (uncooked) | 2 tbsp | 30 | 1% | 1% | 0% |
| ★   Oat Bran | 1 cup | 90 | 3% | 2% | 0% |
| ★   Wheat Bran | 1/4 cup | 30 | 1% | 0% | 0% |
| ★ Oatmeal | 1 cup | 150 | 4% | 2% | 0% |
| ★ Oats (uncooked) | 1/4 cup | 150 | 4% | 2% | 0% |
| ★ Oats, Quick Cooking | 1 cup | 150 | 4% | 2% | 0% |

**Brand Name Foods**

| FOOD | Serving Size | Calories | Tot Fat | Sat Fat | Chol |
|------|--------------|----------|---------|---------|------|
| ★ ALBERS Hominy Quick Grits | | | | | |
|    (uncooked)—NESTLÉ | 1/4 cup | 140 | 1% | 0% | 0% |

★  Foods with this symbol have less than or equal to 5% *Daily Value* for <u>all</u> three nutrients (5% Rule).
❖  Foods with this symbol have <u>at least one</u> of the three nutrients greater than 5% *Daily Value* but less than or equal to 20% *Daily Value.*
☼  Foods with this symbol have <u>at least one</u> of the three nutrients greater than 20% *Daily Value* (20% Rule).

| FOOD | Serving Size | Calories | Tot Fat | Sat Fat | Chol |
|------|--------------|----------|---------|---------|------|
| **ARROWHEAD MILLS Hot Cereal (uncooked)** | | | | | |
| ★ 7 Grain | 1/3 cup | 140 | 2% | 0% | 0% |
| ★ Bear Mush | 1/4 cup | 160 | 2% | 0% | 0% |
| ★ Bits of Barley | 1/3 cup | 140 | 2% | 0% | 0% |
| ★ Bulgur Wheat | 1/4 cup | 150 | 1% | 0% | 0% |
| ★ Corn Grits, White | 1/4 cup | 140 | 0% | 0% | 0% |
| ★ Corn Grits, Yellow | 1/4 cup | 130 | 0% | 0% | 0% |
| ★ Couscous | 1/4 cup | 170 | 0% | 0% | 0% |
| ★ Oat Bran | 1/3 cup | 150 | 4% | 0% | 0% |
| ★ Rice & Shine | 1/4 cup | 150 | 2% | 0% | 0% |
| ★ Soy Grits | 1/4 cup | 140 | 2% | 0% | 0% |
| ★ Steel Cut Oats | 1/4 cup | 170 | 5% | 3% | 0% |
| ★ Wheat-Free 7 Grain Cereal | 1/4 cup | 120 | 2% | 0% | 0% |
| **ARROWHEAD MILLS Instant Oatmeal (prep as dir)** | | | | | |
| ★ Cinnamon Raisin Almond | 1 pkg | 130 | 5% | 0% | 0% |
| ★ Maple Apple Spice | 1 pkg | 130 | 3% | 0% | 0% |
| ★ Regular | 1 pkg | 110 | 3% | 0% | 0% |
| **CREAM OF WHEAT (prep as dir)** | | | | | |
| —NABISCO | | | | | |
| ★ Instant | 1 cup | 120 | 0% | 0% | 0% |
| ★ Instant Mix-Ins: Apple Granola Crunch | 1 cup | 150 | 1% | 0% | 0% |
| ★ Quick | 1 cup | 120 | 0% | 0% | 0% |
| **MALT-O-MEAL (uncooked)** | | | | | |
| ★ Chocolate | 1/3 cup | 220 | 1% | 0% | 0% |
| ★ Maple Brown Sugar | 1/3 cup | 220 | 0% | 0% | 0% |
| ★ Quick | 3 tbsp | 120 | 0% | 0% | 0% |
| **MOTHER'S—QUAKER** | | | | | |
| ★ Instant Oatmeal | 1/2 cup | 150 | 5% | 3% | 0% |
| ★ Multigrain | 1/2 cup | 130 | 2% | 0% | 0% |
| ★ Oat Bran | 1/2 cup | 150 | 5% | 5% | 0% |
| ❖ Whole Wheat | 1/2 cup | 130 | 8% | 5% | 0% |
| ★ NABISCO Cream of Rice | 1 cup | 130 | 0% | 0% | 0% |
| ★ QUAKER Enriched Masa Harina (uncooked) | 1/4 cup | 110 | 2% | 0% | 0% |
| **QUAKER Hominy Grits (uncooked)** | | | | | |
| ★ Quick, White | 1/4 cup | 130 | 1% | 0% | 0% |
| ★ Quick, Yellow | 1/4 cup | 120 | 1% | 0% | 0% |
| ★ Regular, White | 1/4 cup | 140 | 1% | 0% | 0% |
| **QUAKER Instant Grits (prep as dir)** | | | | | |
| ★ Butter Flavor | 1 pkt | 100 | 2% | 0% | 0% |
| ★ Original | 1 pkt | 100 | 0% | 0% | 0% |
| ★ w/Bacon Bits | 1 pkt | 100 | 1% | 0% | 0% |
| ★ w/Ham Bits | 1 pkt | 90 | 1% | 0% | 0% |
| ★ w/Real Cheddar Cheese Flavor | 1 pkt | 100 | 2% | 3% | 0% |
| ★ w/Sausage Bits | 1 pkt | 100 | 2% | 0% | 0% |
| ★ Zesty Cheddar | 1 pkt | 100 | 2% | 3% | 0% |

| FOOD | Serving Size | Calories | Tot Fat | Sat Fat | Chol |
|---|---|---|---|---|---|
| QUAKER Instant Oatmeal (prep as dir) | | | | | |
| ★ Apple, Raisin & Walnut | 1 pkt | 140 | 4% | 3% | 0% |
| ★ Apples & Cinnamon | 1 pkt | 130 | 2% | 3% | 0% |
| ★ Blueberries & Cream | 1 pkt | 130 | 4% | 3% | 0% |
| ★ Cinnamon Toast | 1 pkt | 130 | 3% | 0% | 0% |
| ★ Cinnamon-Spice | 1 pkt | 170 | 3% | 0% | 0% |
| ★ Cinnamon Graham Cookie | 1 pkt | 150 | 4% | 3% | 0% |
| ★ Honey Nut | 1 pkt | 130 | 5% | 3% | 0% |
| ★ Maple/Brown Sugar | 1 pkt | 160 | 3% | 3% | 0% |
| ★ Peaches & Cream | 1 pkt | 130 | 3% | 3% | 0% |
| ★ Radical Raspberry | 1 pkt | 150 | 5% | 3% | 0% |
| ★ Raisin, Date & Walnut | 1 pkt | 130 | 4% | 3% | 0% |
| ★ Raisin-Spice | 1 pkt | 160 | 3% | 3% | 0% |
| ★ Regular | 1 pkt | 130 | 4% | 3% | 0% |
| ★ Strawberries & Cream | 1 pkt | 130 | 3% | 3% | 0% |
| ★ Strawberries 'N Stuff | 1 pkt | 150 | 3% | 3% | 0% |
| ★ QUAKER Oat Bran | 1/2 cup | 150 | 5% | 5% | 0% |
| QUAKER Oats | | | | | |
| ★ Old Fashioned | 1/2 cup | 150 | 5% | 3% | 0% |
| ★ Quick | 1/2 cup | 150 | 5% | 3% | 0% |
| ★ QUAKER Scotch Barley, Regular medium pearled (uncooked) | 1/4 cup | 170 | 2% | 0% | 0% |
| ★ QUAKER Unprocessed Bran | 1/3 cup | 30 | 0% | 0% | 0% |
| ★ RALSTON | 1 cup | 130 | 1% | 0% | 0% |
| ★ WHEAT HEARTS (uncooked)— GENERAL MILLS | 1/4 cup | 130 | 2% | 0% | 0% |

### READY-TO-EAT CEREALS

**Generic Foods**

| FOOD | Serving Size | Calories | Tot Fat | Sat Fat | Chol |
|---|---|---|---|---|---|
| ★ Bran Flakes | 3/4 cup | 100 | 1% | 0% | 0% |
| ★ Corn Chex | 1 cup | 110 | 0% | 0% | 0% |
| ★ Corn Flakes | 1 cup | 110 | 0% | 0% | 0% |
| ★ Frosted Wheat Flakes | 1 cup | 100 | 0% | 0% | 0% |
| ★ Puffed Rice | 1 cup | 60 | 0% | 0% | 0% |
| ★ Puffed Wheat | 1 cup | 40 | 0% | 0% | 0% |
| ★ Raisin Bran | 1 cup | 190 | 2% | 0% | 0% |
| ★ Rice Chex | 1 cup | 100 | 0% | 0% | 0% |
| ★ Shredded Wheat Biscuit | 2 biscuits | 170 | 1% | 0% | 0% |
| ★ Wheat Chex | 1 cup | 170 | 2% | 3% | 0% |
| ★ Wheat Germ, Toasted | 2 tbsp | 60 | 2% | 1% | 0% |

★ Foods with this symbol have less than or equal to 5% *Daily Value* for <u>all</u> three nutrients (5% Rule).
❖ Foods with this symbol have <u>at least one</u> of the three nutrients greater than 5% *Daily Value* but less than or equal to 20% *Daily Value*.
Ⓐ Foods with this symbol have <u>at least one</u> of the three nutrients greater than 20% *Daily Value* (20% Rule).

| FOOD | Serving Size | Calories | Tot Fat | Sat Fat | Chol |
|---|---|---|---|---|---|
| **Brand Name Foods** | | | | | |
| ★ 100% BRAN—NABISCO | 1/3 cup | 80 | 1% | 0% | 0% |
| 100% NATURAL—QUAKER | | | | | |
| ★ Low Fat w/Raisins | 1/2 cup | 190 | 5% | 5% | 0% |
| ❖ Oats & Honey | 1/2 cup | 220 | 12% | 18% | 0% |
| ❖ Oats, Honey & Raisins | 1/2 cup | 220 | 12% | 18% | 0% |
| ★ ALL BRAN—KELLOGG'S | 1/2 cup | 80 | 2% | 0% | 0% |
| ★ w/Extra Fiber | 1/2 cup | 50 | 2% | 0% | 0% |
| ★ ALPHA-BITS—POST | 1 cup | 130 | 1% | 0% | 0% |
| ★ Marshmallow | 1 cup | 120 | 1% | 0% | 0% |
| ★ APPLE CINNAMON RICE | | | | | |
| KRISPIES—KELLOGG'S | 3/4 cup | 110 | 0% | 0% | 0% |
| ★ APPLE CINNAMON SQUARES | | | | | |
| —KELLOGG'S | 3/4 cup | 180 | 2% | 0% | 0% |
| ★ APPLE JACKS—KELLOGG'S | 1 cup | 110 | 0% | 0% | 0% |
| ★ APPLE RAISIN CRISP—KELLOGG'S | 1 cup | 180 | 0% | 0% | 0% |
| ARROWHEAD MILLS | | | | | |
| ★ Amaranth Flakes | 1 cup | 130 | 3% | 0% | 0% |
| ★ Apple Corns | 1 cup | 150 | 2% | 0% | 0% |
| ★ Bran Flakes | 1 cup | 100 | 2% | 0% | 0% |
| ★ Corn Flakes | 1 cup | 130 | 0% | 0% | 0% |
| ★ Crispy Puffs | 1 cup | 80 | 2% | 0% | 0% |
| ★ Kamut Flakes | 1 cup | 120 | 2% | 0% | 0% |
| ★ Maple Corns | 1 cup | 190 | 5% | 3% | 0% |
| ★ Multigrain Flakes | 1 cup | 140 | 2% | 0% | 0% |
| ★ Nature O's | 1 cup | 130 | 3% | 3% | 0% |
| ★ Oat Bran Flakes | 1 cup | 110 | 3% | 5% | 0% |
| ★ Puffed Corn | 1 cup | 80 | 0% | 0% | 0% |
| ★ Puffed Kamut | 1 cup | 50 | 0% | 0% | 0% |
| ★ Puffed Millet | 1 cup | 90 | 1% | 0% | 0% |
| ★ Puffed Rice | 1 cup | 90 | 0% | 0% | 0% |
| ★ Puffed Wheat | 1 cup | 90 | 1% | 0% | 0% |
| ★ Spelt Flakes | 1 cup | 100 | 2% | 0% | 0% |
| ★ Wheat Bran | 1/4 cup | 30 | 1% | 0% | 0% |
| ★ Wheat Germ, Raw | 3 tbsp | 50 | 1% | 0% | 0% |
| ❖ BANANA NUT CRUNCH—POST | 1 cup | 250 | 9% | 5% | 0% |
| BARBARA'S BAKERY | | | | | |
| ★ Corn Flakes | 1 cup | 110 | 0% | 0% | 0% |
| ★ Raisin Bran | 1 cup | 170 | 2% | 0% | 0% |
| ★ Shredded Wheat | 2 biscuits | 140 | 2% | 0% | 0% |
| ★ BASIC 4—GENERAL MILLS | 1 1/4 cups | 210 | 5% | 0% | 0% |
| ❖ BLUEBERRY MORNING—POST | 1 1/4 cups | 230 | 6% | 3% | 0% |
| ★ BLUEBERRY SQUARES—KELLOGG'S | 3/4 cup | 180 | 2% | 0% | 0% |
| ★ BODY BUDDIES Natural Fruit— | | | | | |
| GENERAL MILLS | 1 cup | 120 | 2% | 0% | 0% |
| ★ BOO BERRY—GENERAL MILLS | 1 cup | 120 | 1% | 0% | 0% |
| ★ BRAN BUDS—KELLOGG'S | 1/3 cup | 70 | 2% | 0% | 0% |
| BRAN'NOLA—POST | | | | | |

| FOOD | Serving Size | Calories | Tot Fat | Sat Fat | Chol |
|---|---|---|---|---|---|
| ★ Original | 1/2 cup | 200 | 4% | 3% | 0% |
| ★ Raisin | 1/2 cup | 200 | 5% | 3% | 0% |
| ★ BREAKFAST O'S—BARBARA'S BAKERY | 1 cup | 120 | 3% | 0% | 0% |
| ★ BROWN RICE CRISPS— | | | | | |
|    BARBARA'S BAKERY | 1 cup | 120 | 2% | 0% | 0% |
| ❖ C.W. POST Hearty Granola—POST | 2/3 cup | 280 | 13% | 6% | 0% |
| CAP'N CRUNCH—QUAKER | | | | | |
| ★ Deep Sea Crunch | 1 cup | 130 | 3% | 3% | 0% |
| ★ Original | 3/4 cup | 110 | 2% | 0% | 0% |
| ★ Peanut Butter | 3/4 cup | 110 | 4% | 3% | 0% |
| ★ With Crunchberries | 3/4 cup | 100 | 2% | 0% | 0% |
| CHEERIOS—GENERAL MILLS | | | | | |
| ★ Apple Cinnamon | 3/4 cup | 120 | 4% | 0% | 0% |
| ★ CHEERIOS | 1 cup | 110 | 3% | 0% | 0% |
| ★ Honey Nut | 1 cup | 120 | 2% | 0% | 0% |
| ★ Multi-Grain | 1 cup | 110 | 2% | 0% | 0% |
| ★ CINNAMON OAT SQUARES— | | | | | |
|    QUAKER | 1 cup | 230 | 4% | 3% | 0% |
| ★ CINNAMON MINI BUNS— | | | | | |
|    KELLOGG'S | 3/4 cup | 120 | 1% | 0% | 0% |
| ❖ CINNAMON TOAST CRUNCH— | | | | | |
|    GENERAL MILLS | 3/4 cup | 130 | 6% | 3% | 0% |
| ❖ CLUSTERS—GENERAL MILLS | 1 cup | 220 | 6% | 3% | 0% |
| ★ COCOA KRISPIES—KELLOGG'S | 3/4 cup | 120 | 1% | 0% | 0% |
| ★ Cocoa PEBBLES—POST | 3/4 cup | 120 | 2% | 5% | 0% |
| ★ COCOA PUFFS—GENERAL MILLS | 1 cup | 120 | 1% | 0% | 0% |
| COMMON SENSE—KELLOGG'S | | | | | |
| ★ Oat Bran | 3/4 cup | 110 | 2% | 0% | 0% |
| ★ Oat Bran w/Raisins | 1 1/4 cup | 200 | 4% | 3% | 0% |
| ★ COMPLETE Bran Flakes—KELLOGG'S | 3/4 cup | 100 | 1% | 0% | 0% |
| ★ CORN POPS—KELLOGG'S | 1 cup | 110 | 0% | 0% | 0% |
| ★ COUNT CHOCULA—GENERAL MILLS | 1 cup | 120 | 1% | 0% | 0% |
| ★ COUNTRY Corn Flakes— | | | | | |
|    GENERAL MILLS | 1 cup | 120 | 1% | 0% | 0% |
| ❖ CRACKLIN' OAT BRAN—KELLOGG'S | 3/4 cup | 230 | 12% | 15% | 0% |
| ★ CRISPIX—KELLOGG'S | 1 cup | 110 | 0% | 0% | 0% |
| ★ CRISPY WHEATS 'N RAISINS— | | | | | |
|    GENERAL MILLS | 1 cup | 190 | 2% | 0% | 0% |
| ★ CRUNCHY BRAN—QUAKER | 3/4 cup | 90 | 2% | 0% | 0% |
| ★ DOUBLE DIP CRUNCH—KELLOGG'S | 3/4 cup | 110 | 0% | 0% | 0% |
| ★ FEATHERWEIGHT Corn Flakes | 1 cup | 110 | 0% | 0% | 0% |
| ★ FIBER ONE—GENERAL MILLS | 1/2 cup | 60 | 2% | 0% | 0% |
| ★ FRANKENBERRY—GENERAL MILLS | 1 cup | 120 | 1% | 0% | 0% |
| ★ FROOT LOOPS—KELLOGG'S | 1 cup | 120 | 2% | 3% | 0% |

★ Foods with this symbol have less than or equal to 5% *Daily Value* for <u>all</u> three nutrients (5% Rule).
❖ Foods with this symbol have <u>at least one</u> of the three nutrients greater than 5% *Daily Value* but less than or equal to 20% *Daily Value*.
Ⓐ Foods with this symbol have <u>at least one</u> of the three nutrients greater than 20% *Daily Value* (20% Rule).

| FOOD | Serving Size | Calories | Tot Fat | Sat Fat | Chol |
|------|------|------|------|------|------|
| ★ FROSTED BRAN—KELLOGG'S | 3/4 cup | 100 | 0% | 0% | 0% |
| ★ FROSTED BRAN FLAKES—KELLOGG'S | 3/4 cup | 100 | 0% | 0% | 0% |
| ★ FROSTED FUNNIES— | | | | | |
|    BARBARA'S BAKERY | 1 cup | 110 | 0% | 0% | 0% |
| ★ FROSTED KRISPIES—KELLOGG'S | 3/4 cup | 110 | 0% | 0% | 0% |
| FROSTED MINI WHEATS—KELLOGG'S | | | | | |
| ★   Bite Size | 1 cup | 190 | 2% | 0% | 0% |
| ★   Regular | 1 cup | 190 | 2% | 0% | 0% |
| ★ FROSTED WHEAT BITES—NABISCO | 1 cup | 190 | 2% | 0% | 0% |
| FRUIT & FIBRE—POST | | | | | |
| ★   Dates, Raisins & Walnuts | 1 cup | 210 | 5% | 3% | 0% |
| ★   Peaches, Raisins & Almonds | 1 cup | 210 | 5% | 3% | 0% |
| FRUIT WHEATS—NABISCO | | | | | |
| ★   Blueberry | 3/4 cup | 170 | 1% | 0% | 0% |
| ★   Raspberry | 3/4 cup | 160 | 1% | 0% | 0% |
| ★   Strawberry | 3/4 cup | 170 | 1% | 0% | 0% |
| ★ FRUITFUL BRAN—KELLOGG'S | 1 1/4 cup | 170 | 2% | 0% | 0% |
| ★ FRUITY MARSHMALLOW | | | | | |
|    KRISPIES—KELLOGG'S | 3/4 cup | 110 | 0% | 0% | 0% |
| ★ Fruity PEBBLES—POST | 3/4 cup | 110 | 2% | 3% | 0% |
| ❖ GENERAL MILLS Raisin Nut Bran | 1 cup | 210 | 7% | 3% | 0% |
| ★ GOLDEN CRISP—POST | 3/4 cup | 110 | 0% | 0% | 0% |
| ★ GOLDEN GRAHAMS—GENERAL MILLS | 3/4 cup | 120 | 2% | 0% | 0% |
| ★ GRAPE-NUTS—POST | 1/2 cup | 200 | 2% | 0% | 0% |
| ★ GRAPE-NUTS Flakes—POST | 3/4 cup | 100 | 1% | 0% | 0% |
| GREAT GRAINS—POST | | | | | |
| ❖   Crunchy Pecan | 2/3 cup | 220 | 10% | 4% | 0% |
| ❖   Raisins, Dates & Pecans | 2/3 cup | 210 | 7% | 3% | 0% |
| HEALTH VALLEY Fat Free Cereals | | | | | |
| ★   Crisp Brown Rice | | | | | |
|     (Honey Sweetened) | 1 cup | 110 | 0% | 0% | 0% |
| ★   Puffed Corn (Honey Sweetened) | 1 cup | 80 | 0% | 0% | 0% |
| HEALTH VALLEY Fat Free Granola | | | | | |
| ★   Date & Almond Flavor | 2/3 cup | 180 | 0% | 0% | 0% |
| ★   Raisin Cinnamon | 2/3 cup | 180 | 0% | 0% | 0% |
| ★   Tropical Fruit | 2/3 cup | 180 | 0% | 0% | 0% |
| HEALTH VALLEY Fat Free | | | | | |
|   *Granola O's* | | | | | |
| ★   Almond Flavor | 3/4 cup | 120 | 0% | 0% | 0% |
| ★   Apple Cinnamon | 3/4 cup | 120 | 0% | 0% | 0% |
| ★   Honey Crunch | 3/4 cup | 120 | 0% | 0% | 0% |
| HEALTH VALLEY Fat Free | | | | | |
|   Honey Clusters & Flakes | | | | | |
| ★   Almond Flavor | 3/4 cup | 130 | 0% | 0% | 0% |
| ★   Apple Cinnamon | 3/4 cup | 130 | 0% | 0% | 0% |
| ★   Honey Crunch | 3/4 cup | 130 | 0% | 0% | 0% |
| HEALTHY CHOICE Multi-Grain | | | | | |
|   Cereal—KELLOGG'S | | | | | |
| ★   Flakes | 1 cup | 100 | 0% | 0% | 0% |

| FOOD | Serving Size | Calories | Tot Fat | Sat Fat | Chol |
|---|---|---|---|---|---|
| ★ Squares | 1 1/4 cups | 190 | 2% | 0% | 0% |
| ★ Raisins, Crunchy Oat Clusters & Almonds | 1 1/4 cups | 200 | 3% | 0% | 0% |
| HEARTLAND Granola—PET | | | | | |
| ★ Lowfat | 1/2 cup | 210 | 5% | 5% | 0% |
| ❖ Original | 1/2 cup | 290 | 16% | 17% | 0% |
| ❖ Raisin | 1/2 cup | 290 | 15% | 6% | 0% |
| ★ HIDDEN TREASURES— GENERAL MILLS | 3/4 cup | 130 | 3% | 0% | 0% |
| ★ HIGH 5—BARBARA'S BAKERY | 3/4 cup | 100 | 1% | 0% | 0% |
| ★ HONEY BUNCHES OF OATS— POST | 3/4 cup | 120 | 3% | 3% | 0% |
| ★ w/Almonds | 3/4 cup | 130 | 5% | 3% | 0% |
| ★ HONEYCOMB—POST | 1 1/3 cups | 110 | 0% | 0% | 0% |
| JUST RIGHT—KELLOGG'S | | | | | |
| ★ Fruit & Nut | 1 cup | 200 | 3% | 0% | 0% |
| ★ w/Crunchy Nuggets | 1 cup | 210 | 2% | 0% | 0% |
| ★ KABOOM—GENERAL MILLS | 1 1/4 cups | 120 | 2% | 0% | 0% |
| KASHI Cereals | | | | | |
| ★ Breakfast Pilaf | 1/2 cup | 170 | 5% | 0% | 0% |
| ★ Puffed | 1 cup | 70 | 1% | 0% | 0% |
| KASHI Seven Whole Grains & Sesame | | | | | |
| ★ Honey Puffed | 1 cup | 120 | 2% | 0% | 0% |
| ❖ Medley | 1/2 cup | 100 | 6% | 0% | 0% |
| KELLOGG'S | | | | | |
| ★ CORN FLAKES | 1 cup | 110 | 0% | 0% | 0% |
| ★ FROSTED FLAKES | 3/4 cup | 120 | 0% | 0% | 0% |
| ★ Low Fat Granola (w/or w/o Raisins) | 1/2 cup | 210 | 5% | 0% | 0% |
| ★ Raisin Bran | 1 cup | 170 | 2% | 0% | 0% |
| ★ Raisin Squares | 3/4 cup | 180 | 2% | 0% | 0% |
| ★ Strawberry Squares | 3/4 cup | 180 | 2% | 0% | 0% |
| ★ KENMEI Rice Bran—KELLOGG'S | 3/4 cup | 110 | 2% | 0% | 0% |
| KIDS FAVORITES—QUAKER | | | | | |
| ★ Marshmallow Stars | 3/4 cup | 120 | 2% | 3% | 0% |
| ★ Sugar Frosted Flakes | 3/4 cup | 110 | 0% | 0% | 0% |
| ★ KING VITAMIN—QUAKER | 1 1/2 cups | 120 | 2% | 0% | 0% |
| ★ KIX—GENERAL MILLS | 1 1/3 cups | 120 | 1% | 0% | 0% |
| ★ Berry Berry | 3/4 cup | 120 | 2% | 0% | 0% |
| KRETSCHMER—QUAKER | | | | | |
| ★ Wheat Bran, Toasted | 1/4 cup | 30 | 2% | 0% | 0% |
| ★ Wheat Germ | 2 tbsp | 50 | 2% | 0% | 0% |
| ★ Wheat Germ, Honey Crunch | 1 2/3 tbsp | 50 | 2% | 0% | 0% |

★ Foods with this symbol have less than or equal to 5% *Daily Value* for <u>all</u> three nutrients (5% Rule).
❖ Foods with this symbol have <u>at least one</u> of the three nutrients greater than 5% *Daily Value* but less than or equal to 20% *Daily Value.*
Ⓐ Foods with this symbol have <u>at least one</u> of the three nutrients greater than 20% *Daily Value* (20% Rule).

| FOOD | Serving Size | Calories | Tot Fat | Sat Fat | Chol |
|------|------|------|------|------|------|
| KRUSTEAZ—CONTINENTAL MILLS | | | | | |
| ★ Corn Flakes | 1 cup | 130 | 0% | 0% | 0% |
| ★ Crisp Rice | 1 cup | 130 | 0% | 0% | 0% |
| ★ Frosted Flakes | 3/4 cup | 110 | 0% | 0% | 0% |
| ★ Fruit Whirls | 3/4 cup | 120 | 2% | 0% | 0% |
| ★ Raisin Bran | 3/4 cup | 210 | 2% | 0% | 0% |
| KRUSTEAZ Toasted Oats— CONTINENTAL MILLS | | | | | |
| ★ Apple Cinnamon | 3/4 cup | 130 | 3% | 0% | 0% |
| ★ Honey Nut | 3/4 cup | 120 | 3% | 0% | 0% |
| ★ Regular | 1 cup | 120 | 3% | 0% | 0% |
| ★ LIFE—QUAKER | 3/4 cup | 120 | 2% | 0% | 0% |
| ★ Oat Cinnamon | 1 cup | 190 | 3% | 0% | 0% |
| ★ LUCKY CHARMS—GENERAL MILLS | 1 cup | 120 | 2% | 0% | 0% |
| MUESLIX—KELLOGG'S | | | | | |
| ★ Crispy Blend | 2/3 cup | 200 | 5% | 0% | 0% |
| ❖ Golden Crunch | 3/4 cup | 210 | 8% | 5% | 0% |
| ★ NABISCO Shredded Wheat | 2 biscuits | 160 | 1% | 0% | 0% |
| ★ *Spoon Size* | 1 cup | 170 | 1% | 0% | 0% |
| ★ NATURE VALLEY Low Fat Fruit Granola—GENERAL MILLS | 2/3 cup | 210 | 4% | 0% | 0% |
| NATURE VALLEY 100% Natural Oat—GENERAL MILLS | | | | | |
| ❖ Cinnamon & Raisin | 3/4 cup | 240 | 12% | 5% | 0% |
| ❖ Fruit & Nut | 2/3 cup | 250 | 17% | 10% | 0% |
| ❖ Toasted Oats & Honey | 3/4 cup | 250 | 15% | 6% | 0% |
| ★ NINJA TURTLES—RALSTON | 1 cup | 110 | 0% | 0% | 0% |
| ★ NUT & HONEY CRUNCH—KELLOGG'S | 2/3 cup | 120 | 3% | 0% | 0% |
| ★ NUT & HONEY CRUNCH O'S —KELLOGG'S | 3/4 cup | 120 | 4% | 0% | 0% |
| NUTRI-GRAIN—KELLOGG'S | | | | | |
| ★ Almond Raisin | 1 1/4 cups | 200 | 5% | 0% | 0% |
| ★ Golden Wheat | 3/4 cup | 100 | 1% | 0% | 0% |
| ★ Golden Wheat & Raisin | 1 1/4 cups | 180 | 2% | 0% | 0% |
| ★ Nuggets | 1/2 cup | 180 | 2% | 0% | 0% |
| ★ OAT BRAN—QUAKER | 1 1/4 cups | 210 | 5% | 3% | 0% |
| ★ OAT SQUARES—QUAKER | 1 cup | 220 | 5% | 3% | 0% |
| OATMEAL CRISP—GENERAL MILLS | | | | | |
| ❖ Almond | 1 cup | 230 | 9% | 4% | 0% |
| ★ Apple Cinnamon | 1 cup | 210 | 4% | 0% | 0% |
| ★ Raisin | 1 cup | 210 | 5% | 0% | 0% |
| ★ OH!S, Honey Graham—QUAKER | 3/4 cup | 110 | 3% | 3% | 0% |
| POP-EYE—QUAKER | | | | | |
| ★ Cocoa Blasts | 1 cup | 130 | 2% | 3% | 0% |
| ★ Fruit Curls | 1 cup | 120 | 2% | 0% | 0% |
| ★ Jeepers | 1 1/3 cups | 110 | 2% | 0% | 0% |
| ★ Jeepers Crispy Corn Puffs | 1 1/3 cups | 110 | 1% | 0% | 0% |
| ★ *Oat'mmms* | 1 cup | 120 | 3% | 3% | 0% |
| ★ *Oat'mmms* Toasted Oat | 1 cup | 110 | 2% | 0% | 0% |

| FOOD | Serving Size | Calories | Tot Fat | Sat Fat | Chol |
|---|---|---|---|---|---|
| POST | | | | | |
| ★ Bran Flakes | 2/3 cup | 90 | 1% | 0% | 0% |
| ★ Raisin Bran | 1 cup | 190 | 1% | 0% | 0% |
| ★ POST TOASTIES | 1 cup | 100 | 0% | 0% | 0% |
| ★ PRODUCT 19—KELLOGG'S | 1 cup | 110 | 0% | 0% | 0% |
| ★ PUFFED RICE—QUAKER | 1 cup | 50 | 0% | 0% | 0% |
| ★ PUFFED WHEAT—QUAKER | 1 1/4 cups | 50 | 0% | 0% | 0% |
| RALSTON | | | | | |
| ★ Bran Flakes | 1 cup | 180 | 0% | 0% | 0% |
| ★ Corn Chex | 1 cup | 110 | 0% | 0% | 0% |
| ★ Corn Flakes | 1 cup | 100 | 0% | 0% | 0% |
| ★ Frosted Flakes | 1 cup | 150 | 1% | 0% | 0% |
| ★ Rice Chex | 1 cup | 100 | 0% | 0% | 0% |
| ★ Wheat Chex | 1 cup | 170 | 2% | 3% | 0% |
| ★ REESE'S PEANUT BUTTER PUFFS—GENERAL MILLS | 3/4 cup | 130 | 5% | 3% | 0% |
| ★ RICE KRISPIES—KELLOGG'S | 1 1/4 cups | 110 | 0% | 0% | 0% |
| ★ RICE KRISPIES TREATS Cereal—KELLOGG'S | 3/4 cup | 120 | 2% | 0% | 0% |
| RIPPLE CRISP—GENERAL MILLS | | | | | |
| ★ Honey Bran | 1 1/4 cups | 190 | 1% | 0% | 0% |
| ★ Honey Corn | 3/4 cup | 110 | 1% | 0% | 0% |
| ★ S'MORES GRAHAMS—GENERAL MILLS | 3/4 cup | 120 | 2% | 0% | 0% |
| ★ SHREDDED SPOONFULS—BARBARA'S BAKERY | 3/4 cup | 120 | 2% | 0% | 0% |
| ★ SHREDDED WHEAT—QUAKER | 3 biscuits | 220 | 2% | 3% | 0% |
| ★ SHREDDED WHEAT 'N BRAN—NABISCO | 1 1/4 cups | 200 | 1% | 0% | 0% |
| ★ SMACKS—KELLOGG'S | 3/4 cup | 110 | 1% | 0% | 0% |
| ★ SPECIAL K—KELLOGG'S | 1 cup | 110 | 0% | 0% | 0% |
| ★ SPRINKLE SPANGLES—GENERAL MILLS | 1 cup | 120 | 2% | 0% | 0% |
| STARTOONS—BARBARA'S BAKERY | | | | | |
| ★ Cocoa | 1 cup | 110 | 1% | 0% | 0% |
| ★ Honey | 1 cup | 110 | 0% | 0% | 0% |
| SUN COUNTRY GRANOLA—QUAKER | | | | | |
| ❖ Almonds | 1/2 cup | 270 | 14% | 8% | 0% |
| ❖ Raisin & Date | 1/2 cup | 260 | 12% | 5% | 0% |
| ★ SUN CRUNCHERS—GENERAL MILLS | 1 cup | 210 | 5% | 0% | 0% |
| ★ SWEET PUFFS—QUAKER | 1 cup | 130 | 1% | 0% | 0% |
| ★ TEAM Flakes—NABISCO | 1 1/4 cups | 220 | 0% | 0% | 0% |
| TOASTED OATMEAL—QUAKER | | | | | |
| ❖ Honey Nut | 1 cup | 200 | 7% | 5% | 0% |
| ★ Original | 1 cup | 120 | 2% | 0% | 0% |

★ Foods with this symbol have less than or equal to 5% *Daily Value* for all three nutrients (5% Rule).
❖ Foods with this symbol have at least one of the three nutrients greater than 5% *Daily Value* but less than or equal to 20% *Daily Value*.
Ⓐ Foods with this symbol have at least one of the three nutrients greater than 20% *Daily Value* (20% Rule).

| FOOD | Serving Size | Calories | Tot Fat | Sat Fat | Chol |
|------|------|------|------|------|------|
| TOTAL—GENERAL MILLS | | | | | |
| ★ Corn Flakes | 1 1/3 cups | 110 | 1% | 0% | 0% |
| ★ Raisin Bran | 1 cup | 180 | 2% | 0% | 0% |
| ★ Whole Grain | 3/4 cup | 110 | 1% | 0% | 0% |
| ★ TRIPLES—GENERAL MILLS | 1 cup | 120 | 2% | 0% | 0% |
| ★ TRIX—GENERAL MILLS | 1 cup | 120 | 2% | 0% | 0% |
| ★ WHEATIES—GENERAL MILLS | 1 cup | 110 | 2% | 0% | 0% |
| ★ Dunk-A-Balls | 3/4 cup | 110 | 1% | 0% | 0% |
| ★ Honey Gold | 3/4 cup | 110 | 1% | 0% | 0% |

# Condiments

## BARBECUE SAUCES

**Brand Name Foods**

| FOOD | Serving Size | Calories | Tot Fat | Sat Fat | Chol |
|------|------|------|------|------|------|
| HEALTHY CHOICE Barbecue Sauces—CONAGRA | | | | | |
| ★ Hickory | 2 tbsp | 25 | 0% | 0% | 0% |
| ★ Hot & Spicy | 2 tbsp | 25 | 0% | 0% | 0% |
| ★ Original | 2 tbsp | 25 | 0% | 0% | 0% |
| ★ HEINZ Old Fashioned *Thick Rich* Barbecue Sauce | 2 tbsp | 40 | 0% | 0% | 0% |
| HUNT'S Barbecue Sauce | | | | | |
| ★ Bold Hickory | 2 tbsp | 45 | 1% | 0% | 0% |
| ★ Bold Original | 2 tbsp | 45 | 0% | 0% | 0% |
| ★ Hickory | 2 tbsp | 40 | 0% | 0% | 0% |
| ★ Hickory & Brown Sugar | 2 tbsp | 70 | 0% | 0% | 0% |
| ★ Honey Hickory | 2 tbsp | 40 | 0% | 0% | 0% |
| ★ Honey Mustard | 2 tbsp | 50 | 0% | 0% | 0% |
| ★ Hot & Spicy | 2 tbsp | 50 | 0% | 0% | 0% |
| ★ Light | 2 tbsp | 25 | 0% | 0% | 0% |
| ★ Mesquite | 2 tbsp | 40 | 1% | 0% | 0% |
| ★ Mild Barbecue | 2 tbsp | 40 | 0% | 0% | 0% |
| ★ Mild Dijon | 2 tbsp | 40 | 0% | 0% | 0% |
| ★ Original | 2 tbsp | 40 | 0% | 0% | 0% |
| ★ Teriyaki | 2 tbsp | 50 | 0% | 0% | 0% |
| KRAFT Barbecue Sauce | | | | | |
| ★ Char-Grill | 2 tbsp | 60 | 2% | 0% | 0% |
| ★ Extra Rich Original | 2 tbsp | 50 | 0% | 0% | 0% |
| ★ Garlic | 2 tbsp | 40 | 0% | 0% | 0% |
| ★ Hickory Smoke | 2 tbsp | 40 | 0% | 0% | 0% |
| ★ Hickory Smoke Onion Bits | 2 tbsp | 50 | 0% | 0% | 0% |
| ★ Honey | 2 tbsp | 50 | 0% | 0% | 0% |
| ★ Hot | 2 tbsp | 40 | 0% | 0% | 0% |
| ★ Hot Hickory Smoke | 2 tbsp | 40 | 0% | 0% | 0% |
| ★ Italian Seasonings | 2 tbsp | 45 | 1% | 0% | 0% |
| ★ Kansas City Style | 2 tbsp | 45 | 0% | 0% | 0% |

| FOOD | Serving Size | Calories | Tot Fat | Sat Fat | Chol |
|------|:---:|:---:|:---:|:---:|:---:|
| ★ Mesquite Smoke | 2 tbsp | 40 | 0% | 0% | 0% |
| ★ Onion Bits | 2 tbsp | 50 | 0% | 0% | 0% |
| ★ Original | 2 tbsp | 40 | 0% | 0% | 0% |
| ★ Salsa Style | 2 tbsp | 40 | 0% | 0% | 0% |
| ★ Teriyaki | 2 tbsp | 60 | 2% | 0% | 0% |
| KRAFT *Thick 'N Spicy* Barbecue Sauce | | | | | |
| ★ Hickory Smoke | 2 tbsp | 50 | 0% | 0% | 0% |
| ★ Honey | 2 tbsp | 60 | 0% | 0% | 0% |
| ★ Kansas City Style | 2 tbsp | 60 | 0% | 0% | 0% |
| ★ Mesquite Smoke | 2 tbsp | 50 | 0% | 0% | 0% |
| ★ Original | 2 tbsp | 50 | 0% | 0% | 0% |

## COCKTAIL SAUCES

**Brand Name Foods**

| FOOD | Serving Size | Calories | Tot Fat | Sat Fat | Chol |
|------|:---:|:---:|:---:|:---:|:---:|
| ★ DEL MONTE Seafood Cocktail Sauce | 1/4 cup | 100 | 0% | 0% | 0% |
| GOLDEN DIPT Cocktail Sauce— MCCORMICK | | | | | |
| ★ Extra Hot | 1/4 cup | 100 | 0% | 0% | 0% |
| ★ Regular | 1/4 cup | 110 | 0% | 0% | 0% |
| ★ HEINZ Seafood Cocktail Sauce | 1/4 cup | 60 | 0% | 0% | 0% |
| ★ SAUCEWORKS Cocktail Sauce— KRAFT | 1/4 cup | 60 | 1% | 0% | 0% |

## CRANBERRY AND CHUTNEY SAUCES

**Brand Name Foods**

| FOOD | Serving Size | Calories | Tot Fat | Sat Fat | Chol |
|------|:---:|:---:|:---:|:---:|:---:|
| ★ S & W Cranberry Sauce (jellied & whole) | 1/4 cup | 100 | 0% | 0% | 0% |
| ★ SMUCKER'S Cranberry Sauce | 1 tbsp | 25 | 0% | 0% | 0% |
| TAJ *Creative Condiments* Chutney | | | | | |
| ★ Mango, Sweet | 1 tbsp | 20 | 0% | 0% | 0% |
| ★ Mint, Hot | 1 tbsp | 0 | 0% | 0% | 0% |
| ★ Tamarind, Tangy | 1 tbsp | 25 | 1% | 0% | 0% |

★ Foods with this symbol have less than or equal to 5% *Daily Value* for <u>all</u> three nutrients (5% Rule).
❖ Foods with this symbol have <u>at least one</u> of the three nutrients greater than 5% *Daily Value* but less than or equal to 20% *Daily Value*.
⊛ Foods with this symbol have <u>at least one</u> of the three nutrients greater than 20% *Daily Value* (20% Rule).

| FOOD | Serving Size | Calories | Tot Fat | Sat Fat | Chol |
|---|---|---|---|---|---|

### HORSERADISH

**Brand Name Foods**

KRAFT Horseradish

| | | | | | |
|---|---|---|---|---|---|
| ★ Cream Style Horseradish | 1 tsp | 0 | 0% | 0% | 0% |
| ★ Horseradish Mustard | 1 tsp | 0 | 0% | 0% | 0% |
| ★ Prepared Horseradish | 1 tsp | 0 | 0% | 0% | 0% |
| ★ SAUCEWORKS Horseradish Sauce—KRAFT | 1 tsp | 20 | 2% | 0% | 2% |

### KETCHUP AND STEAK SAUCES

**Brand Name Foods**

A-1 Steak Sauce—NABISCO

| | | | | | |
|---|---|---|---|---|---|
| ★ Bold | 1 tbsp | 20 | 0% | 0% | 0% |
| ★ Steak Sauce | 1 tbsp | 15 | 0% | 0% | 0% |
| ★ Thick & Hearty | 1 tbsp | 25 | 0% | 0% | 0% |
| ★ DEL MONTE Ketchup | 1 tbsp | 15 | 0% | 0% | 0% |
| ★ HEALTHY CHOICE Ketchup—CONAGRA | 1 tbsp | 10 | 0% | 0% | 0% |
| ★ HEINZ 57 Ketchup | 1 tbsp | 15 | 0% | 0% | 0% |
| ★ HEINZ 57 Steak Sauce | 1 tbsp | 15 | 0% | 0% | 0% |
| ★ HUNT'S Ketchup | 1 tbsp | 15 | 0% | 0% | 0% |
| ★ HUNT'S Steak Sauce | 1 tbsp | 10 | 0% | 0% | 0% |
| ★ SMUCKER'S Ketchup | 1 tbsp | 25 | 0% | 0% | 0% |

### MUSTARDS

**Brand Name Foods**

| | | | | | |
|---|---|---|---|---|---|
| ★ BEST FOODS *Dijonnaise* Creamy Mustard Blend | 1 tsp | 12 | 2% | 0% | 0% |
| ★ GREY POUPON—NABISCO | 1 tsp | 5 | 0% | 0% | 0% |
| GULDEN'S Mustard—AMERICAN HOME FOODS | | | | | |
| ★ Diablo | 1 tsp | 5 | 0% | 0% | 0% |
| ★ Dijon Style | 1 tsp | 0 | 0% | 0% | 0% |
| ★ Special Blend Yellow | 1 tsp | 0 | 0% | 0% | 0% |
| ★ Spicy Brown | 1 tsp | 10 | 0% | 0% | 0% |
| ★ HELLMAN'S *Dijonnaise* Creamy Mustard Blend | 1 tsp | 12 | 2% | 0% | 0% |
| ★ KRAFT Pure Prepared Mustard | 1 tsp | 0 | 0% | 0% | 0% |

| FOOD | Serving Size | Calories | Tot Fat | Sat Fat | Chol |
|---|---|---|---|---|---|

## OLIVES

**Generic Foods**

| FOOD | Serving Size | Calories | Tot Fat | Sat Fat | Chol |
|---|---|---|---|---|---|
| ★ Pickled Green Olives | 4 olives | 15 | 3% | 1% | 0% |
| ★ Ripe Mission Olives | 5 olives | 25 | 5% | 2% | 0% |
| ★ Ripe Olives (canned, large) | 3 olives | 15 | 2% | 1% | 0% |

**Brand Name Foods**

| FOOD | Serving Size | Calories | Tot Fat | Sat Fat | Chol |
|---|---|---|---|---|---|
| ❖ PROGRESSO Oil Cured Olives—PET | 6 olives | 80 | 9% | 3% | 0% |
| ★ PROGRESSO Olive Salad (drained)—PET | 2 tbsp | 25 | 4% | 2% | 0% |
| VLASIC *Early California* Ripe Black Olives—CAMPBELL'S | | | | | |
| ★ Chopped or Sliced | 1 tsp | 25 | 4% | 0% | 0% |
| ★ Colossal | 2 olives | 20 | 3% | 0% | 0% |
| ★ Extra Large | 3 olives | 25 | 4% | 0% | 0% |
| ★ Small, Medium, or Large | 4–6 olives | 25 | 4% | 0% | 0% |
| VLASIC *Early California* Spanish Olives—CAMPBELL'S | | | | | |
| ★ Alcaparrado | 1 tsp | 20 | 2% | 0% | 0% |
| ★ Sliced Salad | 1 tsp | 20 | 2% | 0% | 0% |
| ★ Stuffed Queen | 2 olives | 20 | 2% | 0% | 0% |
| ★ Stuffed Spanish | 6 olives | 20 | 3% | 0% | 0% |

## PEPPERS AND CHILIES

**Brand Name Foods**

| FOOD | Serving Size | Calories | Tot Fat | Sat Fat | Chol |
|---|---|---|---|---|---|
| ★ DEL MONTE Hot Chili Peppers | 4 peppers | 10 | 0% | 0% | 0% |
| DEL MONTE Jalapenos | | | | | |
| ★ Chilpotle Peppers in Spice Sauce | 2 tbsp | 20 | 1% | 0% | 0% |
| ★ Pickled Sliced | 2 tbsp | 5 | 0% | 0% | 0% |
| ★ Pickled Sliced Jalapeno Nachos | 2 tbsp | 5 | 0% | 0% | 0% |
| ★ Pickled Whole | 2–3 peppers | 5 | 0% | 0% | 0% |
| ★ Whole | 1 pepper | 3 | 0% | 0% | 0% |
| OLD EL PASO Chilies/Jalapenos —PET | | | | | |
| ★ Green Chilies, Chopped | 2 tbsp | 5 | 0% | 0% | 0% |
| ★ Green Chilies, Whole | 1 chile | 10 | 0% | 0% | 0% |
| ★ Peeled Jalapenos | 3 pcs | 10 | 0% | 0% | 0% |
| ★ Pickled Jalapenos | 2 pcs | 5 | 0% | 0% | 0% |
| ★ Pickled Jalapeno Slices | 2 tbsp | 15 | 0% | 0% | 0% |
| ★ Tomatoes & Green Chilies | 1/4 cup | 10 | 0% | 0% | 0% |

★ Foods with this symbol have less than or equal to 5% *Daily Value* for <u>all</u> three nutrients (5% Rule).

❖ Foods with this symbol have <u>at least one</u> of the three nutrients greater than 5% *Daily Value* but less than or equal to 20% *Daily Value*.

⊛ Foods with this symbol have <u>at least one</u> of the three nutrients greater than 20% *Daily Value* (20% Rule).

| FOOD | Serving Size | Calories | Tot Fat | Sat Fat | Chol |
|---|---|---|---|---|---|
| ★ Tomatoes & Jalapenos | 1/4 cup | 15 | 0% | 0% | 0% |
| ★ PANCHO VILLA Diced Green Chiles—PET | 2 tbsp | 5 | 0% | 0% | 0% |
| PROGRESSO Peppers—PET | | | | | |
| ★ Cherry Peppers (drained) | 2 tbsp | 30 | 3% | 2% | 0% |
| ❖ Fried Peppers (drained) | 2 tbsp | 60 | 8% | 2% | 0% |
| ★ Hot Cherry Peppers | 1 pepper | 15 | 0% | 0% | 0% |
| ★ Pepper Salad (drained) | 2 tbsp | 25 | 3% | 1% | 0% |
| ★ Roasted Peppers | 1/2 pc | 10 | 0% | 0% | 0% |
| ★ Tuscan Peppers (drained) | 3 peppers | 10 | 0% | 0% | 0% |
| ★ RO-TEL Diced Tomatoes & Green Chilies—AMERICAN HOME FOODS | 1/2 cup | 20 | 0% | 0% | 0% |
| ROSARITA Chiles—HUNT WESSON | | | | | |
| ★ Diced Jalapenos | 2 tbsp | 5 | 0% | 0% | 0% |
| ★ Diced or Whole Green | 2 tbsp | 5 | 0% | 0% | 0% |
| ★ Nacho Sliced Jalapenos | 2 tbsp | 5 | 0% | 0% | 0% |
| ★ Whole Jalapenos | 2 tbsp | 10 | 0% | 0% | 0% |
| VLASIC Peppers—CAMPBELL'S | | | | | |
| ★ Hot Banana | 1 oz | 5 | 0% | 0% | 0% |
| ★ Hot Jalapeno | 1/4 cup | 10 | 0% | 0% | 0% |
| ★ Mild/Hot Cherry | 1 oz | 10 | 0% | 0% | 0% |
| ★ Mild/Hot Ringsor Chunks | 1 oz | 5 | 0% | 0% | 0% |
| ★ Pepperoncini Salad | 1 oz | 5 | 0% | 0% | 0% |
| ★ Sweet Pepper Rings | 1 oz | 25 | 0% | 0% | 0% |
| ★ Tiny Mexican Hot | 1 oz | 10 | 0% | 0% | 0% |

## PICKLES AND PICKLED VEGETABLES

**Generic Foods**

| | | | | | |
|---|---|---|---|---|---|
| ★ Bread and Butter Pickles | 1/4 cup | 30 | 0% | 0% | 0% |
| ★ Chowchow, Sour | 2 tbsp | 10 | 1% | 0% | 0% |
| ★ Chowchow, Sweet | 2 tbsp | 40 | 0% | 0% | 0% |
| ★ Cucumber Dill Pickle | 1 pickle | 5 | 0% | 0% | 0% |
| ★ Cucumber Dill Pickle, Kosher | 1 pickle | 10 | 0% | 0% | 0% |
| ★ Pimiento (canned) | 1 tsp | 1 | 0% | 0% | 0% |
| ★ Sauerkraut | 1/2 cup | 20 | 0% | 0% | 0% |
| ★ Sour Cucumber Pickle | 1 pickle | 4 | 0% | 0% | 0% |
| ★ Sweet Cucumber Pickle | 1 pickle | 40 | 0% | 0% | 0% |
| ★ Sweet Gherkin Pickle | 2 pickles | 40 | 0% | 0% | 0% |

**Brand Name Foods**

| | | | | | |
|---|---|---|---|---|---|
| CLAUSSEN Pickles—OSCAR MAYER | | | | | |
| ★ Bread 'N Butter Chips | 4 slices | 20 | 0% | 0% | 0% |
| ★ Half Sours New York Deli Style | 1 oz | 5 | 0% | 0% | 0% |
| ★ Hamburger Dills, Slices, or Chips | 10 slices | 5 | 0% | 0% | 0% |
| ★ Kosher Dills, Halves | 1 oz | 5 | 0% | 0% | 0% |
| ★ Kosher Dills, Slices | 4 slices | 5 | 0% | 0% | 0% |

| FOOD | Serving Size | Calories | Tot Fat | Sat Fat | Chol |
|---|---|---|---|---|---|
| ★ Kosher Dills, Spears | 1 spear | 5 | 0% | 0% | 0% |
| ★ Kosher Dills, Whole | 1 oz | 5 | 0% | 0% | 0% |
| ★ Kosher Mini Dills | 1 pickle | 5 | 0% | 0% | 0% |
| ★ Sauerkraut | 1/4 cup | 5 | 0% | 0% | 0% |
| ★ Tomatoes, Halves | 1 oz | 5 | 0% | 0% | 0% |
| DEL MONTE Dill Pickles | | | | | |
| ★ Hamburger Chips | 5 chips | 5 | 0% | 0% | 0% |
| ★ Pickle Halves | 1/4 pickle | 5 | 0% | 0% | 0% |
| ★ Tiny Kosher | 1 1/2 pickles | 5 | 0% | 0% | 0% |
| ★ Whole | 1 1/2 pickles | 5 | 0% | 0% | 0% |
| ★ DEL MONTE Sauerkraut | 1/2 cup | 15 | 0% | 0% | 0% |
| DEL MONTE Sweet Pickles | | | | | |
| ★ Chips | 5 chips | 40 | 0% | 0% | 0% |
| ★ Gherkin | 2 pickles | 40 | 0% | 0% | 0% |
| ★ Midget | 3 pickles | 40 | 0% | 0% | 0% |
| ★ Whole | 1 pickle | 40 | 0% | 0% | 0% |
| PROGRESSO—PET | | | | | |
| ★ Capers (drained) | 1 tsp | 0 | 0% | 0% | 0% |
| ★ Eggplant Appetizer | 2 tbsp | 30 | 3% | 1% | 0% |
| ⦿ Marinated Artichoke Hearts | 1/3 cup | 160 | 22% | 10% | 0% |
| ★ VLASIC Cocktail Onions— | | | | | |
| CAMPBELL'S | 1 oz | 4 | 0% | 0% | 0% |
| ★ VLASIC Garden Mix, Hot & Spicy | | | | | |
| —CAMPBELL'S | 1 oz | 4 | 0% | 0% | 0% |
| VLASIC Pickles—CAMPBELL'S | | | | | |
| ★ Baby Kosher Dills | 1 pickle | 4 | 0% | 0% | 0% |
| ★ Bread & Butter Chips | 1 pickle | 30 | 0% | 0% | 0% |
| ★ Bread & Butter Chunks | 1 pickle | 25 | 0% | 0% | 0% |
| ★ Bread & Butter Stixs | 1 pickle | 20 | 0% | 0% | 0% |
| ★ Crunchy Kosher Dills | 1 pickle | 4 | 0% | 0% | 0% |
| ★ Deli Dill Halves | 1 oz | 4 | 0% | 0% | 0% |
| ★ Kosher Dill Gherkins | 1 oz | 4 | 0% | 0% | 0% |
| ★ Kosher Dill Spears | 1 oz | 4 | 0% | 0% | 0% |
| ★ Kosher Snack Chunks | 1 oz | 4 | 0% | 0% | 0% |
| ★ Original Dill | 1 oz | 2 | 0% | 0% | 0% |
| ★ Polish Snack Chunks | 1 oz | 4 | 0% | 0% | 0% |
| ★ Sweet Chips | 1 oz | 30 | 0% | 0% | 0% |
| ★ Zesty Crunchy Dill | 1 oz | 2 | 0% | 0% | 0% |
| ★ Zesty Dill Snack Chunks | 1 oz | 4 | 0% | 0% | 0% |
| ★ Zesty Dill Spears | 1 oz | 4 | 0% | 0% | 0% |

★ Foods with this symbol have less than or equal to 5% *Daily Value* for all three nutrients (5% Rule).
❖ Foods with this symbol have at least one of the three nutrients greater than 5% *Daily Value* but less than or equal to 20% *Daily Value*.
⦿ Foods with this symbol have at least one of the three nutrients greater than 20% *Daily Value* (20% Rule).

| FOOD | Serving Size | Calories | Tot Fat | Sat Fat | Chol |
|------|------|------|------|------|------|
| **RELISHES** | | | | | |
| **Brand Name Foods** | | | | | |
| DEL MONTE Relishes | | | | | |
| ★ Hamburger Pickle | 1 tbsp | 20 | 0% | 0% | 0% |
| ★ Hot Dog Pickle | 1 tbsp | 15 | 0% | 0% | 0% |
| ★ Sweet Pickle | 1 tbsp | 20 | 0% | 0% | 0% |
| HEINZ Relishes | | | | | |
| ★ Hamburger Pickle Relish | 1 tbsp | 20 | 0% | 0% | 0% |
| ★ Hot Dog Pickle Relish | 1 tbsp | 20 | 0% | 0% | 0% |
| ★ OLD EL PASO Jalapeno Relish—PET | 1 tbsp | 5 | 0% | 0% | 0% |
| VLASIC Relishes—CAMPBELL'S | | | | | |
| ★ Dill Pickle Relish | 1 tbsp | 1 | 0% | 0% | 0% |
| ★ Hamburger Pickle Relish | 1 tbsp | 20 | 0% | 0% | 0% |
| ★ Hot Dog Pickle Relish | 1 tbsp | 20 | 1% | 0% | 0% |
| ★ Sweet Pickle Relish | 1 tbsp | 20 | 0% | 0% | 0% |
| **TARTAR SAUCES** | | | | | |
| **Generic Foods** | | | | | |
| ⊛ Tartar Sauce | 2 tbsp | 150 | 26% | 16% | 5% |
| ❖ Tartar Sauce, Low calorie | 2 tbsp | 60 | 10% | 6% | 5% |
| **Brand Name Foods** | | | | | |
| BEST FOODS Tartar Sauce—CPC | | | | | |
| ★ Reduced Fat | 1 tbsp | 30 | 3% | 0% | 0% |
| ❖ Regular | 1 tbsp | 70 | 12% | 5% | 2% |
| GOLDEN DIPT Tartar Sauce— MCCORMICK | | | | | |
| ★ Fat-Free | 2 tbsp | 35 | 0% | 0% | 0% |
| ⊛ Regular | 2 tbsp | 160 | 24% | 11% | 8% |
| HELLMAN'S Tartar Sauce—CPC | | | | | |
| ★ Reduced Fat | 1 tbsp | 30 | 3% | 0% | 0% |
| ❖ Regular | 1 tbsp | 70 | 12% | 5% | 2% |
| ★ KRAFT Nonfat Tartar Sauce | 2 tbsp | 25 | 0% | 0% | 0% |
| SAUCEWORKS Tartar Sauce— KRAFT | | | | | |
| ⊛ Natural Lemon & Herb Tartar | 2 tbsp | 150 | 25% | 13% | 5% |
| ❖ Tartar Sauce | 2 tbsp | 100 | 15% | 20% | 3% |

| FOOD | Serving Size | Calories | Tot Fat | Sat Fat | Chol |
|---|---|---|---|---|---|

# Cookies

## BUTTER AND SHORTBREAD COOKIES

**Generic Foods**

| FOOD | Serving Size | Calories | Tot Fat | Sat Fat | Chol |
|---|---|---|---|---|---|
| ❖ Pecan Shortbread | 2 cookies | 160 | 15% | 11% | 4% |
| ❖ Shortbread | 3 cookies | 160 | 14% | 17% | 4% |

**Brand Name Foods**

| FOOD | Serving Size | Calories | Tot Fat | Sat Fat | Chol |
|---|---|---|---|---|---|
| ❖ ESTEE Shortbread | 4 cookies | 130 | 6% | 5% | 0% |
| ❖ FAMILY FAVORITES Fudge Striped Shortbread—NABISCO | 3 cookies | 160 | 12% | 8% | 0% |
| FUDGE SHOPPE—KEEBLER | | | | | |
| ❖ *Fudge 'N Caramel* Shortbread w/ Fudge 'n Real Caramel | 2 cookies | 120 | 9% | 20% | 1% |
| Ⓐ *Fudge Stripes* Fudge Covered Shortbread | 3 cookies | 160 | 12% | 23% | 0% |
| ❖ *P.B. Fudgebutters* Fudge Covered Shortbread w/Real Peanut Butter | 2 cookies | 130 | 11% | 20% | 1% |
| ❖ KEEBLER *Sweet Spots* Shortbread w/Chocolate | 1 pkg | 120 | 9% | 15% | 1% |
| ❖ LORNA DOONE Shortbread— NABISCO | 4 cookies | 140 | 11% | 6% | 2% |
| MOTHER'S—M.C.COOKIE | | | | | |
| ❖ Almond Shortbread | 3 cookies | 180 | 17% | 20% | 0% |
| ❖ Butter Cookies | 5 cookies | 140 | 9% | 15% | 3% |
| ❖ English Tea | 2 cookies | 180 | 11% | 20% | 0% |
| Ⓐ Striped Shortbread | 3 cookies | 170 | 12% | 25% | 0% |
| ❖ NABISCO Imported Danish Cookies | 5 cookies | 170 | 13% | 10% | 0% |
| ❖ PECAN PASSION Pecan Shortbread—NABISCO | 1 cookie | 90 | 8% | 4% | 1% |
| ❖ PECAN SANDIES, Rich Shortbread w/Crunchy Pecan Pieces—KEEBLER | 1 cookie | 80 | 8% | 5% | 1% |
| ★ 25% Reduced Fat | 1 cookie | 70 | 5% | 3% | 0% |
| ❖ *Bite Size Pecan Sandies* | 8 cookies | 170 | 15% | 10% | 1% |
| ❖ Sandwich w/Praline Creme | 1 cookie | 80 | 9% | 8% | 0% |
| ❖ *Toffee Sandies* w/Crunchy Toffee Pieces | 1 cookie | 80 | 7% | 5% | 1% |
| ❖ PEPPERIDGE FARM *Distinctive* Butter Chessman—CAMPBELL'S | 3 cookies | 120 | 8% | 15% | 7% |
| PEPPERIDGE FARM *International Collection*—CAMPBELL'S | | | | | |
| ❖ Biarritz | 6 cookies | 160 | 12% | 20% | 0% |

★ Foods with this symbol have less than or equal to 5% *Daily Value* for <u>all</u> three nutrients (5% Rule).

❖ Foods with this symbol have <u>at least one</u> of the three nutrients greater than 5% *Daily Value* but less than or equal to 20% *Daily Value*.

Ⓐ Foods with this symbol have <u>at least one</u> of the three nutrients greater than 20% *Daily Value* (20% Rule).

| FOOD | Serving Size | Calories | Tot Fat | Sat Fat | Chol |
|---|---|---|---|---|---|
| ❖ Esprit, Blanc | 1 cookie | 80 | 7% | 13% | 3% |
| ❖ Highland Shortbread | 2 cookies | 140 | 5% | 3% | 6% |
| ❖ Madaillon au Beurre | 4 cookies | 150 | 8% | 15% | 5% |
| ❖ Selection de Choix | 5 cookies | 150 | 11% | 20% | 1% |
| ❖ Pecan Shortbread | 2 cookies | 140 | 14% | 13% | 1% |
| ❖ Shortbread | 2 cookies | 140 | 11% | 13% | 3% |
| ❖ SOCIAL TEA Biscuits—NABISCO | 6 cookies | 120 | 6% | 4% | 2% |
| � SUNSHINE BISCUITS Fudge Striped Shortbread | 3 cookies | 160 | 14% | 25% | 0% |

### CHOCOLATE COOKIES

**Generic Foods**

| | | | | | |
|---|---|---|---|---|---|
| ❖ Chocolate Wafer | 5 wafers | 130 | 7% | 5% | 0% |

**Brand Name Foods**

| ARCHWAY | | | | | |
|---|---|---|---|---|---|
| ❖ Dutch Cocoa | 1 cookie | 120 | 6% | 5% | 1% |
| ★ Fat Free Chocolate | 1 cookie | 90 | 0% | 0% | 0% |
| ❖ Fudge Nut Bar | 1 cookie | 110 | 7% | 5% | 1% |
| ❖ Mud Pie | 1 cookie | 110 | 6% | 5% | 2% |
| ❖ Rocky Road | 1 cookie | 120 | 7% | 5% | 3% |
| BARBARA'S BAKERY Fat Free Mini Cookies | | | | | |
| ★ Cocoa Mocha | 6 cookies | 100 | 0% | 0% | 0% |
| ★ Double Chocolate | 6 cookies | 90 | 0% | 0% | 0% |
| ❖ DUNKAROOS Chocolate w/ Vanilla Frosting—GENERAL MILLS | 1 tray | 120 | 7% | 6% | 0% |
| EAGLE—ANHEUSER BUSCH | | | | | |
| ❖ Fudge Brownie w/Chocolate Chip | 1 cookie | 260 | 17% | 20% | 7% |
| � Gourmet Chocolate Fudge Brownie Style | 1 cookie | 330 | 25% | 25% | 5% |
| ★ ELFIN DELIGHTS Fat Free Devil's Food—KEEBLER | 1 cookie | 70 | 0% | 0% | 0% |
| ★ ENTENMANN'S Fat Free, Cholesterol Free Chocolate Brownie—KRAFT | 2 cookies | 80 | 0% | 0% | 0% |
| ESTEE | | | | | |
| ❖ Fudge | 4 cookies | 150 | 11% | 8% | 0% |
| ★ *Snack Crisp* Chocolate | 30 crisps | 130 | 5% | 3% | 0% |
| GRANDMA'S—FRITO-LAY | | | | | |
| ❖ Big Cookies: Nutty Fudge | 1 cookie | 190 | 12% | 8% | 0% |
| ❖ Mini Cookies: Chocolate | 1 pkg | 170 | 12% | 10% | 0% |
| HEALTH VALLEY Fat Free Centers | | | | | |
| ★ Chocolate Caramel | 2 cookies | 70 | 0% | 0% | 0% |
| ★ Chocolate Cherry | 2 cookies | 70 | 0% | 0% | 0% |
| ★ Chocolate Fudge | 2 cookies | 70 | 0% | 0% | 0% |

| FOOD | Serving Size | Calories | Tot Fat | Sat Fat | Chol |
|------|--------------|----------|---------|---------|------|
| ★ Chocolate Mint Fudge | 2 cookies | 70 | 0% | 0% | 0% |
| ★ Chocolate Raspberry | 2 cookies | 70 | 0% | 0% | 0% |
| ★ Chocolate Strawberry | 2 cookies | 70 | 0% | 0% | 0% |
| MOTHER'S—M.C. COOKIE | | | | | |
| ❖ Double Fudge | 3 cookies | 170 | 12% | 20% | 0% |
| Ⓐ Flaky Flix Fudge | 2 cookies | 140 | 11% | 25% | 0% |
| ❖ Fudge Bowl Crowns | 2 cookies | 140 | 9% | 20% | 0% |
| ❖ Fudge Bowl Nuggets | 2 cookies | 140 | 9% | 20% | 0% |
| ❖ Walnut Fudge | 2 cookies | 130 | 11% | 13% | 0% |
| NABISCO | | | | | |
| ❖ Chocolate Snaps | 7 cookies | 140 | 8% | 10% | 0% |
| ❖ Famous Chocolate Wafers | 5 cookies | 140 | 6% | 7% | 1% |
| PEPPERIDGE FARM *Old Fashioned*—CAMPBELL'S | | | | | |
| ❖ Brownie Chocolate Nut | 3 cookies | 160 | 14% | 15% | 5% |
| ❖ Chocolate Chocolate Walnut | 1 cookie | 130 | 9% | 10% | 2% |
| PEPPERIDGE FARM *Tiny Goldfish* —CAMPBELL'S | | | | | |
| ❖ Chocolate | 19 pcs | 140 | 8% | 8% | 3% |
| ❖ Chocolate Chunk | 19 pcs | 150 | 11% | 13% | 7% |
| ★ SNACKWELL'S Fat Free Devil's Food Cookie Cakes—NABISCO | 1 cookie | 50 | 0% | 0% | 0% |

## CHOCOLATE CHIP COOKIES

### Generic Foods

| | | | | | |
|------|--------------|----------|---------|---------|------|
| ❖ Chocolate Chip | 2 cookies | 140 | 11% | 12% | 3% |

### Brand Name Foods

| ARCHWAY | | | | | |
|------|--------------|----------|---------|---------|------|
| ❖ Chocolate Chip | 1 cookie | 130 | 9% | 8% | 1% |
| ❖ Chocolate Chip & Toffee | 1 cookie | 140 | 11% | 8% | 2% |
| ❖ Chocolate Chip Drop | 1 cookie | 140 | 15% | 15% | 4% |
| ❖ Chocolate Chip Ice Box | 1 cookie | 140 | 11% | 13% | 2% |
| ❖ Chocolate Chip Supreme | 1 cookie | 120 | 7% | 8% | 1% |
| BARBARA'S BAKERY | | | | | |
| ❖ Chocolate Chip | 2 cookies | 170 | 11% | 8% | 0% |
| ❖ Chocolate Chocolate Chip | 2 cookies | 150 | 11% | 8% | 0% |
| ❖ *Small Indulgences* Chocolate Chip Crisps | 6 cookies | 140 | 11% | 20% | 5% |
| CHIPS AHOY!—NABISCO | | | | | |
| ❖ Chewy Chocolate Chip | 3 cookies | 170 | 12% | 14% | 1% |
| ❖ Chunky Chocolate Chip | 1 cookie | 80 | 7% | 14% | 3% |

★ Foods with this symbol have less than or equal to 5% *Daily Value* for <u>all</u> three nutrients (5% Rule).
❖ Foods with this symbol have <u>at least one</u> of the three nutrients greater than 5% *Daily Value* but less than or equal to 20% *Daily Value*.
Ⓐ Foods with this symbol have <u>at least one</u> of the three nutrients greater than 20% *Daily Value* (20% Rule).

| FOOD | Serving Size | Calories | Tot Fat | Sat Fat | Chol |
|---|---|---|---|---|---|
| ❖ Mini Bite Size Chocolate Chip | 14 cookies | 150 | 11% | 14% | 0% |
| ❖ Real Chocolate Chip | 3 cookies | 160 | 12% | 12% | 0% |
| ❖ Reduced Fat | 3 cookies | 150 | 9% | 8% | 0% |
| ❖ Sprinkled Real Chocolate Chip | 3 cookies | 170 | 12% | 13% | 0% |
| ❖ Striped Pure Chocolate Chip | 1 cookie | 80 | 6% | 6% | 0% |
| ❖ CHIPS DELUXE Chocolate Chip —KEEBLER | 1 cookie | 80 | 7% | 8% | 0% |
| ★ 25% Reduced Fat | 1 cookie | 70 | 5% | 5% | 0% |
| ❖ Bakery Crisp Chips Deluxe | 3 cookies | 180 | 14% | 15% | 3% |
| ❖ Bite Size Chips Deluxe | 8 cookies | 160 | 14% | 15% | 1% |
| ❖ Bite Size Rainbow Chips Deluxe | 7 cookies | 140 | 11% | 13% | 1% |
| ❖ Chocolate Lovers Chips Deluxe | 1 cookie | 90 | 8% | 13% | 3% |
| ❖ Rainbow Chips Deluxe | 1 cookie | 80 | 6% | 10% | 1% |
| ❖ DUNCAN HINES Mixes: Chocolate Chip (prep as dir) —PROCTER & GAMBLE | 1 cookie | 150 | 11% | 10% | 4% |
| ❖ DUNKAROOS Chocolate Chip w/ Chocolate Frosting—GENERAL MILLS | 1 tray | 120 | 7% | 6% | 0% |
| EAGLE—ANHEUSER BUSCH ❖ Chocolate Chip | 1 cookie | 190 | 12% | 13% | 5% |
| ⊛ Gourmet: Peanut Butter Chocolate Chip | 1 cookie | 360 | 31% | 30% | 5% |
| ❖ ENTENMANN'S Chocolate Chip —KRAFT | 3 cookies | 140 | 11% | 11% | 4% |
| ESTEE ❖ Chocolate Chip | 4 cookies | 150 | 11% | 10% | 0% |
| ★ Chocolate Chip Cookie Mix | 1/9 pkg | 90 | 3% | 5% | 0% |
| FEATHERWEIGHT ❖ Chocolate Chip | 4 cookies | 140 | 8% | 10% | 0% |
| ❖ Double Chocolate Chip | 4 cookies | 140 | 8% | 10% | 0% |
| GRANDMA'S Big Cookies—FRITO-LAY ❖ Chocolate Chip | 1 cookie | 190 | 14% | 13% | 0% |
| ❖ Fudge Chocolate Chip | 1 cookie | 170 | 9% | 10% | 0% |
| ❖ GRANDMA'S Rich N' Chewey Chocolate Chip—FRITO-LAY | 2 cookies | 270 | 17% | 20% | 0% |
| HEALTH VALLEY Fat Free Healthy Chips ★ Double Chocolate Flavor | 3 cookies | 100 | 0% | 0% | 0% |
| ★ Old Fashioned Flavor | 3 cookies | 100 | 0% | 0% | 0% |
| ★ Original Flavor | 3 cookies | 100 | 0% | 0% | 0% |
| ★ KEEBLER Soft Batch Chocolate Chip | 1 cookie | 80 | 5% | 5% | 0% |
| ❖ LITTLE DEBBIE Individual Snacks: Chocolate Chip—MCKEE | 1/2 pkg (38 g) | 180 | 15% | 14% | 2% |
| MOTHER'S—M.C.COOKIE ❖ Chocolate Chip | 2 cookies | 160 | 12% | 15% | 3% |
| ❖ Chocolate Chip Angel | 3 cookies | 180 | 14% | 20% | 0% |
| ❖ Chocolate Chip Parade | 4 cookies | 130 | 8% | 10% | 0% |
| ❖ NABISCO Chocolate Chip Snaps | 7 cookies | 150 | 8% | 7% | 0% |

| FOOD | Serving Size | Calories | Tot Fat | Sat Fat | Chol |
|------|--------------|----------|---------|---------|------|
| PEPPERIDGE FARM *American Collection*—CAMPBELL'S | | | | | |
| ❖ Beacon Hill (chocolate walnut) | 1 cookie | 130 | 11% | 10% | 2% |
| ❖ Charleston (milk chocolate toffee pecan) | 1 cookie | 130 | 11% | 13% | 7% |
| ❖ Chesapeake (chocolate chunk pecan) | 1 cookie | 140 | 12% | 8% | 3% |
| ❖ Nantucket (chocolate chunk) | 1 cookie | 130 | 11% | 15% | 3% |
| ❖ Sausalito (milk chocolate macadamia) | 1 cookie | 140 | 11% | 10% | 3% |
| ❖ Tahoe (white chunk macadamia) | 1 cookie | 130 | 11% | 15% | 5% |
| ❖ PEPPERIDGE FARM *Old Fashioned* Chocolate Chip—CAMPBELL'S | 3 cookies | 140 | 11% | 13% | 3% |
| PEPPERIDGE FARM *Soft Baked* —CAMPBELL'S | | | | | |
| ❖ Chocolate Chunk | 1 cookie | 130 | 9% | 13% | 3% |
| ❖ Milk Chocolate Macadamia | 1 cookie | 130 | 9% | 13% | 3% |
| PILLSBURY | | | | | |
| ❖ Chocolate Chip | 1 cookie | 130 | 9% | 8% | 1% |
| ❖ Chocolate Chocolate Chip | 1 cookie | 130 | 9% | 8% | 0% |
| ❖ SMART SNACKERS: Chocolate Chip—WEIGHT WATCHERS | 2 cookies | 140 | 8% | 10% | 0% |
| ❖ SNACKWELL'S Reduced Fat Chocolate Chip—NABISCO | 13 cookies | 130 | 5% | 8% | 0% |
| SUNSHINE BISCUITS | | | | | |
| ❖ *Chip-A-Roos* | 3 cookies | 190 | 15% | 18% | 0% |
| ❖ Mini Chocolate Chip | 5 cookies | 160 | 12% | 15% | 0% |
| WESTBRAE NATURAL Chocolate Chip Classics | | | | | |
| ❖ Bach | 1 cookie | 90 | 5% | 9% | 2% |
| ❖ Brahms | 1 cookie | 110 | 8% | 13% | 2% |
| ❖ Chopin | 1 cookie | 110 | 7% | 14% | 2% |
| ❖ Mozart | 1 cookie | 110 | 6% | 12% | 3% |
| ❖ Verdi | 1 cookie | 110 | 8% | 15% | 3% |

## CHOCOLATE-COATED COOKIES

### Brand Name Foods

| FOOD | Serving Size | Calories | Tot Fat | Sat Fat | Chol |
|------|--------------|----------|---------|---------|------|
| FAMILY FAVORITES—NABISCO | | | | | |
| ❖ Fudge Covered Grahams | 3 cookies | 140 | 10% | 8% | 0% |
| ❖ Fudge Striped Shortbread | 3 cookies | 160 | 12% | 8% | 0% |
| FUDGE SHOPPE—KEEBLER | | | | | |
| Ⓐ *Deluxe Grahams* | 3 cookies | 140 | 11% | 23% | 0% |

★ Foods with this symbol have less than or equal to 5% *Daily Value* for all three nutrients (5% Rule).

❖ Foods with this symbol have at least one of the three nutrients greater than 5% *Daily Value* but less than or equal to 20% *Daily Value*.

Ⓐ Foods with this symbol have at least one of the three nutrients greater than 20% *Daily Value* (20% Rule).

| FOOD | Serving Size | Calories | Tot Fat | Sat Fat | Chol |
|---|---|---|---|---|---|
| ❖ *Fudge 'N Caramel* Shortbread w/Fudge 'n Real Caramel | 2 cookies | 120 | 9% | 20% | 1% |
| Ⓐ *Fudge Sticks* Fudge Covered Creme Wafers | 3 cookies | 150 | 12% | 23% | 0% |
| Ⓐ *Fudge Stripes* Fudge Covered Shortbread | 3 cookies | 160 | 12% | 23% | 0% |
| ❖ *P.B. Fudgebutters* Fudge Covered Shortbread w/Real Peanut Butter | 2 cookies | 130 | 11% | 20% | 1% |
| ❖ HEYDAY Bars, Fudge, Caramel, and Peanut—NABISCO | 1 bar | 110 | 8% | 6% | 0% |
| ❖ MALLOMARS Chocolate Sandwich —NABISCO | 2 cookies | 120 | 8% | 14% | 0% |
| ❖ MYSTIC MINT Sandwich—NABISCO | 1 cookie | 90 | 6% | 5% | 0% |
| NABISCO Marshmallow Fudge | | | | | |
| ❖ Puffs | 1 cookie | 90 | 6% | 5% | 0% |
| ❖ Twirls | 1 cookie | 130 | 8% | 6% | 0% |
| OREO Sandwich—NABISCO | | | | | |
| ❖ Fudge Covered | 1 cookie | 110 | 9% | 7% | 0% |
| ❖ White Fudge Covered | 1 cookie | 110 | 9% | 7% | 0% |
| PEPPERIDGE FARM *Distinctive* —CAMPBELL'S | | | | | |
| ❖ Bordeaux | 4 cookies | 130 | 8% | 13% | 3% |
| ❖ Geneva | 3 cookies | 160 | 14% | 18% | 0% |
| ❖ Milk Chocolate Bordeaux | 3 cookies | 160 | 14% | 18% | 0% |
| PEPPERIDGE FARM *International Collection*—CAMPBELL'S | | | | | |
| ❖ Delice Dark Chocolate | 2 cookies | 110 | 6% | 10% | 0% |
| ❖ Esprit, Noir | 1 cookie | 90 | 8% | 18% | 3% |
| ❖ Biarritz | 6 cookies | 160 | 12% | 20% | 0% |
| ❖ Selection de Choix | 5 cookies | 150 | 11% | 20% | 1% |
| ❖ PINWHEELS Pure Chocolate and Marshmallow—NABISCO | 1 cookie | 130 | 8% | 13% | 0% |
| ❖ RITZ, Chocolate Covered—NABISCO | 3 wafers | 150 | 10% | 20% | 0% |
| SUNSHINE BISCUITS | | | | | |
| Ⓐ Fudge Dipped Grahams | 4 cookies | 170 | 14% | 30% | 0% |
| ❖ Fudge Dipped *Oh! Berry* Wafers | 3 cookies | 120 | 7% | 5% | 0% |
| ❖ Fudge Mint Patties | 2 cookies | 130 | 11% | 18% | 0% |
| Ⓐ Fudge Striped Shortbread | 3 cookies | 160 | 14% | 25% | 0% |

## FRUIT AND FRUIT-FILLED COOKIES

**Brand Name Foods**

| ARCHWAY | | | | | |
|---|---|---|---|---|---|
| ★ Apple Filled Oatmeal | 1 cookie | 110 | 5% | 3% | 1% |
| ❖ Apple N' Raisin | 1 cookie | 130 | 7% | 5% | 2% |
| ❖ Apricot Filled | 1 cookie | 110 | 6% | 5% | 2% |
| ❖ Blueberry Filled | 1 cookie | 110 | 6% | 5% | 2% |

| FOOD | Serving Size | Calories | Tot Fat | Sat Fat | Chol |
|---|---|---|---|---|---|
| ❖ Cherry Filled | 1 cookie | 110 | 6% | 5% | 3% |
| ❖ Cherry Nougat | 3 cookies | 150 | 14% | 8% | 0% |
| ★ Cinnamon Apple | 1 cookie | 110 | 5% | 3% | 2% |
| ★ Fat Free Apple Bar | 1 bar | 60 | 0% | 0% | 0% |
| ★ Fat Free Cranberry Bar | 1 bar | 70 | 0% | 0% | 0% |
| ★ Fat Free Fig Bar | 1 bar | 80 | 0% | 0% | 0% |
| ❖ Fruit and Honey Bar | 1 bar | 110 | 6% | 3% | 2% |
| ❖ Fruit Cake | 3 cookies | 140 | 11% | 8% | 1% |
| ❖ Raspberry Filled | 1 cookie | 110 | 6% | 5% | 2% |
| ★ Strawberry Filled | 1 cookie | 100 | 5% | 3% | 1% |
| BAKERY WAGON—M.C. COOKIE | | | | | |
| ★ Apple Filled Oatmeal | 1 cookie | 90 | 5% | 5% | 0% |
| ❖ Apple Walnut Raisin | 1 cookie | 100 | 6% | 5% | 0% |
| ★ Fat Free Apple Cobbler | 1 cookie | 70 | 0% | 0% | 0% |
| ★ Fat Free Raspberry Cobbler | 1 cookie | 70 | 0% | 0% | 0% |
| ★ Honey Fruit Bars | 1 cookie | 100 | 4% | 5% | 2% |
| ★ BARBARA'S BAKERY Fat Free Mini Cookies: Caramel Apple | 6 cookies | 110 | 0% | 0% | 0% |
| ESTEE Cookies | | | | | |
| ★ Fig Bar, Low fat | 2 bars | 100 | 2% | 0% | 0% |
| ★ Fig Bars: All flavors | 2 bars | 100 | 2% | 0% | 0% |
| ★ *Snack Crisps* Apple Cinnamon | 27 crisps | 130 | 5% | 0% | 0% |
| HEALTH VALLEY Fat Free *Bakes* | | | | | |
| ★ Apple | 1 bar | 70 | 0% | 0% | 0% |
| ★ Date | 1 bar | 70 | 0% | 0% | 0% |
| ★ Raisin | 1 bar | 70 | 0% | 0% | 0% |
| HEALTH VALLEY Fat Free *Bakes* Fruit Bars | | | | | |
| ★ Blueberry Apple | 1 bar | 110 | 0% | 0% | 0% |
| ★ Raspberry | 1 bar | 110 | 0% | 0% | 0% |
| ★ Strawberry | 1 bar | 110 | 0% | 0% | 0% |
| HEALTH VALLEY Fat Free | | | | | |
| ★ Apple Spice | 3 cookies | 100 | 0% | 0% | 0% |
| ★ Apricot Delight | 3 cookies | 100 | 0% | 0% | 0% |
| ★ Banana Spice | 3 cookies | 100 | 0% | 0% | 0% |
| ★ Date Delight | 3 cookies | 100 | 0% | 0% | 0% |
| ★ Date Granola | 3 cookies | 100 | 0% | 0% | 0% |
| ★ Hawaiian Fruit | 3 cookies | 100 | 0% | 0% | 0% |
| ★ Raspberry Apple | 3 cookies | 100 | 0% | 0% | 0% |
| HEALTH VALLEY Fat Free Fruit Bars | | | | | |
| ★ Apple | 1 bar | 140 | 0% | 0% | 0% |
| ★ Apricot | 1 bar | 140 | 0% | 0% | 0% |
| ★ Date | 1 bar | 140 | 0% | 0% | 0% |

★ Foods with this symbol have less than or equal to 5% *Daily Value* for all three nutrients (5% Rule).

❖ Foods with this symbol have at least one of the three nutrients greater than 5% *Daily Value* but less than or equal to 20% *Daily Value*.

Ⓐ Foods with this symbol have at least one of the three nutrients greater than 20% *Daily Value* (20% Rule).

| FOOD | Serving Size | Calories | Tot Fat | Sat Fat | Chol |
|------|------|------|------|------|------|
| ★ Raisin | 1 bar | 140 | 0% | 0% | 0% |
| HEALTH VALLEY Fat Free *Fruit Centers* | | | | | |
| ★ Apple | 1 cookie | 70 | 0% | 0% | 0% |
| ★ Apricot | 1 cookie | 70 | 0% | 0% | 0% |
| ★ Date | 1 cookie | 70 | 0% | 0% | 0% |
| ★ Raisin Apple | 1 cookie | 70 | 0% | 0% | 0% |
| ★ Raspberry | 1 cookie | 70 | 0% | 0% | 0% |
| ★ Tropical Fruit | 1 cookie | 70 | 0% | 0% | 0% |
| HEALTH VALLEY Fat Free *Fruit Centers* (Mini Cookies) | | | | | |
| ★ Apple-Cinnamon | 2 cookies | 70 | 0% | 0% | 0% |
| ★ Orange-Pineapple | 2 cookies | 70 | 0% | 0% | 0% |
| ★ Peach-Apricot | 2 cookies | 70 | 0% | 0% | 0% |
| ★ Raspberry | 2 cookies | 70 | 0% | 0% | 0% |
| ★ Strawberry | 2 cookies | 70 | 0% | 0% | 0% |
| HEALTH VALLEY Fat Free Jumbo | | | | | |
| ★ Apple Raisin | 1 cookie | 80 | 0% | 0% | 0% |
| ★ Raisin-Raisin | 1 cookie | 80 | 0% | 0% | 0% |
| ★ Raspberry | 1 cookie | 80 | 0% | 0% | 0% |
| MOTHER'S—M.C. COOKIE | | | | | |
| ★ Fat Free Fig Bar | 1 cookie | 70 | 0% | 0% | 0% |
| ★ Fat Free Whole Wheat Fig Bar | 1 cookie | 70 | 0% | 0% | 0% |
| ❖ Fig Bar | 2 cookies | 130 | 6% | 5% | 0% |
| ⦿ Iced Raisin | 2 cookies | 180 | 12% | 35% | 0% |
| ❖ Whole Wheat Fig Bar | 2 cookies | 130 | 8% | 8% | 0% |
| NEWTONS—NABISCO | | | | | |
| ★ Fat Free: All flavors | 2 cookies | 100 | 0% | 0% | 0% |
| ★ Fig | 2 cookies | 110 | 4% | 4% | 0% |
| ★ OH! BERRY Fat Free Strawberry Wafer—SUNSHINE BISCUITS | 8 cookies | 100 | 0% | 0% | 0% |
| PEPPERIDGE FARM *Distinctive* —CAMPBELL'S | | | | | |
| ★ Chantilly Hazelnut Raspberry | 1 cookie | 80 | 5% | 3% | 2% |
| ❖ Linzer Raspberry Filled | 1 cookie | 100 | 6% | 5% | 2% |
| PEPPERIDGE FARM *Fruit Cookies* —CAMPBELL'S | | | | | |
| ❖ Apricot Raspberry | 3 cookies | 140 | 9% | 10% | 2% |
| ★ Cherry Cobbler | 1 cookie | 70 | 4% | 5% | 1% |
| ★ Fig Bars | 2 bars | 120 | 5% | 0% | 0% |
| ★ Peach Tart | 2 cookies | 120 | 5% | 5% | 0% |
| ❖ Strawberry | 3 cookies | 140 | 8% | 10% | 3% |
| SMART SNACKERS— WEIGHT WATCHERS | | | | | |
| ★ Apple Raisin Bars | 1 bar | 70 | 3% | 3% | 0% |
| ★ Fruit Filled, Fig | 1 bar | 70 | 0% | 0% | 0% |
| ★ Fruit Filled, Raspberry | 1 bar | 70 | 0% | 0% | 0% |
| SUNSHINE BISCUITS | | | | | |
| ★ Fig Bars | 2 cookies | 110 | 4% | 3% | 0% |

| FOOD | Serving Size | Calories | Tot Fat | Sat Fat | Chol |
|------|--------------|----------|---------|---------|------|
| ★ Golden Fruit Apple | 1 cookie | 80 | 2% | 0% | 0% |
| ★ Golden Fruit Apple Cinnamon Bar | 1 cookie | 60 | 0% | 0% | 0% |
| ★ Golden Fruit Raisin | 1 cookie | 80 | 2% | 0% | 0% |
| ★ Low Fat Golden Fruit Cranberry | 1 cookie | 70 | 2% | 0% | 0% |
| ★ ULTRA SLIM-FAST Fig | 1 cookie | 60 | 1% | 0% | 0% |
| WESTBRAE NATURAL Cookie Jar Classics | | | | | |
| ❖ Dutch Apple Cinnamon | 1 cookie | 110 | 6% | 12% | 4% |
| ★ Fruit Bar | 1 bar | 90 | 0% | 0% | 0% |

## GRAHAM CRACKERS

**Generic Foods**

Graham Cracker

| FOOD | Serving Size | Calories | Tot Fat | Sat Fat | Chol |
|------|--------------|----------|---------|---------|------|
| ❖ Chocolate coated | 2 crackers | 140 | 10% | 15% | 0% |
| ★ Cinnamon | 4 crackers | 120 | 4% | 3% | 0% |
| ★ Honey | 4 crackers | 120 | 4% | 3% | 0% |
| ★ Plain | 4 crackers | 120 | 4% | 3% | 0% |

**Brand Name Foods**

BUGS BUNNY—NABISCO

| FOOD | Serving Size | Calories | Tot Fat | Sat Fat | Chol |
|------|--------------|----------|---------|---------|------|
| ❖ Chocolate Graham | 13 pcs | 140 | 7% | 5% | 0% |
| ❖ Cinnamon Graham | 13 pcs | 140 | 7% | 4% | 0% |
| ❖ Graham | 10 cookies | 140 | 7% | 4% | 0% |
| DUNKAROOS—GENERAL MILLS | | | | | |
| ❖ Chocolate Graham w/Chocolate Chip Frosting | 1 tray | 130 | 7% | 6% | 0% |
| ❖ Cinnamon Graham w/Vanilla Frosting & Sprinkles | 1 tray | 130 | 7% | 6% | 0% |
| ❖ EAGLE Peanut Butter & Graham —ANHEUSER BUSCH | 6 cookies | 250 | 15% | 13% | 0% |
| Ⓐ FUDGE SHOPPE *Deluxe* Grahams —KEEBLER | 3 cookies | 140 | 11% | 23% | 0% |
| GRAHAMS—SUNSHINE BISCUITS | | | | | |
| ❖ Cinnamon | 2 crackers | 140 | 9% | 8% | 0% |
| ❖ Honey | 2 crackers | 120 | 6% | 5% | 0% |
| ★ HAIN Animal Grahams | 15 crackers | 80 | 5% | 0% | 0% |
| ★ HAIN Honey Grahams: Regular or Cinnamon | 2 crackers | 80 | 5% | 0% | 0% |
| HEALTH VALLEY Fat Free | | | | | |
| ★ Amaranth Graham | 8 crackers | 100 | 0% | 0% | 0% |
| ★ Oat Bran Graham | 8 crackers | 100 | 0% | 0% | 0% |

★ Foods with this symbol have less than or equal to 5% *Daily Value* for <u>all</u> three nutrients (5% Rule).

❖ Foods with this symbol have <u>at least one</u> of the three nutrients greater than 5% *Daily Value* but less than or equal to 20% *Daily Value*.

Ⓐ Foods with this symbol have <u>at least one</u> of the three nutrients greater than 20% *Daily Value* (20% Rule).

| FOOD | Serving Size | Calories | Tot Fat | Sat Fat | Chol |
|------|--------------|----------|---------|---------|------|
| HONEY MAID—NABISCO | | | | | |
| ★ Cinnamon Grahams | 10 crackers | 140 | 4% | 2% | 0% |
| ★ Honey Grahams | 8 crackers | 120 | 4% | 2% | 0% |
| GRAHAM SELECTS—KEEBLER | | | | | |
| ❖ Apple Cinnamon | 8 crackers | 130 | 6% | 5% | 0% |
| ★ Cinnamon *Crisp*, Low Fat | 8 crackers | 110 | 2% | 3% | 0% |
| ❖ Honey | 8 crackers | 150 | 9% | 8% | 0% |
| ★ Honey, Low Fat | 9 crackers | 120 | 2% | 3% | 0% |
| ★ Original | 8 crackers | 130 | 5% | 5% | 0% |
| ★ MOTHER'S Dinosaur Grrrahams —M.C. COOKIE | 2 cookies | 130 | 5% | 5% | 0% |
| NABISCO | | | | | |
| ★ Grahams | 8 crackers | 120 | 5% | 3% | 0% |
| ⊛ Pure Chocolate Grahams | 3 cookies | 160 | 12% | 23% | 0% |
| PEPPERIDGE FARM *Tiny Goldfish*—CAMPBELL'S | | | | | |
| ❖ Cinnamon Graham | 19 pcs | 150 | 11% | 13% | 3% |
| ❖ Graham | 19 pcs | 150 | 11% | 13% | 5% |
| RALSTON—BREMNER | | | | | |
| ❖ Cinnamon Grahams | 2 whole | 130 | 8% | 5% | 0% |
| ★ Graham Crackers | 2 whole | 120 | 5% | 3% | 0% |
| ★ SNACKWELL'S Fat Free Cinnamon Grahams Snacks—NABISCO | 20 pcs | 110 | 0% | 0% | 0% |
| TEDDY GRAHAMS Snacks —NABISCO | | | | | |
| ❖ Chocolate | 24 pcs | 140 | 7% | 5% | 0% |
| ❖ Cinnamon | 24 pcs | 140 | 7% | 4% | 0% |
| ❖ Honey | 24 pcs | 140 | 7% | 5% | 0% |
| ★ ULTRA SLIM-FAST Cinnamon Grahams | 40 cookies | 120 | 2% | 0% | 0% |

### OATMEAL COOKIES

**Generic Foods**

| FOOD | Serving Size | Calories | Tot Fat | Sat Fat | Chol |
|------|--------------|----------|---------|---------|------|
| ❖ Oatmeal | 2 cookies | 130 | 9% | 6% | 2% |
| ❖ Oatmeal Raisin | 2 cookies | 140 | 9% | 6% | 2% |

**Brand Name Foods**

| FOOD | Serving Size | Calories | Tot Fat | Sat Fat | Chol |
|------|--------------|----------|---------|---------|------|
| ARCHWAY | | | | | |
| ❖ Date Filled Oatmeal | 1 cookie | 110 | 6% | 5% | 1% |
| ★ Oatmeal Raisin, Fat Free | 1 cookie | 100 | 0% | 0% | 0% |
| ★ Oatmeal Raspberry, Fat Free | 1 cookie | 100 | 0% | 0% | 0% |
| ❖ Iced Oatmeal | 1 cookie | 120 | 8% | 5% | 1% |
| ★ Oatmeal | 1 cookie | 110 | 5% | 5% | 1% |
| ❖ Oatmeal Pecan | 1 cookie | 120 | 8% | 8% | 1% |
| ❖ Oatmeal Raisin | 1 cookie | 110 | 6% | 5% | 1% |
| ★ Oatmeal Raisin Bran | 1 cookie | 110 | 5% | 5% | 1% |

| FOOD | Serving Size | Calories | Tot Fat | Sat Fat | Chol |
|---|---|---|---|---|---|
| ❖ Ruth's Golden Oatmeal | 1 cookie | 120 | 8% | 5% | 1% |
| ❖ Ruth's Oatmeal | 1 cookie | 120 | 7% | 5% | 1% |
| BAKERY WAGON—M.C. COOKIE | | | | | |
| ★ Chocolate Chunk Oatmeal | 1 cookie | 100 | 5% | 5% | 0% |
| ★ Date Filled Oatmeal | 1 cookie | 90 | 4% | 5% | 0% |
| ❖ Oatmeal Walnut Raisin | 1 cookie | 100 | 6% | 5% | 0% |
| ★ Raspberry Filled Oatmeal | 1 cookie | 100 | 5% | 5% | 0% |
| ❖ Soft Oatmeal | 1 cookie | 100 | 6% | 5% | 0% |
| BARBARA'S BAKERY | | | | | |
| ★ Fat Free Oatmeal Raisin | 6 cookies | 110 | 0% | 0% | 0% |
| ❖ Oatmeal Raisin | 2 cookies | 160 | 11% | 3% | 0% |
| ❖ DUNCAN HINES Mixes: Oatmeal Raisin (prep as dir)— | | | | | |
| PROCTER & GAMBLE | 1 cookie | 140 | 10% | 7% | 4% |
| EAGLE—ANHEUSER BUSCH | | | | | |
| ⊛ Gourmet: Oatmeal Raisin | 1 cookie | 330 | 26% | 20% | 3% |
| ❖ Iced Oatmeal | 1 cookie | 170 | 8% | 5% | 0% |
| ❖ Oatmeal Creme Pie | 1 cookie | 310 | 18% | 15% | 2% |
| ENTENMANN'S Fat Free, Cholesterol Free—KRAFT | | | | | |
| ★ Oatmeal Chocolatey Chip | 2 cookies | 80 | 0% | 0% | 0% |
| ★ Oatmeal Raisin | 2 cookies | 80 | 0% | 0% | 0% |
| ❖ ENTENMANN'S Oatmeal Raisin | | | | | |
| —KRAFT | 4 cookies | 130 | 8% | 5% | 0% |
| ★ FAMILY FAVORITES Oatmeal | | | | | |
| —NABISCO | 1 cookie | 80 | 5% | 3% | 0% |
| ❖ FEATHERWEIGHT Oatmeal Raisin | 4 cookies | 140 | 8% | 5% | 0% |
| ❖ GRANDMA'S Big Cookies: Oatmeal Apple Spice—FRITO-LAY | 1 cookie | 170 | 9% | 8% | 0% |
| ★ HEALTH VALLEY Fat Free Raisin Oatmeal | 3 cookies | 100 | 0% | 0% | 0% |
| ★ KEEBLER Soft Batch Oatmeal Raisin | 1 cookie | 70 | 5% | 5% | 0% |
| ★ KRUSTEAZ Lowfat Oatmeal Cookie Mix (prep as dir) (2 1/2")—CONTINENTAL MILLS | 1 cookie | 110 | 3% | 0% | 3% |
| ❖ LITTLE DEBBIE Individual Snacks: Oatmeal Raisin Cookie—MCKEE | 1/2 pkg (38 g) | 160 | 10% | 8% | 0% |
| MOTHER'S—M.C. COOKIE | | | | | |
| ❖ Iced Oatmeal | 2 cookies | 120 | 6% | 8% | 0% |
| ❖ Oatmeal | 2 cookies | 110 | 8% | 8% | 0% |
| ❖ Oatmeal Chocolate Chip | 2 cookies | 150 | 8% | 10% | 0% |
| ❖ Oatmeal Raisin | 5 cookies | 150 | 11% | 10% | 2% |
| ❖ Oatmeal Walnut Chocolate Chip | 2 cookies | 130 | 9% | 10% | 0% |

★ Foods with this symbol have less than or equal to 5% *Daily Value* for all three nutrients (5% Rule).
❖ Foods with this symbol have at least one of the three nutrients greater than 5% *Daily Value* but less than or equal to 20% *Daily Value*.
⊛ Foods with this symbol have at least one of the three nutrients greater than 20% *Daily Value* (20% Rule).

| FOOD | Serving Size | Calories | Tot Fat | Sat Fat | Chol |
|------|-------------|----------|---------|---------|------|
| ❖ PEPPERIDGE FARM *American Collection* Santa Fe (oatmeal raisin)—CAMPBELL'S | 1 cookie | 120 | 7% | 5% | 1% |
| PEPPERIDGE FARM *Old Fashioned*—CAMPBELL'S | | | | | |
| ❖ Butterscotch Oatmeal | 3 cookies | 170 | 14% | 15% | 3% |
| ❖ Irish Oatmeal | 3 cookies | 130 | 9% | 8% | 1% |
| ❖ Oatmeal Raisin | 3 cookies | 160 | 9% | 8% | 3% |
| ❖ PEPPERIDGE FARM *Soft Baked* Oatmeal Raisin—CAMPBELL'S | 1 cookie | 110 | 6% | 5% | 5% |
| ❖ PILLSBURY Oatmeal Chocolate Chip | 1 cookie | 120 | 9% | 8% | 1% |
| ★ SMART SNACKERS Oatmeal Raisin—WEIGHT WATCHERS | 2 cookies | 120 | 3% | 0% | 0% |
| SUNSHINE BISCUITS | | | | | |
| ❖ Country Style Oatmeal | 3 cookies | 170 | 11% | 8% | 0% |
| ❖ Iced Oatmeal | 2 cookies | 120 | 8% | 5% | 0% |
| ❖ Oatmeal Chocolate Chip | 3 cookies | 170 | 12% | 15% | 0% |
| ❖ WESTBRAE NATURAL Oatmeal Raisin | 1 cookie | 100 | 3% | 7% | 2% |

## PLAIN, SUGAR, AND WAFER COOKIES

### Generic Foods

| FOOD | Serving Size | Calories | Tot Fat | Sat Fat | Chol |
|------|-------------|----------|---------|---------|------|
| ❖ Sugar | 2 cookies | 140 | 10% | 10% | 4% |
| ❖ Vanilla Wafer | 8 cookies | 140 | 7% | 4% | 6% |
| ★ Fat Free Sugar | 1 cookie | 70 | 0% | 0% | 0% |
| ❖ Soft Sugar | 1 cookie | 110 | 6% | 5% | 2% |
| ❖ Sugar | 1 cookie | 120 | 6% | 5% | 1% |

### Brand Name Foods

| FOOD | Serving Size | Calories | Tot Fat | Sat Fat | Chol |
|------|-------------|----------|---------|---------|------|
| ❖ BAKERY WAGON Vanilla Wafers, Cholesterol Free—M.C. COOKIE | 6 cookies | 130 | 9% | 10% | 0% |
| BARBARA'S BAKERY Animal Cookies | | | | | |
| ❖ Cinnamon | 8 cookies | 130 | 8% | 13% | 0% |
| ❖ Vanilla | 8 cookies | 130 | 8% | 13% | 0% |
| ❖ BARNUM'S ANIMALS Crackers —NABISCO | 12 crackers | 140 | 6% | 4% | 0% |
| ❖ DUNCAN HINES Mixes: Golden Sugar (prep as basic recipe)—PROCTER & GAMBLE | 1 cookie | 120 | 9% | 7% | 4% |
| ❖ ESTEE Vanilla | 4 cookies | 140 | 9% | 5% | 0% |
| ❖ FEATHERWEIGHT Vanilla Natural Flavor | 4 cookies | 140 | 8% | 8% | 0% |
| ❖ GRANDMA'S Mini Cookies: Vanilla—FRITO-LAY | 1 pkg | 170 | 12% | 10% | 0% |

| FOOD | Serving Size | Calories | Tot Fat | Sat Fat | Chol |
|------|-------------|----------|---------|---------|------|
| KEEBLER | | | | | |
| ❖   Golden Vanilla Wafers (artificially flavored) | 8 cookies | 150 | 11% | 10% | 0% |
| ★   Golden Vanilla Wafers 30% Reduced Fat (artificially flavored) | 8 cookies | 130 | 5% | 3% | 0% |
| ❖   Iced Animal | 6 cookies | 140 | 7% | 10% | 0% |
| MOTHER'S—M.C. COOKIE | | | | | |
| Ⓐ   Circus Animals | 6 cookies | 140 | 9% | 25% | 0% |
| ❖   Sugar | 2 cookies | 140 | 9% | 10% | 0% |
| ❖   Vanilla Wafers | 6 cookies | 150 | 9% | 10% | 1% |
| ❖   Zoo Pals | 14 cookies | 140 | 8% | 8% | 0% |
| ❖ NABISCO Brown Edge Wafers | 5 cookies | 140 | 9% | 8% | 1% |
| ★ NATIONAL Arrowroot Biscuit | | | | | |
|     —NABISCO | 1 cookie | 20 | 0% | 0% | 0% |
| ❖ NILLA Wafers—NABISCO | 8 cookies | 140 | 7% | 5% | 2% |
| ❖ PEPPERIDGE FARM Old Fashioned Sugar—CAMPBELL'S | 3 cookies | 140 | 9% | 8% | 5% |
| ❖ PEPPERIDGE FARM Tiny Goldfish Vanilla—CAMPBELL'S | 19 pcs | 150 | 11% | 13% | 7% |
| ❖ RALSTON Vanilla Wafers | 7 wafers | 150 | 9% | 5% | 0% |
| SUNSHINE BISCUITS | | | | | |
| ❖   Animal Crackers | 14 crackers | 140 | 6% | 5% | 0% |
| ❖   Vanilla Wafers | 7 cookies | 150 | 11% | 8% | 1% |

## SANDWICH COOKIES

### Generic Foods

| | | | | | |
|------|-------------|----------|---------|---------|------|
| ❖ Chocolate Sandwich w/Vanilla Filling | 3 cookies (30 g) | 150 | 10% | 8% | 0% |
| ❖ Vanilla Sandwich w/Creme Filling | 3 cookies | 140 | 9% | 5% | 0% |

### Brand Name Foods

| | | | | | |
|------|-------------|----------|---------|---------|------|
| ❖ BARBARA'S BAKERY Cookies & Creme: All flavors | 2 cookies | 120 | 8% | 20% | 5% |
| BISCOS—NABISCO | | | | | |
| ❖   Sugar Wafers | 8 cookies | 140 | 8% | 6% | 0% |
| ❖   Waffle Cremes | 4 cookies | 180 | 14% | 11% | 0% |
| ❖ CAMEO Creme Sandwich—NABISCO | 2 cookies | 130 | 7% | 5% | 0% |
| ❖ COOKIE BREAK Vanilla Artificially Flavored Creme Sandwich—NABISCO | 3 cookies | 160 | 10% | 7% | 0% |

★   Foods with this symbol have less than or equal to 5% *Daily Value* for all three nutrients (5% Rule).
❖   Foods with this symbol have at least one of the three nutrients greater than 5% *Daily Value* but less than or equal to 20% *Daily Value*.
Ⓐ   Foods with this symbol have at least one of the three nutrients greater than 20% *Daily Value* (20% Rule).

| FOOD | Serving Size | Calories | Tot Fat | Sat Fat | Chol |
|---|---|---|---|---|---|
| E.L. FUDGE Sandwich—KEEBLER | | | | | |
| ❖ Butter Flavored w/Fudge Creme Filling | 3 cookies | 170 | 12% | 10% | 1% |
| ❖ Chocolate w/Vanilla Creme Filling | 3 cookies | 170 | 12% | 10% | 0% |
| ❖ Fudge w/Fudge Creme Filling | 3 cookies | 160 | 11% | 10% | 0% |
| ❖ EAGLE Vanilla Creme —ANHEUSER BUSCH | 6 cookies | 260 | 17% | 13% | 0% |
| ELFIN DELIGHTS 50% Reduced Fat Chocolate Sandwich—KEEBLER | | | | | |
| ★ w/Fudge Creme | 2 cookies | 110 | 4% | 3% | 0% |
| ★ w/Vanilla Creme | 2 cookies | 110 | 4% | 3% | 0% |
| ESTEE | | | | | |
| ❖ Chocolate Creme Wafers | 7 wafers | 160 | 12% | 8% | 0% |
| ❖ Chocolate Sandwich | 3 cookies | 160 | 9% | 8% | 0% |
| ❖ Double Decker Lemon Creme | 5 wafers | 170 | 12% | 8% | 0% |
| ❖ Original Sandwich | 3 cookies | 160 | 9% | 8% | 0% |
| ❖ Peanut Butter Sandwich | 3 cookies | 160 | 11% | 5% | 0% |
| ❖ Triple Decker Banana/Chocolate/ Strawberry Wafers | 3 wafers | 140 | 11% | 5% | 0% |
| ❖ Vanilla & Strawberry Creme Wafers | 5 wafers | 170 | 12% | 5% | 0% |
| ❖ Vanilla Creme Wafers | 7 wafers | 160 | 11% | 5% | 0% |
| ❖ Vanilla Sandwich | 3 cookies | 160 | 8% | 5% | 0% |
| ❖ FAMILY FAVORITES Vanilla Sandwich—NABISCO | 3 cookies | 170 | 12% | 8% | 0% |
| FEATHERWEIGHT Creme Wafers | | | | | |
| ❖ Chocolate | 7 wafers | 160 | 12% | 8% | 0% |
| ❖ Vanilla | 7 wafers | 160 | 11% | 5% | 0% |
| FUDGE SHOPPE—KEEBLER | | | | | |
| Ⓐ *Fudge Sticks* Fudge Covered Creme Wafers | 3 cookies | 150 | 12% | 23% | 0% |
| Ⓐ *Grasshopper* Chocolatey Fudge Mint | 4 cookies | 150 | 11% | 25% | 0% |
| ❖ GRANDMA'S Mini Cookies: Vanilla Cream—FRITO-LAY | 1 pkg | 150 | 11% | 8% | 0% |
| HYDROX—SUNSHINE BISCUITS | | | | | |
| ❖ Original | 3 cookies | 150 | 11% | 10% | 0% |
| ❖ Reduced Fat | 3 cookies | 130 | 6% | 5% | 0% |
| KEEBLER Cookies | | | | | |
| ★ French Vanilla Creme (Vanilla Creme Filled) | 1 cookie | 80 | 5% | 5% | 0% |
| ❖ *Krisp Kreem* Sugar Wafers | 5 pcs | 140 | 11% | 8% | 0% |
| ★ *Opera Creme* (Lemon Creme Filled) | 1 cookie | 80 | 5% | 5% | 0% |
| ❖ *Pitter Patter* Peanut Butter Creme | 1 cookie | 90 | 6% | 5% | 0% |
| ❖ LITTLE DEBBIE Individual Snacks: Creme Filled Chocolate (51 g) —MCKEE | 1 pkg | 260 | 18% | 13% | 0% |
| ❖ MYSTIC MINT Sandwich—NABISCO | 1 cookie | 90 | 6% | 5% | 0% |

| FOOD | Serving Size | Calories | Tot Fat | Sat Fat | Chol |
|------|--------------|----------|---------|---------|------|
| MOO TOWN SNACKERS Cookies & Creme—SARGENTO | | | | | |
| ❖ Vanilla Sticks & Chocolate Fudge Creme | 1 unit | 140 | 11% | 10% | 0% |
| ❖ Honey Graham Sticks & Vanilla Creme w/Rainbow Sprinkles | 1 unit | 140 | 11% | 5% | 0% |
| MOTHER'S | | | | | |
| ❖ Duplex Creme | 3 cookies | 170 | 12% | 20% | 0% |
| ❖ Taffy | 2 cookies | 180 | 12% | 10% | 0% |
| NUTTER BUTTER Sandwich —NABISCO | | | | | |
| ❖ *Bites* Peanut Butter | 10 cookies | 150 | 10% | 7% | 1% |
| ❖ Peanut Butter | 2 cookies | 130 | 9% | 6% | 1% |
| ❖ Peanut Creme Patties | 5 patties | 160 | 10% | 6% | 0% |
| OREO Sandwich—NABISCO | | | | | |
| ❖ Chocolate | 3 cookies | 160 | 11% | 8% | 0% |
| ❖ *Double Stuf* | 2 cookies | 140 | 11% | 8% | 0% |
| ❖ Fudge Covered | 1 cookie | 110 | 9% | 7% | 0% |
| ❖ Reduced Fat | 3 cookies | 140 | 8% | 6% | 0% |
| ❖ White Fudge Covered | 1 cookie | 110 | 9% | 7% | 0% |
| PEPPERIDGE FARM *Distinctive* —CAMPBELL'S | | | | | |
| ❖ Brussels | 3 cookies | 150 | 11% | 15% | 2% |
| ❖ Brussels Mint | 3 cookies | 190 | 15% | 18% | 0% |
| ❖ Double Chocolate Milano | 2 cookies | 150 | 12% | 15% | 3% |
| ❖ Hazelnut Milano | 2 cookies | 130 | 11% | 10% | 2% |
| ❖ Lido | 1 cookie | 90 | 7% | 8% | 2% |
| ❖ Milano | 3 cookies | 180 | 15% | 18% | 3% |
| ❖ Milk Chocolate Milano | 3 cookies | 180 | 15% | 18% | 3% |
| ❖ Mint Milano | 2 cookies | 140 | 12% | 18% | 2% |
| ❖ Orange Milano | 2 cookies | 140 | 12% | 13% | 2% |
| RALSTON Sandwich—BREMNER | | | | | |
| ❖ Chocolate | 2 cookies | 130 | 10% | 5% | 0% |
| ❖ Duplex | 2 cookies | 130 | 9% | 5% | 0% |
| ❖ Lemon | 2 cookies | 120 | 8% | 4% | 0% |
| ❖ Vanilla | 2 cookies | 130 | 9% | 5% | 0% |
| SMART SNACKERS Sandwich —WEIGHT WATCHERS | | | | | |
| ★ Chocolate | 2 cookies | 140 | 5% | 5% | 0% |
| ★ Vanilla | 2 cookies | 140 | 5% | 5% | 0% |
| SNACKWELL'S Reduced Fat —NABISCO | | | | | |
| ★ Chocolate Sandwich w/ Chocolate Creme | 2 cookies | 100 | 4% | 3% | 0% |

★ Foods with this symbol have less than or equal to 5% *Daily Value* for all three nutrients (5% Rule).
❖ Foods with this symbol have at least one of the three nutrients greater than 5% *Daily Value* but less than or equal to 20% *Daily Value*.
Ⓐ Foods with this symbol have at least one of the three nutrients greater than 20% *Daily Value* (20% Rule).

| FOOD | Serving Size | Calories | Tot Fat | Sat Fat | Chol |
|---|---|---|---|---|---|
| ★ Vanilla Creme Sandwich w/ Vanilla Creme | 2 cookies | 110 | 4% | 3% | 0% |
| SUNSHINE BISCUITS Sugar Wafers | | | | | |
| ❖ Chocolate | 3 wafers | 130 | 11% | 10% | 0% |
| ❖ Peanut Butter | 4 wafers | 170 | 14% | 10% | 0% |
| ❖ Vanilla | 3 wafers | 130 | 9% | 8% | 0% |
| SUNSHINE BISCUITS Vienna Fingers | | | | | |
| ★ Chocolate | 2 cookies | 120 | 5% | 5% | 0% |
| ★ Low Fat | 2 cookies | 130 | 5% | 3% | 0% |
| ❖ Vanilla | 2 cookies | 140 | 9% | 8% | 0% |
| ULTRA SLIM-FAST Sandwich | | | | | |
| ★ Chocolate | 3 cookies | 130 | 5% | 5% | 0% |
| ★ Vanilla | 3 cookies | 130 | 5% | 5% | 0% |

## OTHER COOKIES

### Generic Foods

| FOOD | Serving Size | Calories | Tot Fat | Sat Fat | Chol |
|---|---|---|---|---|---|
| ★ Fortune | 5 cookies | 80 | 1% | 1% | 0% |
| ★ Gingersnap | 4 cookies | 120 | 5% | 3% | 0% |
| ☮ Ladyfinger | 3 cookies | 110 | 4% | 4% | 36% |
| ❖ Macaroon | 1 cookie | 120 | 6% | 17% | 0% |
| ❖ Molasses | 2 cookies | 130 | 6% | 3% | 0% |
| ❖ Peanut Butter | 2 cookies | 140 | 11% | 7% | 2% |

### Brand Name Foods

| FOOD | Serving Size | Calories | Tot Fat | Sat Fat | Chol |
|---|---|---|---|---|---|
| ARCHWAY | | | | | |
| ★ Almond Crescents | 2 cookies | 100 | 5% | 3% | 1% |
| ❖ Aunt Bea's Pound Cake Cookie | 1 cookie | 110 | 6% | 5% | 3% |
| ❖ Bells and Stars | 3 cookies | 150 | 11% | 8% | 2% |
| ❖ Black Walnut Ice Box | 1 cookie | 120 | 9% | 8% | 2% |
| ❖ Carrot Cake | 1 cookie | 120 | 8% | 5% | 1% |
| ★ Cinnamon Honey Heart, Fat Free | 3 cookies | 100 | 0% | 0% | 0% |
| ❖ Cinnamon Snaps | 5 cookies | 150 | 11% | 8% | 2% |
| ❖ Coconut Macaroon | 1 cookie | 90 | 8% | 20% | 0% |
| ★ Cookie Jar Hermits | 1 cookie | 110 | 5% | 3% | 1% |
| ★ Dark Molasses | 1 cookie | 110 | 5% | 3% | 1% |
| ❖ Frosty Lemon | 1 cookie | 120 | 8% | 5% | 0% |
| ❖ Gingersnaps | 5 cookies | 140 | 8% | 5% | 0% |
| ★ Granola, Fat Free | 2 cookies | 100 | 0% | 0% | 0% |
| ❖ Iced Gingerbread | 3 cookies | 140 | 8% | 5% | 2% |
| ★ Iced Molasses | 1 cookie | 110 | 5% | 5% | 0% |
| ★ Lemon Drop | 1 cookie | 110 | 5% | 3% | 2% |
| ★ Lemon Nuggets, Fat Free | 5 cookies | 100 | 0% | 0% | 0% |
| ❖ Lemon Snaps | 5 cookies | 150 | 11% | 8% | 2% |
| ★ Molasses | 1 cookie | 110 | 5% | 3% | 3% |
| ❖ New Orleans Cake | 1 cookie | 110 | 6% | 5% | 1% |
| ❖ Nutty Nougat | 3 cookies | 160 | 15% | 10% | 0% |

| % DAILY VALUE | | | | | |
|---|---|---|---|---|---|
| FOOD | Serving Size | Calories | Tot Fat | Sat Fat | Chol |
| Ol' Fashion Peanut Butter | 1 cookie | 130 | 9% | 5% | 3% |
| Old Fashion Molasses | 1 cookie | 120 | 5% | 5% | 2% |
| Old Fashion Windmill | 1 cookie | 100 | 6% | 3% | 0% |
| Party Treats | 3 cookies | 140 | 11% | 10% | 5% |
| Peanut Butter | 1 cookie | 140 | 11% | 8% | 3% |
| Peanut Butter n' Chips | 1 cookie | 140 | 11% | 8% | 2% |
| Peanut Jumble | 1 cookie | 130 | 11% | 8% | 1% |
| Pecan Crunch | 6 cookies | 150 | 12% | 10% | 3% |
| Pecan Ice Box | 1 cookie | 140 | 12% | 8% | 3% |
| Pecan Malted Nougat | 3 cookies | 160 | 15% | 10% | 0% |
| Pfeffernusse | 2 cookies | 140 | 2% | 0% | 0% |
| Soft Molasses Drop | 1 cookie | 110 | 5% | 5% | 1% |
| Wedding Cakes | 3 cookies | 160 | 12% | 8% | 0% |
| BAKERY WAGON—M.C. COOKIE | | | | | |
| Ginger Snaps | 5 cookies | 160 | 11% | 10% | 0% |
| Iced Molasses | 1 cookie | 100 | 4% | 5% | 1% |
| Mini Iced Molasses | 3 cookies | 130 | 5% | 5% | 0% |
| BARBARA'S BAKERY Small Indulgences | | | | | |
| Butter Pecan Bites | 6 cookies | 140 | 12% | 40% | 7% |
| Coffee Cake Crunch | 6 cookies | 130 | 9% | 30% | 7% |
| Lemon Almond Delights | 6 cookies | 140 | 9% | 30% | 7% |
| DUNCAN HINES Mixes: Peanut Butter (prep as dir) —PROCTER & GAMBLE | 1 cookie | 140 | 12% | 9% | 4% |
| EAGLE—ANHEUSER BUSCH | | | | | |
| Fudge Stripe Creme Pie | 1 cookie | 310 | 18% | 20% | 2% |
| Lemon Creme | 6 cookies | 260 | 17% | 13% | 0% |
| Peanut Butter Bars | 1 bar | 170 | 15% | 15% | 0% |
| EAGLE Gourmet—ANHEUSER BUSCH | | | | | |
| Ginger | 1 cookie | 240 | 5% | 5% | 7% |
| Macadamia Coconut | 1 cookie | 330 | 25% | 25% | 7% |
| ESTEE | | | | | |
| Coconut | 4 cookies | 140 | 9% | 10% | 0% |
| Lemon | 4 cookies | 140 | 9% | 5% | 0% |
| Snack Crisps Lemon | 30 crisps | 130 | 5% | 3% | 0% |
| FEATHERWEIGHT | | | | | |
| Lemon | 4 cookies | 140 | 8% | 8% | 0% |
| Peanut Butter | 4 cookies | 140 | 8% | 8% | 0% |
| GRANDMA'S Big Cookies—FRITO-LAY | | | | | |
| Old Time Molasses | 1 cookie | 160 | 6% | 5% | 0% |
| Peanut Butter | 1 cookie | 190 | 14% | 10% | 0% |
| GRANDMA'S Mini Cookies: Peanut Butter—FRITO-LAY | 1 pkg | 170 | 11% | 8% | 0% |

★ Foods with this symbol have less than or equal to 5% *Daily Value* for all three nutrients (5% Rule).
❖ Foods with this symbol have at least one of the three nutrients greater than 5% *Daily Value* but less than or equal to 20% *Daily Value*.
Ⓐ Foods with this symbol have at least one of the three nutrients greater than 20% *Daily Value* (20% Rule).

COOKIES—*OTHER* COOKIES     125

| FOOD | Serving Size | Calories | Tot Fat | Sat Fat | Chol |
|------|--------------|----------|---------|---------|------|
| HAIN Fat Free Mini Munchies | | | | | |
| ★ Banana Split | 5 minis | 60 | 0% | 0% | 0% |
| ★ Chocolate Mint Crunch | 5 minis | 60 | 0% | 0% | 0% |
| ★ Peach Cobbler | 5 minis | 60 | 0% | 0% | 0% |
| ★ Peanut Butter Crunch | 5 minis | 50 | 1% | 0% | 0% |
| ★ Strawberry Cheesecake | 5 minis | 60 | 0% | 0% | 0% |
| ❖ KEEBLER Danish Wedding | 4 cookies | 120 | 8% | 10% | 0% |
| ★ LA CHOY Fortune Cookies— | | | | | |
| HUNT WESSON | 4 cookies | 110 | 0% | 0% | 0% |
| MOTHER'S—M.C. COOKIE | | | | | |
| Ⓐ Checkerboard Wafers | 8 cookies | 150 | 12% | 25% | 0% |
| ❖ Cocadas | 5 cookies | 150 | 11% | 15% | 2% |
| ❖ Cookie Parade | 4 cookies | 140 | 11% | 15% | 0% |
| Ⓐ Flaky Flix Vanilla | 2 cookies | 140 | 12% | 25% | 0% |
| Ⓐ Frosted Holiday | 4 cookies | 130 | 9% | 25% | 0% |
| ❖ Gaucho Peanut Butter | 2 cookies | 190 | 15% | 13% | 0% |
| ❖ Gingerbread Man | 6 cookies | 140 | 9% | 10% | 2% |
| ❖ Macaroon | 2 cookies | 150 | 12% | 20% | 0% |
| ❖ Marias | 3 cookies | 170 | 9% | 8% | 2% |
| ❖ MLB Double Header Duplex | 3 cookies | 170 | 12% | 20% | 0% |
| Ⓐ North Poles | 2 cookies | 140 | 11% | 30% | 0% |
| ❖ Pecan Goldens | 2 cookies | 170 | 17% | 8% | 0% |
| Ⓐ Rainbow Wafers | 8 cookies | 150 | 12% | 25% | 0% |
| ❖ Triplet Assortment | 2 cookies | 140 | 11% | 15% | 0% |
| ★ Old Fashion Ginger Snaps | 4 cookies | 120 | 4% | 2% | 0% |
| PEPPERIDGE FARM Distinctive Selection—CAMPBELL'S | | | | | |
| ❖ Cafe Favorites | 4 cookies | 140 | 11% | 13% | 3% |
| ❖ Chocolate Laced Pirouette | 5 cookies | 180 | 15% | 13% | 2% |
| ❖ Dessert Favorites | 3 cookies | 170 | 14% | 15% | 2% |
| ❖ Party Favorites | 3 cookies | 170 | 12% | 15% | 3% |
| ❖ Personal Favorites | 4 cookies | 170 | 14% | 15% | 3% |
| ❖ Toy Chest Butter Assortment | 3 cookies | 120 | 8% | 15% | 7% |
| PEPPERIDGE FARM Old Fashioned—CAMPBELL'S | | | | | |
| ★ Gingerman | 4 cookies | 120 | 5% | 5% | 3% |
| ❖ Hazelnut | 3 cookies | 160 | 12% | 10% | 0% |
| ❖ Lemon Nut Crunch | 3 cookies | 170 | 14% | 10% | 5% |
| ❖ Molasses Crisps | 5 cookies | 150 | 9% | 8% | 0% |
| ❖ PEPPERIDGE FARM Soft Baked Caramel Pecan—CAMPBELL'S | 1 cookie | 130 | 11% | 8% | 7% |
| PEPPERIDGE FARM Biscotti —CAMPBELL'S | | | | | |
| ❖ Almond (5 1/2") | 1 cookie | 160 | 9% | 8% | 3% |
| ❖ Almond Chocolate Dipped (5 1/2") | 1 cookie | 210 | 15% | 18% | 7% |
| ❖ Anise (5 1/2") | 1 cookie | 160 | 8% | 10% | 5% |
| ★ Caruso (Almond) | 1 cookie | 90 | 5% | 5% | 2% |
| ❖ Chocolate Dipped Almond | 1 cookie | 110 | 6% | 10% | 3% |

| FOOD | Serving Size | Calories | Tot Fat | Sat Fat | Chol |
|---|---|---|---|---|---|
| ❖ Chocolate Dipped Orange | 1 cookie | 110 | 7% | 8% | 3% |
| ❖ Chocolate Hazelnut (5 1/2") | 1 cookie | 160 | 14% | 10% | 8% |
| ❖ Cinnamon Chip (5 1/2") | 1 cookie | 160 | 9% | 10% | 8% |
| ❖ Cranberry Pistachio (5 1/2") | 1 cookie | 160 | 9% | 10% | 3% |
| ❖ Figaro (Chocolate Dipped Almond) | 1 cookie | 110 | 6% | 10% | 3% |
| ★ La Scala (Anise) | 1 cookie | 90 | 5% | 5% | 2% |
| ❖ Orange Chocolate Dipped (5 1/2") | 1 cookie | 200 | 12% | 15% | 5% |
| ★ Tosca (Cranberry Pistachio) | 1 cookie | 90 | 5% | 5% | 2% |
| PILLSBURY | | | | | |
| ❖ Candy | 1 cookie | 130 | 9% | 10% | 1% |
| ❖ Dinosaurs | 2 cookies | 120 | 8% | 8% | 1% |
| ❖ Holiday | 2 cookies | 130 | 11% | 10% | 0% |
| ❖ Peanut Butter | 1 cookie | 110 | 8% | 5% | 1% |
| ❖ Sugar | 2 cookies | 130 | 8% | 8% | 1% |
| ❖ Teddy Bears | 2 cookies | 120 | 8% | 5% | 1% |
| SNACKWELL'S—NABISCO | | | | | |
| ★ Double Fudge Cookie Cakes, Fat Free | 1 cookie | 50 | 0% | 0% | 0% |
| ★ Oatmeal with Raisins, Reduced Fat | 2 cookies | 110 | 4% | 0% | 0% |
| SUNSHINE BISCUITS | | | | | |
| ❖ Almond Crescents | 4 cookies | 150 | 9% | 8% | 0% |
| ❖ Ginger Snaps | 7 cookies | 130 | 7% | 5% | 0% |
| ❖ Iced Gingerbread | 5 cookies | 130 | 9% | 8% | 2% |
| ❖ Jingles | 6 cookies | 150 | 8% | 5% | 0% |
| ❖ Lemon Coolers | 5 cookies | 140 | 9% | 8% | 0% |
| WESTBRAE NATURAL Cookie Jar | | | | | |
| ❖ Honey Almond | 1 cookie | 110 | 7% | 12% | 3% |
| ❖ Peanut Butter Nut | 1 cookie | 110 | 6% | 7% | 2% |
| ❖ Raspberry Vanilla Flavored | 1 cookie | 110 | 6% | 12% | 3% |

# Crackers

## BAGEL CHIPS

**Brand Name Foods**

PEPPERIDGE FARM Bagel Chips
—CAMPBELL'S

| | | | | | |
|---|---|---|---|---|---|
| ★ Onion Multigrain | 1 oz | 120 | 5% | 0% | 0% |
| ❖ Three Cheese | 1 oz | 140 | 11% | 5% | 0% |
| ❖ Toasted Onion & Garlic | 1 oz | 110 | 7% | 5% | 0% |

★ Foods with this symbol have less than or equal to 5% *Daily Value* for all three nutrients (5% Rule).
❖ Foods with this symbol have at least one of the three nutrients greater than 5% *Daily Value* but less than or equal to 20% *Daily Value*.
Ⓐ Foods with this symbol have at least one of the three nutrients greater than 20% *Daily Value* (20% Rule).

| FOOD | Serving Size | Calories | Tot Fat | Sat Fat | Chol |
|------|------|------|------|------|------|
| **CRACKERS** | | | | | |
| **Generic Foods** | | | | | |
| ❖ Cheese Cracker | 30 crackers | 150 | 14% | 14% | 0% |
| ❖ Cheese Filled Sandwich Cracker | 4 crackers | 140 | 10% | 7% | 0% |
| ★ Crispbread, Rye | 3 crackers | 110 | 0% | 0% | 0% |
| ★ Matzo | 1 board | 120 | 1% | 0% | 0% |
| ★ Melba Toast | 3 slcs | 60 | 1% | 0% | 0% |
| ❖ Peanut Butter Filled Sandwich Cracker | 4 crackers | 140 | 10% | 7% | 0% |
| ★ Rye Wafer | 2 wafers | 90 | 1% | 1% | 0% |
| ★ Saltines | 10 crackers | 130 | 4% | 2% | 0% |
| ❖ Soda Cracker | 10 crackers | 130 | 6% | 3% | 0% |
| ❖ Whole Wheat Cracker | 8 crackers | 140 | 9% | 5% | 0% |
| **Brand Name Foods** | | | | | |
| BETTER CHEDDARS Baked Snack Crackers—NABISCO | | | | | |
| ❖ Low Sodium | 22 crackers | 150 | 12% | 8% | 1% |
| ❖ Original | 22 crackers | 150 | 12% | 10% | 0% |
| ❖ Reduced Fat | 24 crackers | 140 | 9% | 8% | 1% |
| CHEEZ-IT—SUNSHINE BISCUITS | | | | | |
| ❖ Hot & Spicy | 26 crackers | 160 | 12% | 8% | 0% |
| ❖ Low-Sodium | 27 crackers | 160 | 12% | 10% | 0% |
| ❖ Original | 27 crackers | 160 | 12% | 10% | 0% |
| ❖ Reduced Fat | 30 crackers | 130 | 7% | 5% | 0% |
| ❖ White Cheddar | 26 crackers | 160 | 14% | 10% | 1% |
| ❖ CHICKEN IN A BISKIT Flavored Crackers—NABISCO | 14 crackers | 160 | 15% | 8% | 0% |
| CLUB Partners Crackers—KEEBLER | | | | | |
| ★ 50% Reduced Sodium | 4 crackers | 70 | 5% | 5% | 0% |
| ★ Garlic Bread Flavored | 4 crackers | 70 | 5% | 5% | 0% |
| ★ Original | 4 crackers | 70 | 5% | 5% | 0% |
| ★ Touch of Cheddar | 4 crackers | 70 | 4% | 5% | 1% |
| CRACKER PAKS Cracker Sandwiches—KEEBLER | | | | | |
| ❖ Cheese & Peanut Butter | 1 pkg | 190 | 14% | 10% | 1% |
| ❖ Club & Cheddar | 1 pkg | 190 | 17% | 13% | 3% |
| ❖ Toast & Peanut Butter | 1 pkg | 190 | 14% | 10% | 0% |
| ❖ Town House & Cheddar | 1 pkg | 200 | 20% | 13% | 3% |
| ❖ EAGLE Baked Shamu Shapes —ANHEUSER BUSCH | 1 cup | 160 | 15% | 10% | 0% |
| EAGLE—ANHEUSER BUSCH | | | | | |
| ❖ Cheese on Cheese | 6 crackers | 210 | 17% | 15% | 1% |
| ❖ Honey Roast Peanut Butter Cheese | 6 crackers | 230 | 18% | 10% | 0% |
| ❖ Peanut Butter on Toast | 6 crackers | 210 | 15% | 13% | 0% |
| ❖ Wheat and Cheddar Cheese | 6 crackers | 200 | 15% | 15% | 1% |

| FOOD | Serving Size | Calories | Tot Fat | Sat Fat | Chol |
|---|---|---|---|---|---|
| ESTEE Snack Crisps | | | | | |
| ★ Ranch | 30 crisps | 130 | 5% | 3% | 1% |
| ★ White Cheddar | 27 crisps | 130 | 5% | 5% | 2% |
| ★ ESTEE Unsalted Crackers | 1 cracker | 70 | 0% | 0% | 0% |
| FEATHERWEIGHT Snack Crackers | | | | | |
| ★ Cheddar Cheese | 24 crackers | 120 | 3% | 3% | 0% |
| ★ Onion Poppy | 15 crackers | 120 | 3% | 0% | 0% |
| ★ Sesame Wheat | 18 crackers | 120 | 3% | 0% | 0% |
| ★ Unsalted | 1 cracker | 70 | 3% | 3% | 0% |
| ★ GARDEN CRISPS Vegetable Crackers—NABISCO | 15 crackers | 130 | 5% | 3% | 0% |
| HAIN Crackers | | | | | |
| ❖ Cheese | 11 crackers | 130 | 7% | 3% | 0% |
| ★ Herb, 98% Fat Free | 11 crackers | 110 | 0% | 0% | 0% |
| ★ Onion, 98% Fat Free | 11 crackers | 110 | 0% | 0% | 0% |
| ❖ Rich | 11 crackers | 130 | 9% | 0% | 0% |
| ❖ Sesame | 11 crackers | 140 | 9% | 3% | 0% |
| ❖ Vegetable | 11 crackers | 140 | 9% | 3% | 0% |
| ★ Vegetable, 98% Fat Free | 11 crackers | 110 | 0% | 0% | 0% |
| ★ Whole wheat, 98% Fat Free | 11 crackers | 110 | 0% | 0% | 0% |
| HARVEST CRISPS—NABISCO | | | | | |
| ❖ Five Grain | 13 crackers | 130 | 6% | 3% | 0% |
| ❖ Oat | 13 crackers | 140 | 7% | 4% | 0% |
| HEALTH VALLEY Fat Free Whole Wheat | | | | | |
| ★ Cheese | 5 crackers | 50 | 0% | 0% | 0% |
| ★ Herb | 5 crackers | 50 | 0% | 0% | 0% |
| ★ Onion | 5 crackers | 50 | 0% | 0% | 0% |
| ★ Regular | 5 crackers | 50 | 0% | 0% | 0% |
| ★ Vegetable: Regular or No Salt | 5 crackers | 50 | 0% | 0% | 0% |
| HEALTH VALLEY Fat Free Fire Crackers | | | | | |
| ★ Hot 3 Chilies & Cheese | 6 crackers | 50 | 0% | 0% | 0% |
| ★ Medium Jalapeno & Cheese | 6 crackers | 50 | 0% | 0% | 0% |
| ★ Mild Chili & Cheese | 6 crackers | 50 | 0% | 0% | 0% |
| HEALTH VALLEY Fat Free Pizza Crackers | | | | | |
| ★ Garlic & Herb | 6 crackers | 50 | 0% | 0% | 0% |
| ★ Pizza Italiano | 6 crackers | 50 | 0% | 0% | 0% |
| ★ Zesty Cheese | 6 crackers | 50 | 0% | 0% | 0% |
| HI HO—SUNSHINE BISCUITS | | | | | |
| ❖ Butter Flavored | 9 crackers | 160 | 14% | 8% | 0% |
| ❖ Cracked Pepper | 9 crackers | 160 | 14% | 8% | 0% |
| ❖ Multi-Grain | 9 crackers | 160 | 14% | 8% | 0% |
| ❖ Original | 9 crackers | 160 | 14% | 8% | 0% |

★ Foods with this symbol have less than or equal to 5% *Daily Value* for all three nutrients (5% Rule).
❖ Foods with this symbol have at least one of the three nutrients greater than 5% *Daily Value* but less than or equal to 20% *Daily Value*.
Ⓐ Foods with this symbol have at least one of the three nutrients greater than 20% *Daily Value* (20% Rule).

| FOOD | Serving Size | Calories | Tot Fat | Sat Fat | Chol |
|------|--------------|----------|---------|---------|------|
| ❖ Reduced Fat | 10 crackers | 140 | 8% | 5% | 0% |
| ❖ Whole Wheat | 9 crackers | 150 | 12% | 8% | 0% |
| KRISPY—SUNSHINE BISCUITS | | | | | |
| ★ Cracked Pepper | 5 crackers | 60 | 2% | 0% | 0% |
| ★ Fat Free | 5 crackers | 60 | 0% | 0% | 0% |
| ★ Mild Cheddar | 5 crackers | 60 | 3% | 3% | 0% |
| ★ Original | 5 crackers | 60 | 2% | 0% | 0% |
| ★ Soup & Oyster Crackers | 17 crackers | 60 | 2% | 0% | 0% |
| ★ Unsalted Tops | 5 crackers | 60 | 2% | 0% | 0% |
| ★ Whole Wheat | 5 crackers | 60 | 2% | 0% | 0% |
| LITTLE DEBBIE Individual Snacks (40 g)—MCKEE | | | | | |
| ❖ Cheese Crackers w/Peanut Butter | 1 pkg | 210 | 15% | 13% | 0% |
| ❖ Cheese on Cheese Crackers | 1 pkg | 200 | 17% | 13% | 2% |
| ❖ Toasty Crackers w/Peanut Butter | 1 pkg | 210 | 15% | 13% | 0% |
| MANISCHEWITZ Matzos | | | | | |
| ★ 100% Whole Wheat | 1 board | 90 | 1% | 0% | 0% |
| ★ Garlic | 1 board | 100 | 0% | 0% | 0% |
| ★ Miniatures | 13 crackers | 110 | 0% | 0% | 0% |
| ★ Passover | 1 board | 120 | 0% | 0% | 0% |
| ★ Thins/Dietetic | 1 board | 90 | 1% | 0% | 0% |
| ★ Unsalted | 1 board | 110 | 1% | 1% | 0% |
| MANISCHEWITZ *Tams* | | | | | |
| ❖ Garlic | 10 crackers | 140 | 8% | 10% | 0% |
| ❖ Onion | 10 crackers | 140 | 8% | 9% | 0% |
| ❖ Sodium Free | 10 crackers | 140 | 7% | 11% | 0% |
| ❖ Wheat | 10 crackers | 130 | 8% | 10% | 0% |
| MR. PHIPPS Pretzel Chips—NABISCO | | | | | |
| ★ Lower Sodium | 16 chips | 120 | 4% | 0% | 0% |
| ★ Original | 16 chips | 120 | 4% | 0% | 0% |
| ★ Original, Fat Free | 16 chips | 100 | 0% | 0% | 0% |
| MR. PHIPPS Tater Crisps Snacks —NABISCO | | | | | |
| ❖ Bar-B-Que | 21 crisps | 130 | 6% | 3% | 0% |
| ❖ Original | 23 crisps | 120 | 7% | 4% | 0% |
| ❖ Sour Cream 'n Onion | 22 crisps | 130 | 6% | 3% | 0% |
| MR. PHIPPS Tortilla Crisps—NABISCO | | | | | |
| ❖ Nacho | 28 crisps | 130 | 7% | 4% | 0% |
| ❖ Original | 28 crisps | 130 | 7% | 3% | 0% |
| MR. SALTY—NABISCO | | | | | |
| ★ Pretzel Chips | 16 chips | 110 | 4% | 0% | 0% |
| ★ Pretzel Chips, Fat Free | 16 chips | 100 | 0% | 0% | 0% |
| MUNCH'EMS Crackers—KEEBLER | | | | | |
| ❖ Cheddar | 28 crackers | 140 | 9% | 5% | 0% |
| ❖ Ranch | 28 crackers | 130 | 8% | 5% | 0% |
| ❖ Seasoned Original | 30 crackers | 130 | 8% | 5% | 0% |
| ❖ Sour Cream & Onion | 28 crackers | 140 | 9% | 5% | 0% |
| ❖ NABISCO Bacon Flavored Crackers —NABISCO | 15 crackers | 160 | 13% | 7% | 0% |

| FOOD | Serving Size | Calories | Tot Fat | Sat Fat | Chol |
|---|---|---|---|---|---|
| NABS—NABISCO | | | | | |
| ❖ Cheese Peanut Butter Sandwich | 6 sandwiches | 190 | 15% | 10% | 0% |
| ❖ Peanut Butter Toast Sandwich | 6 sandwiches | 190 | 15% | 10% | 0% |
| ❖ NIPS Cheese Snack Crackers | | | | | |
| —NABISCO | 29 crackers | 150 | 10% | 8% | 0% |
| ❖ OAT THINS Snack Crackers | | | | | |
| —NABISCO | 18 crackers | 140 | 9% | 5% | 0% |
| ★ OYSTERETTES Soup and Oyster | | | | | |
| Crackers—NABISCO | 19 crackers | 60 | 4% | 3% | 0% |
| PEPPERIDGE FARM Distinctive | | | | | |
| —CAMPBELL'S | | | | | |
| ★ Butter Flavored Thins | 4 crackers | 70 | 5% | 5% | 3% |
| ★ Cracked Wheat | 2 crackers | 70 | 4% | 5% | 0% |
| ★ Hearty Wheat | 3 crackers | 80 | 5% | 0% | 0% |
| ★ Sesame | 3 crackers | 70 | 4% | 0% | 0% |
| PEPPERIDGE FARM Tiny Goldfish | | | | | |
| —CAMPBELL'S | | | | | |
| ❖ Cheddar Cheese | 55 pcs | 140 | 9% | 8% | 3% |
| ❖ Cheddar Cheese, Reduced Sodium | 60 pcs | 150 | 9% | 8% | 3% |
| ❖ Original | 55 pcs | 140 | 9% | 10% | 0% |
| ❖ Parmesan Cheese | 60 pcs | 140 | 8% | 8% | 0% |
| ❖ Pizza | 55 pcs | 140 | 9% | 8% | 0% |
| ★ Pretzel | 45 pcs | 120 | 4% | 3% | 0% |
| PEPPERIDGE FARM Tortilla Crisps—CAMPBELL'S | | | | | |
| ❖ Chili Cheese | 36 pcs | 130 | 11% | 5% | 1% |
| ❖ Original | 36 pcs | 130 | 9% | 5% | 1% |
| ❖ Salsa | 36 pcs | 130 | 11% | 5% | 1% |
| PREMIUM Saltines—NABISCO | | | | | |
| ★ Fat Free | 5 crackers | 50 | 0% | 0% | 0% |
| ★ Low Sodium | 5 crackers | 60 | 2% | 0% | 0% |
| ❖ Mini Bits | 34 crackers | 150 | 10% | 6% | 0% |
| ★ Original | 5 crackers | 60 | 3% | 0% | 0% |
| ★ PREMIUM Soup and Oyster | | | | | |
| Crackers—NABISCO | 23 crackers | 60 | 2% | 0% | 0% |
| RALSTON—BREMNER | | | | | |
| ❖ Animal Crackers | 12 crackers | 130 | 6% | 4% | 0% |
| ❖ Big Cheese Cracker | 25 crackers | 140 | 10% | 6% | 1% |
| ❖ Cheddar Snacks | 18 crackers | 150 | 11% | 6% | 0% |
| ★ Oyster Crackers | 35 crackers | 70 | 3% | 0% | 0% |
| ★ Rich & Crisp | 1 whole | 70 | 5% | 0% | 0% |
| ❖ Sesame & Wheat Snacks | 17 crackers | 150 | 10% | 5% | 0% |
| ❖ Snackers | 9 crackers | 140 | 9% | 5% | 0% |
| ❖ Snackers, Unsalted | 9 crackers | 150 | 12% | 5% | 0% |

★ Foods with this symbol have less than or equal to 5% *Daily Value* for all three nutrients (5% Rule).
❖ Foods with this symbol have at least one of the three nutrients greater than 5% *Daily Value* but less than or equal to 20% *Daily Value*.
Ⓐ Foods with this symbol have at least one of the three nutrients greater than 20% *Daily Value* (20% Rule).

| FOOD | Serving Size | Calories | Tot Fat | Sat Fat | Chol |
|---|---|---|---|---|---|
| ❖ Thin Wheat: Regular or Unsalted | 16 crackers | 140 | 6% | 3% | 0% |
| ❖ Wheat Snacks: Regular or Unsalted Tops | 16 crackers | 140 | 6% | 3% | 0% |
| RITZ BITS—NABISCO | | | | | |
| ❖ Mini Crackers | 48 crackers | 160 | 14% | 8% | 0% |
| ❖ Sandwiches with Real Cheese | 14 crackers | 160 | 15% | 12% | 1% |
| ❖ Sandwiches with Real Peanut Butter | 13 crackers | 150 | 12% | 7% | 0% |
| ❖ RITZ: Regular or Low Sodium —NABISCO | 5 crackers | 80 | 6% | 4% | 0% |
| ★ ROYAL LUNCH Milk Crackers —NABISCO | 1 cracker | 50 | 3% | 0% | 0% |
| RY-KRISP—BREMNER | | | | | |
| ★ Original | 2 crackers | 60 | 0% | 0% | 0% |
| ★ Seasoned | 2 crackers | 60 | 2% | 0% | 0% |
| ★ Sesame | 2 crackers | 60 | 2% | 0% | 0% |
| SALTINES—BREMNER | | | | | |
| ★ Deluxe | 5 crackers | 60 | 3% | 0% | 0% |
| ★ Deluxe Unsalted | 5 crackers | 70 | 3% | 0% | 0% |
| ★ Fat Free | 5 crackers | 60 | 0% | 0% | 0% |
| ★ Wheat | 5 crackers | 60 | 3% | 0% | 0% |
| SNACKWELL'S Crackers—NABISCO | | | | | |
| ★ Cheese, Reduced Fat | 36 crackers | 130 | 3% | 3% | 0% |
| ★ Classic Golden, Reduced Fat | 6 crackers | 60 | 1% | 0% | 0% |
| ★ Cracked Pepper | 7 crackers | 60 | 0% | 0% | 0% |
| ★ Wheat, Fat Free | 5 crackers | 60 | 0% | 0% | 0% |
| ❖ SNORKELS Cheddar Snack Crackers—NABISCO | 56 crackers | 140 | 8% | 7% | 1% |
| ❖ SOCIABLES—NABISCO | 7 crackers | 80 | 6% | 3% | 0% |
| ❖ SWISS Cheese Naturally Flavored Snack Crackers—NABISCO | 15 crackers | 140 | 10% | 7% | 0% |
| ❖ TID-BIT Cheese Baked Snack Crackers—NABISCO | 32 crackers | 150 | 13% | 8% | 0% |
| TOASTED COMPLEMENTS —KEEBLER | | | | | |
| ❖ Onion | 9 crackers | 140 | 9% | 5% | 0% |
| ❖ Sesame | 9 crackers | 140 | 9% | 5% | 0% |
| ❖ Wheat | 9 crackers | 140 | 9% | 8% | 0% |
| TOWN HOUSE Classic Crackers —KEEBLER | | | | | |
| ❖ 50% Reduced Sodium | 5 crackers | 80 | 7% | 5% | 0% |
| ❖ Original | 5 crackers | 80 | 7% | 5% | 0% |
| ❖ Wheat | 5 crackers | 80 | 6% | 5% | 0% |
| TRISCUIT Wafers—NABISCO | | | | | |
| ❖ Deli-Style Rye Whole Wheat 'n Rye | 7 wafers | 140 | 8% | 4% | 0% |
| ❖ Garden Herb | 6 wafers | 130 | 7% | 4% | 0% |
| ❖ Low Sodium | 7 wafers | 150 | 8% | 5% | 0% |

| FOOD | Serving Size | Calories | Tot Fat | Sat Fat | Chol |
|---|---|---|---|---|---|
| ❖    Original | 7 wafers | 140 | 8% | 4% | 0% |
| ★    Reduced Fat | 8 wafers | 130 | 4% | 3% | 0% |
| ❖    Whole Wheat 'n Bran | 7 wafers | 140 | 8% | 4% | 0% |
| ❖  TWIGS Sesame and Cheese Snack Sticks—NABISCO | 15 sticks | 150 | 11% | 9% | 0% |
| ★  UNEEDA Biscuits Unsalted Tops —NABISCO | 2 crackers | 60 | 3% | 0% | 0% |
| ❖  VEGETABLE THINS Snack Crackers—NABISCO | 14 crackers | 160 | 13% | 7% | 0% |
| ★  WAVERLY Crackers—NABISCO | 5 crackers | 70 | 5% | 4% | 0% |
|    WHEAT THINS Snack Crackers —NABISCO | | | | | |
| ❖    Low Salt | 16 crackers | 140 | 9% | 5% | 0% |
| ❖    Multi-Grain | 17 crackers | 130 | 6% | 2% | 0% |
| ❖    Original | 16 crackers | 140 | 9% | 6% | 0% |
| ❖    Reduced Fat | 18 crackers | 120 | 6% | 3% | 0% |
|    WHEATABLES Wheat Snack Crackers—KEEBLER | | | | | |
| ❖    50% Reduced Sodium | 25 crackers | 150 | 11% | 10% | 0% |
| ❖    French Onion | 25 crackers | 150 | 11% | 10% | 0% |
| ❖    Original | 25 crackers | 150 | 11% | 10% | 0% |
| ❖    Ranch | 25 crackers | 150 | 11% | 10% | 0% |
| ❖    White Cheddar Flavor | 25 crackers | 150 | 11% | 10% | 0% |
| ★    Reduced Fat | 29 crackers | 130 | 5% | 5% | 0% |
|    WHEATINES—BARBARA'S BAKERY | | | | | |
| ★    Cracked Pepper | 1 lg. square | 60 | 2% | 5% | 0% |
| ★    Lightly Salted Tops | 1 lg. square | 60 | 2% | 0% | 0% |
| ★    Sesame | 1 lg. square | 60 | 2% | 0% | 0% |
| ★  WHEATKRISP—BREMNER | 2 crackers | 70 | 2% | 0% | 0% |
| ★  WHEATSWORTH Stoned Ground Wheat Crackers—NABISCO | 5 crackers | 80 | 5% | 3% | 0% |
|    ZESTA Saltine Crackers—KEEBLER | | | | | |
| ★    50% Reduced Sodium | 5 crackers | 60 | 3% | 3% | 0% |
| ★    Fat Free | 5 crackers | 50 | 0% | 0% | 0% |
| ★    Original | 5 crackers | 60 | 3% | 3% | 0% |
| ★    Soup & Oyster Crackers | 42 crackers | 70 | 4% | 5% | 0% |
| ★    Unsalted Tops | 5 crackers | 60 | 3% | 3% | 0% |
| ❖  ZINGS Snack Chips—NABISCO | 1 bag | 240 | 17% | 10% | 0% |
| ★  ZWIEBACK Teething Toast —NABISCO | 1 toast | 35 | 0% | 0% | 0% |

★  Foods with this symbol have less than or equal to 5% *Daily Value* for <u>all</u> three nutrients (5% Rule).

❖  Foods with this symbol have <u>at least one</u> of the three nutrients greater than 5% *Daily Value* but less than or equal to 20% *Daily Value.*

Ⓐ  Foods with this symbol have <u>at least one</u> of the three nutrients greater than 20% *Daily Value* (20% Rule).

| FOOD | Serving Size | Calories | Tot Fat | Sat Fat | Chol |
|------|-------------|----------|---------|---------|------|

## RICE, POPCORN, AND GRAIN CAKES

### Generic Foods

| FOOD | Serving Size | Calories | Tot Fat | Sat Fat | Chol |
|------|-------------|----------|---------|---------|------|
| ★ Corn Cake | 1 cake | 35 | 0% | 1% | 0% |
| ★ Multigrain Cake | 1 cake | 35 | 0% | 1% | 0% |
| ★ Popcorn Cake | 1 cake | 40 | 0% | 0% | 0% |
| ★ Rice Cake | 1 cake | 35 | 0% | 1% | 0% |
| ★ Rye Cake | 1 cake | 35 | 0% | 1% | 0% |
| ★ Sesame Seed Cake | 1 cake | 35 | 0% | 1% | 0% |

### Brand Name Foods

| FOOD | Serving Size | Calories | Tot Fat | Sat Fat | Chol |
|------|-------------|----------|---------|---------|------|
| **HAIN Popcorn Rice Cakes** | | | | | |
| ★ Butter Flavored | 1 cake | 40 | 0% | 0% | 0% |
| ★ White Cheddar Flavored | 1 cake | 40 | 1% | 0% | 1% |
| **HAIN Mini Popcorn Rice Cakes** | | | | | |
| ★ Apple Cinnamon Flavored | 6 minis | 60 | 0% | 0% | 0% |
| ★ Honey Nut | 6 minis | 60 | 0% | 0% | 0% |
| ★ Mild Cheddar Flavored | 6 minis | 70 | 3% | 0% | 1% |
| ★ White Cheddar Flavored | 6 minis | 70 | 4% | 0% | 1% |
| **HAIN Rice Cakes** | | | | | |
| ★ Apple Cinnamon Flavored | 1 cake | 50 | 0% | 0% | 0% |
| ★ Honey Nut | 1 cake | 50 | 1% | 0% | 0% |
| **HAIN Mini Rice Cakes** | | | | | |
| ★ Butter Flavored | 7 minis | 60 | 0% | 0% | 0% |
| ★ Caramel Flavored | 5 minis | 60 | 0% | 0% | 0% |
| ★ Cheese Flavored | 6 minis | 70 | 4% | 2% | 1% |
| ★ Ranch | 6 minis | 80 | 5% | 0% | 0% |
| **LUNDBERG Brown Rice Cakes** | | | | | |
| ★ Buckwheat | 1 cake | 60 | 1% | 0% | 0% |
| ★ Caraway | 1 cake | 60 | 0% | 0% | 0% |
| ★ Dill | 5 cakes | 60 | 2% | 0% | 1% |
| ★ Mini Sesame | 5 cakes | 50 | 0% | 0% | 0% |
| ★ Plain | 1 cake | 60 | 1% | 0% | 0% |
| ★ Popcorn | 1 cake | 60 | 1% | 0% | 0% |
| **ORVILLE REDENBACHER'S Mini Popcorn Cakes—HUNT WESSON** | | | | | |
| ★ Apple Cinnamon | 11 minis | 100 | 0% | 0% | 0% |
| ★ Butter | 13 minis | 100 | 3% | 1% | 0% |
| ★ Caramel | 11 minis | 100 | 0% | 0% | 0% |
| ★ Honey Nut | 11 minis | 100 | 0% | 0% | 0% |
| ★ White Cheddar Cheese | 13 minis | 100 | 2% | 1% | 0% |
| **ORVILLE REDENBACHER'S Popcorn Cakes—HUNT WESSON** | | | | | |
| ★ Butter | 3 cakes | 110 | 3% | 2% | 0% |
| ★ Caramel | 2 cakes | 80 | 0% | 0% | 0% |
| ★ White Cheddar Cheese | 3 cakes | 110 | 3% | 1% | 0% |

| FOOD | Serving Size | Calories | Tot Fat | Sat Fat | Chol |
|------|------|------|------|------|------|
| QUAKER Corn Cakes | | | | | |
| ★ Butter Popped Corn | 1 cake | 35 | 0% | 0% | 0% |
| ★ Caramel Corn | 1 cake | 50 | 0% | 0% | 0% |
| ★ Mild White Cheddar | 1 cake | 40 | 0% | 0% | 0% |
| ★ Mild White Cheddar, Mini | 6 cakes | 50 | 0% | 0% | 0% |
| ★ Nacho | 1 cake | 40 | 0% | 0% | 0% |
| QUAKER Mini Rice Cakes | | | | | |
| ★ Apple Cinnamon | 5 cakes | 50 | 0% | 0% | 0% |
| ★ Buttered Popped Corn | 6 cakes | 50 | 0% | 0% | 0% |
| ★ Caramel Corn | 5 cakes | 50 | 0% | 0% | 0% |
| ★ Cinnamon Crunch | 5 cakes | 50 | 0% | 0% | 0% |
| ★ Honey Nut | 5 cakes | 50 | 0% | 0% | 0% |
| ★ White Cheddar | 6 cakes | 50 | 0% | 0% | 0% |
| QUAKER Rice Cakes | | | | | |
| ★ Apple Cinnamon | 1 cake | 50 | 0% | 0% | 0% |
| ★ Cinnamon Crunch | 1 cake | 50 | 0% | 0% | 0% |
| ★ QUAKER Wheat Grain Cakes | 1 cake | 35 | 0% | 0% | 0% |

# Dairy and Dairy Substitutes

## AMERICAN CHEESE

### Generic Foods

| | | | | | |
|------|------|------|------|------|------|
| ⊛ American Pasteurized Process Cheese | 1 oz | 110 | 14% | 28% | 9% |
| ❖ American Processed Cheese Spread | 1 oz | 80 | 9% | 19% | 5% |

### Brand Name Foods

| | | | | | |
|------|------|------|------|------|------|
| ALPINE LACE | | | | | |
| ❖ American Flavor Pasteurized Process Cheese: Plain or Hot Pepper | 1 oz | 80 | 9% | 20% | 7% |
| ★ American Fat Free Pasteurized Process Skim Milk Cheese | 1 oz | 45 | 0% | 0% | 1% |
| ★ HEALTHY CHOICE Singles: American (White or Yellow) —CONAGRA | 1 slc | 30 | 0% | 0% | 1% |
| KRAFT | | | | | |
| ⊛ Deluxe American Pasteurized Processed Cheese | 1 oz | 100 | 14% | 30% | 8% |
| ❖ Singles American Flavor Pasteurized Process Cheese Product | 3/4 oz | 70 | 8% | 18% | 5% |

★ Foods with this symbol have less than or equal to 5% *Daily Value* for all three nutrients (5% Rule).
❖ Foods with this symbol have at least one of the three nutrients greater than 5% *Daily Value* but less than or equal to 20% *Daily Value*.
⊛ Foods with this symbol have at least one of the three nutrients greater than 20% *Daily Value* (20% Rule).

| FOOD | Serving Size | Calories | Tot Fat | Sat Fat | Chol |
|---|---|---|---|---|---|
| LAND O'LAKES American Pasteurized Process Cheese | | | | | |
| ✍ American | 1 oz | 110 | 14% | 31% | 10% |
| ✍ American & Swiss | 1 oz | 100 | 13% | 29% | 11% |
| ✍ American, Sharp | 1 oz | 110 | 14% | 30% | 9% |
| ✍ Less Salt | 1 oz | 110 | 14% | 32% | 9% |
| ❖ *Light*, Reduced Fat | 1 oz | 70 | 7% | 15% | 6% |
| ✍ OLD ENGLISH Sharp American Pasteurized Process—KRAFT | 1 oz | 100 | 14% | 30% | 8% |

CHEDDAR CHEESE

**Generic Foods**

| | | | | | |
|---|---|---|---|---|---|
| ✍ Cheddar | 1 oz | 110 | 14% | 30% | 10% |
| ✍ Cheddar, shredded | 1/4 cup | 110 | 14% | 30% | 10% |

**Brand Name Foods**

| | | | | | |
|---|---|---|---|---|---|
| ALPINE LACE | | | | | |
| ❖ Cheddar, Reduced Fat | 1 oz | 80 | 7% | 15% | 5% |
| ★ Cheddar Pasteurized Process Skim Milk, Fat Free | 1 oz | 45 | 0% | 0% | 1% |
| ❖ CRACKER BARREL Cheddar Cheese, Reduced Fat—KRAFT | 1 oz | 80 | 8% | 15% | 7% |
| HEALTHY CHOICE Shreds—CONAGRA | | | | | |
| ★ Cheddar | 1/4 cup | 45 | 0% | 0% | 1% |
| ★ Fancy Cheddar | 1/4 cup | 45 | 0% | 0% | 1% |
| KRAFT Pasteurized Process Cheese Product | | | | | |
| ★ *Free* Fat Free Singles Sharp Cheddar Artificially Flavored Nonfat | 2/3 oz | 30 | 0% | 0% | 1% |
| ★ *Healthy Favorites* Fat Free Cheddar Cheese, shredded | 1/4 cup | 45 | 0% | 0% | 1% |
| ❖ Singles Sharp Cheddar Flavor | 3/4 oz | 70 | 8% | 18% | 5% |
| KRAFT Natural Reduced Fat Cheese | | | | | |
| ❖ Mild Cheddar, shredded | 1/4 cup | 80 | 8% | 18% | 7% |
| ❖ Mild or Sharp Cheddar | 1 oz | 80 | 8% | 18% | 7% |
| LAND O'LAKES | | | | | |
| ✍ *Chedarella* | 1 oz | 100 | 12% | 26% | 8% |
| ❖ *Light* Cheddar, Reduced Fat | 1 oz | 70 | 6% | 13% | 4% |
| MOO TOWN SNACKERS—SARGENTO | | | | | |
| ✍ Cheddar | 1 piece | 100 | 12% | 25% | 8% |
| ❖ Light Mild Cheddar | 1 piece | 60 | 6% | 13% | 3% |

| FOOD | Serving Size | Calories | Tot Fat | Sat Fat | Chol |
|------|------|------|------|------|------|
| **SARGENTO** | | | | | |
| ❖ Imitation Cheddar Cheese, shredded | 1/4 cup | 90 | 10% | 6% | 0% |
| ❖ *Preferred Light* Mild Cheddar, shredded | 1/4 cup | 70 | 7% | 14% | 3% |
| Ⓐ Cheddar Cheese, shredded | 1/4 cup | 110 | 14% | 31% | 10% |
| Ⓐ Cheddar Cheese, sliced | 1 slc | 110 | 14% | 31% | 10% |
| ❖ SPREADERY Cheddar Cheese Snack—KRAFT | 2 tbsp | 80 | 7% | 15% | 5% |
| ❖ Medium | 2 tbsp | 80 | 7% | 15% | 5% |
| ❖ Sharp | 2 tbsp | 80 | 7% | 15% | 5% |
| ❖ Vermont Sharp White | 2 tbsp | 80 | 7% | 15% | 5% |

### CHEESE SPREADS

**Brand Name Foods**

| FOOD | Serving Size | Calories | Tot Fat | Sat Fat | Chol |
|------|------|------|------|------|------|
| Ⓐ CHEEZ WHIZ Pasteurized Process Cheese Spread—KRAFT | 2 tbsp | 90 | 11% | 25% | 7% |
| Ⓐ Hot Salsa | 2 tbsp | 90 | 11% | 25% | 8% |
| Ⓐ Mild Salsa | 2 tbsp | 90 | 11% | 25% | 8% |
| Ⓐ w/Jalapeno Peppers | 2 tbsp | 90 | 11% | 25% | 8% |
| KRAFT Spreads | | | | | |
| Ⓐ Pasteurized Process Cheese Spread w/Bacon | 2 tbsp | 90 | 12% | 25% | 8% |
| ❖ Pimento | 2 tbsp | 80 | 9% | 20% | 7% |
| ❖ Pineapple | 2 tbsp | 70 | 8% | 18% | 5% |
| Ⓐ *Roka* Brand Blue | 2 tbsp | 80 | 11% | 23% | 7% |
| PRICE'S Cheese Spread —FROMAGERIE BEL | | | | | |
| ★ Light Pimiento | 2 tbsp | 60 | 5% | 5% | 3% |
| ❖ Pimiento | 2 tbsp | 80 | 10% | 13% | 6% |
| VELVEETA Pasteurized Process Cheese Spread—KRAFT | | | | | |
| ❖ *Italiana* | 1 oz | 80 | 9% | 20% | 7% |
| ❖ Original | 1 oz | 80 | 9% | 20% | 7% |
| ❖ w/Jalapeno Pepper (Mild or Hot) | 1 oz | 80 | 9% | 20% | 7% |

### COTTAGE CHEESE

**Generic Foods**

| FOOD | Serving Size | Calories | Tot Fat | Sat Fat | Chol |
|------|------|------|------|------|------|
| ★ Cottage Cheese (dry curd) | 1/4 cup | 30 | 0% | 0% | 1% |
| ★ Cottage Cheese, 1% Lowfat | 1/2 cup | 80 | 2% | 4% | 2% |
| ❖ Cottage Cheese, 2% Lowfat | 1/2 cup | 100 | 3% | 7% | 3% |

★ Foods with this symbol have less than or equal to 5% *Daily Value* for <u>all</u> three nutrients (5% Rule).
❖ Foods with this symbol have <u>at least one</u> of the three nutrients greater than 5% *Daily Value* but less than or equal to 20% *Daily Value*.
Ⓐ Foods with this symbol have <u>at least one</u> of the three nutrients greater than 20% *Daily Value* (20% Rule).

| FOOD | Serving Size | Calories | Tot Fat | Sat Fat | Chol |
|---|---|---|---|---|---|
| ❖ Cottage Cheese, 4% Fat (large curd) | 1/2 cup | 120 | 8% | 16% | 6% |
| ❖ Cottage Cheese, 4% Fat (small curd) | 1/2 cup | 110 | 7% | 15% | 5% |
| ❖ Ricotta, Part Skim Milk | 1/4 cup | 80 | 7% | 14% | 6% |
| Ⓐ Ricotta, Whole Milk | 1/4 cup | 100 | 11% | 23% | 9% |
| **Brand Name Foods** | | | | | |
| ★ BREAKSTONE'S Dry Curd Cottage Cheese—KRAFT | 1/4 cup | 45 | 0% | 0% | 2% |
| BREAKSTONE'S Low Fat Cottage Cheese, 2% Milk Fat—KRAFT | | | | | |
| ❖ Large Curd | 1/2 cup | 90 | 4% | 8% | 5% |
| ❖ Small Curd | 1/2 cup | 90 | 4% | 8% | 5% |
| Ⓐ BREAKSTONE'S Ricotta Cheese —KRAFT | 1/4 cup | 110 | 12% | 25% | 8% |
| KNUDSEN Cottage Cheese, 4% Milk Fat—KRAFT | | | | | |
| ❖ Large Curd | 1/2 cup | 130 | 8% | 18% | 10% |
| ❖ Small Curd | 1/2 cup | 120 | 8% | 18% | 8% |
| ★ KNUDSEN *Free* Fat Free Cottage Cheese—KRAFT | 1/2 cup | 80 | 0% | 0% | 3% |
| KNUDSEN Lowfat Cottage Cheese & Fruit, 1.5% Milk Fat—KRAFT | | | | | |
| ★ Peach | 4 oz | 110 | 2% | 5% | 3% |
| ★ Pineapple | 4 oz | 110 | 2% | 5% | 3% |
| ★ Strawberry | 4 oz | 110 | 2% | 5% | 3% |
| ❖ Tropical Fruit | 4 oz | 120 | 3% | 8% | 3% |
| LIGHT N' LIVELY Lowfat Cottage Cheese, 1% Milk Fat—KRAFT | | | | | |
| ★ Plain | 1/2 cup | 80 | 2% | 5% | 5% |
| ★ w/Garden Salad | 1/2 cup | 90 | 2% | 5% | 5% |
| ★ w/Peach & Pineapple | 1/2 cup | 120 | 2% | 5% | 3% |
| ★ LIGHT N' LIVELY *Free* Nonfat Cottage Cheese—KRAFT | 1/2 cup | 80 | 0% | 0% | 3% |
| SARGENTO Ricotta | | | | | |
| ❖ Light | 1/4 cup | 60 | 4% | 4% | 8% |
| ❖ Old Fashioned | 1/4 cup | 90 | 9% | 20% | 9% |
| ❖ Part-Skim | 1/4 cup | 80 | 8% | 17% | 7% |
| WEIGHT WATCHERS Cottage Cheese | | | | | |
| ★ 1% Milk Fat | 1/2 cup | 90 | 2% | 3% | 2% |
| ❖ 2% Milk Fat | 1/2 cup | 90 | 3% | 8% | 5% |

## CREAM CHEESE

**Generic Foods**

| | | | | | |
|---|---|---|---|---|---|
| Ⓐ Cream Cheese | 1 oz | 100 | 15% | 32% | 10% |
| Ⓐ Neufchâtel | 1 oz | 70 | 10% | 21% | 7% |

| FOOD | Serving Size | Calories | Tot Fat | Sat Fat | Chol |
|------|------|------|------|------|------|
| **Brand Name Foods** | | | | | |
| HEALTHY CHOICE Cream Cheese —CONAGRA | | | | | |
| ★ Herbs & Garlic | 2 tbsp | 25 | 0% | 0% | 1% |
| ★ Plain | 2 tbsp | 25 | 0% | 0% | 1% |
| ★ Strawberry | 2 tbsp | 35 | 0% | 0% | 1% |
| PHILADELPHIA BRAND Cream Cheese—KRAFT | | | | | |
| ❖ Neufchatel | 1 oz | 70 | 9% | 20% | 7% |
| ☻ Plain | 1 oz | 100 | 15% | 30% | 10% |
| ☻ w/Chives | 1 oz | 90 | 14% | 30% | 10% |
| ☻ w/Pimentos | 1 oz | 90 | 14% | 30% | 10% |
| ☻ Whipped | 3 tbsp | 110 | 17% | 35% | 12% |
| ☻ Whipped w/Smoked Salmon | 3 tbsp | 100 | 14% | 30% | 10% |
| PHILADELPHIA BRAND *Free* Fat Free Cream Cheese—KRAFT | | | | | |
| ★ Plain | 1 oz | 25 | 0% | 0% | 1% |
| ★ Soft | 2 tbsp | 30 | 0% | 0% | 1% |
| ❖ PHILADELPHIA BRAND *Light* Cream Cheese—KRAFT | 2 tbsp | 70 | 8% | 18% | 5% |
| PHILADELPHIA BRAND Soft Cream Cheese—KRAFT | | | | | |
| ☻ Plain | 2 tbsp | 100 | 15% | 35% | 10% |
| ☻ w/Chives & Onion | 2 tbsp | 110 | 15% | 35% | 10% |
| ☻ w/Herb & Garlic | 2 tbsp | 110 | 15% | 35% | 10% |
| ☻ w/Olive & Pimento | 2 tbsp | 100 | 14% | 30% | 10% |
| ☻ w/Pineapple | 2 tbsp | 100 | 14% | 30% | 10% |
| ☻ w/Smoked Salmon | 2 tbsp | 100 | 14% | 30% | 10% |
| ☻ w/Strawberry | 2 tbsp | 100 | 14% | 30% | 10% |
| SPREADERY Cheese Snack Neufchâtel Cheese—KRAFT | | | | | |
| ☻ w/Classic Ranch Flavor | 2 tbsp | 80 | 11% | 25% | 7% |
| ❖ w/Garden Vegetables | 2 tbsp | 70 | 9% | 20% | 7% |
| ☻ w/Garlic & Herb | 2 tbsp | 80 | 11% | 25% | 7% |
| ❖ WEIGHT WATCHERS Light Cream Cheese | 2 tbsp | 40 | 4% | 8% | 3% |

## MONTEREY JACK CHEESE

**Generic Foods**

| FOOD | Serving Size | Calories | Tot Fat | Sat Fat | Chol |
|------|------|------|------|------|------|
| ☻ Monterey Jack | 1 oz | 110 | 13% | 27% | 8% |

★ Foods with this symbol have less than or equal to 5% *Daily Value* for <u>all</u> three nutrients (5% Rule).

❖ Foods with this symbol have <u>at least one</u> of the three nutrients greater than 5% *Daily Value* but less than or equal to 20% *Daily Value*.

☻ Foods with this symbol have <u>at least one</u> of the three nutrients greater than 20% *Daily Value* (20% Rule).

| FOOD | Serving Size | Calories | Tot Fat | Sat Fat | Chol |
|------|-------------|----------|---------|---------|------|
| **Brand Name Foods** | | | | | |
| ❖ ALPINE LACE Reduced Fat | | | | | |
|     Monterey Jack | 1 oz | 70 | 7% | 15% | 5% |
|   KRAFT Natural Reduced Fat Cheese | | | | | |
| ❖   Monterey Jack | 1 oz | 80 | 8% | 18% | 7% |
| ★   Monterey Jack w/Peppers | 1 oz | 80 | 8% | 18% | 7% |
| Ⓐ LAND O'LAKES Monterey Jack | 1 oz | 110 | 14% | 25% | 10% |
|   SARGENTO Monterey Jack Cheese | | | | | |
| Ⓐ   Shredded | 1/4 cup | 100 | 13% | 27% | 10% |
| Ⓐ   Sliced | 1 slc | 100 | 13% | 27% | 10% |

MOZZARELLA CHEESE

| FOOD | Serving Size | Calories | Tot Fat | Sat Fat | Chol |
|------|-------------|----------|---------|---------|------|
| **Generic Foods** | | | | | |
| ❖ Mozzarella, Skim milk | 1 oz | 70 | 7% | 14% | 5% |
| ❖ Mozzarella, Whole milk | 1 oz | 80 | 9% | 19% | 7% |
| **Brand Name Foods** | | | | | |
| ALPINE LACE | | | | | |
| ❖   Low Moisture Part-Skim | | | | | |
|     Mozzarella (50% less sodium) | 1 oz | 70 | 8% | 15% | 5% |
| ★   Mozzarella Fat Free Pasteurized | | | | | |
|     Process Skim Milk Cheese | 1 oz | 45 | 0% | 0% | 1% |
|   HEALTHY CHOICE—CONAGRA | | | | | |
| ★   Fancy Mozzarella Shreds | 1/4 cup | 45 | 0% | 0% | 1% |
| ★   Mozzarella Shreds | 1/4 cup | 45 | 0% | 0% | 1% |
| ★   Mozzarella String Cheese | 1 stick | 45 | 0% | 0% | 1% |
|   KRAFT | | | | | |
| ★   *Healthy Favorites* Fat Free | | | | | |
|     Mozzarella Cheese, shredded | 1/4 cup | 50 | 0% | 0% | 1% |
| ❖   Natural Reduced Fat Low- | | | | | |
|     Moisture Part-Skim | | | | | |
|     Mozzarella, shredded | 1/4 cup | 80 | 8% | 18% | 7% |
| ❖ LAND O'LAKES Mozzarella | 1 oz | 80 | 9% | 18% | 5% |
|   SARGENTO | | | | | |
| ❖   Imitation Mozzarella Cheese, | | | | | |
|     shredded | 1/4 cup | 80 | 10% | 6% | 0% |
| ❖   Mozzarella Cheese, shredded | 1/4 cup | 80 | 9% | 18% | 6% |
| Ⓐ   Mozzarella Cheese, sliced | 1 slc | 130 | 13% | 29% | 9% |
| ❖   *Preferred Light* Mozzarella, | | | | | |
|     shredded | 1/4 cup | 70 | 6% | 12% | 3% |
| ❖   *Preferred Light* Mozzarella, sliced | 1 slc | 100 | 8% | 15% | 5% |

| FOOD | Serving Size | Calories | Tot Fat | Sat Fat | Chol |
|------|-------------|----------|---------|---------|------|

### PARMESAN AND ROMANO CHEESES

**Generic Foods**

| FOOD | Serving Size | Calories | Tot Fat | Sat Fat | Chol |
|------|-------------|----------|---------|---------|------|
| ★ Parmesan, grated | 2 tsp | 25 | 2% | 5% | 1% |
| Ⓐ Romano | 1 oz | 110 | 12% | 24% | 10% |

**Brand Name Foods**

| FOOD | Serving Size | Calories | Tot Fat | Sat Fat | Chol |
|------|-------------|----------|---------|---------|------|
| DI GIORNO Parmesan & Romano Cheeses—KRAFT | | | | | |
| ★ Parmesan | 2 tsp | 20 | 2% | 5% | 2% |
| ★ 100% Parmesan, grated | 2 tsp | 20 | 2% | 5% | 2% |
| ★ 100% Parmesan, shredded | 2 tsp | 20 | 2% | 5% | 1% |
| ★ Romano | 2 tsp | 20 | 2% | 5% | 2% |
| ★ 100% Romano, grated | 2 tsp | 25 | 2% | 5% | 2% |
| ★ 100% Romano, shredded | 2 tsp | 20 | 2% | 5% | 2% |
| ★ KRAFT *Free* Nonfat Grated Topping | 2 tsp | 15 | 0% | 0% | 0% |
| SARGENTO | | | | | |
| Ⓐ Parmesan & Romano Cheeses, shredded | 1/4 cup | 110 | 11% | 24% | 8% |
| Ⓐ Parmesan Cheese, shredded | 1/4 cup | 110 | 12% | 26% | 8% |

### SWISS CHEESE

**Generic Foods**

| FOOD | Serving Size | Calories | Tot Fat | Sat Fat | Chol |
|------|-------------|----------|---------|---------|------|
| Ⓐ Swiss | 1 oz | 110 | 12% | 25% | 9% |
| Ⓐ Swiss Pasteurized Process | 1 oz | 100 | 11% | 23% | 8% |

**Brand Name Foods**

| FOOD | Serving Size | Calories | Tot Fat | Sat Fat | Chol |
|------|-------------|----------|---------|---------|------|
| ALPINE LACE Swiss, Reduced Fat | | | | | |
| ❖ Baby Swiss | 1 oz | 90 | 9% | 20% | 7% |
| ❖ Swiss | 1 oz | 90 | 9% | 20% | 7% |
| KRAFT | | | | | |
| Ⓐ Deluxe Swiss Pasteurized Processed Cheese | 1 oz | 90 | 11% | 25% | 8% |
| ★ *Free* Singles Swiss Artificially Flavored Nonfat Pasteurized Process Cheese Product | 2/3 oz | 30 | 0% | 0% | 1% |
| ❖ Singles Swiss Flavor Pasteurized Process Cheese Product | 3/4 oz | 70 | 8% | 18% | 5% |
| LAND O'LAKES | | | | | |
| Ⓐ Baby Swiss | 1 oz | 110 | 13% | 25% | 9% |
| ❖ *Light Swiss*, Reduced Fat | 1 oz | 80 | 6% | 15% | 5% |

★  Foods with this symbol have less than or equal to 5% *Daily Value* for all three nutrients (5% Rule).

❖  Foods with this symbol have at least one of the three nutrients greater than 5% *Daily Value* but less than or equal to 20% *Daily Value*.

Ⓐ  Foods with this symbol have at least one of the three nutrients greater than 20% *Daily Value* (20% Rule).

| FOOD | Serving Size | Calories | Tot Fat | Sat Fat | Chol |
|------|--------------|----------|---------|---------|------|
| ⊛ Swiss | 1 oz | 110 | 12% | 28% | 9% |
| ⊛ SARGENTO Swiss Cheese, shredded | 1/4 cup | 110 | 13% | 27% | 9% |
| SARGENTO Swiss Cheese, sliced | | | | | |
| ⊛ Jarlsberg | 1 slc | 120 | 14% | 25% | 7% |
| ❖ *Preferred Light* Swiss | 1 slc | 80 | 6% | 13% | 6% |
| ❖ Swiss | 1 slc | 80 | 10% | 20% | 7% |
| ⊛ *Wafer Thin* Swiss | 2 slcs | 110 | 13% | 27% | 9% |

## *OTHER* CHEESES

**Generic Foods**

| FOOD | Serving Size | Calories | Tot Fat | Sat Fat | Chol |
|------|--------------|----------|---------|---------|------|
| ⊛ Blue | 1 oz | 100 | 13% | 27% | 7% |
| ⊛ Brie | 1 oz | 100 | 12% | 25% | 9% |
| ⊛ Camembert | 1 oz | 90 | 11% | 22% | 7% |
| ⊛ Caraway | 1 oz | 110 | 13% | 26% | 9% |
| ⊛ Cheshire | 1 oz | 110 | 13% | 28% | 10% |
| ⊛ Colby | 1 oz | 110 | 14% | 29% | 9% |
| ⊛ Edam | 1 oz | 100 | 12% | 25% | 8% |
| ⊛ Feta | 1 oz | 80 | 9% | 21% | 8% |
| ⊛ Fontina | 1 oz | 110 | 14% | 27% | 11% |
| ⊛ Goat, hard | 1 oz | 130 | 16% | 35% | 10% |
| ⊛ Goat, semisoft | 1 oz | 100 | 13% | 29% | 7% |
| ⊛ Goat, soft | 1 oz | 80 | 9% | 21% | 4% |
| ⊛ Gouda | 1 oz | 100 | 12% | 25% | 11% |
| ⊛ Gruyere | 1 oz | 120 | 14% | 27% | 10% |
| ⊛ Havarti | 1 oz | 120 | 16% | 33% | 11% |
| ⊛ Limburger | 1 oz | 90 | 12% | 24% | 9% |
| ⊛ Muenster | 1 oz | 100 | 13% | 27% | 9% |
| ⊛ Pimento Processed | 1 oz | 110 | 14% | 28% | 9% |
| ⊛ Port du Salut | 1 oz | 100 | 12% | 24% | 12% |
| ⊛ Provolone | 1 oz | 100 | 12% | 24% | 7% |
| ⊛ Roquefort | 1 oz | 110 | 13% | 27% | 9% |
| ⊛ Tilsit | 1 oz | 100 | 11% | 24% | 10% |

**Brand Name Foods**

| FOOD | Serving Size | Calories | Tot Fat | Sat Fat | Chol |
|------|--------------|----------|---------|---------|------|
| ALPINE LACE Reduced Fat Cheeses | | | | | |
| ❖ Colby | 1 oz | 80 | 8% | 15% | 5% |
| ⊛ Havarti | 1 oz | 90 | 12% | 25% | 8% |
| ❖ Lightly Smoked Provolone | 1 oz | 70 | 8% | 15% | 5% |
| ⊛ Muenster, Reduced Sodium | 1 oz | 100 | 14% | 25% | 8% |
| CHEEZ WHIZ—KRAFT | | | | | |
| ❖ *Light* Pasteurized Process Cheese Product | 2 tbsp | 80 | 5% | 10% | 5% |
| ❖ Squeezable Pasteurized Process Cheese Sauce | 2 tbsp | 100 | 12% | 20% | 5% |
| HEALTHY CHOICE—CONAGRA | | | | | |
| ★ Process Cheese Loaf | 1 oz | 35 | 0% | 0% | 1% |

| FOOD | Serving Size | Calories | Tot Fat | Sat Fat | Chol |
|------|------|------|------|------|------|
| ★ Mexican Shreds | 1/4 cup | 45 | 0% | 0% | 1% |
| ★ Pizza Shreds | 1/4 cup | 45 | 0% | 0% | 1% |
| ★ Pizza String Cheese | 1 stick | 45 | 0% | 0% | 1% |
| KRAFT | | | | | |
| ⊛ Deluxe Pimento Pasteurized Processed Cheese | 1 oz | 100 | 12% | 30% | 8% |
| ❖ Natural Reduced Fat Colby Cheese | 1 oz | 80 | 8% | 18% | 7% |
| LAND O'LAKES | | | | | |
| ⊛ Brick | 1 oz | 100 | 13% | 26% | 9% |
| ❖ *Light* Reduced Fat Jalapeno | 1 oz | 70 | 6% | 13% | 5% |
| ⊛ Muenster | 1 oz | 100 | 13% | 26% | 8% |
| ⊛ Provolone | 1 oz | 100 | 12% | 22% | 7% |
| MOO TOWN SNACKERS—SARGENTO | | | | | |
| ⊛ Colby-Jack | 1 pc | 90 | 12% | 25% | 7% |
| ❖ Light String | 1 pc | 60 | 4% | 10% | 3% |
| ❖ String | 1 pc | 70 | 7% | 16% | 4% |
| ⊛ SARGENTO Blue Cheese, crumbled | 1/4 cup | 100 | 13% | 26% | 7% |
| SARGENTO Cheeses, shredded | | | | | |
| ⊛ 4 Cheese Mexican Recipe Blend | 1/4 cup | 110 | 14% | 28% | 8% |
| ⊛ 6 Cheese Italian Recipe Blend | 1/4 cup | 90 | 10% | 21% | 7% |
| ⊛ Colby-Jack | 1/4 cup | 10 | 14% | 30% | 9% |
| ⊛ For Nachos & Tacos | 1/4 cup | 110 | 13% | 27% | 8% |
| ⊛ For Pizza | 1/4 cup | 90 | 10% | 21% | 6% |
| ⊛ For Tacos | 1/4 cup | 110 | 13% | 28% | 9% |
| ⊛ Pizza Double Cheese | 1/4 cup | 90 | 10% | 22% | 7% |
| ❖ *Preferred Light* For Tacos | 1/4 cup | 70 | 7% | 13% | 5% |
| SARGENTO Sliced Cheeses | | | | | |
| ⊛ Colby | 1 slc | 110 | 15% | 33% | 10% |
| ⊛ Muenster | 1 slc | 100 | 13% | 29% | 8% |
| ⊛ Provolone | 1 slc | 100 | 13% | 25% | 8% |
| ⊛ SPREADERY Cheese Snack Pimento Spread—KRAFT | 2 tbsp | 100 | 12% | 25% | 7% |
| THE LAUGHING COW— FROMAGERIE BEL | | | | | |
| ⊛ Bonbel | 1 oz | 100 | 12% | 25% | 8% |
| ❖ Mini Babybel | 1 pc | 70 | 9% | 20% | 5% |
| ❖ Original Wedge | 1 pc | 70 | 9% | 19% | 6% |
| ❖ VELVEETA *Light* Pasteurized Process Cheese Product—KRAFT | 1 oz | 60 | 5% | 10% | 3% |
| VELVEETA Shredded Pasteurized Process Cheese Food—KRAFT | | | | | |
| ⊛ Hot or Mild Mexican w/ Jalapeno Peppers | 1/4 cup | 130 | 14% | 30% | 10% |
| ⊛ Plain | 1/4 cup | 130 | 14% | 30% | 10% |

★ Foods with this symbol have less than or equal to 5% *Daily Value* for <u>all</u> three nutrients (5% Rule).

❖ Foods with this symbol have <u>at least one</u> of the three nutrients greater than 5% *Daily Value* but less than or equal to 20% *Daily Value*.

⊛ Foods with this symbol have <u>at least one</u> of the three nutrients greater than 20% *Daily Value* (20% Rule).

| FOOD | Serving Size | Calories | Tot Fat | Sat Fat | Chol |
|------|-------------|----------|---------|---------|------|
| WISPRIDE Port Wine Cup— FROMAGERIE BEL | | | | | |
| ❖ Light | 2 tbsp | 80 | 5% | 10% | 4% |
| ❖ Regular | 2 tbsp | 100 | 11% | 20% | 7% |
| ❖ WISPRIDE Sharp Cheese Log— FROMAGERIE BEL | 2 tbsp | 100 | 12% | 20% | 7% |

## COFFEE CREAMERS

### Brand Name Foods

| FOOD | Serving Size | Calories | Tot Fat | Sat Fat | Chol |
|------|-------------|----------|---------|---------|------|
| CARNATION *Coffee-Mate* Flavored Non-Dairy Creamers—NESTLÉ | | | | | |
| ★ Amaretto | 1 tbsp | 40 | 3% | 0% | 0% |
| ★ French Vanilla | 1 tbsp | 40 | 3% | 0% | 0% |
| ★ French Vanilla, Fat Free | 1 tbsp | 25 | 0% | 0% | 0% |
| ★ Hazelnut | 1 tbsp | 40 | 3% | 0% | 0% |
| ★ Hazelnut, Fat Free | 1 tbsp | 25 | 0% | 0% | 0% |
| ★ Irish Creme | 1 tbsp | 40 | 3% | 0% | 0% |
| CARNATION *Coffee-Mate* Non-Dairy Creamer—NESTLÉ | | | | | |
| ★ Fat Free | 1 tbsp | 10 | 0% | 0% | 0% |
| ★ Lite | 1 tbsp | 10 | 1% | 0% | 0% |
| ★ Regular | 1 tbsp | 20 | 2% | 0% | 0% |
| CREMORA—BORDEN | | | | | |
| ★ 35% Fat | 1 tsp | 10 | 1% | 3% | 0% |
| ★ Lite | 1 tsp | 10 | 0% | 0% | 0% |
| INTERNATIONAL DELIGHT— M STAR INC. | | | | | |
| ★ Cinnamon Hazelnut | 1 tbsp | 45 | 2% | 0% | 0% |
| ★ Irish Creme | 1 tbsp | 45 | 2% | 0% | 0% |
| ★ Suisse Chocolate Mocha | 1 tbsp | 45 | 2% | 0% | 0% |
| INTERNATIONAL DELIGHT Cappuccino, No Fat—M STAR INC. | | | | | |
| ★ Hazelnut | 1 tbsp | 25 | 0% | 0% | 0% |
| ★ Italian Style | 1 tbsp | 25 | 0% | 0% | 0% |
| ★ Raspberry | 1 tbsp | 25 | 0% | 0% | 0% |
| MOCHA MIX Non-Dairy Creamer —PRESTO FOODS | | | | | |
| ★ Fat Free | 1 tbsp | 10 | 0% | 0% | 0% |
| ★ Lite | 1 tbsp | 10 | 1% | 0% | 0% |
| ★ Original | 1 tbsp | 20 | 2% | 0% | 0% |
| SIGNATURE FLAVORS, Fat Free —PRESTO FOODS | | | | | |
| ★ French Vanilla | 1 tbsp | 35 | 0% | 0% | 0% |
| ★ Irish Creme | 1 tbsp | 35 | 0% | 0% | 0% |
| ★ *Kahlua* | 1 tbsp | 35 | 0% | 0% | 0% |
| ★ *Mauna Loa* Macadamia Nut | 1 tbsp | 35 | 0% | 0% | 0% |

| FOOD | Serving Size | Calories | Tot Fat | Sat Fat | Chol |
|------|------|------|------|------|------|
| SIGNATURE FLAVORS Half and Half—PRESTO FOODS | | | | | |
| ❖ Almond Roca Buttercrunch | 2 tbsp | 80 | 5% | 10% | 3% |
| ❖ French Vanilla | 2 tbsp | 80 | 5% | 10% | 3% |
| ❖ Irish Creme | 2 tbsp | 80 | 5% | 10% | 3% |
| ★ SWISS MISS N-Rich Coffee Creamer—HUNT WESSON | 1 tsp | 10 | 1% | 1% | 0% |

## CREAM

**Generic Foods**

| FOOD | Serving Size | Calories | Tot Fat | Sat Fat | Chol |
|------|------|------|------|------|------|
| ★ Cream, Half & Half | 1 tbsp | 20 | 3% | 5% | 2% |
| ❖ Cream, Light | 1 tbsp | 30 | 4% | 9% | 3% |
| ❖ Cream, Whipping, Heavy (unwhipped) | 1 tbsp | 50 | 8% | 17% | 7% |
| ❖ Cream, Whipping, Light (unwhipped) | 1 tbsp | 45 | 7% | 14% | 6% |

## DAIRY SUBSTITUTES: CHEESE

**Brand Name Foods**

| FOOD | Serving Size | Calories | Tot Fat | Sat Fat | Chol |
|------|------|------|------|------|------|
| ❖ BETTER THAN CREAM CHEESE (nondairy)—TOFUTTI | 1 oz | 80 | 12% | 10% | 0% |
| NUTOFU Soy Cheese Products | | | | | |
| ❖ Cheddar | 1 oz | 70 | 6% | 3% | 0% |
| ★ Cheddar, fat free | 1 oz | 40 | 0% | 0% | 0% |
| ❖ Herb Spice | 1 oz | 70 | 6% | 3% | 0% |
| ❖ Jalapeno | 1 oz | 70 | 6% | 3% | 0% |
| ❖ Monterey Jack | 1 oz | 70 | 6% | 3% | 0% |
| ❖ Mozzarella | 1 oz | 70 | 6% | 3% | 0% |
| ★ Mozzarella, fat free | 1 oz | 40 | 0% | 0% | 0% |

## DAIRY SUBSTITUTES: DRINKS

**Generic Foods**

| FOOD | Serving Size | Calories | Tot Fat | Sat Fat | Chol |
|------|------|------|------|------|------|
| ❖ Soy Milk | 1 oz | 80 | 7% | 3% | 0% |

**Brand Name Foods**

| FOOD | Serving Size | Calories | Tot Fat | Sat Fat | Chol |
|------|------|------|------|------|------|
| ★ HEALTH VALLEY Fat Free Soy Moo Soy Drink | 1 cup | 110 | 0% | 0% | 0% |

★ Foods with this symbol have less than or equal to 5% *Daily Value* for <u>all</u> three nutrients (5% Rule).

❖ Foods with this symbol have <u>at least one</u> of the three nutrients greater than 5% *Daily Value* but less than or equal to 20% *Daily Value*.

Ⓐ Foods with this symbol have <u>at least one</u> of the three nutrients greater than 20% *Daily Value* (20% Rule).

| FOOD | Serving Size | Calories | Tot Fat | Sat Fat | Chol |
|------|------|------|------|------|------|
| ❖ LOMA LINDA *Soyagen*— | | | | | |
|    WORTHINGTON FOODS | 1/4 cup | 130 | 9% | 5% | 0% |
| RICE DREAM—IMAGINE FOODS | | | | | |
| ★   Carob Lite | 1 cup | 150 | 5% | 0% | 0% |
| ★   Chocolate | 1 cup | 190 | 5% | 0% | 0% |
| ★   Organic Original Lite | 1 cup | 120 | 3% | 1% | 0% |
| ★   Vanilla Lite | 1 cup | 120 | 3% | 1% | 0% |
| WESTBRAE Rice Drinks | | | | | |
| ★   Plain | 8 fl oz | 100 | 5% | 3% | 0% |
| ★   Vanilla | 8 fl oz | 120 | 5% | 3% | 0% |
| WESTSOY Beverages— | | | | | |
|    WESTBRAE NATURAL | | | | | |
| ❖   100% Organic, Original | 8 fl oz | 140 | 8% | 5% | 0% |
| ❖   100% Organic, Unsweetened | 8 fl oz | 80 | 6% | 3% | 0% |
| ★   Non Fat, Plain | 8 fl oz | 80 | 0% | 0% | 0% |
| ★   Non Fat, Vanilla | 8 fl oz | 80 | 0% | 0% | 0% |
| ★   Soy Drink, Plain | 8 fl oz | 90 | 3% | 3% | 0% |
| ★   Soy Drink, Vanilla | 8 fl oz | 120 | 3% | 3% | 0% |
| WESTSOY Lite Beverages— | | | | | |
|    WESTBRAE NATURAL | | | | | |
| ★   Cocoa | 8 fl oz | 150 | 4% | 2% | 0% |
| ★   Plain | 8 fl oz | 100 | 3% | 2% | 0% |
| ★   Vanilla | 8 fl oz | 120 | 4% | 2% | 0% |
| WESTSOY Malteds— | | | | | |
|    WESTBRAE NATURAL | | | | | |
| ❖   Almond | 1 pkg | 240 | 18% | 13% | 0% |
| ❖   Carob | 1 pkg | 270 | 18% | 13% | 0% |
| ❖   Java | 1 pkg | 270 | 18% | 13% | 0% |
| WESTSOY Plus Beverages— | | | | | |
|    WESTBRAE NATURAL | | | | | |
| ❖   Cocoa | 8 fl oz | 190 | 6% | 5% | 0% |
| ❖   Plain | 8 fl oz | 130 | 6% | 2% | 0% |
| ❖   Vanilla | 8 fl oz | 150 | 6% | 2% | 0% |

## MILK

**Generic Foods**

| FOOD | Serving Size | Calories | Tot Fat | Sat Fat | Chol |
|------|------|------|------|------|------|
| ❖ Buttermilk | 1 cup | 100 | 3% | 7% | 3% |
| ❖ Condensed, Sweetened (canned) | 2 tbsp | 120 | 5% | 11% | 4% |
| ★ Evaporated, Skim (canned) | 2 tbsp | 25 | 0% | 0% | 0% |
| ❖ Evaporated, Whole (canned) | 2 tbsp | 40 | 4% | 7% | 3% |
| ⊛ Goat, Whole | 1 oz | 170 | 16% | 33% | 9% |
| ❖ Lowfat, 1% Milk Fat | 1 cup | 100 | 4% | 8% | 3% |
| ❖ Lowfat, 2% Milk Fat | 1 cup | 120 | 7% | 15% | 6% |
| ★ Skim/Nonfat | 1 cup | 90 | 1% | 1% | 1% |
| ⊛ Whole, 3.3% Milk Fat | 1 cup | 150 | 13% | 25% | 11% |

| FOOD | Serving Size | Calories | Tot Fat | Sat Fat | Chol |
|---|---|---|---|---|---|
| **Brand Name Foods** | | | | | |
| CARNATION Evaporated Milk —NESTLÉ | | | | | |
| ★ Lowfat | 2 tbsp | 25 | 1% | 0% | 2% |
| ★ Skim | 2 tbsp | 25 | 0% | 0% | 0% |
| ❖ Whole | 2 tbsp | 40 | 4% | 7% | 3% |
| CARNATION Milk—NESTLÉ | | | | | |
| ★ Nonfat Dry Milk Powder | 1/3 cup dry | 80 | 0% | 0% | 1% |
| ❖ Sweetened Condensed | 2 tbsp | 130 | 5% | 10% | 3% |
| EAGLE Brand Sweetened Condensed Milk—BORDEN | | | | | |
| ★ Fat Free | 2 tbsp | 110 | 0% | 0% | 1% |
| ★ Low Fat | 2 tbsp | 120 | 2% | 5% | 2% |
| ❖ Regular (8% Milk Fat) | 2 tbsp | 130 | 5% | 10% | 3% |
| PET Evaporated Milk | | | | | |
| ❖ Regular | 2 tbsp | 40 | 3% | 6% | 2% |
| ★ Skim | 2 tbsp | 25 | 0% | 0% | 1% |

### SOUR CREAM

| FOOD | Serving Size | Calories | Tot Fat | Sat Fat | Chol |
|---|---|---|---|---|---|
| **Generic Foods** | | | | | |
| ❖ Sour Cream | 2 tbsp | 60 | 9% | 19% | 4% |
| ❖ Sour Cream, Half and Half | 1 oz | 40 | 6% | 11% | 4% |
| Ⓐ Sour Cream, Imitation | 1 oz | 60 | 9% | 27% | 0% |
| **Brand Name Foods** | | | | | |
| BREAKSTONE'S Sour Cream—KRAFT | | | | | |
| ★ *Free* Fat Free | 2 tbsp | 35 | 0% | 0% | 1% |
| ❖ Regular | 2 tbsp | 60 | 8% | 20% | 8% |
| Ⓐ IMO Sour Cream Substitute | 1 oz | 60 | 9% | 26% | 0% |
| KNUDSEN Sour Cream—KRAFT | | | | | |
| ★ *Free* Fat Free | 2 tbsp | 35 | 0% | 0% | 0% |
| ❖ *Hampshire* | 2 tbsp | 60 | 9% | 20% | 8% |
| ❖ *Light* | 2 tbsp | 40 | 4% | 10% | 3% |
| ★ NATURALLY YOURS Real Dairy No Fat Sour Cream | 2 tbsp | 20 | 0% | 0% | 0% |
| ❖ SOUR SUPREME Better Than Sour Cream (nondairy)—TOFUTTI | 1 oz | 50 | 8% | 10% | 0% |
| STONYFIELD FARM Sour Cream | | | | | |
| ❖ Light | 2 tbsp | 45 | 5% | 10% | 3% |
| ❖ Regular | 2 tbsp | 60 | 9% | 18% | 7% |

★ Foods with this symbol have less than or equal to 5% *Daily Value* for all three nutrients (5% Rule).
❖ Foods with this symbol have at least one of the three nutrients greater than 5% *Daily Value* but less than or equal to 20% *Daily Value*.
Ⓐ Foods with this symbol have at least one of the three nutrients greater than 20% *Daily Value* (20% Rule).

| FOOD | Serving Size | Calories | Tot Fat | Sat Fat | Chol |
|------|-------------|----------|---------|---------|------|

## WHIPPED TOPPINGS

**Generic Foods**

| FOOD | Serving Size | Calories | Tot Fat | Sat Fat | Chol |
|------|-------------|----------|---------|---------|------|
| ❖ Cream, Whipped, Imitation (frozen) | 2 tbsp | 30 | 4% | 10% | 0% |
| ★ Cream, Whipped, Imitation (pressurized) | 2 tbsp | 20 | 3% | 5% | 2% |
| ❖ Cream, Whipped, Imitation (pressurized) | 2 tbsp | 25 | 3% | 8% | 0% |

**Brand Name Foods**

| FOOD | Serving Size | Calories | Tot Fat | Sat Fat | Chol |
|------|-------------|----------|---------|---------|------|
| ❖ BORDEN Heavy Whipping Cream | 1 tbsp | 50 | 9% | 15% | 7% |
| COOL WHIP Whipped Topping —KRAFT | | | | | |
| ❖   Extra Creamy | 2 tbsp | 30 | 3% | 10% | 0% |
| ★   Lite | 2 tbsp | 20 | 2% | 5% | 0% |
| ❖   Non-Dairy | 2 tbsp | 25 | 2% | 8% | 0% |
| ★ D-ZERTA Reduced Calorie Whipped Topping Mix (prep as dir)—KRAFT | 2 tbsp | 10 | 1% | 4% | 0% |
| ★ DREAM WHIP Whipped Topping Mix (prep w/2% milk)—KRAFT | 2 tbsp | 20 | 1% | 4% | 0% |
| ★ ESTEE Whipped Topping Mix | 3/4 tsp mix | 10 | 1% | 0% | 0% |
| KRAFT Toppings | | | | | |
| ★   Real Cream | 2 tbsp | 20 | 2% | 5% | 2% |
| ★   Whipped | 2 tbsp | 20 | 2% | 5% | 0% |
| ★ LA CREME Lite Whipped Topping—PET | 2 tbsp | 15 | 2% | 5% | 0% |
| ❖ PET Whip Non-Dairy Topping | 2 tbsp | 30 | 3% | 10% | 0% |
| ❖ REDDI WIP—BEATRICE CHEESE | 2 tbsp | 20 | 2% | 6% | 2% |

## YOGURT

**Brand Name Foods**

| FOOD | Serving Size | Calories | Tot Fat | Sat Fat | Chol |
|------|-------------|----------|---------|---------|------|
| BREYER'S Lowfat Yogurt—KRAFT | | | | | |
| ❖   1% Milk Fat: All flavors | 8 oz | 250 | 4% | 8% | 5% |
| ❖   1.5% Milk Fat: All flavors | 8 oz | 220 | 5% | 10% | 7% |
| DANNON | | | | | |
| ❖   *Double Delights* Lowfat Yogurt w/Fruit Toppings: All flavors | 6 oz | 170 | 4% | 7% | 4% |
| ❖   Fruit On The Bottom Lowfat Yogurt: All flavors | 8 oz | 240 | 5% | 8% | 5% |
| ★   *Light* Nonfat Yogurt: All flavors | 8 oz | 100 | 0% | 0% | 2% |
| ★   Nonfat Yogurt, Plain | 8 oz | 110 | 0% | 0% | 2% |
| ❖   *Sprinkl'ins* Lowfat Yogurt w/ Sprinkles: All flavors | 4.1 oz | 140 | 4% | 8% | 3% |
| ★   *Tropifruta* Nonfat Yogurt: All flavors | 6 oz | 150 | 0% | 0% | 1% |

| FOOD | Serving Size | Calories | Tot Fat | Sat Fat | Chol |
|---|---|---|---|---|---|
| DANNON Blended Nonfat Yogurt | | | | | |
| ★ Blueberry | 6 oz | 160 | 0% | 0% | 0% |
| ★ French Vanilla | 6 oz | 160 | 0% | 0% | 0% |
| ★ Lemon Chiffon | 6 oz | 150 | 0% | 0% | 0% |
| ★ Peach | 6 oz | 150 | 0% | 0% | 0% |
| ★ Raspberry | 6 oz | 160 | 0% | 0% | 0% |
| ★ Strawberry | 6 oz | 150 | 0% | 0% | 0% |
| ★ Strawberry Banana | 6 oz | 150 | 0% | 0% | 0% |
| DANNON *Danimals* Lowfat Yogurt | | | | | |
| ❖ All flavors except Grape Lemonade; Wild Raspberry | 4.4 oz | 140 | 3% | 6% | 3% |
| ❖ Grape Lemonade | 4.4 oz | 130 | 3% | 6% | 3% |
| ❖ Wild Raspberry | 4.4 oz | 130 | 3% | 6% | 3% |
| DANNON *Light 'n Crunchy* Nonfat Yogurt | | | | | |
| ★ All flavors except Lemon Chiffon w/Blueberry | 8 oz | 150 | 0% | 0% | 1% |
| ★ Lemon Chiffon w/Blueberry | 8 oz | 140 | 0% | 0% | 1% |
| DANNON Lowfat Yogurt | | | | | |
| ❖ All flavors except Coffee; Lemon; Plain; Vanilla | 8 oz | 210 | 5% | 10% | 5% |
| ❖ Coffee | 8 oz | 230 | 5% | 10% | 7% |
| ❖ Lemon | 8 oz | 230 | 5% | 10% | 7% |
| ❖ Plain | 8 oz | 140 | 6% | 11% | 6% |
| ❖ Vanilla | 8 oz | 230 | 5% | 10% | 7% |
| DANNON *Sprinkl'ins Crazy Crunch* Lowfat Yogurt | | | | | |
| ❖ Cherry w/Honey Grahams | 4.4 oz | 170 | 4% | 8% | 3% |
| ❖ Grape w/Chocolate Grahams | 4.4 oz | 160 | 4% | 7% | 3% |
| ❖ Vanilla w/Chocolate Grahams | 4.4 oz | 160 | 4% | 7% | 3% |
| ❖ Vanilla w/Honey Grahams | 4.4 oz | 170 | 4% | 8% | 3% |
| ★ KNUDSEN *Cal 70* Nonfat Yogurt w/Aspartame: All flavors—KRAFT | 6 oz | 70 | 0% | 0% | 2% |
| KNUDSEN *Free* Nonfat Yogurt—KRAFT | | | | | |
| ★ Lemon | 6 oz | 160 | 0% | 0% | 2% |
| ★ Mixed Berry | 6 oz | 170 | 0% | 0% | 2% |
| ★ Peach | 6 oz | 170 | 0% | 0% | 2% |
| ★ Red Raspberry | 6 oz | 160 | 0% | 0% | 2% |
| ★ Strawberry | 6 oz | 160 | 0% | 0% | 2% |
| ★ Vanilla | 6 oz | 170 | 0% | 0% | 2% |
| LIGHT N' LIVELY—KRAFT | | | | | |
| ★ *Free 50 Calories* Nonfat Yogurt w/Aspartame: All flavors | 4.4 oz | 50 | 0% | 0% | 1% |
| ★ *Free 70 Calories* Nonfat Yogurt w/Aspartame: All flavors | 6 oz | 70 | 0% | 0% | 2% |

★ Foods with this symbol have less than or equal to 5% *Daily Value* for all three nutrients (5% Rule).
❖ Foods with this symbol have at least one of the three nutrients greater than 5% *Daily Value* but less than or equal to 20% *Daily Value*.
Ⓐ Foods with this symbol have at least one of the three nutrients greater than 20% *Daily Value* (20% Rule).

| FOOD | Serving Size | Calories | Tot Fat | Sat Fat | Chol |
|---|---|---|---|---|---|
| LIGHT N' LIVELY *Free* Nonfat Yogurt—KRAFT | | | | | |
| ★ Blueberry | 6 oz | 190 | 0% | 0% | 2% |
| ★ Lemon Flavored | 6 oz | 170 | 0% | 0% | 2% |
| ★ Mixed Berry | 6 oz | 170 | 0% | 0% | 2% |
| ★ Peach | 6 oz | 170 | 0% | 0% | 2% |
| ★ Red Raspberry | 6 oz | 180 | 0% | 0% | 2% |
| ★ Strawberry | 6 oz | 180 | 0% | 0% | 2% |
| ★ Strawberry Fruit Cup | 6 oz | 170 | 0% | 0% | 2% |
| ★ Vanilla | 6 oz | 160 | 0% | 0% | 2% |
| ★ MOUNTAIN HIGH Honey De-Lite 0.5% Lowfat Yogurt: All flavors—BORDEN | 8 oz | 190 | 2% | 3% | 3% |
| STONYFIELD FARM Nonfat Yogurt | | | | | |
| ★ Apricot Mango | 1 cup | 150 | 0% | 0% | 1% |
| ★ Plain | 1 cup | 100 | 0% | 0% | 1% |
| ★ Wild Blueberry | 1 cup | 160 | 0% | 0% | 1% |
| ★ WEIGHT WATCHERS *Ultimate 90*: All flavors | 1 cup | 90 | 0% | 0% | 2% |
| YOPLAIT—GENERAL MILLS | | | | | |
| ★ Fruit-on-the-Bottom Fat Free Yogurt: All flavors | 6 oz | 160 | 0% | 0% | 1% |
| ★ Light Yogurt: All flavors | 6 oz | 90 | 0% | 0% | 0% |
| ❖ Original Nonfat Yogurt, Plain | 6 oz | 100 | 0% | 0% | 2% |
| ❖ *Trix* Yogurt: All flavors | 6 oz | 180 | 4% | 7% | 3% |
| YOPLAIT Crunch 'n Yogurt—GENERAL MILLS | | | | | |
| ★ Peach w/Granola | 7 oz | 220 | 3% | 0% | 1% |
| ★ Strawberry w/Cereal Nuggets | 7 oz | 200 | 1% | 0% | 1% |
| ★ Strawberry w/Granola | 7 oz | 220 | 3% | 0% | 1% |
| ★ Vanilla w/Chocolate Flavored Crunchies | 7 oz | 220 | 3% | 2% | 1% |
| ★ Vanilla w/Granola | 7 oz | 220 | 3% | 0% | 1% |
| YOPLAIT Crunch 'n Yogurt Light—GENERAL MILLS | | | | | |
| ★ Cappuccino w/Chocolate Nuggets | 7 oz | 130 | 2% | 0% | 1% |
| ★ Cherry Cheesecake w/Graham Crunch | 7 oz | 130 | 2% | 0% | 1% |
| ★ Raspberry w/Granola | 7 oz | 130 | 2% | 0% | 1% |
| ★ Strawberry w/Granola | 7 oz | 130 | 2% | 0% | 1% |
| YOPLAIT Custard Style Yogurt—GENERAL MILLS | | | | | |
| ❖ Fruit flavors | 6 oz | 170 | 4% | 8% | 4% |
| ❖ Vanilla | 6 oz | 170 | 4% | 9% | 4% |
| YOPLAIT Extra Creamy Non-Fat Yogurt—GENERAL MILLS | | | | | |
| ★ Plain | 1 cup | 140 | 0% | 0% | 2% |
| ★ Vanilla | 1 cup | 210 | 0% | 0% | 2% |

| | FOOD | Serving Size | Calories | Tot Fat | Sat Fat | Chol |
|---|---|---|---|---|---|---|
| ★ | All fruit flavors | | | | | |
| ★ | Custard Style | 6 oz | 90 | 0% | 0% | 0% |
| | YOPLAIT Low-Fat Breakfast Yogurt—GENERAL MILLS | | | | | |
| ★ | Mixed Berry | 6 oz | 200 | 3% | 4% | 3% |
| ★ | Strawberry Banana | 6 oz | 200 | 3% | 5% | 3% |
| ★ | Tropical Fruit | 6 oz | 210 | 4% | 5% | 3% |
| | YOPLAIT Original 99% Fat Free Yogurt—GENERAL MILLS | | | | | |
| ★ | All fruit flavors | 6 oz | 180 | 3% | 5% | 3% |
| ❖ | Vanilla | 6 oz | 170 | 3% | 6% | 3% |

# Desserts

## BARS

### Generic Foods

| | FOOD | Serving Size | Calories | Tot Fat | Sat Fat | Chol |
|---|---|---|---|---|---|---|
| ❖ | Date Squares | 1 square | 200 | 7% | 6% | 13% |
| ❖ | Rice Krispie Square w/Almonds | 1 oz bar | 130 | 9% | 5% | 0% |
| ❖ | Rice Krispie Square w/Chocolate Chips | 1 oz bar | 150 | 6% | 7% | 0% |

### Brand Name Foods

| | FOOD | Serving Size | Calories | Tot Fat | Sat Fat | Chol |
|---|---|---|---|---|---|---|
| | BETTY CROCKER Supreme Dessert Bar & Cookie Mixes (prep as dir)—GENERAL MILLS | | | | | |
| ★ | Caramel Oatmeal | 1 bar | 180 | 12% | 9% | 0% |
| ❖ | Chocolate Chunk | 1 bar | 180 | 13% | 13% | 4% |
| ❖ | Chocolate Peanut Butter | 1 bar | 170 | 11% | 11% | 4% |
| ❖ | Easy Layer | 1 bar | 170 | 12% | 19% | 0% |
| ❖ | *M&M's* Cookie | 1 bar | 170 | 12% | 12% | 4% |
| ❖ | Raspberry | 1 bar | 170 | 9% | 7% | 0% |
| ❖ | Strawberry Swirl Cheese Cake | 1 bar | 180 | 16% | 14% | 6% |
| ❖ | *Sunkist* Lemon | 1 bar | 140 | 6% | 6% | 12% |
| | DELUXE Bar Mixes (prep as dir) —PILLSBURY | | | | | |
| ❖ | Apple Streusel | 1/24 pan | 150 | 9% | 8% | 0% |
| ❖ | *Chips Ahoy!* | 1/18 pan | 180 | 11% | 10% | 3% |
| ❖ | Fudge Swirl Cookie | 1/20 pan | 180 | 12% | 8% | 3% |
| ❖ | Lemon Cheesecake | 1/24 pan | 180 | 15% | 18% | 8% |
| ❖ | *Nutter Butter* | 1/18 pan | 180 | 11% | 8% | 5% |
| ❖ | *Oreo* | 1/24 pan | 150 | 9% | 8% | 3% |

★ Foods with this symbol have less than or equal to 5% *Daily Value* for all three nutrients (5% Rule).
❖ Foods with this symbol have at least one of the three nutrients greater than 5% *Daily Value* but less than or equal to 20% *Daily Value*.
✇ Foods with this symbol have at least one of the three nutrients greater than 20% *Daily Value* (20% Rule).

| FOOD | Serving Size | Calories | Tot Fat | Sat Fat | Chol |
|------|--------------|----------|---------|---------|------|
| **LITTLE DEBBIE Individual Snacks** | | | | | |
| —MCKEE | | | | | |
| ✺ *Nutty Bars* Wafer Bars | 1 pkg | 270 | 24% | 14% | 0% |
| ✺ Peanut Butter Bars | 1 pkg | 250 | 21% | 11% | 0% |

<u>BROWNIES</u>

**Generic Foods**

| | | | | | |
|------|--------------|----------|---------|---------|------|
| ❖ Brownie (large) | 1 brownie | 230 | 14% | 12% | 3% |
| ❖ Brownie (small, 1 3/4" × 3/4") | 1 brownie | 120 | 7% | 6% | 2% |

**Brand Name Foods**

| | | | | | |
|------|--------------|----------|---------|---------|------|
| ARROWHEAD MILLS Brownie Mixes | | | | | |
| ★ Fat Free | 1 brownie | 120 | 0% | 0% | 0% |
| ★ Regular | 1 brownie | 110 | 1% | 0% | 0% |
| BETTY CROCKER Brownie Mixes | | | | | |
| (prep as dir)—GENERAL MILLS | | | | | |
| ❖ Caramel | 1 brownie | 190 | 13% | 9% | 8% |
| ❖ Chocolate Chip | 1 brownie | 200 | 16% | 14% | 8% |
| ❖ Cookies & Cream | 1 brownie | 200 | 15% | 10% | 8% |
| ❖ Dark Chocolate Fudge | 1 brownie | 190 | 13% | 9% | 8% |
| ❖ Frosted | 1 brownie | 230 | 15% | 12% | 8% |
| ❖ Fudge | 1 brownie | 190 | 12% | 8% | 6% |
| ❖ German Chocolate | 1 brownie | 220 | 14% | 12% | 8% |
| ❖ Hot Fudge | 1 brownie | 190 | 13% | 13% | 8% |
| ❖ Original | 1 brownie | 200 | 13% | 9% | 8% |
| ❖ Peanut Butter Candies w/ | | | | | |
| *Reese's Pieces* | 1 brownie | 210 | 16% | 14% | 8% |
| ❖ Walnut | 1 brownie | 200 | 17% | 10% | 8% |
| ❖ White-Chocolate Swirl | 1 brownie | 210 | 15% | 15% | 8% |
| DELUXE Brownie Mixes | | | | | |
| (prep as dir)—PILLSBURY | | | | | |
| ❖ Chocolate Deluxe | 1/20 cake | 180 | 11% | 8% | 3% |
| ❖ Cream Cheese Swirl | 1/20 cake | 180 | 14% | 13% | 8% |
| ❖ Fudge (21.5 oz) | 1/20 cake | 180 | 12% | 8% | 3% |
| ❖ Hot Fudge | 1/24 cake | 160 | 11% | 10% | 3% |
| ★ *Lovin' Lites* Fudge | 1/16 cake | 160 | 5% | 5% | 5% |
| ❖ Walnut | 1/18 cake | 180 | 14% | 8% | 3% |
| DUNCAN HINES Brownie Mixes | | | | | |
| (prep as basic recipe)— | | | | | |
| PROCTER & GAMBLE | | | | | |
| ❖ Chewy Recipe Fudge | 1 brownie | 160 | 11% | 6% | 3% |
| ❖ Dark Choc. Flavor Fudge w/ | | | | | |
| Milk Choc. Chunks | 1 brownie | 160 | 11% | 8% | 3% |
| ❖ Dark Chocolate Flavor Fudge | 1 brownie | 170 | 11% | 7% | 4% |
| ❖ Double Fudge | 1 brownie | 170 | 11% | 7% | 7% |
| ❖ Milk Chocolate Chunk | 1 brownie | 170 | 10% | 6% | 7% |
| ❖ Peanut Butter | 1 brownie | 160 | 13% | 7% | 3% |

| FOOD | Serving Size | Calories | Tot Fat | Sat Fat | Chol |
|---|---|---|---|---|---|
| ❖ Turtle | 1 brownie | 160 | 9% | 7% | 3% |
| ❖ Walnut | 1 brownie | 170 | 13% | 6% | 3% |
| DUNCAN HINES Microwave Brownies (prep as dir)— PROCTER & GAMBLE | | | | | |
| ❖ Double Choc. Brownie w/ Choc. Flavored Chips | 1 brownie | 180 | 10% | 9% | 0% |
| ❖ Frosted Brownie | 1 brownie | 210 | 12% | 8% | 0% |
| ★ ENTENMANN'S Fat Free, Cholesterol Free Fudge Brownies—KRAFT | 1/10 strip | 110 | 0% | 0% | 0% |
| ❖ ESTEE Brownie Mix | 1/8 pkg | 100 | 6% | 10% | 0% |
| HEALTH VALLEY Fat Free Brownie Bars | | | | | |
| ★ w/Caramel Topping | 1 bar | 110 | 0% | 0% | 0% |
| ★ w/Cherry Topping | 1 bar | 110 | 0% | 0% | 0% |
| ★ w/Fudge Topping | 1 bar | 110 | 0% | 0% | 0% |
| ★ w/Raspberry Topping | 1 bar | 110 | 0% | 0% | 0% |
| ★ w/Strawberry Topping | 1 bar | 110 | 0% | 0% | 0% |
| ❖ KRUSTEAZ Fudge Brownie Mix (prep as dir) (2" sq.)— CONTINENTAL MILLS | 1 pc | 190 | 11% | 8% | 7% |
| LITTLE DEBBIE Individual Snacks—MCKEE | | | | | |
| ⓐ Fudge Brownie | 1 pkg | 310 | 23% | 14% | 5% |
| ❖ Fudge Rounds | 1 pkg | 290 | 18% | 15% | 2% |
| ❖ PILLSBURY Fudge Brownie Mix | 1/20 pkg | 160 | 9% | 8% | 0% |

## CAKES AND CUPCAKES

**Generic Foods**

| FOOD | Serving Size | Calories | Tot Fat | Sat Fat | Chol |
|---|---|---|---|---|---|
| ★ Angel Food | 1 slc | 160 | 0% | 0% | 0% |
| ⓐ Carrot | 1 slc | 350 | 32% | 20% | 14% |
| ⓐ Cheesecake | 1 slc | 420 | 47% | 81% | 37% |
| ⓐ Chocolate w/Chocolate Icing | 1 slc | 300 | 20% | 26% | 13% |
| ❖ Chocolate w/o Icing | 1 slc | 240 | 14% | 11% | 0% |
| ⓐ Cupcake w/Chocolate Icing | 1 cupcake | 290 | 17% | 22% | 11% |
| ❖ Cupcake w/o Icing | 1 cupcake | 290 | 15% | 13% | 0% |
| ❖ Devil's Food | 1 slc | 340 | 19% | 14% | 0% |
| ⓐ Devil's Food Cupcake w/ Chocolate Icing | 1 cupcake | 270 | 14% | 18% | 30% |
| ❖ Devil's Food w/Icing | 1 slc | 270 | 14% | 18% | 13% |
| ❖ Fruitcake | 1 slc | 280 | 15% | 8% | 4% |
| ❖ Fudge | 1 slc | 340 | 19% | 14% | 0% |

★ Foods with this symbol have less than or equal to 5% *Daily Value* for all three nutrients (5% Rule).
❖ Foods with this symbol have at least one of the three nutrients greater than 5% *Daily Value* but less than or equal to 20% *Daily Value*.
ⓐ Foods with this symbol have at least one of the three nutrients greater than 20% *Daily Value* (20% Rule).

| FOOD | Serving Size | Calories | Tot Fat | Sat Fat | Chol |
|---|---|---|---|---|---|
| ❧ German Chocolate w/Icing | 1 slc | 290 | 23% | 19% | 13% |
| ❖ Gingerbread | 1 slc | 280 | 14% | 12% | 5% |
| ❖ Marble Pudding | 1 slc | 330 | 14% | 9% | 0% |
| ❧ Pineapple Upside Down | 1 slc | 400 | 23% | 18% | 9% |
| ❧ Pound | 1 slc | 320 | 25% | 33% | 24% |
| ❖ Shortcake Biscuit | 1 biscuit | 280 | 17% | 15% | 1% |
| ❧ Sponge | 1 slc | 140 | 2% | 2% | 21% |
| ❧ Walnut Slice | 1 slc | 460 | 54% | 28% | 16% |
| ❖ White w/Chocolate Icing | 1 slc | 310 | 19% | 17% | 1% |
| ❖ White w/Coconut Icing | 1 slc | 290 | 13% | 16% | 0% |
| ❖ Yellow | 1 slc | 300 | 15% | 10% | 10% |
| ❧ Yellow w/Chocolate Icing | 1 slc | 300 | 22% | 19% | 15% |

**Brand Name Foods**

AUNT FANNY'S Cup Cakes—PET

| | | | | | |
|---|---|---|---|---|---|
| ❧ Chocolate | 2 cupcakes | 310 | 18% | 25% | 7% |
| ❖ Orange | 2 cupcakes | 310 | 18% | 20% | 5% |

ENTENMANN'S Cakes—KRAFT

| | | | | | |
|---|---|---|---|---|---|
| ❧ All Butter French Crumb Cake | 1/8 cake | 210 | 15% | 30% | 19% |
| ❧ All Butter Loaf | 1/6 loaf | 220 | 15% | 31% | 27% |
| ❖ Banana Crunch Cake | 1/8 cake | 220 | 15% | 11% | 13% |
| ❧ Carrot Cake | 1/8 cake | 290 | 24% | 17% | 12% |
| ❧ Chocolate Fudge Cake | 1/6 cake | 310 | 22% | 24% | 14% |
| ❧ Louisiana Crunch Cake | 1/9 cake | 310 | 21% | 18% | 17% |
| ❧ Marble Loaf | 1/8 loaf | 200 | 16% | 29% | 21% |
| ❧ Marshmallow Iced Devil's Food Cake | 1/6 cake | 350 | 28% | 24% | 15% |
| ❖ Raisin Loaf | 1/8 loaf | 220 | 14% | 10% | 17% |
| ❧ Sour Cream Chip & Nut Loaf | 1/8 loaf | 240 | 21% | 19% | 16% |
| ❧ Thick Fudge Golden Cake | 1/6 cake | 330 | 24% | 20% | 17% |

ENTENMANN'S Fat Free, Cholesterol Free Cakes—KRAFT

| | | | | | |
|---|---|---|---|---|---|
| ★ Apple Spice Crumb | 1/8 cake | 130 | 0% | 0% | 0% |
| ★ Banana Crunch | 1/8 cake | 140 | 0% | 0% | 0% |
| ★ Banana Loaf | 1/8 loaf | 150 | 0% | 0% | 0% |
| ★ Blueberry Crunch | 1/8 cake | 140 | 0% | 0% | 0% |
| ★ Carrot | 1/8 cake | 170 | 0% | 0% | 0% |
| ★ Chocolate Crunch | 1/8 cake | 130 | 0% | 0% | 0% |
| ★ Chocolate Loaf | 1/8 loaf | 130 | 0% | 0% | 0% |
| ★ Fudge Iced Chocolate | 1/6 cake | 210 | 0% | 0% | 0% |
| ★ Fudge Iced Golden | 1/6 cake | 220 | 0% | 0% | 0% |
| ★ Golden Chocolatey Chip Loaf | 1/8 loaf | 130 | 0% | 0% | 0% |
| ★ Golden French Crumb | 1/8 cake | 140 | 0% | 0% | 0% |
| ★ Golden Loaf | 1/8 loaf | 120 | 0% | 0% | 0% |
| ★ Louisiana Crunch | 1/6 cake | 220 | 0% | 0% | 0% |
| ★ Marble Loaf | 1/8 loaf | 130 | 0% | 0% | 0% |
| ★ Mocha Iced Chocolate | 1/6 cake | 200 | 0% | 0% | 0% |
| ★ Raisin Loaf | 1/8 loaf | 140 | 0% | 0% | 0% |

| FOOD | Serving Size | Calories | Tot Fat | Sat Fat | Chol |
|---|---|---|---|---|---|
| AUNT FANNY'S *Fingers*—PET | | | | | |
| ❖   Chocolate | 2 fingers | 290 | 15% | 20% | 7% |
| ❖   Raspberry | 2 fingers | 280 | 12% | 20% | 2% |
| ❖   Vanilla | 2 fingers | 290 | 15% | 20% | 3% |
| LITTLE DEBBIE Individual Snacks—MCKEE | | | | | |
| ❖   *Banana Twins* Cakes | 1 pkg | 250 | 16% | 9% | 3% |
| Ⓐ   Chocolate Chip Cake | 1 pkg | 270 | 22% | 15% | 3% |
| Ⓐ   Coconut Cake | 1 pkg | 290 | 21% | 17% | 1% |
| Ⓐ   Devil *Cremes* Cakes | 1 pkg | 370 | 24% | 14% | 1% |
| ★   Fat Free *Figaroos* Snack Squares | 1 pkg | 180 | 0% | 0% | 0% |
| Ⓐ   Frosted Fudge Cake | 1 pkg | 270 | 21% | 14% | 3% |
| ❖   Golden *Cremes* Cakes | 1 pkg | 280 | 19% | 13% | 2% |
| Ⓐ   Snack Cake, Chocolate | 1 pkg | 360 | 27% | 19% | 0% |
| Ⓐ   Snack Cake, Vanilla | 1 pkg | 370 | 28% | 20% | 0% |
| ❖   Spice Cake | 1 pkg | 270 | 20% | 16% | 3% |
| ❖   Strawberry Shortcake Rolls | 1 pkg | 290 | 17% | 13% | 5% |
| Ⓐ   Swiss Rolls | 1 pkg | 320 | 23% | 16% | 6% |
| Ⓐ   Zebra Cake | 1 pkg | 370 | 28% | 20% | 0% |
| Ⓐ  PEPPERIDGE FARM All Butter Pound Cake—CAMPBELL'S | 1/5 cake | 290 | 20% | 35% | 37% |
| PEPPERIDGE FARM Layer Cakes —CAMPBELL'S | | | | | |
| Ⓐ   Chocolate Fudge | 1/6 cake | 300 | 24% | 25% | 11% |
| Ⓐ   Chocolate Fudge Stripe | 1/6 cake | 290 | 22% | 15% | 12% |
| Ⓐ   Coconut | 1/6 cake | 300 | 22% | 20% | 13% |
| Ⓐ   Devil's Food | 1/6 cake | 290 | 21% | 25% | 11% |
| Ⓐ   German Chocolate | 1/6 cake | 300 | 25% | 20% | 12% |
| Ⓐ   Golden | 1/6 cake | 290 | 22% | 15% | 17% |
| Ⓐ   Strawberry Stripe | 1/6 cake | 310 | 20% | 20% | 22% |
| ❖   Vanilla | 1/6 cake | 290 | 20% | 13% | 15% |
| PEPPERIDGE FARM *Special Recipe* Cakes—CAMPBELL'S | | | | | |
| ❖   Boston Creme | 1/8 cake | 260 | 14% | 13% | 15% |
| ❖   Chocolate Mousse | 1/8 cake | 250 | 15% | 15% | 8% |
| Ⓐ   Deluxe Carrot | 1/8 cake | 310 | 25% | 20% | 13% |
| ❖   Lemon Mousse | 1/8 cake | 250 | 18% | 20% | 15% |
| ❖   Pineapple Cream w/Toasted Coconut | 1/9 cake | 240 | 15% | 15% | 10% |
| ❖   Strawberry Cream w/Coconut | 1/9 cake | 230 | 14% | 15% | 10% |
| SARA LEE Cakes | | | | | |
| Ⓐ   Carrot | 1/6 cake | 320 | 26% | 18% | 10% |
| Ⓐ   Chocolate Mousse | 1/5 cake | 400 | 38% | 100% | 10% |
| Ⓐ   Chocolate Swirl | 1/4 cake | 330 | 22% | 30% | 22% |

★   Foods with this symbol have less than or equal to 5% *Daily Value* for <u>all</u> three nutrients (5% Rule).

❖   Foods with this symbol have <u>at least one</u> of the three nutrients greater than 5% *Daily Value* but less than or equal to 20% *Daily Value.*

Ⓐ   Foods with this symbol have <u>at least one</u> of the three nutrients greater than 20% *Daily Value* (20% Rule).

| FOOD | Serving Size | Calories | Tot Fat | Sat Fat | Chol |
|---|---|---|---|---|---|
| ⊛ Pound | 1/4 cake | 320 | 25% | 45% | 28% |
| SARA LEE Cream Cheesecakes | | | | | |
| ⊛ Cherry | 1/4 cake | 350 | 18% | 25% | 12% |
| ⊛ French | 1/6 cake | 350 | 32% | 65% | 7% |
| ⊛ Original | 1/4 cake | 350 | 28% | 45% | 17% |
| ⊛ Strawberry | 1/4 cake | 330 | 18% | 25% | 13% |
| ⊛ Strawberry French | 1/6 cake | 320 | 22% | 45% | 7% |
| SARA LEE Layer Cakes | | | | | |
| ⊛ Double Chocolate | 1/8 cake | 260 | 20% | 55% | 8% |
| ⊛ Flaky Coconut | 1/8 cake | 280 | 22% | 60% | 10% |
| ⊛ Fudge Golden | 1/8 cake | 270 | 20% | 50% | 5% |
| ⊛ German Chocolate | 1/8 cake | 280 | 23% | 55% | 10% |
| AUNT FANNY'S *Twirls*—PET | | | | | |
| ❖ Almond | 1 twirl | 110 | 6% | 3% | 0% |
| ❖ Cinnamon | 1 twirl | 110 | 6% | 3% | 0% |
| ❖ Coconut | 1 twirl | 110 | 6% | 5% | 0% |
| ❖ Pecan | 1 twirl | 100 | 6% | 3% | 0% |

## CAKE MIXES

**Brand Name Foods**

| FOOD | Serving Size | Calories | Tot Fat | Sat Fat | Chol |
|---|---|---|---|---|---|
| BETTY CROCKER Classic Dessert Mixes (prep as dir)—GENERAL MILLS | | | | | |
| ❖ Chocolate Pudding Cake | 1/8 cake | 170 | 6% | 5% | 9% |
| ❖ Date Bar | 1/12 pkg | 160 | 10% | 11% | 0% |
| ❖ Gingerbread Cake and Cookie Mix | 1/8 pkg | 230 | 11% | 9% | 9% |
| ❖ Golden Pound Cake | 1/8 cake | 290 | 19% | 17% | 18% |
| ❖ Lemon Chiffon Cake | 1/16 cake | 140 | 5% | 3% | 9% |
| ❖ Lemon Pudding Cake | 1/8 cake | 180 | 6% | 5% | 12% |
| ⊛ Pineapple Upside Down Cake | 1/6 cake | 400 | 23% | 19% | 12% |
| BETTY CROCKER *Super Moist* Angel Food Cake Mixes (prep as dir)—GENERAL MILLS | | | | | |
| ★ Chocolate Swirl | 1/12 cake | 150 | 0% | 0% | 0% |
| ★ Confetti | 1/12 cake | 150 | 0% | 0% | 0% |
| ★ Lemon Custard | 1/12 cake | 140 | 0% | 0% | 0% |
| ★ One-Step White | 1/12 cake | 140 | 0% | 0% | 0% |
| ★ Traditional | 1/12 cake | 130 | 0% | 0% | 0% |
| BETTY CROCKER *Super Moist* Cake Mixes (prep as dir)— GENERAL MILLS | | | | | |
| ⊛ Butter Chocolate | 1/12 cake | 270 | 21% | 34% | 25% |
| ❖ Butter Pecan | 1/12 cake | 250 | 17% | 13% | 18% |
| ⊛ Butter Yellow | 1/12 cake | 260 | 17% | 30% | 25% |
| ⊛ Carrot Cake | 1/10 cake | 300 | 20% | 14% | 22% |
| ❖ Cherry Chip | 1/10 cake | 280 | 18% | 14% | 0% |
| ⊛ Chocolate Chip | 1/12 cake | 280 | 22% | 16% | 18% |
| ❖ Chocolate Fudge | 1/12 cake | 250 | 18% | 14% | 18% |

| FOOD | Serving Size | Calories | Tot Fat | Sat Fat | Chol |
|---|---|---|---|---|---|
| ❖ Devil's Food | 1/12 cake | 250 | 18% | 14% | 18% |
| ❖ Double Chocolate Swirl | 1/12 cake | 250 | 18% | 15% | 18% |
| ❖ French Vanilla | 1/12 cake | 250 | 16% | 12% | 18% |
| ❖ Fudge Marble | 1/12 cake | 250 | 17% | 12% | 18% |
| ❖ German Chocolate | 1/12 cake | 250 | 17% | 14% | 18% |
| Ⓐ Golden Vanilla | 1/12 cake | 280 | 22% | 15% | 18% |
| ❖ Lemon | 1/12 cake | 250 | 17% | 13% | 18% |
| ❖ Milk Chocolate | 1/12 cake | 250 | 16% | 18% | 18% |
| ❖ Party Swirl | 1/12 cake | 250 | 17% | 12% | 18% |
| ❖ Peanut Butter Chocolate Swirl | 1/12 cake | 240 | 15% | 11% | 18% |
| ❖ Rainbow Chip | 1/12 cake | 250 | 17% | 15% | 18% |
| ❖ Sour Cream White | 1/10 cake | 280 | 19% | 15% | 0% |
| ❖ Spice | 1/12 cake | 250 | 17% | 12% | 18% |
| Ⓐ Strawberry Swirl | 1/10 cake | 290 | 18% | 14% | 22% |
| ❖ White | 1/12 cake | 240 | 15% | 12% | 0% |
| ❖ White w/Chocolate Swirl | 1/12 cake | 250 | 17% | 13% | 18% |
| ❖ Yellow | 1/12 cake | 250 | 15% | 12% | 18% |
| BETTY CROCKER *Super Moist* Light Cake Mixes (prep as dir) —GENERAL MILLS | | | | | |
| Ⓐ Devil's Food | 1/10 cake | 230 | 7% | 10% | 22% |
| ❖ White | 1/10 cake | 210 | 5% | 7% | 0% |
| Ⓐ Yellow | 1/10 cake | 230 | 7% | 9% | 22% |
| BUNDT Cake Mixes (prep as dir) —PILLSBURY | | | | | |
| Ⓐ Chocolate Caramel Nut | 1/16 cake | 290 | 28% | 18% | 13% |
| Ⓐ Double Hot Fudge | 1/16 cake | 280 | 25% | 25% | 13% |
| Ⓐ Strawberry Cream Cheese | 1/16 cake | 300 | 26% | 23% | 20% |
| DUNCAN HINES Cake Mixes (prep as basic recipe)— PROCTER & GAMBLE | | | | | |
| ★ Angel Food | 1/12 cake | 140 | 0% | 0% | 0% |
| Ⓐ Butter Recipe Fudge | 1/10 cake | 320 | 26% | 38% | 27% |
| Ⓐ Butter Recipe Golden | 1/10 cake | 320 | 24% | 37% | 27% |
| ❖ Caramel | 1/12 cake | 250 | 17% | 11% | 16% |
| Ⓐ Devil's Food | 1/12 cake | 290 | 22% | 15% | 16% |
| Ⓐ Dutch Dark Fudge | 1/12 cake | 290 | 22% | 15% | 16% |
| ❖ French Vanilla | 1/12 cake | 250 | 17% | 11% | 16% |
| ❖ Fudge Marble | 1/12 cake | 250 | 17% | 11% | 16% |
| ❖ Raspberry | 1/12 cake | 250 | 17% | 11% | 16% |
| ❖ Spice | 1/12 cake | 250 | 17% | 11% | 16% |
| ❖ Supreme Cakes: All flavors | 1/12 cake | 250 | 17% | 11% | 16% |
| Ⓐ Swiss Chocolate | 1/12 cake | 290 | 22% | 15% | 16% |
| ❖ White | 1/12 cake | 240 | 16% | 10% | 0% |

★ Foods with this symbol have less than or equal to 5% *Daily Value* for <u>all</u> three nutrients (5% Rule).

❖ Foods with this symbol have <u>at least one</u> of the three nutrients greater than 5% *Daily Value* but less than or equal to 20% *Daily Value*.

Ⓐ Foods with this symbol have <u>at least one</u> of the three nutrients greater than 20% *Daily Value* (20% Rule).

| FOOD | Serving Size | Calories | Tot Fat | Sat Fat | Chol |
|---|---|---|---|---|---|
| ❖ Yellow | 1/12 cake | 250 | 17% | 11% | 16% |
| DUNCAN HINES *DeLights* Cake Mixes (prep as dir)— PROCTER & GAMBLE | | | | | |
| ❖ Devil's Food | 1/10 cake | 220 | 8% | 9% | 13% |
| ❖ Fudge Marble | 1/10 cake | 220 | 8% | 9% | 13% |
| ❖ Yellow | 1/10 cake | 220 | 7% | 7% | 10% |
| DUNCAN HINES Microwave Cakes—PROCTER & GAMBLE | | | | | |
| ❖ Blueberry Crumbcake | 1/8 cake | 160 | 9% | 6% | 0% |
| ❖ Cinnamon Crumbcake | 1/8 cake | 170 | 11% | 7% | 0% |
| ❖ Devil's Food Cupcake w/ Choc. Frosting | 1 cupcake | 180 | 10% | 8% | 0% |
| ❖ Yellow Cupcake w/Choc. Frosting | 1 cupcake | 200 | 13% | 10% | 0% |
| ESTEE Cake Mixes | | | | | |
| ❖ Chocolate | 1/5 pkg | 190 | 6% | 10% | 0% |
| ❖ Lemon | 1/5 pkg | 200 | 6% | 10% | 0% |
| ❖ Pound | 1/5 pkg | 200 | 6% | 10% | 0% |
| ❖ White | 1/5 pkg | 200 | 6% | 10% | 0% |
| JELL-O Brand No Bake Desserts (prep as dir)—KRAFT | | | | | |
| Ⓐ Blueberry Cheesecake | 1/8 cake | 320 | 19% | 21% | 2% |
| Ⓐ Cherry Cheesecake | 1/8 cake | 330 | 19% | 21% | 2% |
| Ⓐ Homestyle Cheesecake | 1/6 cake | 360 | 24% | 19% | 2% |
| Ⓐ Real Cheesecake | 1/6 cake | 350 | 25% | 27% | 2% |
| Ⓐ Strawberry Cheesecake | 1/8 cake | 340 | 19% | 21% | 2% |
| ❖ Scone & Shortcake Mix— CONTINENTAL MILLS | 1 scone | 180 | 14% | 10% | 0% |
| MOIST SUPREME Cake Mixes (prep as dir)—PILLSBURY | | | | | |
| ★ Angel Food | 1/10 cake | 150 | 0% | 0% | 0% |
| ❖ Banana | 1/12 cake | 260 | 17% | 13% | 18% |
| Ⓐ Butter Recipe | 1/12 cake | 260 | 18% | 30% | 25% |
| Ⓐ Butter Recipe Chocolate | 1/12 cake | 270 | 20% | 35% | 25% |
| ❖ Carrot | 1/12 cake | 260 | 18% | 13% | 18% |
| ❖ Chocolate | 1/12 cake | 250 | 17% | 13% | 12% |
| ❖ Chocolate Chip | 1/12 cake | 240 | 15% | 15% | 12% |
| ❖ Dark Chocolate | 1/12 cake | 250 | 17% | 13% | 18% |
| Ⓐ Devil's Food | 1/12 cake | 270 | 22% | 15% | 18% |
| ❖ French Vanilla | 1/12 cake | 300 | 20% | 15% | 15% |
| ❖ Fudge Swirl | 1/12 cake | 250 | 15% | 13% | 18% |
| ❖ *Funfetti* | 1/12 cake | 240 | 14% | 10% | 0% |
| ❖ German Chocolate | 1/12 cake | 250 | 17% | 13% | 12% |
| Ⓐ Lemon | 1/10 cake | 300 | 20% | 15% | 22% |
| ❖ *Lovin' Lites* Devil's Food | 1/10 cake | 230 | 8% | 10% | 15% |
| ❖ *Lovin' Lites* White | 1/10 cake | 230 | 8% | 8% | 15% |
| ❖ *Lovin' Lites* Yellow | 1/10 cake | 230 | 8% | 8% | 15% |
| ❖ Strawberry | 1/12 cake | 260 | 17% | 13% | 18% |

| FOOD | Serving Size | Calories | Tot Fat | Sat Fat | Chol |
|------|------|------|------|------|------|
| ❖ Sunshine Vanilla | 1/12 cake | 260 | 18% | 15% | 18% |
| ❖ White | 1/10 cake | 280 | 17% | 13% | 0% |
| ❖ White 'N Fudge Swirl | 1/12 cake | 250 | 15% | 13% | 12% |
| ❖ Yellow | 1/12 cake | 240 | 15% | 13% | 18% |
| ROBIN HOOD Pouch Cake Mixes (prep as dir)—GENERAL MILLS | | | | | |
| ⊛ Devil's Food | 1/5 cake | 310 | 26% | 18% | 14% |
| ❖ Yellow | 1/5 cake | 280 | 20% | 14% | 14% |
| ❖ STREUSEL SWIRL Cinnamon Streusel Cake Mix (prep as dir) —PILLSBURY | 1/16 cake | 260 | 17% | 13% | 13% |

## Donuts

**Generic Foods**

| FOOD | Serving Size | Calories | Tot Fat | Sat Fat | Chol |
|------|------|------|------|------|------|
| ❖ Cake Donut | 1 donut | 230 | 19% | 12% | 6% |
| ⊛ Creme-Filled Yeast Donut | 1 donut | 200 | 21% | 19% | 4% |
| ❖ French Cruller | 1 donut | 230 | 15% | 13% | 2% |
| ❖ Glazed Yeast Donut | 1 donut | 220 | 19% | 16% | 3% |
| ❖ Jelly-Filled Yeast Donut | 1 donut | 190 | 16% | 13% | 5% |
| ❖ Old-Fashioned | 1 donut | 230 | 19% | 10% | 7% |

**Brand Name Foods**

| FOOD | Serving Size | Calories | Tot Fat | Sat Fat | Chol |
|------|------|------|------|------|------|
| AUNT FANNY'S *Dunkin Stix*—PET | | | | | |
| ❖ Cherry | 1 stick | 180 | 17% | 15% | 2% |
| ❖ Chocolate | 1 stick | 180 | 18% | 15% | 2% |
| ❖ Regular (1.4 oz) | 1 stick | 190 | 17% | 20% | 3% |
| ENTENMANN'S Donuts—KRAFT | | | | | |
| ❖ Crumb Topped Donuts | 1 donut | 260 | 19% | 14% | 5% |
| ❖ Devil's Food Crumb Donuts | 1 donut | 250 | 19% | 18% | 5% |
| ⊛ Frosted Mini Donuts | 2 donuts | 270 | 31% | 32% | 3% |
| ❖ Glazed Buttermilk Donuts | 1 donut | 270 | 20% | 15% | 3% |
| ❖ Glazed Chocolate *Popems* | 4 pcs | 200 | 15% | 12% | 4% |
| ❖ Glazed *Popems* | 6 pcs | 240 | 17% | 13% | 5% |
| ⊛ Rich Frosted Donuts | 1 donut | 280 | 30% | 31% | 4% |
| ENTENMANN'S Variety Donuts —KRAFT | | | | | |
| ⊛ Cinnamon Sugar | 1 donut | 310 | 29% | 21% | 7% |
| ⊛ Crumb Topped | 1 donut | 420 | 34% | 25% | 7% |
| ⊛ Rich Frosted | 1 donut | 400 | 42% | 42% | 5% |
| ⊛ LITTLE DEBBIE Individual Snacks: Donut Sticks—MCKEE | 1 pkg | 250 | 23% | 18% | 2% |

★ Foods with this symbol have less than or equal to 5% *Daily Value* for <u>all</u> three nutrients (5% Rule).
❖ Foods with this symbol have <u>at least one</u> of the three nutrients greater than 5% *Daily Value* but less than or equal to 20% *Daily Value*.
⊛ Foods with this symbol have <u>at least one</u> of the three nutrients greater than 20% *Daily Value* (20% Rule).

| FOOD | Serving Size | Calories | Tot Fat | Sat Fat | Chol |
|---|---|---|---|---|---|

FROSTINGS

**Brand Name Foods**

BETTY CROCKER *Creamy Deluxe*
Light Ready-to-Spread Frostings
—GENERAL MILLS

| FOOD | Serving Size | Calories | Tot Fat | Sat Fat | Chol |
|---|---|---|---|---|---|
| ★ Chocolate | 2 tbsp | 120 | 1% | 3% | 0% |
| ★ Milk Chocolate | 2 tbsp | 120 | 2% | 4% | 0% |
| ★ Vanilla | 2 tbsp | 120 | 1% | 2% | 0% |

BETTY CROCKER *Creamy Deluxe*
Ready-to-Spread Frostings—
GENERAL MILLS

| FOOD | Serving Size | Calories | Tot Fat | Sat Fat | Chol |
|---|---|---|---|---|---|
| ❖ Butter Cream | 2 tbsp | 160 | 9% | 9% | 0% |
| ❖ Butter Pecan | 2 tbsp | 150 | 9% | 7% | 0% |
| ❖ Caramel Chocolate Chip | 2 tbsp | 140 | 9% | 8% | 0% |
| ❖ Cherry | 2 tbsp | 140 | 8% | 6% | 0% |
| ❖ Chocolate | 2 tbsp | 150 | 9% | 7% | 0% |
| ❖ Chocolate Chip | 2 tbsp | 160 | 10% | 12% | 0% |
| ❖ Chocolate Chip Cookie Dough | 2 tbsp | 160 | 9% | 9% | 0% |
| ❖ Chocolate Chocolate Chip | 2 tbsp | 150 | 10% | 13% | 0% |
| ❖ Chocolate Swiss Almond | 2 tbsp | 150 | 9% | 7% | 0% |
| ❖ Coconut Pecan | 2 tbsp | 150 | 13% | 17% | 0% |
| ❖ Cream Cheese | 2 tbsp | 140 | 8% | 6% | 0% |
| ❖ Dark Chocolate | 2 tbsp | 150 | 9% | 8% | 0% |
| ❖ French Vanilla | 2 tbsp | 140 | 8% | 7% | 0% |
| ❖ Lemon | 2 tbsp | 140 | 8% | 6% | 0% |
| ❖ Milk Chocolate | 2 tbsp | 150 | 9% | 7% | 0% |
| ❖ Rainbow Chip | 2 tbsp | 160 | 9% | 14% | 0% |
| ❖ Sour Cream Chocolate | 2 tbsp | 150 | 9% | 7% | 0% |
| ❖ Sour Cream White | 2 tbsp | 150 | 8% | 7% | 0% |
| ❖ Strawberry Cream Cheese | 2 tbsp | 150 | 9% | 7% | 0% |
| ❖ Vanilla | 2 tbsp | 140 | 8% | 6% | 0% |
| ❖ White Chocolate | 2 tbsp | 140 | 8% | 7% | 0% |

BETTY CROCKER *Creamy Deluxe*
Ready-to-Spread Party Frostings
—GENERAL MILLS

| FOOD | Serving Size | Calories | Tot Fat | Sat Fat | Chol |
|---|---|---|---|---|---|
| ❖ Chocolate w/Dinosaurs | 2 tbsp | 150 | 8% | 7% | 0% |
| ❖ Vanilla w/Bears | 2 tbsp | 140 | 8% | 6% | 0% |

BETTY CROCKER Creamy Frosting
Mixes (prep as dir)—GENERAL MILLS

| FOOD | Serving Size | Calories | Tot Fat | Sat Fat | Chol |
|---|---|---|---|---|---|
| ❖ Chocolate Fudge | 2 tbsp | 140 | 7% | 5% | 0% |
| ❖ Coconut Pecan | 2 tbsp | 160 | 12% | 14% | 0% |
| ❖ Creamy Vanilla | 2 tbsp | 130 | 6% | 5% | 0% |
| ★ BETTY CROCKER Fluffy White Frosting Mix (prep as dir)— GENERAL MILLS | 6 tbsp | 100 | 0% | 0% | 0% |

| FOOD | Serving Size | Calories | Tot Fat | Sat Fat | Chol |
|------|------|------|------|------|------|
| BETTY CROCKER *Whipped Deluxe* Ready-to-Spread Frostings—GENERAL MILLS | | | | | |
| ❖ Cream Cheese | 2 tbsp | 110 | 7% | 8% | 0% |
| ❖ Lemon | 2 tbsp | 110 | 7% | 7% | 0% |
| ❖ Strawberry | 2 tbsp | 110 | 7% | 8% | 0% |
| ❖ Vanilla Cream | 2 tbsp | 110 | 7% | 7% | 0% |
| CREAMY SUPREME/FROSTING SUPREME—PILLSBURY | | | | | |
| ❖ Caramel Pecan | 2 tbsp | 150 | 12% | 10% | 0% |
| ❖ Chocolate | 2 tbsp | 140 | 9% | 8% | 0% |
| ❖ Chocolate Fudge | 2 tbsp | 140 | 9% | 8% | 0% |
| ❖ Coconut Pecan | 2 tbsp | 160 | 15% | 20% | 0% |
| ❖ Cream Cheese | 2 tbsp | 150 | 9% | 8% | 0% |
| ❖ Creamy Candy | 2 tbsp | 150 | 11% | 10% | 0% |
| ❖ Dark Chocolate | 2 tbsp | 130 | 9% | 8% | 0% |
| ❖ French Vanilla | 2 tbsp | 150 | 9% | 8% | 0% |
| ❖ *Funfetti* Chocolate | 2 tbsp | 140 | 9% | 8% | 0% |
| ❖ *Funfetti* Pink Vanilla | 2 tbsp | 150 | 9% | 8% | 0% |
| ❖ *Funfetti* Vanilla | 2 tbsp | 150 | 9% | 8% | 0% |
| ❖ Lemon Creme | 2 tbsp | 150 | 9% | 8% | 0% |
| ★ *Lovin' Lites* Milk Chocolate | 2 tbsp | 130 | 5% | 5% | 0% |
| ★ *Lovin' Lites* Vanilla | 2 tbsp | 140 | 5% | 5% | 0% |
| ❖ Milk Chocolate | 2 tbsp | 140 | 9% | 8% | 0% |
| ❖ *Oreo* | 2 tbsp | 150 | 9% | 8% | 0% |
| ★ Reduced Fat Chocolate Fudge | 2 tbsp | 140 | 5% | 5% | 0% |
| ❖ Strawberry Creme | 2 tbsp | 150 | 9% | 8% | 0% |
| ❖ Swirl Milk Chocolate w/Fudge Glaze | 2 tbsp | 140 | 9% | 8% | 0% |
| ❖ Swirl Vanilla w/Fudge Glaze | 2 tbsp | 150 | 9% | 8% | 0% |
| ❖ Vanilla | 2 tbsp | 150 | 9% | 8% | 0% |
| DUNCAN HINES Frostings (prep as dir)—PROCTER & GAMBLE | | | | | |
| ❖ Buttercream | 2 tbsp | 140 | 8% | 7% | 0% |
| ❖ Caramel | 2 tbsp | 140 | 8% | 7% | 0% |
| ❖ Chocolate | 2 tbsp | 130 | 8% | 7% | 0% |
| ❖ Chocolate Buttercream | 2 tbsp | 130 | 8% | 7% | 0% |
| ❖ Cream Cheese | 2 tbsp | 140 | 8% | 7% | 0% |
| ❖ Dark Chocolate | 2 tbsp | 130 | 8% | 7% | 0% |
| ❖ Lemon Cream | 2 tbsp | 140 | 8% | 7% | 0% |
| ❖ Milk Chocolate | 2 tbsp | 130 | 8% | 7% | 0% |
| ❖ Raspberries 'n Cream | 2 tbsp | 140 | 8% | 7% | 0% |
| ❖ Vanilla | 2 tbsp | 140 | 8% | 7% | 0% |
| ★ ESTEE Frosting | 1/5 pkg | 80 | 0% | 0% | 0% |

★ Foods with this symbol have less than or equal to 5% *Daily Value* for <u>all</u> three nutrients (5% Rule).

❖ Foods with this symbol have <u>at least one</u> of the three nutrients greater than 5% *Daily Value* but less than or equal to 20% *Daily Value*.

Ⓐ Foods with this symbol have <u>at least one</u> of the three nutrients greater than 20% *Daily Value* (20% Rule).

| FOOD | Serving Size | Calories | Tot Fat | Sat Fat | Chol |
|---|---|---|---|---|---|
| ❖ ROBIN HOOD Chocolate Frosting Mix (prep as dir)—GENERAL MILLS | 2 tbsp | 140 | 7% | 5% | 0% |

## GELATIN

### Generic Foods

| | | | | | |
|---|---|---|---|---|---|
| ★ Gelatin: All flavors | 1/2 cup | 70 | 0% | 0% | 0% |
| ★ Low-Calorie Gelatin: All flavors | 1/2 cup | 10 | 0% | 0% | 0% |

### Brand Name Foods

| | | | | | |
|---|---|---|---|---|---|
| ★ D-ZERTA Low Calorie Strawberry Gelatin—KRAFT | 1/2 cup | 10 | 0% | 0% | 0% |
| ★ DEL MONTE Gel Snack Cups: All flavors | 1 snack cup | 100 | 0% | 0% | 0% |
| ★ HAIN Super Fruits Dessert Mixes: All flavors (prep as dir)—HAIN | 1/2 cup | 90 | 0% | 0% | 0% |
| ★ HUNT'S Snack Pack Juicy Gels: All flavors—HUNT WESSON | 1 each | 100 | 0% | 0% | 0% |
| JELL-O Brand—KRAFT | | | | | |
| ★ Gelatin Snacks: All flavors | 1 snack cup | 80 | 0% | 0% | 0% |
| ★ Gelatin: All flavors | 1/2 cup | 80 | 0% | 0% | 0% |
| ★ Sugar Free Low Calorie Gelatin Snacks: All flavors | 1 snack cup | 10 | 0% | 0% | 0% |
| ★ Sugar Free Low Calorie Gelatin: All flavors | 1/2 cup | 10 | 0% | 0% | 0% |
| ★ KRAFT *Handi-Snacks* Gel Snacks: All flavors | 1 snack cup | 80 | 0% | 0% | 0% |
| ★ SWISS MISS Gels: All flavors—HUNT WESSON | 1 each | 80 | 0% | 0% | 0% |

## PASTRIES

### Generic Foods

| | | | | | |
|---|---|---|---|---|---|
| ⊛ Cream Puff Shell | 1 puff | 240 | 26% | 19% | 43% |
| ⊛ Cream Puff w/Custard | 1 puff | 340 | 31% | 24% | 58% |
| ⊛ Eclair | 1 eclair | 210 | 19% | 16% | 34% |
| ★ Phyllo Dough (raw) | 20 g | 60 | 2% | 1% | 0% |
| ⊛ Puff Pastry Shell | 2 shells | 440 | 47% | 22% | 0% |

### Brand Name Foods

| | | | | | |
|---|---|---|---|---|---|
| ENTENMANN'S Fat Free, Cholesterol Free Pastries—KRAFT | | | | | |
| ★ Black Forest Pastry | 1/9 danish | 130 | 0% | 0% | 0% |
| ★ Raspberry Cheese Pastry | 1/9 danish | 140 | 0% | 0% | 0% |
| ENTENMANN'S Pastries—KRAFT | | | | | |
| ❖ Apple Puffs | 1 puff | 260 | 19% | 16% | 0% |

| | FOOD | Serving Size | Calories | Tot Fat | Sat Fat | Chol |
|---|---|---|---|---|---|---|
| Ⓐ | Apple Strudel | 1/4 strudel | 310 | 21% | 18% | 0% |
| Ⓐ | Chocolate Eclairs | 1 eclair | 250 | 13% | 10% | 24% |
| Ⓐ | Blueberry Turnovers | 1 turnover | 340 | 25% | 15% | 0% |
| | PEPPERIDGE FARM Puff Pastries —CAMPBELL'S | | | | | |
| ❖ | Apple Dumplings | 1 dumpling | 290 | 17% | 13% | 0% |
| Ⓐ | Apple Turnovers | 1 turnover | 330 | 22% | 15% | 0% |
| ❖ | Apple Turnovers, Mini | 1 turnover | 140 | 12% | 10% | 0% |
| Ⓐ | Apple Turnovers w/Vanilla Icing | 1 turnover | 360 | 22% | 15% | 0% |
| ❖ | Cherry Turnovers | 1 turnover | 320 | 20% | 15% | 0% |
| ❖ | Cherry Turnovers, Mini | 1 turnover | 140 | 12% | 10% | 0% |
| ❖ | Cherry Turnovers w/Vanilla Icing | 1 turnover | 340 | 20% | 15% | 0% |
| Ⓐ | Dark Chocolate Clouds | 2 pastries | 580 | 58% | 75% | 8% |
| ❖ | Dough Sheets | 1/6 sheet | 200 | 17% | 13% | 0% |
| Ⓐ | Milk Chocolate Clouds | 2 pastries | 580 | 58% | 75% | 18% |
| Ⓐ | Patty Shells | 1 shell | 230 | 22% | 15% | 0% |
| ❖ | Peach Cobbler Turnovers, Mini | 1 turnover | 160 | 12% | 10% | 1% |
| ❖ | Peach Dumplings | 1 dumpling | 300 | 17% | 13% | 0% |
| Ⓐ | Peach Turnovers | 1 turnover | 340 | 23% | 15% | 0% |
| Ⓐ | Raspberry Turnovers | 1 turnover | 330 | 22% | 15% | 0% |
| ❖ | Raspberry Turnovers, Mini | 1 turnover | 140 | 11% | 8% | 0% |
| Ⓐ | Raspberry Turnovers w/Vanilla Icing | 1 turnover | 360 | 22% | 15% | 0% |
| ❖ | Strawberry Turnovers, Mini | 1 turnover | 140 | 11% | 8% | 0% |
| | PILLSBURY Turnovers | | | | | |
| Ⓐ | Apple | 2 turnovers | 350 | 26% | 18% | 0% |
| Ⓐ | Cherry | 2 turnovers | 350 | 26% | 18% | 0% |

## PIES

**Generic Foods**

*Note: All pies are 9" unless otherwise noted*

| | | | | | | |
|---|---|---|---|---|---|---|
| Ⓐ | Apple | 1/8 pie | 300 | 21% | 13% | 0% |
| Ⓐ | Apple (2 crust) | 1/8 pie | 490 | 33% | 28% | 0% |
| Ⓐ | Banana Cream | 1/8 pie | 400 | 31% | 28% | 25% |
| Ⓐ | Blackberry (2 crust) | 1/8 pie | 470 | 32% | 26% | 0% |
| ❖ | Blueberry | 1/8 pie | 290 | 19% | 12% | 0% |
| Ⓐ | Blueberry (2 crust) | 1/8 pie | 470 | 32% | 26% | 0% |
| ❖ | Boston Cream | 1/12 pie | 290 | 19% | 20% | 14% |
| Ⓐ | Cherry | 1/8 pie | 490 | 34% | 27% | 0% |
| Ⓐ | Cherry (2 crust) | 1/8 pie | 500 | 33% | 29% | 0% |

---

★ Foods with this symbol have less than or equal to 5% *Daily Value* for <u>all</u> three nutrients (5% Rule).

❖ Foods with this symbol have <u>at least one</u> of the three nutrients greater than 5% *Daily Value* but less than or equal to 20% *Daily Value*.

Ⓐ Foods with this symbol have <u>at least one</u> of the three nutrients greater than 20% *Daily Value* (20% Rule).

| FOOD | Serving Size | Calories | Tot Fat | Sat Fat | Chol |
|---|---|---|---|---|---|
| ✤ Chocolate Cream | 1/6 (8" pie) | 340 | 34% | 30% | 2% |
| ✤ Chocolate Meringue | 1/8 pie | 470 | 35% | 42% | 35% |
| ✤ Coconut Cream | 1/8 pie | 400 | 33% | 38% | 26% |
| ✤ Coconut Custard | 1/8 pie | 420 | 34% | 45% | 61% |
| ✤ Custard | 1/8 pie | 260 | 18% | 18% | 29% |
| ✤ Fried Fruit Pie | 1 pie | 270 | 22% | 33% | 4% |
| ✤ Lemon Chiffon | 1/8 pie | 450 | 28% | 25% | 82% |
| ✤ Lemon Meringue | 1/8 pie | 360 | 25% | 20% | 23% |
| ✤ Mince | 1/8 pie | 480 | 27% | 22% | 0% |
| ❖ Peach | 1/6 (8" pie) | 260 | 18% | 11% | 0% |
| ✤ Peach (2 crust) | 1/8 pie | 490 | 32% | 25% | 0% |
| ✤ Pecan | 1/8 pie | 500 | 42% | 24% | 35% |
| ✤ Pineapple Custard | 1/8 pie | 390 | 24% | 24% | 33% |
| ✤ Pumpkin | 1/8 pie | 320 | 22% | 25% | 22% |
| ✤ Raisin (2 crust) | 1/8 pie | 520 | 32% | 25% | 0% |
| ✤ Rhubarb (2 crust) | 1/8 pie | 490 | 32% | 25% | 0% |
| ✤ Strawberry | 1/8 pie | 350 | 21% | 17% | 0% |
| ✤ Sweet Potato | 1/8 pie | 380 | 31% | 36% | 32% |
| ✤ Turnover, Apple | 1 turnover | 380 | 32% | 27% | 2% |
| ✤ Turnover, Cherry | 1 turnover | 370 | 32% | 23% | 6% |
| ✤ Turnover, Lemon | 1 turnover | 410 | 34% | 25% | 10% |
| ✤ Vanilla Cream | 1/8 pie | 350 | 28% | 25% | 26% |

**Brand Name Foods**

AUNT FANNY'S/McMILLIN's
Pies (4 oz)—PET

| | | | | | |
|---|---|---|---|---|---|
| ✤ Apple | 1 pie | 460 | 35% | 50% | 10% |
| ✤ Berry | 1 pie | 440 | 35% | 50% | 8% |
| ✤ Boston Creme | 1 pie | 440 | 34% | 55% | 8% |
| ✤ Cherry | 1 pie | 400 | 34% | 50% | 10% |
| ✤ Chocolate Creme Pudding | 1 pie | 450 | 40% | 55% | 10% |
| ✤ Coconut Creme Pudding | 1 pie | 440 | 35% | 55% | 8% |
| ✤ Lemon Creme | 1 pie | 420 | 34% | 50% | 10% |
| ✤ Peach | 1 pie | 430 | 34% | 50% | 10% |
| ✤ Pumpkin | 1 pie | 420 | 32% | 40% | 7% |
| ✤ Strawberry | 1 pie | 420 | 32% | 45% | 7% |
| ✤ Vanilla Creme Pudding | 1 pie | 400 | 32% | 50% | 8% |
| BANQUET Cream Pies—CONAGRA | | | | | |
| ✤ Banana | 1/3 pie | 350 | 32% | 25% | 1% |
| ✤ Chocolate | 1/3 pie | 360 | 31% | 25% | 1% |
| ✤ Coconut | 1/3 pie | 350 | 31% | 30% | 1% |
| ✤ Lemon | 1/3 pie | 360 | 31% | 25% | 1% |
| ✤ Strawberry | 1/3 pie | 340 | 26% | 20% | 1% |
| BANQUET Fruit Pies—CONAGRA | | | | | |
| ✤ Apple | 1/5 pie | 300 | 20% | 30% | 2% |
| ✤ Blackberry | 1/5 pie | 300 | 18% | 25% | 2% |
| ✤ Blueberry | 1/5 pie | 260 | 18% | 25% | 2% |
| ✤ Cherry | 1/5 pie | 290 | 22% | 30% | 2% |

| FOOD | Serving Size | Calories | Tot Fat | Sat Fat | Chol |
|---|---|---|---|---|---|
| ⊛ Mincemeat | 1/5 pie | 310 | 20% | 30% | 3% |
| ⊛ Peach | 1/5 pie | 260 | 18% | 25% | 2% |
| ❖ Pumpkin | 1/5 pie | 250 | 12% | 15% | 7% |
| ❖ BETTY CROCKER Classic Dessert Mixes: Boston Cream Pie (prep as dir)—GENERAL MILLS | 1/10 pie | 200 | 7% | 8% | 8% |
| ENTENMANN'S Fat Free, Cholesterol Free Pies—KRAFT | | | | | |
| ★ Apple Beehive Pie | 1/5 pie | 270 | 0% | 0% | 0% |
| ★ Cherry Beehive Pie | 1/5 pie | 270 | 0% | 0% | 0% |
| ENTENMANN'S Pies—KRAFT | | | | | |
| ⊛ Coconut Custard Pie | 1/5 pie | 340 | 29% | 40% | 45% |
| ⊛ Homestyle Apple Pie | 1/6 pie | 300 | 22% | 18% | 0% |
| ⊛ Lemon Pie | 1/6 pie | 340 | 26% | 22% | 16% |
| JELL-O Brand No Bake Desserts (prep as dir)—KRAFT | | | | | |
| ⊛ Chocolate Silk Pie | 1/6 pie | 310 | 25% | 29% | 2% |
| ⊛ Coconut Cream Pie | 1/6 pie | 330 | 29% | 44% | 2% |
| LITTLE DEBBIE Individual Snack Pies—MCKEE | | | | | |
| ⊛ Marshmallow Pie, Banana | 1 pkg | 240 | 13% | 25% | 0% |
| ⊛ Marshmallow Pie, Chocolate | 1 pkg | 240 | 13% | 24% | 0% |
| ❖ Oatmeal Creme Pie | 1 pkg | 300 | 18% | 10% | 0% |
| ❖ Raisin Creme Pie | 1 pkg | 290 | 18% | 15% | 0% |
| MRS. SMITH'S Pies (8")—KELLOGG'S | | | | | |
| ❖ Apple | 1/6 pie | 270 | 17% | 10% | 0% |
| ⊛ Apple Cranberry | 1/6 pie | 280 | 17% | 25% | 0% |
| ❖ Banana Cream | 1/4 pie | 250 | 14% | 13% | 0% |
| ❖ Berry | 1/6 pie | 280 | 17% | 10% | 0% |
| ❖ Blackberry | 1/6 pie | 280 | 17% | 10% | 0% |
| ❖ Blueberry | 1/6 pie | 260 | 17% | 10% | 0% |
| ❖ Boston Cream | 1/8 pie | 170 | 8% | 8% | 8% |
| ❖ Cherry | 1/6 pie | 270 | 17% | 10% | 0% |
| ⊛ Chocolate Cream | 1/4 pie | 290 | 22% | 20% | 0% |
| ⊛ Coconut Cream | 1/4 pie | 280 | 22% | 20% | 0% |
| ⊛ Coconut Custard | 1/5 pie | 280 | 18% | 25% | 25% |
| ❖ Dutch Apple | 1/6 pie | 310 | 20% | 13% | 0% |
| ⊛ French Silk Cream | 1/5 pie | 410 | 32% | 30% | 2% |
| ❖ Hearty Pumpkin | 1/5 pie | 280 | 15% | 15% | 20% |
| ❖ Lemon Cream | 1/4 pie | 270 | 20% | 15% | 0% |
| ⊛ Lemon Meringue | 1/5 pie | 300 | 12% | 10% | 22% |
| ❖ Mince | 1/6 pie | 300 | 17% | 10% | 0% |
| ❖ Peach | 1/6 pie | 260 | 17% | 10% | 0% |
| ⊛ Pecan | 1/5 pie | 520 | 35% | 20% | 23% |

★ Foods with this symbol have less than or equal to 5% *Daily Value* for <u>all</u> three nutrients (5% Rule).

❖ Foods with this symbol have <u>at least one</u> of the three nutrients greater than 5% *Daily Value* but less than or equal to 20% *Daily Value.*

⊛ Foods with this symbol have <u>at least one</u> of the three nutrients greater than 20% *Daily Value* (20% Rule).

| FOOD | Serving Size | Calories | Tot Fat | Sat Fat | Chol |
|------|--------------|----------|---------|---------|------|
| ❖ Pumpkin | 1/5 pie | 270 | 12% | 10% | 15% |
| ❖ Red Raspberry | 1/6 pie | 280 | 17% | 10% | 0% |
| ❖ Strawberry Rhubarb | 1/6 pie | 280 | 17% | 10% | 0% |
| PET-RITZ Pies (4 1/4 oz)—PET | | | | | |
| ➅ Apple | 1 pie | 430 | 31% | 45% | 10% |
| ➅ Blueberry | 1 pie | 450 | 32% | 45% | 10% |
| ➅ Cherry | 1 pie | 450 | 35% | 55% | 10% |
| ➅ Lemon | 1 pie | 450 | 32% | 50% | 10% |
| PET-RITZ Cobblers, frozen—PET | | | | | |
| ➅ Apple | 1/6 cobbler | 280 | 18% | 23% | 1% |
| ❖ Apple Crumb | 1/6 cobbler | 280 | 13% | 18% | 2% |
| ❖ Blackberry | 1/6 cobbler | 260 | 17% | 20% | 1% |
| ❖ Blackberry Crumb | 1/6 cobbler | 260 | 12% | 16% | 2% |
| ➅ Blueberry | 1/6 cobbler | 280 | 17% | 23% | 2% |
| ❖ Cherry | 1/6 cobbler | 300 | 16% | 19% | 1% |
| ❖ Cherry Crumb | 1/6 cobbler | 280 | 9% | 12% | 1% |
| ❖ Peach | 1/6 cobbler | 230 | 14% | 16% | 1% |
| ❖ Peach Crumb | 1/6 cobbler | 230 | 11% | 14% | 2% |
| ❖ Strawberry | 1/6 cobbler | 260 | 15% | 17% | 1% |
| PET-RITZ Cream Pies, frozen—PET | | | | | |
| ➅ Banana Cream | 1/4 pie | 270 | 19% | 42% | 2% |
| ➅ Chocolate | 1/4 pie | 290 | 20% | 40% | 2% |
| ➅ Coconut Cream | 1/4 pie | 270 | 19% | 42% | 2% |
| ➅ Fudge Vanilla Cream | 1/4 pie | 300 | 22% | 43% | 2% |
| ➅ Lemon Cream | 1/4 pie | 270 | 19% | 42% | 2% |
| ➅ Peanut Butter Chocolate | 1/4 pie | 300 | 23% | 42% | 2% |
| ➅ Pumpkin | 1/4 pie | 270 | 19% | 42% | 2% |
| SARA LEE *Homestyle* Pies (9") | | | | | |
| ➅ Apple | 1/8 pie | 330 | 26% | 18% | 0% |
| ➅ Blueberry | 1/8 pie | 350 | 23% | 18% | 0% |
| ➅ Cherry | 1/8 pie | 320 | 25% | 18% | 0% |
| ➅ Chocolate Cream | 1/5 pie | 500 | 49% | 80% | 1% |
| ➅ Coconut Cream | 1/5 pie | 480 | 48% | 70% | 0% |
| ➅ Dutch Apple | 1/8 pie | 350 | 23% | 15% | 0% |
| ❖ Lemon Meringue | 1/6 pie | 350 | 17% | 13% | 0% |
| ➅ Peach | 1/8 pie | 320 | 22% | 15% | 0% |
| ➅ Pecan | 1/8 pie | 520 | 37% | 23% | 15% |
| ❖ Pumpkin | 1/8 pie | 260 | 17% | 13% | 10% |

## PIE CRUSTS

**Brand Name Foods**

| FOOD | Serving Size | Calories | Tot Fat | Sat Fat | Chol |
|------|--------------|----------|---------|---------|------|
| ❖ BETTY CROCKER Pie Crust Mix (9")—GENERAL MILLS | 1/8 crust | 110 | 12% | 11% | 0% |
| ❖ FLAKO Pie Crust Mix—QUAKER | 1/4 cup | 130 | 12% | 15% | 2% |
| ❖ HONEY MAID Graham Pie Crust —NABISCO | 1/6 crust | 140 | 11% | 8% | 0% |

| FOOD | Serving Size | Calories | Tot Fat | Sat Fat | Chol |
|------|------|------|------|------|------|
| ❖ KRUSTEAZ Pie Crust Mix (9")— | | | | | |
|    CONTINENTAL MILLS | 1/8 crust | 90 | 8% | 8% | 0% |
| ❖ NILLA Pie Crust—NABISCO | 1/6 crust | 140 | 12% | 9% | 1% |
| ❖ OREO Pie Crust—NABISCO | 1/6 crust | 140 | 11% | 8% | 0% |
|    ORONOQUE ORCHARDS Pie Crusts—PET | | | | | |
| ❖   Deep Dish (9") | 1/8 crust | 100 | 10% | 7% | 0% |
| ❖   Deep Dish (10") | 1/8 crust | 130 | 13% | 10% | 0% |
| ❖   Graham Cracker crust | 1/8 crust | 110 | 10% | 8% | 0% |
| ❖   Regular (9") | 1/8 crust | 90 | 9% | 7% | 0% |
| ❖   Tart (3") | 1 tart | 140 | 14% | 10% | 0% |
| ❖   Tart (6") | 1/4 crust | 110 | 12% | 8% | 4% |
|    PET-RITZ Pie Crust, frozen—PET | | | | | |
| ❖   Deep Dish (9") | 1/8 crust | 100 | 9% | 11% | 2% |
| ❖   Extra Lg. (9 5/8") | 1/8 crust | 120 | 11% | 14% | 2% |
| ❖   Graham Cracker crust | 1/8 crust | 110 | 10% | 8% | 0% |
| ❖   Regular (9") | 1/8 crust | 80 | 7% | 9% | 1% |
| ❖   Tart (3") | 1 tart | 140 | 14% | 10% | 0% |
| ❖   Tart (6") | 1/4 crust | 110 | 12% | 8% | 0% |
|    PILLSBURY | | | | | |
| ❖   Pie Crust Mix (prep as dir) | 2 tbsp | 100 | 9% | 8% | 0% |
| ❖   Pie Crust | 1/8 crust | 110 | 11% | 15% | 2% |

### PIE FILLINGS: FRUIT

**Brand Name Foods**

| FOOD | Serving Size | Calories | Tot Fat | Sat Fat | Chol |
|------|------|------|------|------|------|
| ★ LIBBY'S Pumpkin Pie Mix—NESTLÉ | 1/2 cup | 100 | 0% | 0% | 0% |
| ★ NONE SUCH Mincemeat—BORDEN | 1/3 cup | 190 | 1% | 0% | 0% |
| ★ SMUCKER'S Strawberry Pie Glaze | 2 oz | 80 | 0% | 0% | 0% |
|    WILDERNESS Pie Filling or Topping—CURTICE BURNS | | | | | |
| ★   All regular varieties | 1/3 cup | 90 | 0% | 0% | 0% |
| ★   Light varieties | 1/3 cup | 60 | 0% | 0% | 0% |

### PUDDING AND PIE FILLINGS

**Generic Foods**

| FOOD | Serving Size | Calories | Tot Fat | Sat Fat | Chol |
|------|------|------|------|------|------|
| ❖ Banana | 1/2 cup | 150 | 4% | 7% | 3% |
| ❖ Chocolate | 1/2 cup | 180 | 7% | 10% | 3% |
| ❖ Chocolate Renin | 1/2 cup | 110 | 4% | 9% | 5% |
| ❖ Coconut | 1/2 cup | 160 | 7% | 14% | 4% |
| ⨀ Custard | 1/2 cup | 150 | 12% | 17% | 46% |
| ❖ Flan | 1/2 cup | 150 | 6% | 13% | 6% |

★   Foods with this symbol have less than or equal to 5% *Daily Value* for <u>all</u> three nutrients (5% Rule).
❖   Foods with this symbol have <u>at least one</u> of the three nutrients greater than 5% *Daily Value* but less than or equal to 20% *Daily Value*.
⨀   Foods with this symbol have <u>at least one</u> of the three nutrients greater than 20% *Daily Value* (20% Rule).

| FOOD | Serving Size | Calories | Tot Fat | Sat Fat | Chol |
|------|--------------|----------|---------|---------|------|
| ❖ Lemon | 1/2 cup | 160 | 4% | 7% | 3% |
| ❖ Rice | 1/2 cup | 160 | 4% | 7% | 3% |
| ❖ Rice w/Raisins | 1/2 cup | 190 | 6% | 11% | 5% |
| ❖ Tapioca | 1/2 cup | 130 | 6% | 8% | 11% |
| ❖ Vanilla | 1/2 cup | 150 | 5% | 6% | 3% |
| ❖ Vanilla Renin | 1/2 cup | 100 | 4% | 7% | 5% |

**Brand Name Foods**

| FOOD | Serving Size | Calories | Tot Fat | Sat Fat | Chol |
|------|--------------|----------|---------|---------|------|
| ★ ALSA *International Desserts* Flan Creme Caramel Mix—CPC | 1/4 pkg | 110 | 0% | 0% | 1% |
| ALSA *International Desserts* Mousse Mixes—CPC | | | | | |
| ❖ Dark Chocolate | 1/4 pkg | 80 | 6% | 20% | 0% |
| ❖ Milk Chocolate | 1/4 pkg | 80 | 7% | 20% | 0% |
| ❖ White Chocolate | 1/4 pkg | 70 | 5% | 16% | 0% |
| BETTY CROCKER Creamy Chilled Dessert Mixes (prep as dir)— GENERAL MILLS | | | | | |
| ★ Banana Cream | 1/9 pkg | 250 | 16% | 14% | 16% |
| ❖ Chocolate French Silk | 1/8 pkg | 270 | 17% | 20% | 2% |
| ❖ Coconut Cream | 1/9 pkg | 290 | 21% | 28% | 19% |
| Ⓐ Cookies & Cream | 1/6 pkg | 380 | 25% | 19% | 2% |
| ❖ *Sunkist* Lemon Supreme | 1/9 pkg | 320 | 19% | 18% | 10% |
| ★ D-ZERTA Reduced Calorie Chocolate Pudding (prep as dir) —KRAFT | 1/2 cup | 60 | 0% | 0% | 0% |
| DEL MONTE Pudding Snack Cups | | | | | |
| ❖ Banana | 1 snack cup | 140 | 6% | 5% | 0% |
| ❖ Butterscotch | 1 snack cup | 140 | 6% | 5% | 0% |
| ❖ Chocolate | 1 snack cup | 160 | 6% | 5% | 0% |
| ❖ Chocolate Fudge | 1 snack cup | 150 | 6% | 5% | 0% |
| ❖ Tapioca | 1 snack cup | 140 | 6% | 5% | 0% |
| ❖ Vanilla | 1 snack cup | 150 | 6% | 5% | 0% |
| DEL MONTE *Lite* Pudding Snack Cups | | | | | |
| ★ Chocolate | 1 snack cup | 100 | 2% | 0% | 0% |
| ★ Vanilla | 1 snack cup | 90 | 2% | 0% | 0% |
| HUNT'S Snack Pack Puddings— HUNT WESSON | | | | | |
| ❖ Banana | 1/2 cup | 160 | 9% | 9% | 0% |
| ❖ Butterscotch | 1/2 cup | 150 | 9% | 8% | 0% |
| ❖ Chocolate | 1 each | 170 | 10% | 8% | 0% |
| ❖ Chocolate Caramel Swirl | 1 each | 170 | 9% | 7% | 0% |
| ❖ Chocolate Fudge | 1 each | 170 | 9% | 7% | 0% |
| ❖ Chocolate Marshmallow | 1/2 cup | 160 | 9% | 10% | 0% |
| ❖ Chocolate Peanut Butter Swirl | 1 each | 170 | 10% | 8% | 0% |
| ❖ Lemon | 1/2 cup | 160 | 5% | 4% | 0% |
| ❖ Milk Chocolate Swirl | 1 each | 160 | 9% | 7% | 0% |
| ❖ S'Mores Swirl | 1 each | 150 | 9% | 8% | 0% |

| FOOD | Serving Size | Calories | Tot Fat | Sat Fat | Chol |
|---|---|---|---|---|---|
| ❖ Tapioca | 1/2 cup | 150 | 9% | 6% | 0% |
| ❖ Vanilla | 1 each | 160 | 9% | 7% | 0% |
| HUNT'S Fat Free Snack Pack Puddings—HUNT WESSON | | | | | |
| ★ Chocolate | 1/2 cup | 100 | 1% | 0% | 0% |
| ★ Tapioca | 1/2 cup | 90 | 1% | 0% | 0% |
| ★ Vanilla | 1/2 cup | 90 | 1% | 0% | 0% |
| JELL-O *Americana* Pudding & Custard Mixes (prep as dir) —KRAFT | | | | | |
| ❖ Custard Dessert | 1/2 cup | 140 | 4% | 7% | 3% |
| ❖ Rice Pudding | 1/2 cup | 160 | 4% | 7% | 3% |
| ❖ Tapioca Pudding | 1/2 cup | 140 | 4% | 7% | 3% |
| JELL-O Brand Cook & Serve Puddings (prep as dir)—KRAFT | | | | | |
| ❖ Banana Cream | 1/2 cup | 140 | 4% | 7% | 3% |
| ❖ Butterscotch | 1/2 cup | 160 | 4% | 7% | 3% |
| ❖ Chocolate | 1/2 cup | 150 | 4% | 8% | 3% |
| ❖ Chocolate Fudge | 1/2 cup | 150 | 4% | 8% | 3% |
| ❖ Coconut Cream | 1/2 cup | 150 | 7% | 18% | 3% |
| ❖ Flan | 1/2 cup | 140 | 4% | 7% | 3% |
| Ⓐ Lemon | 1/2 cup | 140 | 3% | 3% | 24% |
| ❖ Milk Chocolate | 1/2 cup | 150 | 4% | 8% | 3% |
| ❖ Vanilla | 1/2 cup | 140 | 4% | 7% | 3% |
| JELL-O Brand Fat Free Sugar Free Instant Reduced Calorie Pudding & Pie Fillings—KRAFT | | | | | |
| ★ Banana | 1/2 cup | 70 | 0% | 0% | 0% |
| ★ Butterscotch | 1/2 cup | 70 | 0% | 0% | 0% |
| ★ Chocolate | 1/2 cup | 80 | 0% | 0% | 0% |
| ★ Chocolate Fudge | 1/2 cup | 80 | 0% | 0% | 0% |
| ★ Pistachio | 1/2 cup | 70 | 0% | 0% | 0% |
| ★ Vanilla | 1/2 cup | 70 | 0% | 0% | 0% |
| ★ JELL-O Brand *Free* Fat Free Pudding Snacks: All flavors —KRAFT | 1 snack | 100 | 0% | 0% | 0% |
| JELL-O Brand Instant Pudding & Pie Fillings (prep as dir)—KRAFT | | | | | |
| ❖ Banana Cream | 1/2 cup | 150 | 4% | 7% | 3% |
| ❖ Butter Pecan | 1/2 cup | 160 | 5% | 8% | 3% |
| ❖ Butterscotch | 1/2 cup | 150 | 4% | 7% | 3% |
| ❖ Chocolate | 1/2 cup | 160 | 4% | 8% | 3% |
| ❖ Chocolate Fudge | 1/2 cup | 160 | 4% | 8% | 3% |
| ❖ Coconut Cream | 1/2 cup | 160 | 7% | 17% | 3% |
| ❖ French Vanilla | 1/2 cup | 150 | 4% | 7% | 3% |

★ Foods with this symbol have less than or equal to 5% *Daily Value* for all three nutrients (5% Rule).

❖ Foods with this symbol have at least one of the three nutrients greater than 5% *Daily Value* but less than or equal to 20% *Daily Value*.

Ⓐ Foods with this symbol have at least one of the three nutrients greater than 20% *Daily Value* (20% Rule).

| FOOD | Serving Size | Calories | Tot Fat | Sat Fat | Chol |
|---|---|---|---|---|---|
| ❖ Lemon | 1/2 cup | 150 | 4% | 7% | 3% |
| ❖ Milk Chocolate | 1/2 cup | 160 | 4% | 9% | 3% |
| ❖ Pistachio | 1/2 cup | 160 | 5% | 8% | 3% |
| ❖ Vanilla | 1/2 cup | 150 | 4% | 7% | 3% |
| JELL-O Brand Snacks—KRAFT | | | | | |
| ❖ All flavors except Banana and Tapioca | 1 snack | 160 | 8% | 9% | 0% |
| ❖ Banana | 1 snack | 170 | 10% | 11% | 0% |
| ❖ Tapioca | 1 snack | 140 | 6% | 7% | 0% |
| ★ MINUTE Tapioca—KRAFT | 1 1/2 tsp | 20 | 0% | 0% | 0% |
| SWISS MISS Pudding Parfaits —HUNT WESSON | | | | | |
| ❖ Chocolate Chocolate Fudge | 1 each | 160 | 9% | 8% | 0% |
| ❖ Chocolate Vanilla | 1 each | 160 | 9% | 8% | 0% |
| ★ Fat Free Vanilla Chocolate | 1/2 cup | 100 | 1% | 0% | 0% |
| ❖ Milk Chocolate Chocolate Fudge | 1 each | 160 | 9% | 8% | 0% |
| ❖ Vanilla Chocolate | 1 each | 160 | 9% | 8% | 0% |
| SWISS MISS Puddings— HUNT WESSON | | | | | |
| ❖ Butterscotch | 1 each | 160 | 9% | 7% | 0% |
| ❖ Chocolate | 1 each | 170 | 9% | 8% | 0% |
| ❖ Chocolate Caramel Swirl | 1 each | 170 | 10% | 8% | 0% |
| ❖ Chocolate Fudge | 1 each | 180 | 9% | 8% | 0% |
| ❖ Chocolate Vanilla Swirl | 1 each | 170 | 9% | 8% | 0% |
| ❖ Tapioca | 1 each | 140 | 6% | 5% | 0% |
| ❖ Vanilla | 1 each | 160 | 9% | 7% | 0% |
| SWISS MISS Fat Free Puddings— HUNT WESSON | | | | | |
| ★ Chocolate | 1/2 cup | 100 | 1% | 0% | 0% |
| ★ Chocolate Fudge | 1/2 cup | 100 | 0% | 0% | 0% |
| ★ Tapioca | 1/2 cup | 100 | 0% | 0% | 0% |
| ★ Vanilla | 1/2 cup | 100 | 1% | 0% | 0% |

# Eggs and Egg Substitutes

## EGG DISHES

**Brand Name Foods**

| | | | | | |
|---|---|---|---|---|---|
| ❖ BREAKFAST-ON-THE-GO! Handy Ham & Cheese Omelet— WEIGHT WATCHERS | 1 omelet | 230 | 9% | 15% | 12% |
| SWANSON *Great Starts* Breakfast —CAMPBELL'S | | | | | |
| ⊛ *Budget* Scrambled Eggs | 1 pkg | 200 | 18% | 40% | 63% |
| ⊛ Eggs & Silver Dollar Pancakes | 1 pkg | 250 | 22% | 30% | 97% |
| ⊛ Eggs, Bacon & Cheese On a Muffin | 1 pkg | 290 | 23% | 30% | 32% |
| ⊛ Scrambled Eggs & Bacon | 1 pkg | 290 | 29% | 45% | 80% |

| | FOOD | Serving Size | Calories | Tot Fat | Sat Fat | Chol |
|---|---|---|---|---|---|---|
| ⊛ | Scrambled Eggs & Sausage | 1 pkg | 360 | 40% | 50% | 93% |

## EGGS

**Generic Foods**

| | | | | | | |
|---|---|---|---|---|---|---|
| ⊛ | Century | 1 egg | 80 | 7% | 8% | 71% |
| ★ | Chicken, Whites (large, raw) | 1 egg white | 20 | 0% | 0% | 0% |
| ⊛ | Chicken, Whole (large, raw) | 1 egg (50 g) | 80 | 8% | 8% | 71% |
| ⊛ | Chicken, Yolk (large, raw) | 1 yolk | 60 | 8% | 8% | 71% |
| ⊛ | Duck, Whole (raw) | 1 egg (70 g) | 130 | 15% | 13% | 206% |
| ⊛ | Quail, Whole (raw) | 1 egg (9 g) | 15 | 2% | 2% | 25% |

**Brand Name Foods**

| | | | | | | |
|---|---|---|---|---|---|---|
| ⊛ | EGGLAND'S BEST, Whole | 1 egg | 70 | 8% | 8% | 70% |

## EGG SUBSTITUTES

**Generic Foods**

| | | | | | | |
|---|---|---|---|---|---|---|
| ★ | Liquid Egg Substitute | 1/4 cup | 50 | 3% | 2% | 0% |

**Brand Name Foods**

| | | | | | | |
|---|---|---|---|---|---|---|
| ❖ | FEATHERWEIGHT *Egg Magic* | 1 pouch | 110 | 12% | 5% | 1% |
| ★ | FLEISCHMANN'S *Egg Beaters—* NABISCO | 1/4 cup | 30 | 0% | 0% | 0% |
| ★ | HEALTHY CHOICE Cholesterol Free Egg Product (frozen)— CONAGRA | 1/4 cup | 25 | 0% | 0% | 0% |
| | MORNINGSTAR FARMS Egg Substitutes—WORTHINGTON FOODS | | | | | |
| ★ | Better 'N Eggs | 1/4 cup | 20 | 0% | 0% | 0% |
| ★ | Scramblers | 1/4 cup | 35 | 0% | 0% | 0% |
| ★ | SECOND NATURE—M STAR | 1/4 cup | 40 | 0% | 0% | 0% |

# Fats and Oils

## ANIMAL FATS

**Generic Foods**

| | | | | | | |
|---|---|---|---|---|---|---|
| ⊛ | Beef Tallow (lard) | 1 tbsp | 120 | 20% | 32% | 5% |

---

★ Foods with this symbol have less than or equal to 5% *Daily Value* for <u>all</u> three nutrients (5% Rule).

❖ Foods with this symbol have <u>at least one</u> of the three nutrients greater than 5% *Daily Value* but less than or equal to 20% *Daily Value.*

⊛ Foods with this symbol have <u>at least one</u> of the three nutrients greater than 20% *Daily Value* (20% Rule).

| FOOD | Serving Size | Calories | Tot Fat | Sat Fat | Chol |
|------|------|------|------|------|------|
| ❖ Chicken Fat | 1 tbsp | 120 | 20% | 19% | 4% |
| Ⓐ Duck Fat | 1 tbsp | 120 | 20% | 21% | 4% |
| ❖ Goose Fat | 1 tbsp | 120 | 20% | 18% | 4% |
| Ⓐ Pork Fat (lard) | 1 tbsp | 120 | 20% | 25% | 4% |

## BUTTER

### Generic Foods

| | | | | | |
|------|------|------|------|------|------|
| Ⓐ Ghee | 1 tbsp | 120 | 20% | 40% | 11% |
| Ⓐ Regular | 1 tbsp | 100 | 18% | 35% | 10% |
| Ⓐ Whipped | 1 tbsp | 70 | 11% | 23% | 7% |

### Brand Name Foods

| | | | | | |
|------|------|------|------|------|------|
| LAND O'LAKES Butter | | | | | |
| Ⓐ  Stick: Salted or unsalted | 1 tbsp | 100 | 17% | 35% | 10% |
| Ⓐ  Tub: Whipped, Salted or unsalted | 1 tbsp | 70 | 11% | 25% | 7% |
| LAND O'LAKES Light Butter | | | | | |
| ❖  Stick: Salted or unsalted | 1 tbsp | 50 | 8% | 20% | 7% |
| ❖  Tub: Whipped, Salted | 1 tbsp | 35 | 5% | 13% | 3% |

## BUTTER SUBSTITUTES

### Brand Name Foods

| | | | | | |
|------|------|------|------|------|------|
| ★ BEST O' BUTTER Granules— MCCORMICK | 1/2 tsp | 4 | 1% | 0% | 0% |
| ★ MOLLY McBUTTER All Natural Dairy Sprinkles—ALBERTO-CULVER | 1 tsp | 8 | 0% | 0% | 0% |

## COOKING SPRAYS

### Brand Name Foods

| | | | | | |
|------|------|------|------|------|------|
| ★ BAKER'S JOY Vegetable Oil & Flour Baking Spray— ALBERTO-CULVER | 0.25 g | 4 | 2% | 0% | 0% |
| ★ MAZOLA *No Stick* Corn Oil Cooking Spray—CPC | 2.5-second spray | 2 | 0% | 0% | 0% |
| PAM No Stick Cooking Spray— AMERICAN HOME FOODS | | | | | |
| ★  All Natural Olive Oil, aerosol | 1/3-second spray | 0 | 0% | 0% | 0% |
| ★  Butter Flavor, aerosol | 1/3-second spray | 0 | 0% | 0% | 0% |
| ★  Original, aerosol | 1/3-second spray | 0 | 0% | 0% | 0% |
| ★  Pump bottle | 2 pumps | 0 | 0% | 0% | 0% |

| FOOD | Serving Size | Calories | Tot Fat | Sat Fat | Chol |
|------|--------------|----------|---------|---------|------|
| ★ WESSON No Stick Cooking Sprays, Aerosol or Pump— HUNT WESSON | 1 spray (0.25 g) | 2 | 0% | 0% | 0% |

## MARGARINES

### Generic Foods

Stick:

| | | | | | |
|------|--------------|----------|---------|---------|------|
| ❖ Corn oil | 1 tbsp | 100 | 18% | 11% | 0% |
| ❖ Safflower/Soybean | 1 tbsp | 100 | 18% | 9% | 0% |

Tub:

| | | | | | |
|------|--------------|----------|---------|---------|------|
| ❖ Corn oil | 1 tbsp | 100 | 18% | 9% | 0% |
| ❖ Safflower | 1 tbsp | 100 | 18% | 6% | 0% |

### Brand Name Foods

BLUE BONNET Margarine—NABISCO
Stick:

| | | | | | |
|------|--------------|----------|---------|---------|------|
| ❖ 60% vegetable oil | 1 tbsp | 70 | 13% | 8% | 0% |
| ❖ *Better Blend* Spread | 1 tbsp | 90 | 17% | 10% | 0% |

Tub:

| | | | | | |
|------|--------------|----------|---------|---------|------|
| ❖ 48% vegetable oil | 1 tbsp | 60 | 11% | 6% | 0% |
| ❖ *Better Blend* Spread | 1 tbsp | 90 | 17% | 10% | 0% |

CANOLA HARVEST Margarine, Tub—HEARTLIGHT

| | | | | | |
|------|--------------|----------|---------|---------|------|
| ❖ Reduced Fat Spread | 1 tbsp | 60 | 11% | 5% | 0% |
| ❖ Soft | 1 tbsp | 100 | 17% | 5% | 0% |

CHIFFON, Tub—KRAFT

| | | | | | |
|------|--------------|----------|---------|---------|------|
| ❖ Soft Margarine | 1 tbsp | 100 | 17% | 10% | 0% |
| ❖ Whipped Margarine | 1 tbsp | 70 | 11% | 8% | 0% |

FLEISCHMANN'S Margarine— NABISCO
Stick:

| | | | | | |
|------|--------------|----------|---------|---------|------|
| ❖ Light Taste, 56% corn oil | 1 tbsp | 70 | 13% | 8% | 0% |
| ❖ Original | 1 tbsp | 100 | 17% | 10% | 0% |
| Sweet Original, Salted or Unsalted | 1 tbsp | 100 | 17% | 10% | 0% |

Tub:

| | | | | | |
|------|--------------|----------|---------|---------|------|
| ❖ Light Taste, 56% corn oil | 1 tbsp | 70 | 13% | 7% | 0% |
| ❖ Soft, 67% corn oil | 1 tbsp | 80 | 14% | 8% | 0% |

HAIN Safflower Oil Margarines

| | | | | | |
|------|--------------|----------|---------|---------|------|
| ❖ Stick: Regular or Unsalted | 1 tbsp | 100 | 17% | 9% | 0% |
| ❖ Tub: Soft | 1 tbsp | 100 | 17% | 8% | 0% |

★ Foods with this symbol have less than or equal to 5% *Daily Value* for <u>all</u> three nutrients (5% Rule).

❖ Foods with this symbol have <u>at least one</u> of the three nutrients greater than 5% *Daily Value* but less than or equal to 20% *Daily Value*.

Ⓐ Foods with this symbol have <u>at least one</u> of the three nutrients greater than 20% *Daily Value* (20% Rule).

| FOOD | Serving Size | Calories | Tot Fat | Sat Fat | Chol |
|------|--------------|----------|---------|---------|------|
| ❖ HOLLYWOOD Safflower Oil Margarine, Regular or Unsalted —HAIN | 1 tbsp | 100 | 18% | 10% | 0% |
| I CAN'T BELIEVE IT'S NOT BUTTER—VAN DEN BERGH | | | | | |
| ★ Spray bottle | 1 tbsp | 0 | 0% | 0% | 0% |
| ❖ Squeeze bottle, 68% vegetable oil | 1 tbsp | 90 | 15% | 9% | 0% |
| Tub: | | | | | |
| ❖ 70% vegetable oil | 1 tbsp | 90 | 15% | 10% | 0% |
| ❖ Light (40% vegetable oil) | 1 tbsp | 50 | 9% | 5% | 0% |
| IMPERIAL—VAN DEN BERGH | | | | | |
| ❖ Stick, 70% vegetable oil | 1 tbsp | 90 | 16% | 10% | 0% |
| Tub: | | | | | |
| ❖ Diet | 1 tbsp | 50 | 9% | 5% | 0% |
| ❖ Soft, 68% vegetable oil | 1 tbsp | 90 | 15% | 10% | 0% |
| IMPERIAL Delight—VAN DEN BERGH | | | | | |
| ❖ Stick, 25% vegetable oil | 1 tbsp | 70 | 11% | 8% | 0% |
| ❖ Tub | 1 tbsp | 60 | 11% | 7% | 0% |
| KRAFT Touch of Butter | | | | | |
| ❖ Squeeze bottle, 64% oil | 1 tbsp | 80 | 14% | 8% | 0% |
| ❖ Stick, 70% oil | 1 tbsp | 90 | 15% | 10% | 0% |
| ❖ Tub, 47% oil | 1 tbsp | 60 | 11% | 8% | 0% |
| LAND O'LAKES Country Morning Blend | | | | | |
| ❖ Stick, Regular or Unsalted | 1 tbsp | 100 | 17% | 13% | 0% |
| ❖ Tub | 1 tbsp | 100 | 17% | 10% | 0% |
| LAND O'LAKES Country Morning Blend Light | | | | | |
| ❖ Stick, Salted | 1 tbsp | 50 | 9% | 15% | 3% |
| ❖ Tub | 1 tbsp | 50 | 9% | 13% | 2% |
| LAND O'LAKES Margarine | | | | | |
| ❖ Stick | 1 tbsp | 100 | 17% | 10% | 0% |
| ❖ Tub | 1 tbsp | 100 | 17% | 10% | 0% |
| LAND O'LAKES Spread w/ Sweet Cream | | | | | |
| ❖ Stick, Regular or Unsalted | 1 tbsp | 90 | 15% | 10% | 0% |
| ❖ Tub | 1 tbsp | 80 | 12% | 10% | 0% |
| MAZOLA—CPC | | | | | |
| ❖ Stick, Regular or Unsalted | 1 tbsp | 100 | 17% | 10% | 0% |
| Tub: | | | | | |
| ❖ Extra Light Spread | 1 tbsp | 50 | 9% | 5% | 0% |
| ❖ Reduced Calorie Diet | 1 tbsp | 50 | 9% | 5% | 0% |
| ★ NUCOA Margarines—HEART BEAT FOODS | 1 tbsp | 25 | 5% | 3% | 0% |
| ❖ Stick, Real Margarine | 1 tbsp | 100 | 17% | 10% | 0% |
| ★ Tub, Smart Beat, trans fat free | 1 tbsp | 20 | 3% | 0% | 0% |
| PARKAY—KRAFT | | | | | |
| ❖ Squeeze bottle, 64% oil | 1 tbsp | 80 | 14% | 8% | 0% |
| ❖ Stick, 70% oil | 1 tbsp | 90 | 15% | 10% | 0% |

| FOOD | Serving Size | Calories | Tot Fat | Sat Fat | Chol |
|---|---|---|---|---|---|
| Tub: | | | | | |
| ❖   50% oil | 1 tbsp | 60 | 11% | 8% | 0% |
| ❖   *Light*, 40% oil | 1 tbsp | 50 | 9% | 5% | 0% |
| ❖   Soft | 1 tbsp | 100 | 17% | 10% | 0% |
| ❖   Soft Diet | 1 tbsp | 50 | 9% | 5% | 0% |
| ❖   Whipped | 1 tbsp | 70 | 11% | 8% | 0% |
| PROMISE *Ultra*, Tub—VAN DEN BERGH | 1 tbsp | 50 | 9% | 5% | 0% |
| ❖   26% vegetable oil | 1 tbsp | 35 | 6% | 0% | 0% |
| ★   Fat Free | 1 tbsp | 5 | 0% | 0% | 0% |
| SAFFOLA Margarine | | | | | |
| ❖   Stick, Regular or Unsalted | 1 tbsp | 100 | 17% | 10% | 0% |
| Tub: | | | | | |
| ❖   Reduced Fat Margarine | 1 tbsp | 70 | 12% | 5% | 0% |
| ❖   Soft | 1 tbsp | 100 | 17% | 8% | 0% |
| ❖ SHEDD'S SPREAD *Country Crock*, Churn Style or Regular —VAN DEN BERGH | 1 tbsp | 60 | 11% | 7% | 0% |
| WEIGHT WATCHERS Margarine | | | | | |
| ❖   Stick, Reduced Fat | 1 tbsp | 60 | 11% | 8% | 0% |
| Tub: | | | | | |
| ❖   Light | 1 tbsp | 45 | 6% | 5% | 0% |
| ❖   Light, sodium free | 1 tbsp | 45 | 6% | 5% | 0% |

## OILS

**Brand Name Foods**

| FOOD | Serving Size | Calories | Tot Fat | Sat Fat | Chol |
|---|---|---|---|---|---|
| CRISCO—PROCTER & GAMBLE | | | | | |
| Ⓐ   Blend of Canola and Corn Oils | 1 tbsp | 120 | 21% | 7% | 0% |
| Ⓐ   Puritan Oil | 1 tbsp | 120 | 21% | 5% | 0% |
| Ⓐ   Vegetable Oil | 1 tbsp | 120 | 21% | 5% | 0% |
| Ⓐ FLEISCHMANN'S Harvest Blend (Canola/Corn)—HUNT WESSON | 1 tbsp | 120 | 21% | 6% | 0% |
| HAIN Vegetable Oils | | | | | |
| Ⓐ   Almond Oil | 1 tbsp | 120 | 22% | 6% | 0% |
| Ⓐ   Canola Oil | 1 tbsp | 120 | 22% | 4% | 0% |
| Ⓐ   Garlic Flavored Oil | 1 tbsp | 120 | 22% | 11% | 0% |
| Ⓐ   Peanut Oil | 1 tbsp | 120 | 22% | 9% | 0% |
| Ⓐ   Safflower Oil | 1 tbsp | 120 | 22% | 6% | 0% |
| Ⓐ   Sesame Oil | 1 tbsp | 120 | 22% | 11% | 0% |
| Ⓐ   Soybean Oil | 1 tbsp | 120 | 22% | 10% | 0% |
| Ⓐ   Sunflower Oil | 1 tbsp | 120 | 22% | 8% | 0% |
| Ⓐ   Virgin Olive Oil | 1 tbsp | 120 | 22% | 9% | 0% |
| Ⓐ   Walnut Oil | 1 tbsp | 120 | 22% | 7% | 0% |

★  Foods with this symbol have less than or equal to 5% *Daily Value* for <u>all</u> three nutrients (5% Rule).

❖  Foods with this symbol have <u>at least one</u> of the three nutrients greater than 5% *Daily Value* but less than or equal to 20% *Daily Value*.

Ⓐ  Foods with this symbol have <u>at least one</u> of the three nutrients greater than 20% *Daily Value* (20% Rule).

| FOOD | Serving Size | Calories | Tot Fat | Sat Fat | Chol |
|---|---|---|---|---|---|
| | | | % DAILY VALUE | | |
| ⊛ Canola HARVEST Oil— | | | | | |
| VAN DEN BERGH | 1 tbsp | 120 | 22% | 5% | 0% |
| ⊛ HEART BEAT, Canola Oil—NUCOA | 1 tbsp | 120 | 22% | 5% | 0% |
| HOLLYWOOD Vegetable Oils—HAIN | | | | | |
| ⊛ Canola Oil | 1 tbsp | 120 | 22% | 4% | 0% |
| ⊛ Peanut Oil | 1 tbsp | 120 | 22% | 9% | 0% |
| ⊛ Safflower Oil | 1 tbsp | 120 | 22% | 6% | 0% |
| MAZOLA—CPC | | | | | |
| ⊛ Corn Oil | 1 tbsp | 120 | 22% | 10% | 0% |
| ⊛ *Right Blend* (corn and canola) | 1 tbsp | 120 | 22% | 5% | 0% |
| ⊛ ORVILLE REDENBACHER'S | | | | | |
| Popping & Topping Oil— | | | | | |
| HUNT WESSON | 1 tbsp | 120 | 21% | 10% | 0% |
| PROGRESSO Olive Oil—PET | | | | | |
| ⊛ Extra Virgin | 1 tbsp | 120 | 22% | 10% | 0% |
| ⊛ Extra Mild | 1 tbsp | 120 | 22% | 10% | 0% |
| ⊛ Riviera Blend | 1 tbsp | 120 | 22% | 10% | 0% |
| ⊛ SAFFOLA Safflower Oil | 1 tbsp | 120 | 22% | 5% | 0% |
| ❖ SUN LUCK Sesame Oil | 1 tsp | 45 | 8% | 5% | 0% |
| WESSON Oils—HUNT WESSON | | | | | |
| ⊛ *Best Blend* | 1 tbsp | 120 | 21% | 6% | 0% |
| ⊛ Buttery Flavored | 1 tbsp | 120 | 21% | 10% | 0% |
| ⊛ Canola | 1 tbsp | 120 | 21% | 5% | 0% |
| ⊛ Corn | 1 tbsp | 120 | 21% | 9% | 0% |
| ⊛ Olive | 1 tbsp | 120 | 21% | 6% | 0% |
| ⊛ Peanut | 1 tbsp | 120 | 21% | 13% | 0% |
| ⊛ Stir Fry | 1 tbsp | 120 | 21% | 6% | 0% |
| ⊛ Sunflower | 1 tbsp | 120 | 21% | 8% | 0% |
| ⊛ Vegetable | 1 tbsp | 120 | 21% | 10% | 0% |

SHORTENINGS

**Brand Name Foods**

| FOOD | Serving Size | Calories | Tot Fat | Sat Fat | Chol |
|---|---|---|---|---|---|
| CRISCO Shortening—PROCTER & GAMBLE | | | | | |
| ❖ Butter Flavor | 1 tbsp | 110 | 18% | 15% | 0% |
| ❖ Original | 1 tbsp | 110 | 18% | 15% | 0% |
| ❖ WESSON Shortening—HUNT WESSON | 1 tbsp | 110 | 19% | 13% | 0% |

| FOOD | Serving Size | Calories | Tot Fat | Sat Fat | Chol |
|---|---|---|---|---|---|

# Fish and Seafood

## BATTERED AND BREADED FRIED FISH

### Generic Fish

| FOOD | Serving Size | Calories | Tot Fat | Sat Fat | Chol |
|---|---|---|---|---|---|
| ⊛ Catfish | 3 oz | 200 | 17% | 14% | 23% |
| ❖ Clams | 3 oz | 170 | 14% | 11% | 17% |
| ⊛ Crab Cakes | 2 cakes | 320 | 32% | 22% | 55% |
| ⊛ Fish Sticks | 3 oz | 230 | 16% | 13% | 32% |
| ❖ Ocean Perch | 3 oz | 195 | 17% | 14% | 11% |
| ⊛ Oysters | 4 pcs | 250 | 18% | 15% | 24% |
| ❖ Scallops | 3 oz | 180 | 14% | 11% | 17% |
| ❖ Shark | 3 oz | 190 | 18% | 14% | 17% |
| ⊛ Shrimp | 3 oz | 210 | 16% | 9% | 50% |

### Brand Name Foods

| FOOD | Serving Size | Calories | Tot Fat | Sat Fat | Chol |
|---|---|---|---|---|---|
| GORTON'S Crunchy Breaded Fillets & Sticks—GENERAL MILLS | | | | | |
| ⊛ Fish Fillets | 2 fillets | 250 | 21% | 6% | 11% |
| ⊛ Fish Sticks (minced fish) | 6 sticks | 260 | 23% | 7% | 8% |
| ⊛ Garlic 'n Herb Fillet | 2 fillets | 250 | 21% | 7% | 12% |
| ⊛ Hot 'n Spicy Fillets | 2 fillets | 250 | 22% | 7% | 9% |
| ⊛ Southern Fried Country Style Fillets | 2 fillets | 270 | 25% | 9% | 10% |
| GORTON'S Crispy Batter Fillets & Sticks—GENERAL MILLS | | | | | |
| ⊛ Fillets | 2 fillets | 290 | 33% | 22% | 8% |
| ⊛ Haddock Fillets | 2 fillets | 270 | 29% | 22% | 9% |
| ⊛ Lemon Pepper Fillets | 2 fillets | 250 | 25% | 10% | 12% |
| ⊛ Pollock Fillets | 2 fillets | 280 | 30% | 25% | 7% |
| ⊛ Sticks (minced) | 5 sticks | 290 | 30% | 25% | 7% |
| GORTON'S Potato Crisp— GENERAL MILLS | | | | | |
| ⊛ Fillets | 2 fillets | 300 | 29% | 8% | 10% |
| ⊛ Sticks | 6 sticks | 270 | 24% | 21% | 7% |
| GORTON'S Shrimp Products— GENERAL MILLS | | | | | |
| ⊛ Baked Scampi | 6 pcs | 250 | 24% | 15% | 23% |
| ⊛ Beer Batter Shrimp | 6 pcs | 250 | 23% | 12% | 24% |
| ⊛ Marinated and Breaded Original Seasoning | 6 pcs | 230 | 20% | 11% | 26% |
| ⊛ Microwave Crunchy Shrimp | 1 pkg | 300 | 24% | 14% | 34% |
| ⊛ Popcorn Shrimp | 1 cup | 260 | 24% | 16% | 20% |

★ Foods with this symbol have less than or equal to 5% *Daily Value* for <u>all</u> three nutrients (5% Rule).

❖ Foods with this symbol have <u>at least one</u> of the three nutrients greater than 5% *Daily Value* but less than or equal to 20% *Daily Value*.

⊛ Foods with this symbol have <u>at least one</u> of the three nutrients greater than 20% *Daily Value* (20% Rule).

| FOOD | Serving Size | Calories | Tot Fat | Sat Fat | Chol |
|------|-------------|----------|---------|---------|------|
| ✺ Popcorn Shrimp Garlic & Herb | 1 1/4 cups | 270 | 20% | 14% | 33% |
| MRS. PAUL'S—CAMPBELL'S | | | | | |
| ❖ Deviled Crabs | 1 cake | 180 | 14% | 15% | 8% |
| ❖ Fish Sticks | 2 cakes | 210 | 12% | 10% | 5% |
| ✺ Fried Clams | 3 fl oz | 280 | 25% | 15% | 3% |
| ❖ Fried Scallops | 12 scallops | 210 | 12% | 10% | 3% |
| MRS. PAUL'S Batter Dipped Fish —CAMPBELL'S | | | | | |
| ❖ Fillets | 1 fillet | 170 | 15% | 13% | 7% |
| ✺ Portions | 2 fillets | 250 | 25% | 25% | 10% |
| ✺ Sticks | 6 sticks | 270 | 23% | 18% | 8% |
| MRS. PAUL'S Breaded Fish— CAMPBELL'S | | | | | |
| ❖ Portions | 2 portions | 190 | 15% | 15% | 5% |
| ✺ Shrimp, Garlic & Herb | 1 pkg | 340 | 23% | 15% | 37% |
| ✺ Shrimp, Special Recipe | 1 pkg | 350 | 25% | 13% | 32% |
| ❖ Sticks | 6 sticks | 210 | 17% | 10% | 7% |
| ❖ Sticks, Minis | 12 minis | 220 | 17% | 13% | 10% |
| MRS. PAUL'S Crispy Crunchy Batter Dipped Fish—CAMPBELL'S | | | | | |
| ❖ Fillets | 2 fillets | 250 | 20% | 15% | 8% |
| ✺ Flounder Fillets | 2 fillets | 260 | 22% | 15% | 10% |
| ❖ Haddock Fillets | 2 fillets | 250 | 18% | 13% | 8% |
| MRS. PAUL'S Crispy Crunchy Breaded Fish—CAMPBELL'S | | | | | |
| ❖ Deviled Crab Miniatures | 6 minis | 240 | 17% | 15% | 5% |
| ❖ Fillets | 2 fillets | 220 | 15% | 13% | 12% |
| ❖ Sticks | 5 sticks | 210 | 14% | 13% | 7% |
| MRS. PAUL'S *Healthy Treasures* Breaded Fish—CAMPBELL'S | | | | | |
| ❖ Fillets | 1 fillet | 170 | 5% | 8% | 10% |
| ❖ Sticks | 4 sticks | 170 | 5% | 8% | 7% |
| VAN DE KAMP'S *Crisp & Healthy* Breaded Fish—PET | | | | | |
| ❖ Fillets | 2 fillets | 150 | 4% | 3% | 9% |
| ❖ Sticks | 6 sticks | 180 | 4% | 3% | 9% |
| VAN DE KAMP'S Battered Fish —PET | | | | | |
| ❖ Fillets | 1 fillet | 180 | 16% | 9% | 7% |
| ✺ Haddock Fillets | 1 fillet | 260 | 24% | 13% | 10% |
| ✺ Halibut Fillets | 1 fillet | 300 | 32% | 16% | 6% |
| ✺ Nuggets | 8 pcs | 280 | 27% | 14% | 8% |
| ✺ Portions | 2 pcs | 350 | 34% | 18% | 12% |
| ✺ Sticks | 6 sticks | 260 | 25% | 14% | 10% |
| VAN DE KAMP'S Breaded Fish —PET | | | | | |
| ✺ Butterfly Shrimp | 7 shrimp | 280 | 21% | 12% | 19% |
| ✺ Fillets | 2 fillets | 280 | 29% | 14% | 11% |

| FOOD | Serving Size | Calories | Tot Fat | Sat Fat | Chol |
|------|--------------|----------|---------|---------|------|
| ⊛ Fish 'n Fries | 1 pkg | 380 | 28% | 15% | 8% |
| ⊛ Haddock Fillets | 2 fillets | 280 | 26% | 14% | 9% |
| ⊛ Mini Sticks | 13 sticks | 250 | 22% | 11% | 10% |
| ⊛ Perch Fillets | 2 fillets | 300 | 31% | 13% | 9% |
| ❖ Popcorn Shrimp | 20 shrimp | 270 | 19% | 11% | 12% |
| ⊛ Portions | 3 pcs | 330 | 32% | 15% | 11% |
| ⊛ Sticks | 6 sticks | 290 | 26% | 13% | 11% |
| ❖ Whole Shrimp | 7 shrimp | 240 | 15% | 8% | 16% |
| VAN DE KAMP'S Lightly Breaded Fillets—PET | | | | | |
| ❖ Cod | 1 fillet | 220 | 15% | 6% | 11% |
| ❖ Flounder | 1 fillet | 230 | 16% | 9% | 14% |
| ❖ Haddock | 1 fillet | 220 | 16% | 8% | 11% |
| ❖ Sole | 1 fillet | 220 | 17% | 9% | 14% |

## CANNED FISH

### Generic Foods

| FOOD | Serving Size | Calories | Tot Fat | Sat Fat | Chol |
|------|--------------|----------|---------|---------|------|
| ❖ Anchovy Filet | 2 oz | 120 | 8% | 6% | 16% |
| ❖ Clams (solids and liquids) | 2 oz | 30 | 1% | 1% | 12% |
| ❖ Crab, King (canned) | 2 oz | 60 | 2% | 1% | 19% |
| ❖ Crab, Snow (Atlantic) | 2 oz | 40 | 1% | 1% | 17% |
| ❖ Mackerel, Atlantic | 2 oz | 90 | 5% | 5% | 14% |
| ❖ Oyster, Eastern | 2 oz | 40 | 2% | 2% | 10% |
| ❖ Salmon, Chum | 2 oz | 80 | 5% | 4% | 7% |
| ❖ Salmon, Pink (solids and liquids) | 2 oz | 80 | 5% | 4% | 10% |
| ❖ Salmon, Sockeye | 2 oz | 80 | 6% | 5% | 8% |
| ❖ Sardine (in tomato sauce) | 2 pcs | 140 | 14% | 12% | 15% |
| ⊛ Sardine, Atlantic (in oil) | 5 pcs | 130 | 11% | 5% | 28% |
| ⊛ Shrimp meat | 1/2 cup | 80 | 2% | 1% | 37% |
| ❖ Tuna, Light (in oil) | 2 oz (drained) | 110 | 7% | 4% | 3% |
| ❖ Tuna, Light (in water) | 2 oz (drained) | 70 | 1% | 1% | 6% |
| ❖ Tuna, White (in oil) | 2 oz (drained) | 110 | 7% | 4% | 6% |
| ❖ Tuna, White Albacore (in water) | 2 oz (drained) | 80 | 2% | 2% | 8% |

### Brand Name Foods

**Note:** *Values for canned tuna based on drained weight.*

| FOOD | Serving Size | Calories | Tot Fat | Sat Fat | Chol |
|------|--------------|----------|---------|---------|------|
| BUMBLE BEE Tuna | | | | | |
| ❖ Chunk Light (in oil) | 2 oz | 110 | 9% | 5% | 10% |
| ❖ Chunk Light (in water) | 3 oz | 60 | 1% | 0% | 10% |
| ❖ Chunk White (in oil) | 4 oz | 100 | 8% | 5% | 8% |

★ Foods with this symbol have less than or equal to 5% *Daily Value* for <u>all</u> three nutrients (5% Rule).

❖ Foods with this symbol have <u>at least one</u> of the three nutrients greater than 5% *Daily Value* but less than or equal to 20% *Daily Value*.

⊛ Foods with this symbol have <u>at least one</u> of the three nutrients greater than 20% *Daily Value* (20% Rule).

| FOOD | Serving Size | Calories | Tot Fat | Sat Fat | Chol |
|---|---|---|---|---|---|
| ❖ Chunk White (in water) | 5 oz | 60 | 2% | 0% | 8% |
| ❖ Chunk White, Diet (in water) | 8 oz | 70 | 2% | 0% | 8% |
| ❖ Solid White (in oil) | 6 oz | 90 | 5% | 3% | 8% |
| ❖ Solid White (in water) | 7 oz | 70 | 2% | 0% | 8% |
| CHICKEN OF THE SEA Tuna— | | | | | |
| VAN CAMP | | | | | |
| ❖ Chunk Light Tuna in Spring Water | 2 oz | 60 | 1% | 0% | 10% |
| ❖ Chunk Light Tuna w/Canola Oil | 2 oz | 110 | 8% | 0% | 10% |
| ❖ Solid White Tuna in Spring Water | 2 oz | 70 | 2% | 0% | 8% |
| ❖ DEL MONTE Sardines in Tomato Sauce | 1/2 fish w/sauce | 80 | 6% | 7% | 12% |
| FEATHERWEIGHT Canned Fish | | | | | |
| ❖ Chunk Light Tuna (in water) | 1/4 cup | 60 | 1% | 0% | 10% |
| ❖ Pink Salmon | 1/4 cup | 90 | 8% | 5% | 13% |
| GORTON'S CLAMS—GENERAL MILLS | | | | | |
| ⊛ Crunchy Fried | 3 oz | 260 | 26% | 22% | 3% |
| ★ Ocean Chopped & Minced | 1/4 cup | 20 | 0% | 0% | 3% |
| ★ GORTON'S Cod Cakes— GENERAL MILLS | 4 oz | 100 | 1% | 0% | 5% |
| LIBBY'S Salmon—NESTLÉ | | | | | |
| ❖ Pink Salmon | 1/4 cup | 90 | 8% | 6% | 13% |
| ❖ Pink Salmon, Boneless Skinless | 1/3 cup | 70 | 3% | 0% | 13% |
| ❖ Red Salmon | 1/4 cup | 110 | 10% | 8% | 13% |
| MANISCHEWITZ Prepared Fish | | | | | |
| ❖ Fishlets | 7 pcs | 50 | 4% | 0% | 7% |
| ❖ Gefilte Fish in Liquid Broth | 1 pc | 70 | 8% | 8% | 10% |
| ★ Gefilte Fish, Sweet | 1 pc | 35 | 2% | 0% | 3% |
| ❖ Whitefish and Pike in Liquid Broth | 1 pc | 50 | 2% | 5% | 12% |
| ★ Whitefish and Pike, Sweet | 1 pc | 45 | 2% | 0% | 3% |
| PROGRESSO—PET | | | | | |
| ★ Minced Clams | 1/4 cup | 25 | 0% | 0% | 3% |
| ❖ Solid Tuna in Olive Oil | 1/4 cup | 160 | 18% | 10% | 10% |
| S & W Clams | | | | | |
| ★ Fancy Minced/Chopped Clams | 1/4 cup | 20 | 0% | 0% | 3% |
| ❖ Whole Baby Chowder Clams | 1/4 cup | 50 | 2% | 3% | 13% |
| ❖ S & W Fancy Whole Oysters | 2 oz | 70 | 5% | 0% | 7% |
| S & W Tuna | | | | | |
| ❖ Chunk Light Fancy Tuna in Vegetable Oil | 2 oz | 110 | 9% | 5% | 10% |
| ❖ Fancy Tuna in Water | 2 oz | 70 | 1% | 0% | 12% |
| STARKIST Charlie's Lunch Kit (prep as dir)—HEINZ | | | | | |
| ❖ Chunk Light Tuna (in spring water) | 1 serving | 230 | 12% | 8% | 13% |

| FOOD | Serving Size | Calories | Tot Fat | Sat Fat | Chol |
|---|---|---|---|---|---|
| ❖ Chunk White Tuna (in spring water) | 1 serving | 230 | 12% | 8% | 12% |
| STARKIST Light Tuna—HEINZ | | | | | |
| ❖ Chunk Light (in oil) | 2 oz | 110 | 9% | 5% | 10% |
| ❖ Chunk Light (in spring water) | 2 oz | 60 | 1% | 0% | 10% |
| STARKIST Naturally Low Salt/ Low Fat Tuna—HEINZ | | | | | |
| ❖ Chunk Light (in spring water) | 2 oz | 60 | 1% | 0% | 8% |
| ❖ Chunk White (in distilled water) | 2 oz | 60 | 1% | 0% | 8% |
| STARKIST *Select* Tuna—HEINZ | | | | | |
| ❖ Hickory Smoke Solid White (in spring water) | 2 oz | 70 | 2% | 0% | 8% |
| ❖ Prime Catch Solid Light (in spring water) | 2 oz | 60 | 2% | 0% | 10% |
| STARKIST White Tuna—HEINZ | | | | | |
| ❖ Chunk White (in spring water) | 2 oz | 60 | 2% | 0% | 8% |
| ❖ Solid White (in oil) | 2 oz | 90 | 5% | 3% | 8% |
| ❖ Solid White (in spring water) | 2 oz | 70 | 2% | 0% | 8% |
| UNDERWOOD Sardines—PET | | | | | |
| Ⓐ In Mustard Sauce | 1 can | 180 | 18% | 14% | 35% |
| Ⓐ In Soy Oil | 1 can | 220 | 25% | 19% | 34% |
| Ⓐ In Tomato Sauce | 1 can | 180 | 18% | 14% | 38% |

### FRESH OR FROZEN FISH

**Generic Foods**

| FOOD | Serving Size | Calories | Tot Fat | Sat Fat | Chol |
|---|---|---|---|---|---|
| Ⓐ Bass, Freshwater (broiled) | 3 oz | 120 | 6% | 4% | 25% |
| ❖ Bass, Sea (cooked dry heat) | 3 oz | 110 | 3% | 3% | 15% |
| Ⓐ Bass, Striped (broiled) | 3 oz | 110 | 4% | 6% | 29% |
| Ⓐ Bluefish (broiled) | 3 oz | 140 | 7% | 5% | 21% |
| Ⓐ Burbot (broiled) | 3 oz | 100 | 1% | 1% | 22% |
| Ⓐ Carp (cooked dry heat) | 3 oz | 140 | 9% | 6% | 24% |
| ❖ Catfish, Channel (cooked dry heat) | 3 oz | 130 | 11% | 8% | 18% |
| Ⓐ Caviar (Sturgeon Eggs) | 1 tbsp | 40 | 4% | 3% | 31% |
| ❖ Clams (cooked moist heat) | 3 oz | 130 | 3% | 1% | 19% |
| ❖ Cod, Atlantic (broiled) | 3 oz | 90 | 1% | 1% | 16% |
| ❖ Cod, Pacific (broiled) | 3 oz | 90 | 1% | 0% | 14% |
| ❖ Crab (steamed) | 3 oz (meat only) | 80 | 2% | 1% | 15% |
| Ⓐ Crab, Dungeness (cooked moist heat) | 3 oz (meat only) | 90 | 2% | 1% | 21% |
| Ⓐ Crayfish (cooked moist heat) | 3 oz (meat only) | 70 | 2% | 1% | 39% |
| ❖ Flounder (cooked dry heat) | 3 oz | 100 | 2% | 2% | 19% |
| ❖ Grouper (cooked dry heat) | 3 oz | 100 | 2% | 1% | 13% |

★ Foods with this symbol have less than or equal to 5% *Daily Value* for <u>all</u> three nutrients (5% Rule).
❖ Foods with this symbol have <u>at least one</u> of the three nutrients greater than 5% *Daily Value* but less than or equal to 20% *Daily Value*.
Ⓐ Foods with this symbol have <u>at least one</u> of the three nutrients greater than 20% *Daily Value* (20% Rule).

| FOOD | Serving Size | Calories | Tot Fat | Sat Fat | Chol |
|------|--------------|----------|---------|---------|------|
| ⊛ Haddock (broiled) | 3 oz | 100 | 1% | 1% | 21% |
| ❖ Halibut (broiled) | 3 oz | 120 | 4% | 2% | 12% |
| ⊛ Herring, Atlantic (broiled) | 3 oz | 170 | 15% | 11% | 22% |
| ⊛ Herring, Pacific (broiled) | 3 oz | 210 | 23% | 18% | 28% |
| ❖ Lingcod (broiled) | 3 oz | 90 | 2% | 1% | 19% |
| ❖ Lobster (boiled or steamed) | 3 oz (meat only) | 80 | 1% | 0% | 20% |
| ⊛ Mackerel (cooked dry heat) | 3 oz | 220 | 23% | 18% | 21% |
| ❖ Mackerel, King (broiled) | 3 oz | 110 | 3% | 2% | 19% |
| ❖ Mackerel, Pacific (broiled) | 3 oz | 170 | 13% | 12% | 17% |
| ⊛ Mackerel, Spanish (cooked dry heat) | 3 oz | 130 | 8% | 8% | 21% |
| ❖ Ocean Perch (cooked dry heat) | 3 oz | 100 | 3% | 1% | 15% |
| ❖ Orange Roughy (broiled) | 3 oz | 80 | 1% | 0% | 7% |
| ⊛ Oyster, Eastern (cooked moist heat) | 3 oz | 120 | 6% | 5% | 31% |
| ⊛ Perch (cooked dry heat) | 3 oz | 100 | 2% | 1% | 33% |
| ❖ Pike (cooked dry heat) | 3 oz | 100 | 1% | 1% | 14% |
| ⊛ Pollock (cooked dry heat) | 3 oz | 100 | 1% | 1% | 27% |
| ⊛ Pollock, Atlantic (broiled) | 3 oz | 100 | 2% | 1% | 46% |
| ❖ Pompano (cooked dry heat) | 3 oz | 180 | 16% | 19% | 18% |
| ❖ Red Snapper (cooked dry heat) | 3 oz | 110 | 2% | 2% | 13% |
| ❖ Rockfish (cooked dry heat) | 3 oz | 100 | 3% | 2% | 12% |
| ❖ Roe (fish eggs) | 1 tbsp | 20 | 1% | 1% | 19% |
| ⊛ Sablefish (broiled) | 3 oz | 210 | 26% | 17% | 18% |
| ❖ Salmon, Atlantic (broiled) | 3 oz | 160 | 11% | 5% | 20% |
| ❖ Salmon, Atlantic (cooked dry heat) | 3 oz | 180 | 16% | 11% | 18% |
| ⊛ Salmon, Chinook (broiled) | 3 oz | 200 | 17% | 14% | 24% |
| ⊛ Salmon, Chum (broiled) | 3 oz | 130 | 6% | 5% | 27% |
| ❖ Salmon, Coho (cooked dry heat) | 3 oz | 150 | 11% | 8% | 18% |
| ❖ Salmon, Pink (broiled) | 3 oz | 130 | 6% | 3% | 19% |
| ❖ Salmon, Sockeye (cooked dry heat) | 3 oz | 130 | 6% | 3% | 19% |
| ❖ Sheepshead (cooked dry heat) | 3 oz | 110 | 2% | 2% | 19% |
| ⊛ Shrimp (cooked moist heat) | 3 oz | 80 | 1% | 1% | 55% |
| ⊛ Smelt (cooked dry heat) | 3 oz | 110 | 4% | 2% | 26% |
| ❖ Sole (cooked dry heat) | 3 oz | 100 | 2% | 2% | 19% |
| ⊛ Squid (fried) | 3 oz | 150 | 10% | 8% | 74% |
| ⊛ Sturgeon (cooked dry heat) | 3 oz | 120 | 7% | 5% | 21% |
| ❖ Swordfish (cooked dry heat) | 3 oz | 130 | 7% | 6% | 14% |
| ⊛ Trout (broiled) | 3 oz | 160 | 11% | 6% | 21% |
| ⊛ Trout, Rainbow (broiled) | 3 oz | 130 | 6% | 4% | 21% |
| ❖ Tuna, Bluefin (cooked dry heat) | 3 oz | 160 | 8% | 7% | 14% |
| ❖ Tuna, Skipjack (broiled) | 3 oz | 110 | 2% | 2% | 17% |
| ❖ Tuna, Yellowfin (broiled) | 3 oz | 120 | 2% | 1% | 16% |
| ⊛ Whitefish (broiled) | 3 oz | 150 | 10% | 5% | 22% |
| ⊛ Whiting (cooked dry heat) | 3 oz | 100 | 2% | 1% | 24% |

| FOOD | Serving Size | Calories | Tot Fat | Sat Fat | Chol |
|------|-------------|----------|---------|---------|------|

**Brand Name Foods**

GORTON'S Grilled Fillets—
GENERAL MILLS

| | | | | | |
|------|-------------|----------|---------|---------|------|
| ❖ Italian Herb | 1 fillet | 130 | 9% | 5% | 20% |
| ❖ Lemon Pepper | 1 fillet | 120 | 9% | 5% | 20% |

GORTON'S Stir Fry Kits—
GENERAL MILLS

| | | | | | |
|------|-------------|----------|---------|---------|------|
| Ⓐ Scampi | 10 oz | 320 | 21% | 40% | 23% |
| ❖ Sweet & Sour | 10 oz | 280 | 2% | 0% | 15% |
| ❖ Teriyaki | 10 oz | 300 | 2% | 0% | 18% |

LOUIS KEMP *Crab Delights*—
TYSON FOODS

| | | | | | |
|------|-------------|----------|---------|---------|------|
| ★ Chunks | 1/2 cup | 90 | 0% | 0% | 3% |
| ★ Flakes | 1/2 cup | 80 | 2% | 0% | 3% |
| ❖ Legs | 1/2 cup | 130 | 8% | 10% | 2% |

★ LOUIS KEMP *Lobster Delights*

| | | | | | |
|------|-------------|----------|---------|---------|------|
| Chunks—TYSON FOODS | 3 oz | 80 | 0% | 0% | 3% |

★ LOUIS KEMP *Scallop Delights*

| | | | | | |
|------|-------------|----------|---------|---------|------|
| Bay Style—TYSON FOODS | 1/2 cup | 80 | 1% | 0% | 2% |
| ❖ MRS. PAUL'S Kitchen Fillets in Sauce—CAMPBELL'S | 1 fillet | 120 | 8% | 8% | 8% |

MRS. PAUL'S Premium Fillets
—CAMPBELL'S

| | | | | | |
|------|-------------|----------|---------|---------|------|
| ❖ Cod | 1 fillet | 250 | 17% | 15% | 13% |
| ❖ Flounder | 1 fillet | 250 | 20% | 18% | 13% |
| ❖ Haddock | 1 fillet | 230 | 17% | 13% | 12% |
| ❖ Sole | 1 fillet | 250 | 20% | 18% | 13% |

VAN DE KAMP'S Natural Fillets
—PET

| | | | | | |
|------|-------------|----------|---------|---------|------|
| ❖ Flounder | 1 fillet | 110 | 3% | 0% | 15% |
| ❖ Sole | 1 fillet | 110 | 2% | 0% | 17% |

## PROCESSED OR SMOKED FISH

**Generic Foods**

| | | | | | |
|------|-------------|----------|---------|---------|------|
| ❖ Cod, Atlantic (smoked) | 2 oz | 50 | 1% | 0% | 14% |
| ❖ Crab, Imitation (Surimi) | 3 oz | 90 | 2% | 1% | 6% |
| ★ Gefiltefish w/broth | 1 pc | 35 | 1% | 1% | 4% |
| ❖ Haddock (smoked) | 2 oz | 60 | 1% | 0% | 14% |
| ❖ Herring, pickled (Bismarck type) | 2 oz | 130 | 14% | 6% | 2% |
| ❖ Sablefish (smoked) | 2 oz | 140 | 17% | 11% | 12% |
| ★ Salmon (smoked) | 2 oz | 60 | 4% | 3% | 4% |
| ★ Salmon, Chinook (smoked) | 2 oz | 60 | 4% | 3% | 5% |

---

★ Foods with this symbol have less than or equal to 5% *Daily Value* for <u>all</u> three nutrients (5% Rule).

❖ Foods with this symbol have <u>at least one</u> of the three nutrients greater than 5% *Daily Value* but less than or equal to 20% *Daily Value*.

Ⓐ Foods with this symbol have <u>at least one</u> of the three nutrients greater than 20% *Daily Value* (20% Rule).

| FOOD | Serving Size | Calories | Tot Fat | Sat Fat | Chol |
|---|---|---|---|---|---|
| ❖ Sturgeon (smoked) | 2 oz | 100 | 4% | 3% | 19% |
| ❖ Surimi | 3 oz | 80 | 1% | 1% | 9% |
| ❖ Whitefish (smoked) | 2 oz | 60 | 1% | 1% | 6% |

# Frozen Desserts

BARS, CONES, AND POPS

**Brand Name Foods**

| | Serving Size | Calories | Tot Fat | Sat Fat | Chol |
|---|---|---|---|---|---|
| 3 MUSKETEERS (2 fl oz)— M&M/MARS | | | | | |
| ⊛ Chocolate | 1 bar | 140 | 12% | 21% | 4% |
| ❖ Vanilla | 1 bar | 140 | 11% | 20% | 4% |
| BUTTERFINGER—NESTLÉ | | | | | |
| ⊛ Bar | 1 bar | 170 | 18% | 35% | 5% |
| ⊛ Nuggets | 8 pcs | 340 | 37% | 65% | 7% |
| ⊛ CARNATION Strawberry Sundae Cup—NESTLÉ | 1 cup | 200 | 12% | 25% | 10% |
| CHILL UPS | | | | | |
| ★ Burstin' Bubble Gum | 2 pops | 50 | 0% | 0% | 0% |
| ★ Chillin' Cherry | 1 pop | 45 | 0% | 0% | 0% |
| ★ Rompin' Blue Raspberry | 4 pops | 45 | 0% | 0% | 0% |
| ★ Stormin' Strawberry | 3 pops | 50 | 0% | 0% | 0% |
| COOL CREATIONS—NESTLÉ | | | | | |
| ❖ Cookies & Cream Sandwich | 1 sandwich | 240 | 17% | 20% | 5% |
| ★ Ice Pop | 1 pop | 60 | 0% | 0% | 0% |
| ⊛ Lion King Cone | 1 cone | 280 | 22% | 45% | 5% |
| ❖ Mickey Mouse Bar (2.5 oz) | 1 bar | 110 | 11% | 15% | 3% |
| ❖ Mini Sandwich | 1 sandwich | 110 | 8% | 10% | 3% |
| ★ Surprise Pop | 1 pop | 60 | 0% | 0% | 0% |
| ❖ CREAMSICLE Bar—GOOD HUMOR/ BREYERS | 1 bar | 110 | 5% | 10% | 3% |
| ★ CREAMSICLE Frozen Yogurt Bar —GOOD HUMOR/BREYERS | 1 bar | 100 | 2% | 5% | 1% |
| ★ CRYSTAL LIGHT Frozen Pops: All flavors | 1 pop | 15 | 0% | 0% | 0% |
| ★ DOLE Fruit 'n Juice Bars: All flavors—NESTLÉ | 1 bar | 70 | 0% | 0% | 0% |
| ★ DOLE Fruit Juice Bars w/ No Sugar Added: All flavors —NESTLÉ | 1 bar | 25 | 0% | 0% | 0% |
| ★ DOLE Fruit Juice Bars: All flavors—NESTLÉ | 1 bar | 45 | 0% | 0% | 0% |
| DOVE Bite Size—M&M/MARS | | | | | |
| ⊛ Classic Vanilla | 5 bars | 360 | 37% | 80% | 13% |
| ⊛ Double Chocolate | 5 bars | 360 | 35% | 72% | 11% |

| FOOD | Serving Size | Calories | Tot Fat | Sat Fat | Chol |
|---|---|---|---|---|---|
| ⊛ French Vanilla | 5 bars | 370 | 36% | 75% | 20% |
| **DOVEBAR (3 fl oz)**—M&M/MARS | | | | | |
| ⊛ Almond Bar | 1 bar | 280 | 29% | 55% | 10% |
| ⊛ Caramel Creme Swirl | 1 bar | 280 | 25% | 55% | 10% |
| ⊛ Chocolate w/Dark Chocolate | 1 bar | 260 | 26% | 50% | 8% |
| ⊛ Mocha Cashew Crunch | 1 bar | 260 | 26% | 50% | 10% |
| ⊛ Vanilla w/Dark Chocolate | 1 bar | 260 | 26% | 55% | 10% |
| ⊛ Vanilla w/Milk Chocolate | 1 bar | 260 | 26% | 55% | 10% |
| ⊛ Vanilla w/White Coating | 1 bar | 270 | 26% | 55% | 10% |
| **DRUMSTICK Ice Cream Cone** —NESTLÉ | | | | | |
| ⊛ Chocolate | 1 cone | 340 | 29% | 50% | 8% |
| ⊛ Chocolate Dipped | 1 cone | 340 | 26% | 50% | 8% |
| ⊛ Vanilla | 1 cone | 350 | 31% | 55% | 7% |
| ⊛ Vanilla/Caramel | 1 cone | 360 | 31% | 60% | 8% |
| ⊛ Vanilla/Fudge | 1 cone | 370 | 32% | 55% | 7% |
| **ESKIMO PIES** | | | | | |
| ⊛ Original | 1 bar | 180 | 19% | 30% | 3% |
| ⊛ Sweetened w/NutraSweet | 1 bar | 150 | 15% | 30% | 5% |
| **FLINTSTONES**—NESTLÉ | | | | | |
| ★ Cool Cream | 1 bar/pop | 90 | 3% | 5% | 2% |
| ★ Push-Up | 1 bar/pop | 100 | 3% | 5% | 2% |
| ★ Rock Pops | 1 bar/pop | 80 | 0% | 0% | 0% |
| **FUDGSICLE Fudge Bars**— GOOD HUMOR | | | | | |
| ★ Fat Free | 1 pop | 60 | 0% | 0% | 0% |
| ★ Original | 1 pop | 90 | 2% | 5% | 2% |
| ★ Sugar Free | 1 pop | 40 | 1% | 0% | 1% |
| **HÄAGEN-DAZS Frozen Yogurt Bars**—PILLSBURY | | | | | |
| ⊛ Cherry Chocolate Fudge | 1 bar | 240 | 20% | 40% | 12% |
| ★ Peach | 1 bar | 90 | 2% | 3% | 5% |
| ★ Pina Colada | 1 bar | 100 | 2% | 3% | 5% |
| ★ Raspberry & Vanilla | 1 bar | 90 | 1% | 0% | 5% |
| ★ Strawberry Daiquiri | 1 bar | 90 | 2% | 3% | 5% |
| ★ *Tropical Orange Passion* | 1 bar | 100 | 2% | 3% | 5% |
| **HÄAGEN-DAZS Ice Cream Bars** —PILLSBURY | | | | | |
| ⊛ Chocolate & Dark Chocolate | 1 bar | 400 | 42% | 90% | 28% |
| ⊛ Coffee & Almond Crunch | 1 bar | 360 | 40% | 75% | 33% |
| ⊛ Vanilla & Almonds | 1 bar | 370 | 42% | 70% | 30% |
| ⊛ Vanilla & Dark Chocolate | 1 bar | 400 | 42% | 90% | 28% |
| ⊛ Vanilla & Milk Chocolate | 1 bar | 330 | 37% | 70% | 30% |

★ Foods with this symbol have less than or equal to 5% *Daily Value* for <u>all</u> three nutrients (5% Rule).

❖ Foods with this symbol have <u>at least one</u> of the three nutrients greater than 5% *Daily Value* but less than or equal to 20% *Daily Value*.

⊛ Foods with this symbol have <u>at least one</u> of the three nutrients greater than 20% *Daily Value* (20% Rule).

| FOOD | Serving Size | Calories | Tot Fat | Sat Fat | Chol |
|------|--------------|----------|---------|---------|------|
| HÄAGEN-DAZS Ice Cream Bars | | | | | |
| *Extraas*—PILLSBURY | | | | | |
| ✺ *Caramel Cone Explosion* | 1 bar | 350 | 35% | 70% | 22% |
| ✺ *Cookie Dough Dynamo* | 1 bar | 380 | 38% | 70% | 22% |
| ✺ *Ice Cappuccino* | 1 bar | 330 | 37% | 70% | 27% |
| ✺ *Triple Brownie Overload* | 1 bar | 380 | 42% | 70% | 32% |
| HEATH—NESTLÉ | | | | | |
| ✺ Ice Cream Bar | 1 bar | 160 | 18% | 40% | 5% |
| ✺ Nuggets | 8 pcs | 180 | 17% | 35% | 8% |
| ★ JELL-O Frozen Gelatin Pops: | | | | | |
| All flavors—KRAFT | 1 pop | 35 | 0% | 0% | 0% |
| ❖ JELL-O Pudding Pops: All flavors | | | | | |
| —KRAFT | 1 pop | 140 | 6% | 17% | 1% |
| KLONDIKE—GOOD HUMOR | | | | | |
| ❖ *Big Bear* Ice Cream Sandwich | 1 sandwich | 200 | 11% | 15% | 6% |
| ✺ Original Chocolate Coated | | | | | |
| Vanilla Ice Cream | 1 pc | 290 | 31% | 70% | 5% |
| ❖ KLONDIKE Premium Light— | | | | | |
| GOOD HUMOR/BREYERS | 1 bar | 110 | 8% | 20% | 2% |
| LIFESAVERS Ice Pops | | | | | |
| ★ Regular | 1 bar | 35 | 0% | 0% | 0% |
| ★ Sugar Free | 1 bar | 12 | 0% | 0% | 0% |
| MILKY WAY—M&M/MARS | | | | | |
| ❖ Lowfat Chocolate-Malt Milk | | | | | |
| Shake (8 fl oz) | 1 cup | 220 | 5% | 10% | 4% |
| ❖ Reduced Fat (2 fl oz): All flavors | 1 bar | 140 | 10% | 14% | 2% |
| NESTLÉ | | | | | |
| ✺ *Bon Bons* | 5 pcs | 200 | 22% | 40% | 3% |
| ✺ *Crunch* Bar | 1 bar | 200 | 22% | 55% | 5% |
| ✺ *Heath* Bar | 1 bar | 160 | 18% | 40% | 5% |
| ✺ *Quik* Fudge Pops | 2 pops | 160 | 12% | 23% | 8% |
| NESTLÉ *Drumstick* Sundae Cones | | | | | |
| ✺ Cookies 'n Cream | 1 cone | 350 | 29% | 60% | 7% |
| ✺ Vanilla | 1 cone | 340 | 29% | 55% | 7% |
| ✺ Vanilla Caramel | 1 cone | 360 | 31% | 60% | 8% |
| NESTLÉ *Crunch* | | | | | |
| ✺ Cone | 1 cone | 300 | 25% | 50% | 8% |
| ✺ Ice Cream Bar: Vanilla or | | | | | |
| Chocolate | 1 bar | 200 | 22% | 45% | 5% |
| ✺ Nuggets | 8 pcs | 140 | 14% | 25% | 3% |
| ✺ Reduced Fat | 1 bar | 130 | 11% | 25% | 2% |
| POPSICLE—GOOD HUMOR | | | | | |
| ★ Fantastic Fruity! | 1 pop | 60 | 0% | 0% | 0% |
| ★ Firecracker Ice Pops | 1 pop | 40 | 0% | 0% | 0% |
| ★ Ice Pops | 1 pop | 45 | 0% | 0% | 0% |
| ★ Juice Jets | 1 pop | 45 | 0% | 0% | 0% |
| ★ Lick-A-Color | 1 pop | 50 | 0% | 0% | 0% |
| ★ Sherbet Cyclone | 1 pop | 50 | 1% | 0% | 1% |

| FOOD | Serving Size | Calories | Tot Fat | Sat Fat | Chol |
|------|------|------|------|------|------|
| ⊛ REESE'S Peanut Butter Ice Cream Cups—GOOD HUMOR | 1 pc | 160 | 17% | 30% | 3% |
| ⊛ SNICKERS (2 fl oz)—M&M/MARS | 1 bar | 190 | 18% | 21% | 4% |
| STARBURST Lowfat Frozen Yogurt—M&M/MARS | | | | | |
| ★ Bar (1.8 fl oz): All flavors | 1 bar | 70 | 2% | 4% | 2% |
| ★ Cup (3 fl oz) | 1 cup | 80 | 2% | 4% | 2% |
| ★ STARBURST Fruit Juice Bar (1.75 fl oz)—M&M/MARS | 1 bar | 50 | 0% | 0% | 0% |
| WEIGHT WATCHERS Frozen Novelties | | | | | |
| ❖ *Arctic D'Lites* | 1 bar | 130 | 11% | 18% | 2% |
| ★ Berries 'n Creme Mousse | 2 bars | 70 | 2% | 0% | 0% |
| ❖ Caramel Nut Bars | 1 bar | 130 | 12% | 18% | 2% |
| ❖ Chocolate Dip | 1 bar | 100 | 9% | 15% | 2% |
| ★ Chocolate Mousse | 2 bars | 70 | 2% | 3% | 2% |
| ★ *Chocolate Treat* | 1 bar | 100 | 2% | 0% | 3% |
| ❖ Crispy Pralines 'n Creme Bars | 1 bar | 130 | 11% | 18% | 2% |
| ❖ English Toffee Crunch Bars | 1 bar | 120 | 11% | 18% | 2% |
| ★ *Orange Vanilla Treat* | 2 bars | 70 | 2% | 3% | 2% |
| ❖ Vanilla Sandwich Bar | 1 bar | 160 | 5% | 10% | 2% |

<u>CONES</u>

**Generic Foods**

| | | | | | |
|------|------|------|------|------|------|
| ★ Cake | 1 cone | 20 | 0% | 0% | 0% |
| ★ Sugar | 1 cone | 40 | 0% | 0% | 0% |
| ★ Wafer | 1 cone | 20 | 0% | 0% | 0% |

**Brand Name Foods**

| | | | | | |
|------|------|------|------|------|------|
| COMET—NABISCO | | | | | |
| ★ Cups | 1 cone | 20 | 0% | 0% | 0% |
| ★ Sugar Cones | 1 cone | 50 | 0% | 0% | 0% |
| ★ Waffle Cones | 1 cone | 70 | 0% | 0% | 0% |
| ★ OREO Chocolate Cones—NABISCO | 1 cone | 50 | 0% | 0% | 0% |
| ★ TEDDY GRAHAMS Cinnamon Cones—NABISCO | 1 cone | 60 | 1% | 0% | 0% |

---

★ Foods with this symbol have less than or equal to 5% *Daily Value* for <u>all</u> three nutrients (5% Rule).
❖ Foods with this symbol have <u>at least one</u> of the three nutrients greater than 5% *Daily Value* but less than or equal to 20% *Daily Value.*
⊛ Foods with this symbol have <u>at least one</u> of the three nutrients greater than 20% *Daily Value* (20% Rule).

| FOOD | Serving Size | Calories | Tot Fat | Sat Fat | Chol |
|------|-------------|----------|---------|---------|------|

## FROZEN YOGURT

**Generic Foods**

| FOOD | Serving Size | Calories | Tot Fat | Sat Fat | Chol |
|------|-------------|----------|---------|---------|------|
| ❖ Frozen Yogurt: Chocolate; Strawberry; Vanilla | 1/2 cup | 150 | 8% | 17% | 3% |
| Soft Serve | | | | | |
| ❖ Chocolate | 1/2 cup | 120 | 7% | 13% | 1% |
| ❖ Vanilla | 1/2 cup | 110 | 6% | 12% | 1% |

**Brand Name Foods**

| FOOD | Serving Size | Calories | Tot Fat | Sat Fat | Chol |
|------|-------------|----------|---------|---------|------|
| BEN & JERRY'S | | | | | |
| ❖ Apple Pie | 1/2 cup | 150 | 4% | 8% | 3% |
| ★ Banana Strawberry | 1/2 cup | 140 | 3% | 5% | 2% |
| ★ Blueberry | 1/2 cup | 130 | 2% | 5% | 2% |
| ❖ Cherry Garcia | 1/2 cup | 150 | 4% | 10% | 3% |
| ❖ Chocolate Chip Cookie Dough | 1/2 cup | 180 | 6% | 10% | 3% |
| ❖ Chocolate Fudge Brownie | 1/2 cup | 160 | 5% | 8% | 3% |
| ★ Chocolate Raspberry Swirl | 1/2 cup | 170 | 3% | 5% | 2% |
| ❖ Chocolate S'mores | 1/2 cup | 190 | 6% | 13% | 2% |
| ❖ Coffee Almond Fudge | 1/2 cup | 180 | 11% | 10% | 3% |
| ❖ English Toffee Crunch | 1/2 cup | 180 | 8% | 13% | 3% |
| ❖ BIG GURT Vanilla Nonfat Frozen Yogurt & Chocolate Chip Cookie Sandwich—STONYFIELD FARM | 1 sandwich | 230 | 12% | 7% | 0% |
| ❖ BREYERS Lowfat Vanilla Raspberry Twirl | 1/2 cup | 130 | 5% | 10% | 5% |
| DANNON *Light 'N Crunchy* Frozen Yogurt | | | | | |
| ★ *Banana Cream Pie* | 1/2 cup | 110 | 2% | 0% | 0% |
| ★ Mocha Chocolate Chunk | 1/2 cup | 110 | 2% | 0% | 0% |
| ★ Peanut Chocolate Crunch | 1/2 cup | 110 | 0% | 0% | 0% |
| ★ Triple Chocolate | 1/2 cup | 110 | 0% | 0% | 0% |
| ★ Vanilla Blueberry Swirl | 1/2 cup | 110 | 1% | 0% | 0% |
| DANNON *Pure Indulgence* Frozen Yogurt | | | | | |
| ★ Cherry Chocolate Cherry | 1/2 cup | 150 | 5% | 5% | 5% |
| ★ Chunky Chocolate Nut | 1/2 cup | 150 | 5% | 0% | 0% |
| ❖ Coco-Nut Fudge | 1/2 cup | 160 | 5% | 6% | 5% |
| ❖ Cookies 'n Cream | 1/2 cup | 150 | 5% | 10% | 0% |
| ❖ Crunchy Espresso | 1/2 cup | 150 | 5% | 10% | 5% |
| ❖ Heath Toffee Crunch | 1/2 cup | 150 | 5% | 7% | 2% |
| ❖ Vanilla Raspberry Truffle | 1/2 cup | 150 | 5% | 10% | 5% |
| DREYER'S/EDY'S Frozen Yogurt | | | | | |
| ❖ Boysenberry Vanilla Swirl | 1/2 cup | 100 | 4% | 8% | 3% |
| ❖ Chocolate | 1/2 cup | 100 | 5% | 8% | 3% |
| ❖ Chocolate Brownie Chunk | 1/2 cup | 110 | 6% | 8% | 3% |
| ❖ Citrus Heights | 1/2 cup | 80 | 4% | 8% | 3% |
| ❖ Cookies 'N Cream | 1/2 cup | 120 | 6% | 8% | 3% |
| ❖ Expresso Chip | 1/2 cup | 110 | 6% | 13% | 3% |

| | FOOD | Serving Size | Calories | Tot Fat | Sat Fat | Chol |
|---|---|---|---|---|---|---|
| ❖ | *Heath* Toffee Crunch | 1/2 cup | 120 | 6% | 10% | 3% |
| ❖ | Marble Fudge | 1/2 cup | 110 | 5% | 8% | 3% |
| ❖ | Orange Vanilla Swirl | 1/2 cup | 100 | 4% | 8% | 3% |
| ❖ | Perfectly Peach | 1/2 cup | 100 | 4% | 8% | 3% |
| ❖ | Raspberry | 1/2 cup | 100 | 4% | 8% | 3% |
| ❖ | Raspberry Vanilla Swirl | 1/2 cup | 100 | 4% | 8% | 3% |
| ❖ | Strawberry Chocolate Chip | 1/2 cup | 120 | 6% | 10% | 3% |
| ❖ | Vanilla | 1/2 cup | 100 | 4% | 8% | 3% |

HÄAGEN-DAZS Frozen Yogurt
—PILLSBURY

| | FOOD | Serving Size | Calories | Tot Fat | Sat Fat | Chol |
|---|---|---|---|---|---|---|
| ❖ | Chocolate | 1/2 cup | 160 | 4% | 8% | 10% |
| ❖ | Coffee | 1/2 cup | 160 | 4% | 8% | 15% |
| ❖ | *Orange Tango* | 1/2 cup | 130 | 2% | 3% | 7% |
| ❖ | Pina Colada | 1/2 cup | 130 | 2% | 5% | 8% |
| ❖ | *Raspberry Rendezvous* | 1/2 cup | 130 | 2% | 3% | 7% |
| ❖ | *Strawberry Duet* | 1/2 cup | 130 | 3% | 5% | 8% |
| ❖ | Vanilla | 1/2 cup | 160 | 4% | 8% | 15% |

HÄAGEN-DAZS Frozen Yogurt
Extraas—PILLSBURY

| | FOOD | Serving Size | Calories | Tot Fat | Sat Fat | Chol |
|---|---|---|---|---|---|---|
| ❖ | *Brownie Nut Blast* | 1/2 cup | 220 | 12% | 18% | 13% |
| ⓐ | *Strawberry Cheesecake Craze* | 1/2 cup | 220 | 12% | 20% | 22% |

## FROZEN YOGURT: FAT FREE

**Brand Name Foods**

BEN & JERRY'S No Fat Yogurts

| | FOOD | Serving Size | Calories | Tot Fat | Sat Fat | Chol |
|---|---|---|---|---|---|---|
| ★ | Black Raspberry | 1/2 cup | 150 | 0% | 0% | 0% |
| ★ | Blueberry | 1/2 cup | 120 | 0% | 0% | 0% |
| ★ | Cappuccino | 1/2 cup | 140 | 0% | 0% | 0% |
| ★ | Chocolate | 1/2 cup | 120 | 0% | 0% | 0% |
| ★ | Strawberry | 1/2 cup | 140 | 0% | 0% | 0% |
| ★ | Vanilla | 1/2 cup | 120 | 0% | 0% | 0% |
| ★ | Vanilla Fudge Swirl | 1/2 cup | 150 | 0% | 5% | 0% |

DANNON *Light* Frozen Yogurt

| | FOOD | Serving Size | Calories | Tot Fat | Sat Fat | Chol |
|---|---|---|---|---|---|---|
| ★ | Cappuccino | 1/2 cup | 80 | 0% | 0% | 0% |
| ★ | Cherry Vanilla Swirl | 1/2 cup | 90 | 0% | 0% | 0% |
| ★ | Chocolate | 1/2 cup | 80 | 0% | 0% | 0% |
| ★ | Lemon Chiffon | 1/2 cup | 90 | 0% | 0% | 0% |
| ★ | *Peach Raspberry Melba* | 1/2 cup | 90 | 0% | 0% | 0% |
| ★ | *Strawberry Cheesecake* | 1/2 cup | 90 | 0% | 0% | 0% |
| ★ | Vanilla | 1/2 cup | 80 | 0% | 0% | 0% |

DREYER'S/EDY'S Fat Free
Frozen Yogurt

| | FOOD | Serving Size | Calories | Tot Fat | Sat Fat | Chol |
|---|---|---|---|---|---|---|
| ★ | Banana Strawberry | 1/2 cup | 80 | 0% | 0% | 0% |

★ Foods with this symbol have less than or equal to 5% *Daily Value* for <u>all</u> three nutrients (5% Rule).
❖ Foods with this symbol have <u>at least one</u> of the three nutrients greater than 5% *Daily Value* but less than or equal to 20% *Daily Value*.
ⓐ Foods with this symbol have <u>at least one</u> of the three nutrients greater than 20% *Daily Value* (20% Rule).

| FOOD | Serving Size | Calories | Tot Fat | Sat Fat | Chol |
|---|---|---|---|---|---|
| ★ Black Cherry Vanilla Swirl | 1/2 cup | 90 | 0% | 0% | 0% |
| ★ Chocolate | 1/2 cup | 90 | 0% | 0% | 0% |
| ★ Chocolate Fudge | 1/2 cup | 100 | 0% | 0% | 0% |
| ★ Pine-Orange Paradise | 1/2 cup | 90 | 0% | 0% | 0% |
| ★ Raspberry | 1/2 cup | 80 | 0% | 0% | 0% |
| ★ Strawberry | 1/2 cup | 90 | 0% | 0% | 0% |
| ★ Vanilla | 1/2 cup | 90 | 0% | 0% | 0% |
| ★ Vanilla Chocolate Swirl | 1/2 cup | 90 | 0% | 0% | 0% |

### ICE CREAM

**Generic Foods**

| | | | | | |
|---|---|---|---|---|---|
| ⊛ Chocolate | 1/2 cup | 140 | 11% | 22% | 7% |
| ❖ Strawberry | 1/2 cup | 130 | 9% | 18% | 6% |
| ⊛ Vanilla (10% fat) | 1/2 cup | 130 | 11% | 22% | 10% |
| ⊛ Vanilla (16% fat) | 1/2 cup | 180 | 18% | 37% | 15% |
| ❖ Vanilla (soft serve) | 1/2 cup | 110 | 4% | 7% | 3% |

**Brand Name Foods**

BEN & JERRY'S

| | | | | | |
|---|---|---|---|---|---|
| ⊛ Apple Pie | 1/2 cup | 200 | 18% | 35% | 18% |
| ⊛ Banana Walnut | 1/2 cup | 240 | 26% | 35% | 18% |
| ⊛ Butter Pecan | 1/2 cup | 250 | 32% | 45% | 27% |
| ⊛ Cappuccino Chocolate Chunk | 1/2 cup | 220 | 23% | 50% | 22% |
| ⊛ Cherry Garcia | 1/2 cup | 200 | 20% | 40% | 22% |
| ⊛ Cherry Vanilla | 1/2 cup | 180 | 17% | 35% | 22% |
| ⊛ Chocolate | 1/2 cup | 190 | 18% | 35% | 15% |
| ⊛ Chocolate Chip Cookie Dough | 1/2 cup | 230 | 22% | 40% | 22% |
| ⊛ Chocolate Fudge Brownie | 1/2 cup | 200 | 18% | 35% | 13% |
| ⊛ Chocolate Orange Fudge | 1/2 cup | 190 | 18% | 35% | 15% |
| ⊛ Chocolate Peanut Butter Dough | 1/2 cup | 240 | 26% | 35% | 13% |
| ⊛ Chocolate Raspberry Swirl | 1/2 cup | 190 | 15% | 30% | 12% |
| ⊛ Chocolate Raspberry Truffle | 1/2 cup | 220 | 25% | 50% | 23% |
| ⊛ Chocolate Swiss Chocolate Almond | 1/2 cup | 210 | 22% | 40% | 13% |
| ⊛ Chubby Hubby | 1/2 cup | 260 | 26% | 40% | 17% |
| ⊛ Chunky Monkey | 1/2 cup | 240 | 25% | 40% | 18% |
| ⊛ Cinnamon | 1/2 cup | 180 | 20% | 40% | 25% |
| ⊛ Coconut Almond | 1/2 cup | 210 | 25% | 35% | 22% |
| ⊛ Coconut Almond Fudge Chip | 1/2 cup | 260 | 31% | 55% | 20% |
| ⊛ Coffee Toffee Crunch | 1/2 cup | 240 | 25% | 45% | 20% |
| ⊛ English Toffee Crunch | 1/2 cup | 240 | 26% | 45% | 22% |
| ⊛ Maple Walnut | 1/2 cup | 240 | 28% | 40% | 20% |
| ⊛ Mint Chocolate Chunk | 1/2 cup | 220 | 23% | 50% | 22% |
| ⊛ Mint Chocolate Cookie | 1/2 cup | 220 | 22% | 40% | 22% |
| ⊛ Mint Chocolate Fudge Swirl | 1/2 cup | 200 | 20% | 40% | 23% |
| ⊛ Mocha Chunk | 1/2 cup | 220 | 22% | 45% | 20% |

| FOOD | Serving Size | Calories | Tot Fat | Sat Fat | Chol |
|---|---|---|---|---|---|
| ⊛ New York Super Fudge Chunk | 1/2 cup | 240 | 26% | 45% | 13% |
| ⊛ Nutcracker Suite | 1/2 cup | 250 | 29% | 45% | 22% |
| ⊛ Peach | 1/2 cup | 170 | 17% | 35% | 22% |
| ⊛ Peanut Butter Cup | 1/2 cup | 260 | 28% | 45% | 20% |
| ⊛ Pecan Pie | 1/2 cup | 250 | 25% | 40% | 20% |
| ⊛ Peppermint Stick | 1/2 cup | 200 | 18% | 35% | 22% |
| ⊛ Pistachio Pistachio | 1/2 cup | 220 | 26% | 40% | 23% |
| ⊛ Praline Pecan | 1/2 cup | 250 | 26% | 40% | 23% |
| ⊛ Rainforest Crunch | 1/2 cup | 240 | 28% | 45% | 23% |
| ⊛ Reverse Chocolate Chunk | 1/2 cup | 230 | 22% | 50% | 13% |
| ⊛ Strawberry | 1/2 cup | 170 | 15% | 30% | 18% |
| ⊛ Sweet Cream Cookie | 1/2 cup | 220 | 22% | 40% | 22% |
| ⊛ Vanilla Chocolate Chunk | 1/2 cup | 220 | 23% | 50% | 22% |
| ⊛ Vanilla Fudge Swirl | 1/2 cup | 200 | 20% | 40% | 23% |
| ⊛ Vanilla Malted | 1/2 cup | 190 | 20% | 40% | 25% |
| ⊛ Wavy Gravy | 1/2 cup | 260 | 29% | 35% | 18% |
| BEN & JERRY'S *Smooth Line* | | | | | |
| ⊛ Aztec Harvest Coffee | 1/2 cup | 180 | 20% | 40% | 23% |
| ⊛ Deep Dark Chocolate | 1/2 cup | 200 | 18% | 35% | 15% |
| ⊛ Double Chocolate Fudge Swirl | 1/2 cup | 210 | 18% | 35% | 15% |
| ⊛ Mocha Fudge Swirl | 1/2 cup | 210 | 20% | 35% | 22% |
| ⊛ Vanilla | 1/2 cup | 190 | 22% | 40% | 25% |
| ⊛ Vanilla Bean | 1/2 cup | 190 | 20% | 40% | 25% |
| ⊛ Vanilla Caramel Fudge | 1/2 cup | 210 | 20% | 40% | 23% |
| ⊛ White Russian | 1/2 cup | 190 | 20% | 40% | 23% |
| ⊛ BREYER'S Vanilla | 1/2 cup | 150 | 12% | 30% | 12% |
| DREYER'S/EDY'S *Grand* | | | | | |
| ⊛ Almond Affair | 1/2 cup | 140 | 12% | 25% | 10% |
| ❖ Almond Praline | 1/2 cup | 160 | 12% | 20% | 8% |
| ⊛ Biscotti 'N Coffee | 1/2 cup | 150 | 14% | 25% | 8% |
| ⊛ Butter Pecan | 1/2 cup | 160 | 15% | 25% | 8% |
| ⊛ Chocolate | 1/2 cup | 140 | 14% | 25% | 10% |
| ⊛ Chocolate Chips! | 1/2 cup | 160 | 14% | 25% | 8% |
| ⊛ Chocolate Fudge Mousse | 1/2 cup | 160 | 12% | 25% | 8% |
| ⊛ Coffee | 1/2 cup | 140 | 12% | 25% | 8% |
| ⊛ Cookie Dough | 1/2 cup | 170 | 14% | 25% | 8% |
| ⊛ Cookies 'N Cream | 1/2 cup | 160 | 12% | 25% | 8% |
| ⊛ Crunchy Cone | 1/2 cup | 160 | 14% | 30% | 8% |
| ⊛ Expresso Chip | 1/2 cup | 150 | 14% | 30% | 8% |
| ⊛ French Vanilla | 1/2 cup | 160 | 15% | 30% | 18% |
| ⊛ Ice Cream Sandwich | 1/2 cup | 150 | 12% | 25% | 8% |
| ⊛ Marble Fudge | 1/2 cup | 140 | 11% | 25% | 8% |
| ⊛ Mint Chocolate Chips! | 1/2 cup | 160 | 14% | 25% | 8% |
| ❖ Mocha Almond Fudge | 1/2 cup | 150 | 14% | 20% | 8% |

★　Foods with this symbol have less than or equal to 5% *Daily Value* for <u>all</u> three nutrients (5% Rule).
❖　Foods with this symbol have <u>at least one</u> of the three nutrients greater than 5% *Daily Value* but less than or equal to 20% *Daily Value*.
⊛　Foods with this symbol have <u>at least one</u> of the three nutrients greater than 20% *Daily Value* (20% Rule).

| | FOOD | Serving Size | Calories | Tot Fat | Sat Fat | Chol |
|---|---|---|---|---|---|---|
| ✪ | Mud Pie | 1/2 cup | 150 | 12% | 25% | 8% |
| ✪ | Neopolitan | 1/2 cup | 130 | 11% | 25% | 8% |
| ❖ | Real Strawberry | 1/2 cup | 120 | 9% | 20% | 7% |
| ✪ | Rocky Road | 1/2 cup | 170 | 15% | 25% | 8% |
| ✪ | Strawberry Cheesecake | 1/2 cup | 150 | 12% | 25% | 10% |
| ✪ | Toasted Almond | 1/2 cup | 150 | 14% | 25% | 8% |
| ✪ | Vanilla | 1/2 cup | 150 | 15% | 30% | 12% |
| ✪ | Vanilla Bean | 1/2 cup | 150 | 14% | 30% | 10% |
| | DREYER'S/EDY'S *Grand Light* | | | | | |
| ❖ | Almond Praline | 1/2 cup | 110 | 6% | 10% | 5% |
| ❖ | Butter Pecan | 1/2 cup | 120 | 8% | 10% | 5% |
| ❖ | Cafe Au Lait | 1/2 cup | 100 | 6% | 13% | 8% |
| ❖ | Cheesecake Chunk | 1/2 cup | 120 | 8% | 15% | 8% |
| ❖ | Chocolate Almond Fudge | 1/2 cup | 120 | 8% | 13% | 8% |
| ❖ | Chocolate Chip | 1/2 cup | 110 | 8% | 13% | 8% |
| ❖ | Cookie Dough | 1/2 cup | 120 | 6% | 13% | 7% |
| ❖ | Cookies 'N Cream | 1/2 cup | 110 | 6% | 13% | 8% |
| ❖ | *French Silk* | 1/2 cup | 120 | 8% | 15% | 7% |
| ❖ | Marble Fudge | 1/2 cup | 110 | 6% | 13% | 8% |
| ❖ | Mint Fudge | 1/2 cup | 110 | 6% | 13% | 7% |
| ❖ | Mocha Almond Fudge | 1/2 cup | 110 | 8% | 10% | 5% |
| ❖ | Rocky Road | 1/2 cup | 120 | 8% | 13% | 8% |
| ❖ | *Tangerine Dream* | 1/2 cup | 100 | 6% | 10% | 8% |
| ❖ | Vanilla | 1/2 cup | 100 | 6% | 13% | 8% |
| | DREYER'S/EDY'S *Grand*, No Sugar Added | | | | | |
| ❖ | Black Cherry Vanilla Swirl | 1/2 cup | 100 | 6% | 13% | 5% |
| ❖ | Chocolate | 1/2 cup | 100 | 6% | 13% | 5% |
| ❖ | Chocolate Chip | 1/2 cup | 100 | 8% | 13% | 5% |
| ❖ | Marble Fudge | 1/2 cup | 100 | 6% | 13% | 5% |
| ❖ | Mint Fudge | 1/2 cup | 100 | 6% | 13% | 5% |
| ❖ | Mocha Fudge | 1/2 cup | 100 | 6% | 13% | 5% |
| ❖ | Strawberry | 1/2 cup | 90 | 6% | 13% | 5% |
| ❖ | Triple Chocolate | 1/2 cup | 100 | 8% | 13% | 3% |
| ❖ | Vanilla | 1/2 cup | 100 | 6% | 13% | 5% |
| ❖ | Vanilla 'N Caramel | 1/2 cup | 100 | 6% | 13% | 5% |
| | HÄAGEN-DAZS *Cordials*—PILLSBURY | | | | | |
| ✪ | *Baileys* Original Irish Cream | 1/2 cup | 280 | 28% | 55% | 37% |
| ✪ | *DiSaronno* Amaretto | 1/2 cup | 260 | 23% | 45% | 32% |
| | HÄAGEN-DAZS *Extraas*—PILLSBURY | | | | | |
| ✪ | Brownies a la Mode | 1/2 cup | 280 | 28% | 55% | 33% |
| ✪ | *Cappuccino Commotion* | 1/2 cup | 310 | 32% | 60% | 33% |
| ✪ | *Caramel Cone Explosion* | 1/2 cup | 310 | 31% | 60% | 32% |
| ✪ | *Cookie Dough Dynamo* | 1/2 cup | 300 | 29% | 60% | 32% |
| ✪ | *Peanut Butter Burst* | 1/2 cup | 330 | 34% | 55% | 32% |
| ✪ | *Strawberry Cheesecake Craze* | 1/2 cup | 290 | 28% | 50% | 33% |
| ✪ | *Triple Brownie Overload* | 1/2 cup | 300 | 31% | 55% | 30% |

| FOOD | Serving Size | Calories | Tot Fat | Sat Fat | Chol |
|------|------|------|------|------|------|
| HÄAGEN-DAZS—PILLSBURY | | | | | |
| ☉ Butter Pecan | 1/2 cup | 320 | 37% | 55% | 35% |
| ☉ Chocolate | 1/2 cup | 270 | 28% | 55% | 38% |
| ☉ Chocolate Chocolate Chip | 1/2 cup | 300 | 31% | 60% | 33% |
| ☉ Coffee | 1/2 cup | 270 | 28% | 55% | 40% |
| ☉ Cookies & Cream | 1/2 cup | 270 | 26% | 55% | 37% |
| ☉ Macadamia Brittle | 1/2 cup | 300 | 31% | 55% | 37% |
| ☉ Rum Raisin | 1/2 cup | 270 | 26% | 50% | 37% |
| ☉ Strawberry | 1/2 cup | 250 | 25% | 50% | 32% |
| ☉ Vanilla | 1/2 cup | 270 | 28% | 55% | 40% |
| ☉ Vanilla Fudge | 1/2 cup | 280 | 28% | 55% | 35% |
| ☉ Vanilla Swiss Almond | 1/2 cup | 310 | 32% | 55% | 35% |
| SWEET CELEBRATIONS— WEIGHT WATCHERS | | | | | |
| ❖ Brownie a la Mode | 1 brownie | 190 | 6% | 5% | 2% |
| ❖ Brownie Cheesecake | 1 cake | 200 | 9% | 10% | 2% |
| ★ Caramel Fudge a la Mode | 1 cake | 180 | 5% | 5% | 0% |
| ❖ Chocolate Chip Cookie Dough Sundae | 1 sundae | 180 | 6% | 8% | 2% |
| ❖ Chocolate Eclair | 1 eclair | 150 | 8% | 8% | 0% |
| ★ Chocolate Frosted Brownie | 1 brownie | 100 | 4% | 5% | 0% |
| ❖ Chocolate Mocha Pie | 1 pie | 170 | 6% | 5% | 2% |
| ❖ Chocolate Mousse | 1 mousse | 190 | 6% | 8% | 2% |
| ❖ Double Fudge Brownie Parfait | 1 parfait | 190 | 4% | 10% | 2% |
| ❖ Double Fudge Cake | 1 cake | 190 | 7% | 5% | 0% |
| ❖ Mississippi Mud Pie | 1 pie | 180 | 8% | 8% | 2% |
| ★ Peanut Butter Fudge Brownie | 1 brownie | 110 | 4% | 3% | 0% |
| ❖ Praline Pecan Mousse | 1 mousse | 170 | 5% | 5% | 0% |
| ❖ Praline Toffee Crunch Parfait | 1 parfait | 190 | 5% | 10% | 2% |
| ❖ Strawberry Cheesecake | 1 cake | 180 | 8% | 10% | 5% |
| ★ Strawberry Shortcake à la Mode | 1 cake | 180 | 2% | 3% | 2% |
| ❖ Toasted Almond Amaretto Cheesecake | 1 cake | 170 | 8% | 13% | 2% |
| ❖ Triple Chocolate Caramel Mousse | 1 mousse | 200 | 6% | 5% | 2% |
| ❖ Triple Chocolate Cheesecake | 1 cake | 200 | 8% | 13% | 3% |

## ICE CREAM: FAT FREE AND LOW FAT

**Brand Name Foods**

| FOOD | Serving Size | Calories | Tot Fat | Sat Fat | Chol |
|------|------|------|------|------|------|
| ★ BREYER'S Chocolate, Fat Free | 1/2 cup | 95 | 0% | 0% | 1% |
| DREYER'S/EDY'S Fat Free | | | | | |
| ★ Black Cherry Vanilla | 1/2 cup | 100 | 0% | 0% | 0% |
| ★ Chocolate Fudge | 1/2 cup | 100 | 0% | 0% | 0% |
| ★ Marble Fudge | 1/2 cup | 100 | 0% | 0% | 0% |

★ Foods with this symbol have less than or equal to 5% *Daily Value* for <u>all</u> three nutrients (5% Rule).
❖ Foods with this symbol have <u>at least one</u> of the three nutrients greater than 5% *Daily Value* but less than or equal to 20% *Daily Value*.
☉ Foods with this symbol have <u>at least one</u> of the three nutrients greater than 20% *Daily Value* (20% Rule).

| | FOOD | Serving Size | Calories | Tot Fat | Sat Fat | Chol |
|---|---|---|---|---|---|---|
| ★ | Mint Fudge | 1/2 cup | 100 | 0% | 0% | 0% |
| ★ | Raspberry Vanilla Swirl | 1/2 cup | 70 | 0% | 0% | 0% |
| ★ | Strawberry | 1/2 cup | 90 | 0% | 0% | 0% |
| ★ | Vanilla | 1/2 cup | 90 | 0% | 0% | 0% |
| ★ | Vanilla Chocolate Swirl | 1/2 cup | 80 | 0% | 0% | 0% |
| | HEALTHY CHOICE Premium Low Fat—CONAGRA | | | | | |
| ★ | Bananas Foster | 1/2 cup | 110 | 2% | 5% | 2% |
| ★ | Black Forest | 1/2 cup | 120 | 3% | 5% | 3% |
| ❖ | Bordeaux Cherry Chocolate Chip | 1/2 cup | 110 | 3% | 7% | 1% |
| ★ | Butter Pecan Crunch | 1/2 cup | 120 | 3% | 4% | 1% |
| ★ | Cappuccino Chocolate Chunk | 1/2 cup | 120 | 3% | 5% | 3% |
| ★ | Cappuccino Mocha Fudge | 1/2 cup | 120 | 3% | 5% | 1% |
| ★ | Cherry Chocolate Chunk | 1/2 cup | 110 | 3% | 5% | 1% |
| ★ | Cookies 'N Cream | 1/2 cup | 120 | 3% | 5% | 1% |
| ❖ | Double Fudge Swirl | 1/2 cup | 120 | 3% | 6% | 1% |
| ❖ | Fudge Brownie | 1/2 cup | 120 | 3% | 6% | 2% |
| ❖ | Fudge Brownie A La Mode | 1/2 cup | 120 | 3% | 6% | 2% |
| ★ | Malt Caramel Cone | 1/2 cup | 120 | 3% | 5% | 3% |
| ★ | Mint Chocolate Chip | 1/2 cup | 120 | 3% | 5% | 1% |
| ★ | Peanut Butter Cookie Dough 'N Fudge | 1/2 cup | 120 | 3% | 4% | 1% |
| ★ | Praline and Caramel | 1/2 cup | 130 | 3% | 4% | 1% |
| ★ | Praline Caramel Cluster | 1/2 cup | 130 | 3% | 4% | 1% |
| ★ | Rocky Road | 1/2 cup | 140 | 3% | 4% | 1% |
| ★ | Triple Chocolate Chunk | 1/2 cup | 110 | 3% | 5% | 1% |
| ★ | Turtle Fudge Cake | 1/2 cup | 130 | 3% | 5% | 1% |
| ★ | Vanilla | 1/2 cup | 100 | 3% | 5% | 2% |
| | WEIGHT WATCHERS Light | | | | | |
| ❖ | *Cookie Dough Craze* | 1/2 cup | 140 | 5% | 10% | 2% |
| ❖ | *Oh! So Very Vanilla!* | 1/2 cup | 120 | 4% | 8% | 2% |
| ❖ | *Positively Praline Crunch* | 1/2 cup | 140 | 5% | 8% | 2% |
| ❖ | *Reckless Rocky Road* | 1/2 cup | 140 | 5% | 8% | 2% |
| ❖ | *Triple Chocolate Tornado* | 1/2 cup | 150 | 5% | 8% | 2% |

## NONDAIRY FROZEN DESSERTS

**Brand Name Foods**

| | | Serving Size | Calories | Tot Fat | Sat Fat | Chol |
|---|---|---|---|---|---|---|
| | TOFUTTI *Better Than Yogurt* | | | | | |
| ★ | Chocolate Fudge | 1/2 cup | 120 | 3% | 5% | 0% |
| ★ | Coffee Marshmallow Swirl | 1/2 cup | 100 | 2% | 0% | 0% |
| ★ | Passion Island Fruit | 1/2 cup | 100 | 2% | 0% | 0% |
| ★ | Peach Mango | 1/2 cup | 100 | 2% | 0% | 0% |
| ★ | Strawberry Banana | 1/2 cup | 100 | 2% | 0% | 0% |
| ★ | Vanilla Fudge | 1/2 cup | 120 | 3% | 0% | 0% |
| | TOFUTTI | | | | | |
| ★ | Chocolate Fudge Treats | 1 bar | 30 | 0% | 0% | 0% |
| ❖ | *Cuties:* All flavors | 1 sandwich | 120 | 8% | 5% | 0% |

| FOOD | Serving Size | Calories | Tot Fat | Sat Fat | Chol |
|------|--------------|----------|---------|---------|------|
| ★ *Frutti:* All flavors | 1/2 cup | 100 | 0% | 0% | 0% |
| ★ Teddy Fudge | 1 bar | 70 | 2% | 0% | 0% |
| TOFUTTI Frozen Desserts | | | | | |
| ❖ Chocolate Supreme | 1/2 cup | 180 | 17% | 10% | 0% |
| ❖ Vanilla | 1/2 cup | 190 | 17% | 10% | 0% |
| ❖ Vanilla Almond Bark | 1/2 cup | 210 | 20% | 10% | 0% |
| ❖ Wildberry Supreme | 1/2 cup | 190 | 14% | 10% | 0% |

### SHERBETS, SORBETS, AND ICES

**Generic Foods**

| FOOD | Serving Size | Calories | Tot Fat | Sat Fat | Chol |
|------|--------------|----------|---------|---------|------|
| ★ Fruit Ices | 1/2 cup | 120 | 0% | 0% | 0% |
| ❖ Orange Sherbet | 1/2 cup | 130 | 3% | 6% | 2% |
| ★ Pina Colada Sorbet | 1/2 cup | 90 | 4% | 0% | 0% |

**Brand Name Foods**

| FOOD | Serving Size | Calories | Tot Fat | Sat Fat | Chol |
|------|--------------|----------|---------|---------|------|
| BEN & JERRY'S Ices | | | | | |
| ★ Grapefruit | 1/2 cup | 130 | 0% | 0% | 0% |
| ★ Lemon Daiquiri | 1/2 cup | 120 | 0% | 0% | 0% |
| ★ Mandarin | 1/2 cup | 130 | 0% | 0% | 0% |
| ★ Marguerita Lime | 1/2 cup | 120 | 0% | 0% | 0% |
| ★ Raspberry | 1/2 cup | 120 | 0% | 0% | 0% |
| HÄAGEN-DAZS *Sorbet & Cream* —PILLSBURY | | | | | |
| Ⓐ Orange | 1/2 cup | 200 | 14% | 25% | 20% |
| Ⓐ Raspberry | 1/2 cup | 190 | 14% | 25% | 20% |
| HEALTHY CHOICE Premium Low Fat Sorbet—CONAGRA | | | | | |
| ★ Orange Sorbet & Cream | 1/2 cup | 90 | 3% | 5% | 1% |
| ★ Raspberry Sorbet & Cream | 1/2 cup | 90 | 3% | 5% | 1% |
| ★ Strawberry Sorbet & Cream | 1/2 cup | 90 | 3% | 5% | 1% |
| MAMA TISH'S Lite Original Italian Ices | | | | | |
| ★ Lemon | 1/2 cup | 50 | 0% | 0% | 0% |
| ★ Strawberry | 1/2 cup | 40 | 0% | 0% | 0% |
| MAMA TISH'S Original Italian Ices | | | | | |
| ★ Cherry | 1/2 cup | 100 | 0% | 0% | 0% |
| ★ Chocolate | 1/2 cup | 100 | 0% | 0% | 0% |
| ★ Lemon | 1/2 cup | 100 | 0% | 0% | 0% |
| ★ Lemon-Lime | 1/2 cup | 90 | 0% | 0% | 0% |
| ★ Pineapple-Banana-Orange | 1/2 cup | 90 | 0% | 0% | 0% |
| ★ Pineapple-Coconut | 1/2 cup | 90 | 0% | 0% | 0% |
| ★ Strawberry | 1/2 cup | 80 | 0% | 0% | 0% |

★ Foods with this symbol have less than or equal to 5% *Daily Value* for <u>all</u> three nutrients (5% Rule).

❖ Foods with this symbol have <u>at least one</u> of the three nutrients greater than 5% *Daily Value* but less than or equal to 20% *Daily Value.*

Ⓐ Foods with this symbol have <u>at least one</u> of the three nutrients greater than 20% *Daily Value* (20% Rule).

| | FOOD | Serving Size | Calories | Tot Fat | Sat Fat | Chol |
|---|---|---|---|---|---|---|
| ★ | Tropical | 1/2 cup | 90 | 0% | 0% | 0% |

TOPPINGS

**Generic Foods**

| | FOOD | Serving Size | Calories | Tot Fat | Sat Fat | Chol |
|---|---|---|---|---|---|---|
| ★ | Butterscotch | 2 tbsp | 100 | 0% | 0% | 0% |
| ☮ | Butterscotch Sauce | 2 tbsp | 190 | 11% | 22% | 6% |
| ❖ | Chocolate Fudge | 2 tbsp | 100 | 6% | 12% | 0% |
| ★ | Chocolate Syrup | 2 tbsp | 70 | 0% | 1% | 0% |
| ★ | Marshmallow Cream | 2 tbsp | 130 | 0% | 0% | 0% |
| ❖ | Nuts in Syrup | 2 tbsp | 170 | 14% | 4% | 0% |
| ★ | Pineapple | 2 tbsp | 110 | 0% | 0% | 0% |
| ★ | Strawberry | 2 tbsp | 110 | 0% | 0% | 0% |

**Brand Name Foods**

| | FOOD | Serving Size | Calories | Tot Fat | Sat Fat | Chol |
|---|---|---|---|---|---|---|
| ❖ | BARBARA'S BAKERY Chocolate Mountain Chocolate Sauce | 2 tbsp | 120 | 6% | 15% | 1% |
| ★ | ESTEE Chocolate Syrup | 2 tbsp | 50 | 0% | 0% | 0% |
| | HERSHEY's Chocolate Shoppe Ice Cream Toppings | | | | | |
| ★ | Chocolate Malt Syrup | 2 tbsp | 100 | 0% | 0% | 2% |
| ★ | Chocolate Syrup | 2 tbsp | 100 | 0% | 0% | 1% |
| ❖ | Cookies 'n Mint | 2 tbsp | 100 | 9% | 15% | 1% |
| ❖ | Hot Fudge | 2 tbsp | 150 | 9% | 20% | 2% |
| ❖ | Milk Chocolate | 2 tbsp | 140 | 8% | 15% | 2% |
| ❖ | Milk Chocolate w/Almonds | 2 tbsp | 150 | 12% | 15% | 2% |
| ☮ | *Mounds* | 2 tbsp | 140 | 12% | 25% | 1% |
| ❖ | *Reese's* Peanut Butter | 2 tbsp | 160 | 12% | 15% | 2% |
| ★ | Strawberry Syrup | 2 tbsp | 110 | 0% | 0% | 0% |
| ☮ | *York* Peppermint Pattie | 2 tbsp | 170 | 12% | 23% | 1% |
| ★ | KRAFT Marshmallow Creme | 2 tbsp | 40 | 0% | 0% | 0% |
| | KRAFT Toppings | | | | | |
| ★ | Butterscotch (artificially flavored) | 2 tbsp | 130 | 2% | 5% | 2% |
| ★ | Caramel | 2 tbsp | 120 | 0% | 0% | 0% |
| ★ | Chocolate Flavored | 2 tbsp | 110 | 0% | 0% | 0% |
| ❖ | Hot Fudge | 2 tbsp | 140 | 6% | 10% | 0% |
| ★ | Pineapple | 2 tbsp | 110 | 0% | 0% | 0% |
| | MRS. RICHARDSON'S—QUAKER | | | | | |
| ❖ | Butterscotch Caramel Fudge | 2 tbsp | 130 | 2% | 8% | 1% |
| ★ | Caramel, Fat Free | 2 tbsp | 130 | 0% | 0% | 0% |
| ☮ | Hot Fudge | 2 tbsp | 140 | 10% | 30% | 0% |
| ★ | Hot Fudge, Fat Free | 2 tbsp | 110 | 0% | 0% | 0% |
| | SMUCKER'S Special Recipe Toppings | | | | | |
| ★ | Butterscotch Caramel | 2 tbsp | 130 | 2% | 3% | 1% |
| ❖ | Hot Fudge | 2 tbsp | 140 | 6% | 5% | 0% |

| FOOD | Serving Size | Calories | Tot Fat | Sat Fat | Chol |
|---|---|---|---|---|---|
| ★ SMUCKER'S Sundae Syrup: | | | | | |
| All flavors | 2 tbsp | 110 | 0% | 0% | 0% |
| SMUCKER'S Toppings | | | | | |
| ★   Butterscotch & Caramel, Fat Free | 2 tbsp | 130 | 0% | 0% | 0% |
| ★   Chocolate Fudge | 2 tbsp | 130 | 3% | 3% | 0% |
| ★   Hot Caramel | 2 tbsp | 120 | 4% | 3% | 0% |
| ❖   Hot Fudge | 2 tbsp | 140 | 6% | 5% | 0% |
| ★   Light Hot Fudge, Fat Free | 2 tbsp | 90 | 0% | 0% | 0% |
| Ⓐ   *Magic Shell:* All flavors | 2 tbsp | 220 | 25% | 30% | 0% |
| ★   Marshmallow | 2 tbsp | 120 | 0% | 0% | 0% |
| ❖   Peanut Butter Caramel | 2 tbsp | 150 | 7% | 3% | 0% |
| ❖   Pecans in Syrup | 2 tbsp | 190 | 17% | 5% | 0% |
| ★   Pineapple | 2 tbsp | 110 | 0% | 0% | 0% |
| ★   Strawberry | 2 tbsp | 100 | 0% | 0% | 0% |
| ❖   Walnuts in Syrup | 2 tbsp | 190 | 15% | 5% | 0% |

# Fruits

## CANNED FRUIT

### Generic Foods

| FOOD | Serving Size | Calories | Tot Fat | Sat Fat | Chol |
|---|---|---|---|---|---|
| ★ Applesauce (sweetened) | 1/2 cup | 100 | 0% | 0% | 0% |
| ★ Applesauce (unsweetened) | 1/2 cup | 50 | 0% | 0% | 0% |
| ★ Apricots in extra light syrup | 1/2 cup | 70 | 0% | 0% | 0% |
| ★ Apricots in heavy syrup | 1/2 cup | 120 | 0% | 0% | 0% |
| ★ Apricots in juice | 1/2 cup | 70 | 0% | 0% | 0% |
| ★ Blackberries in heavy syrup | 1/2 cup | 130 | 0% | 0% | 0% |
| ★ Blueberries in heavy syrup | 1/2 cup | 120 | 0% | 0% | 0% |
| ★ Boysenberries in heavy syrup | 1/2 cup | 120 | 0% | 0% | 0% |
| ★ Cherries, Sour, in heavy syrup | 1/2 cup | 130 | 0% | 0% | 0% |
| ★ Cherries, Sour, in light syrup | 1/2 cup | 110 | 0% | 0% | 0% |
| ★ Cherries, Sweet, in heavy syrup | 1/2 cup | 120 | 0% | 0% | 0% |
| ★ Cherries, Sweet, in juice | 1/2 cup | 80 | 0% | 0% | 0% |
| ★ Cherries, Sweet, in light syrup | 1/2 cup | 90 | 0% | 0% | 0% |
| ★ Figs in heavy syrup | 1/2 cup | 120 | 0% | 0% | 0% |
| ★ Figs in light syrup | 1/2 cup | 100 | 0% | 0% | 0% |
| ★ Fruit Cocktail in extra light syrup | 1/2 cup | 60 | 0% | 0% | 0% |
| ★ Fruit Cocktail in heavy syrup | 1/2 cup | 100 | 0% | 0% | 0% |
| ★ Fruit Cocktail in juice | 1/2 cup | 60 | 0% | 0% | 0% |
| ★ Mixed Fruit in heavy syrup | 1/2 cup | 100 | 0% | 0% | 0% |
| ★ Peaches in extra light syrup | 1/2 cup | 60 | 0% | 0% | 0% |
| ★ Peaches in heavy syrup | 1/2 cup | 100 | 0% | 0% | 0% |

★   Foods with this symbol have less than or equal to 5% *Daily Value* for <u>all</u> three nutrients (5% Rule).

❖   Foods with this symbol have <u>at least one</u> of the three nutrients greater than 5% *Daily Value* but less than or equal to 20% *Daily Value*.

Ⓐ   Foods with this symbol have <u>at least one</u> of the three nutrients greater than 20% *Daily Value* (20% Rule).

| FOOD | Serving Size | Calories | Tot Fat | Sat Fat | Chol |
|---|---|---|---|---|---|
| ★ Peaches in juice | 1/2 cup | 60 | 0% | 0% | 0% |
| ★ Pears in extra light syrup | 1/2 cup | 70 | 0% | 0% | 0% |
| ★ Pears in heavy syrup | 1/2 cup | 100 | 0% | 0% | 0% |
| ★ Pears in juice | 1/2 cup | 70 | 0% | 0% | 0% |
| ★ Pineapple in heavy syrup | 1/2 cup | 110 | 0% | 0% | 0% |
| ★ Pineapple in juice | 1/2 cup | 80 | 0% | 0% | 0% |
| ★ Pineapple in light syrup | 1/2 cup | 70 | 0% | 0% | 0% |
| ★ Plums in heavy syrup | 1/2 cup | 130 | 0% | 0% | 0% |
| ★ Plums in juice | 1/2 cup | 80 | 0% | 0% | 0% |
| ★ Plums in light syrup | 1/2 cup | 90 | 0% | 0% | 0% |
| ★ Prunes in heavy syrup | 1/2 cup | 150 | 0% | 0% | 0% |
| ★ Raspberries in heavy syrup | 1/2 cup | 130 | 0% | 0% | 0% |

**Brand Name Foods**

| FOOD | Serving Size | Calories | Tot Fat | Sat Fat | Chol |
|---|---|---|---|---|---|
| DEL MONTE Fruit Snack Cups | | | | | |
| ★ Mixed Fruit in heavy syrup | 1 can | 100 | 0% | 0% | 0% |
| ★ *Fruit Naturals* Mixed Fruit in fruit juices | 1 can | 60 | 0% | 0% | 0% |
| ★ *Lite* Mixed Fruit in extra light syrup | 1 can | 60 | 0% | 0% | 0% |
| ★ Diced Peaches in heavy syrup | 1 can | 100 | 0% | 0% | 0% |
| ★ *Fruit Naturals* Diced Peaches in peach juice | 1 can | 60 | 0% | 0% | 0% |
| ★ *Lite* Diced Peaches in extra light syrup | 1 can | 60 | 0% | 0% | 0% |
| ★ Diced Pears in heavy syrup | 1 can | 100 | 0% | 0% | 0% |
| ★ *Lite* Pears in extra light syrup | 1 can | 60 | 0% | 0% | 0% |
| ★ Pineapple Tidbits in pineapple juice | 1 can | 70 | 0% | 0% | 0% |
| DEL MONTE Fruits (canned) | | | | | |
| ★ Apricot Halves in heavy syrup | 1/2 cup | 100 | 0% | 0% | 0% |
| ★ *Lite* Apricot Halves in extra light syrup | 1/2 cup | 60 | 0% | 0% | 0% |
| ★ Cherries (dark) in heavy syrup | 1/2 cup | 100 | 0% | 0% | 0% |
| ★ Chunky Mixed Fruits in heavy syrup | 1/2 cup | 100 | 0% | 0% | 0% |
| ★ *Fruit Naturals* Chunky Mixed fruits in fruit juices | 1/2 cup | 60 | 0% | 0% | 0% |
| ★ *Lite* Chunky Mixed Fruits in extra light syrup | 1/2 cup | 60 | 0% | 0% | 0% |
| ★ Fruit Cocktail in heavy syrup | 1/2 cup | 100 | 0% | 0% | 0% |
| ★ *Fruit Naturals* Fruit Cocktail in fruit juices | 1/2 cup | 60 | 0% | 0% | 0% |
| ★ *Lite* Fruit Cocktail in extra light syrup | 1/2 cup | 60 | 0% | 0% | 0% |
| ★ Mandarin Oranges in light syrup | 1/2 cup | 80 | 0% | 0% | 0% |
| ★ Peaches in heavy syrup | 1/2 cup | 100 | 0% | 0% | 0% |
| ★ *Fruit Naturals* Peaches in peach juice | 1/2 cup | 60 | 0% | 0% | 0% |

| FOOD | Serving Size | Calories | Tot Fat | Sat Fat | Chol |
|---|---|---|---|---|---|
| ★     *Lite* Peaches in extra light syrup | 1/2 cup | 60 | 0% | 0% | 0% |
| ★   Pears in heavy syrup | 1/2 cup | 100 | 0% | 0% | 0% |
| ★   *Fruit Naturals* Pears in pear juice | 1/2 cup | 60 | 0% | 0% | 0% |
| ★   *Lite* Pears in extra light syrup | 1/2 cup | 60 | 0% | 0% | 0% |
| ★   Pineapple (all varieties) in heavy syrup | 1/2 cup | 90 | 0% | 0% | 0% |
| ★   Pineapple (all varieties) in own juices | 1/2 cup | 70 | 0% | 0% | 0% |
| ★   Tropical Fruit Salad in light syrup | 1/2 cup | 80 | 0% | 0% | 0% |
|   DOLE Crushed Pineapple | | | | | |
| ★   In heavy syrup | 1/2 cup | 90 | 0% | 0% | 0% |
| ★   In juice | 1/2 cup | 70 | 0% | 0% | 0% |
|   DOLE Pineapple Slices | | | | | |
| ★   In clarified juice | 2 slcs | 60 | 0% | 0% | 0% |
| ★   In heavy syrup | 2 slcs | 90 | 0% | 0% | 0% |
| ★   In light syrup | 3 1/2 slcs | 60 | 0% | 0% | 0% |
|   DOLE Pineapple Tidbits or Chunks | | | | | |
| ★   In heavy syrup | 1/2 cup | 90 | 0% | 0% | 0% |
| ★   In juice | 1/2 cup | 60 | 0% | 0% | 0% |
| ★   In light syrup | 1/2 cup | 80 | 0% | 0% | 0% |
| ★ DOLE Tropical Fruit Salad in light syrup | 1/2 cup | 80 | 0% | 0% | 0% |
|   HUNT'S—HUNT WESSON | | | | | |
| ★   Fruit Cocktail | 1/2 cup | 90 | 0% | 0% | 0% |
| ★   Peach Halves or Slices | 1/2 cup | 100 | 0% | 0% | 0% |
|   MOTT'S Apple Sauces—CADBURY BEVERAGES | | | | | |
| ★   Chunky | 1/2 cup | 110 | 0% | 0% | 0% |
| ★   Cinnamon | 1/2 cup | 120 | 0% | 0% | 0% |
| ★   Sweetened | 1/2 cup | 110 | 0% | 0% | 0% |
|   MOTT'S Fruit Snacks—CADBURY BEVERAGES | | | | | |
| ★   Cinnamon | 1/2 cup | 90 | 0% | 0% | 0% |
| ★   Dutch Apple Spice | 1/2 cup | 70 | 0% | 0% | 0% |
| ★   Strawberry | 1/2 cup | 80 | 0% | 0% | 0% |
| ★   Sweetened | 1/2 cup | 90 | 0% | 0% | 0% |
|   S & W | | | | | |
| ★   Freestone Peach Halves in heavy syrup | 1/2 cup | 100 | 0% | 0% | 0% |
| ★   Fruit Cocktail in heavy syrup | 1/2 cup | 90 | 0% | 0% | 0% |
| ★   Kadota Figs | 5 pcs | 140 | 2% | 0% | 0% |
| ★   Mandarin Oranges in light syrup | 2/3 cup | 100 | 0% | 0% | 0% |
| ★   Sliced Cling Peaches in heavy syrup | 1/2 cup | 100 | 0% | 0% | 0% |

★  Foods with this symbol have less than or equal to 5% *Daily Value* for <u>all</u> three nutrients (5% Rule).

❖  Foods with this symbol have <u>at least one</u> of the three nutrients greater than 5% *Daily Value* but less than or equal to 20% *Daily Value*.

Ⓐ  Foods with this symbol have <u>at least one</u> of the three nutrients greater than 20% *Daily Value* (20% Rule).

| FOOD | Serving Size | Calories | Tot Fat | Sat Fat | Chol |
|---|---|---|---|---|---|
| ★ Sliced Pineapple | 2 pcs | 90 | 0% | 0% | 0% |
| ★ Thompson Seedless Grapes in heavy syrup | 1/2 cup | 100 | 0% | 0% | 0% |
| S & W Natural Style | | | | | |
| ★ Chunky Mixed Fruit | 1/2 cup | 70 | 0% | 0% | 0% |
| ★ Cling Peaches in Peach Juice | 1/2 cup | 80 | 0% | 0% | 0% |
| ★ Fruit Cocktail | 1/2 cup | 80 | 1% | 0% | 0% |
| ★ Mandarin Oranges | 2/3 cup | 70 | 0% | 0% | 0% |
| SANTA CRUZ Natural Applesauce | | | | | |
| —KNUDSEN | | | | | |
| ★ Apple Sauce | 1/2 cup | 45 | 0% | 0% | 0% |
| ★ Apple Apricot | 1/2 cup | 45 | 0% | 0% | 0% |
| ★ Apple Blackberry | 1/2 cup | 45 | 0% | 0% | 0% |
| ★ Apple Cherry | 1/2 cup | 45 | 0% | 0% | 0% |
| ★ Apple Strawberry | 1/2 cup | 45 | 0% | 0% | 0% |
| ★ Gravenstein | 1/2 cup | 45 | 0% | 0% | 0% |
| ★ SUN LUCK Mandarin Oranges | 2/3 cup | 100 | 0% | 0% | 0% |

## DRIED FRUIT

**Generic Foods**

| FOOD | Serving Size | Calories | Tot Fat | Sat Fat | Chol |
|---|---|---|---|---|---|
| ★ Apples | 1/2 cup | 100 | 0% | 0% | 0% |
| ★ Apricots | 1/3 cup | 100 | 0% | 0% | 0% |
| ★ Dates (whole) | 5 dates | 110 | 0% | 0% | 0% |
| ★ Figs | 1/4 cup | 100 | 1% | 0% | 0% |
| ★ Peaches | 1/4 cup | 100 | 0% | 0% | 0% |
| ★ Prunes | 1/4 cup | 100 | 0% | 0% | 0% |
| ★ Raisins | 1/4 cup | 120 | 0% | 0% | 0% |

**Brand Name Foods**

| FOOD | Serving Size | Calories | Tot Fat | Sat Fat | Chol |
|---|---|---|---|---|---|
| DEL MONTE Dried Fruits | | | | | |
| ★ Apples (sliced) | 1/3 cup | 80 | 0% | 0% | 0% |
| ★ Apricots | 1/3 cup | 80 | 0% | 0% | 0% |
| ★ Dates (chopped) | 1/4 cup | 120 | 0% | 0% | 0% |
| ★ Dates (whole) | 5–6 dates | 120 | 0% | 0% | 0% |
| ★ Mixed Dried Fruits | 1/3 cup | 110 | 0% | 0% | 0% |
| ★ Peaches | 1/3 cup | 90 | 0% | 0% | 0% |
| ★ Prunes (pitted) | 1/4 cup | 120 | 0% | 0% | 0% |
| ★ Raisins | 1/4 cup | 120 | 0% | 0% | 0% |
| ★ Raisins, Golden | 1/4 cup | 120 | 0% | 0% | 0% |
| DOLE Dried Fruits | | | | | |
| ★ Dates (pitted) | 1/2 cup | 280 | 0% | 5% | 0% |
| ❖ Raisins | 1/2 cup | 250 | 0% | 10% | 1% |

| FOOD | Serving Size | Calories | Tot Fat | Sat Fat | Chol |
|------|-------------|----------|---------|---------|------|

### FRESH FRUIT

**Generic Foods**

| FOOD | Serving Size | Calories | Tot Fat | Sat Fat | Chol |
|------|-------------|----------|---------|---------|------|
| ★ Apple (2 3/4" diam) | 1 fruit | 80 | 1% | 0% | 0% |
| ★ Apricot | 3 small | 70 | 1% | 0% | 0% |
| ★ Banana | 1 small | 130 | 1% | 0% | 0% |
| ★ Blackberries | 1 cup | 70 | 1% | 0% | 0% |
| ★ Blueberries | 1 cup | 80 | 1% | 0% | 0% |
| ★ Cantaloupe (cubed) | 1 cup | 50 | 1% | 0% | 0% |
| ★ Cherries, Sweet | 21 cherries | 100 | 2% | 2% | 0% |
| ★ Cranberries | 1/2 cup | 30 | 0% | 0% | 0% |
| ★ Figs | 3 fruits | 100 | 1% | 0% | 0% |
| ★ Grapefruit, Red, Pink, or White | 1/2 fruit | 45 | 0% | 0% | 0% |
| ★ Grapes | 1 cup | 100 | 1% | 1% | 0% |
| ★ Guavas | 2 fruits | 70 | 1% | 1% | 0% |
| ★ Honeydew (cubed) | 1 cup | 40 | 0% | 0% | 0% |
| ★ Kiwifruit | 2 fruits | 90 | 1% | 0% | 0% |
| ★ Lemon (w/o peel) | 1 fruit | 20 | 0% | 0% | 0% |
| ★ Lime | 1 fruit | 20 | 0% | 0% | 0% |
| ★ Mango | 2/3 fruit | 90 | 1% | 0% | 0% |
| ★ Nectarine | 1 fruit | 70 | 1% | 0% | 0% |
| ★ Orange | 1 fruit | 60 | 0% | 0% | 0% |
| ★ Papaya | 1 fruit | 60 | 0% | 0% | 0% |
| ★ Peach | 1 large | 60 | 0% | 0% | 0% |
| ★ Pear | 1 fruit | 80 | 0% | 0% | 0% |
| ★ Pineapple | 1 cup | 70 | 1% | 0% | 0% |
| ★ Plum | 3 fruits | 40 | 0% | 0% | 0% |
| ★ Raspberries | 1 cup | 70 | 1% | 0% | 0% |
| ★ Strawberries | 1 cup | 40 | 1% | 0% | 0% |
| ★ Tangerine | 1 fruit | 50 | 0% | 0% | 0% |
| ★ Watermelon | 1 cup | 45 | 1% | 0% | 0% |

### FROZEN FRUIT

**Generic Foods**

| FOOD | Serving Size | Calories | Tot Fat | Sat Fat | Chol |
|------|-------------|----------|---------|---------|------|
| ★ Berries, sweetened | 1 cup | 130 | 0% | 0% | 0% |
| ★ Berries, unsweetened | 1 cup | 80 | 0% | 0% | 0% |

★ Foods with this symbol have less than or equal to 5% *Daily Value* for <u>all</u> three nutrients (5% Rule).

❖ Foods with this symbol have <u>at least one</u> of the three nutrients greater than 5% *Daily Value* but less than or equal to 20% *Daily Value*.

Ⓐ Foods with this symbol have <u>at least one</u> of the three nutrients greater than 20% *Daily Value* (20% Rule).

| FOOD | Serving Size | Calories | Tot Fat | Sat Fat | Chol |
|------|--------------|----------|---------|---------|------|

# Gravies, Sauces, and Marinades

## COOKING SAUCES AND MARINADES

**Brand Name Foods**

| FOOD | Serving Size | Calories | Tot Fat | Sat Fat | Chol |
|------|--------------|----------|---------|---------|------|
| **BETTY CROCKER** *Dinner Sensations* (prep as dir)— | | | | | |
| GENERAL MILLS | | | | | |
| ⊛ Beef Stroganoff | 1 cup | 320 | 23% | 29% | 17% |
| ❖ Chicken Alfredo | 1 cup | 290 | 17% | 18% | 15% |
| **BETTY CROCKER** *Recipe Sauces* | | | | | |
| —GENERAL MILLS | | | | | |
| ⊛ Alfredo | 1/2 cup | 220 | 31% | 31% | 7% |
| ⊛ Creamy Broccoli | 1/2 cup | 210 | 30% | 35% | 9% |
| ★ Pepper Steak | 1/2 cup | 50 | 3% | 2% | 0% |
| **GOLDEN DIPT** Cooking Sauces | | | | | |
| —MCCORMICK | | | | | |
| ❖ Cajun Style Seafood BBQ Sauce | 1 tbsp | 60 | 7% | 0% | 0% |
| ★ Creole Style Cooking Sauce | 2 tbsp | 25 | 2% | 0% | 0% |
| ★ Lemon Butter Dill Sauce, Fat Free | 2 tbsp | 35 | 0% | 0% | 0% |
| ❖ Lemon Butter Dill Cooking Sauce | 2 tbsp | 120 | 16% | 6% | 0% |
| **GOLDEN DIPT** Marinades— | | | | | |
| MCCORMICK | | | | | |
| ★ Honey Mustard Marinade, Fat Free | 1 tbsp | 25 | 0% | 0% | 0% |
| ★ White Wine Dijon Marinade, Fat Free | 1 tbsp | 10 | 0% | 0% | 0% |
| ❖ Lemon Herb Seafood Marinade | 1 tbsp | 80 | 14% | 6% | 0% |
| **HAIN** Cooking Sauces | | | | | |
| ★ Cacciatore | 1/2 cup | 70 | 2% | 0% | 0% |
| ★ Honey Dijon | 1/2 cup | 90 | 2% | 0% | 0% |
| ★ Honey Ginger | 1/2 cup | 230 | 0% | 0% | 0% |
| **HUNT'S** *Chicken Sensations*— | | | | | |
| HUNT WESSON | | | | | |
| ★ BBQ Flavor | 1 tbsp | 35 | 4% | 1% | 0% |
| ★ Italian Garlic | 1 tbsp | 30 | 4% | 1% | 0% |
| ★ Lemon Herb | 1 tbsp | 30 | 4% | 1% | 0% |
| ★ South Western | 1 tbsp | 30 | 4% | 1% | 0% |
| **HUNT'S** Ready Sauces—HUNT WESSON | | | | | |
| ★ Chunky Chili | 1/4 cup | 21 | 1% | 0% | 0% |
| ★ Chunky Italian | 1/4 cup | 25 | 1% | 0% | 0% |
| ★ Chunky Special | 1/4 cup | 20 | 1% | 0% | 0% |
| ★ Chunky Tomato | 1/4 cup | 15 | 0% | 0% | 0% |
| ★ Country Herb | 1/4 cup | 30 | 2% | 1% | 0% |
| ★ Garlic | 1/4 cup | 30 | 2% | 1% | 0% |
| ★ Garlic & Herb | 1/4 cup | 25 | 1% | 0% | 0% |
| ★ Meatloaf Fixins | 1/4 cup | 25 | 1% | 0% | 0% |
| ★ Original Italian | 1/4 cup | 30 | 2% | 0% | 0% |

| FOOD | Serving Size | Calories | Tot Fat | Sat Fat | Chol |
|---|---|---|---|---|---|
| ★ Salsa | 1/4 cup | 20 | 0% | 0% | 0% |
| ★ KNORR Fresh Gourmet *Stir 'n Sauce* Italian—CPC | 1/2 pouch | 60 | 4% | 2% | 0% |
| KNORR Fresh Gourmet *Toss 'n Sauce*—CPC | | | | | |
| ★ For Carrots: Honey Mustard | 1 tbsp | 30 | 1% | 0% | 0% |
| ★ For Potatoes: Tomato Bacon | 1 tbsp | 30 | 1% | 0% | 0% |
| LAWRY'S Marinades | | | | | |
| ★ Citrus Grill | 1 tbsp | 15 | 0% | 0% | 0% |
| ★ Dijon & Honey | 1 tbsp | 20 | 2% | 0% | 0% |
| ★ Hawaiian | 1 tbsp | 20 | 0% | 0% | 0% |
| ★ Herb & Garlic | 1 tbsp | 10 | 0% | 0% | 0% |
| ★ Lemon Pepper | 1 tbsp | 10 | 1% | 0% | 0% |
| ★ Mesquite | 1 tbsp | 5 | 0% | 0% | 0% |
| ★ Thai Ginger | 1 tbsp | 10 | 1% | 0% | 0% |
| ★ MANISCHEWITZ Tomato & Mushroom Sauce | 1/4 cup | 35 | 2% | 0% | 0% |
| ★ McCORMICK/SCHILLING Seasoning & Sauce Mixes: Meat Marinade | 1/8 pkg | 15 | 0% | 0% | 0% |
| McCORMICK/SCHILLING Sauce Blends for Chicken | | | | | |
| ★ Chicken Dijon | 1/4 pkg | 40 | 2% | 3% | 1% |
| ★ Chicken Italian Marinade | 1/6 pkg | 20 | 0% | 0% | 0% |
| ★ Chicken Mesquite Marinade | 1/6 pkg | 20 | 0% | 0% | 0% |
| ★ Southwest Chicken | 1/6 pkg | 20 | 0% | 0% | 0% |
| ❖ RAGU *Chicken Tonight* Cooking Sauces: Country French—VAN DEN BERGH | 1/2 cup | 120 | 15% | 8% | 5% |
| ★ RAGU *Chicken Tonight* Simmer Sauces—VAN DEN BERGH | | | | | |
| ★ Chicken Cacciatore | 1/2 cup | 80 | 2% | 0% | 0% |
| ❖ Creamy Chicken w/Mushrooms | 1/2 cup | 110 | 14% | 8% | 3% |
| S & W Cooking Sauces | | | | | |
| ★ Herb & Garlic | 1 tbsp | 25 | 0% | 0% | 0% |
| ★ Mesquite | 1 tbsp | 10 | 0% | 0% | 0% |
| ★ Southwestern | 1 tbsp | 10 | 0% | 0% | 0% |
| SIMMER CHEF Cooking Sauces—CAMPBELL'S | 1/2 cup | | | | |
| ❖ Creamy Broccoli | 1/2 cup | 100 | 9% | 10% | 3% |
| ❖ Creamy Mushroom & Herb | 1/2 cup | 90 | 8% | 8% | 2% |
| ❖ Family Style Stroganoff | 1/2 cup | 100 | 9% | 10% | 2% |
| ★ Golden Honey Mustard | 1/2 cup | 150 | 3% | 0% | 0% |
| ★ Hearty Onion & Mushroom | 1/2 cup | 50 | 2% | 0% | 0% |
| ★ Old Country Cacciatore | 1/2 cup | 90 | 5% | 3% | 0% |

★  Foods with this symbol have less than or equal to 5% *Daily Value* for <u>all</u> three nutrients (5% Rule).
❖  Foods with this symbol have <u>at least one</u> of the three nutrients greater than 5% *Daily Value* but less than or equal to 20% *Daily Value*.
☻  Foods with this symbol have <u>at least one</u> of the three nutrients greater than 20% *Daily Value* (20% Rule).

| FOOD | Serving Size | Calories | Tot Fat | Sat Fat | Chol |
|------|-------------|----------|---------|---------|------|
| ★ TAJ Marinade Sauce: Kashmir | | | | | |
| Tandoori | 2 oz | 50 | 5% | 1% | 0% |
| TAJ Simmer Sauce | | | | | |
| ❖ Bombay Sauce | 4 oz | 90 | 8% | 2% | 0% |
| ❖ Calcutta Masala | 4 oz | 100 | 8% | 5% | 1% |

<u>GRAVIES</u>

**Brand Name Foods**

| FOOD | Serving Size | Calories | Tot Fat | Sat Fat | Chol |
|------|-------------|----------|---------|---------|------|
| FRANCO-AMERICAN Gravies— | | | | | |
| CAMPBELL'S | | | | | |
| ★ Au Jus | 1/4 cup | 10 | 1% | 0% | 1% |
| ★ Beef | 1/4 cup | 30 | 3% | 5% | 1% |
| ★ Brown w/Onions | 1/4 cup | 25 | 2% | 0% | 1% |
| ★ Cheese | 1/4 cup | 40 | 3% | 5% | 2% |
| ❖ Chicken | 1/4 cup | 45 | 6% | 5% | 2% |
| ★ Chicken Giblet | 1/4 cup | 30 | 3% | 0% | 3% |
| ★ Creamy Mushroom | 1/4 cup | 20 | 2% | 0% | 1% |
| ❖ Golden Pork | 1/4 cup | 45 | 6% | 8% | 1% |
| ★ Mushroom | 1/4 cup | 20 | 2% | 0% | 1% |
| ★ Turkey | 1/4 cup | 25 | 2% | 0% | 1% |
| ★ HAIN Brown Gravy Mix | 2 tsp mix | 15 | 0% | 0% | 0% |
| ★ HEINZ Fat Free Turkey Gravy | 1/4 cup | 15 | 0% | 0% | 0% |
| HEINZ Home Style Gravies | | | | | |
| ★ Classic Chicken | 1/4 cup | 30 | 3% | 0% | 0% |
| ★ Rich Mushroom | 1/4 cup | 20 | 1% | 0% | 0% |
| ★ Roasted Turkey | 1/4 cup | 25 | 2% | 0% | 0% |
| ★ Savory Brown | 1/4 cup | 25 | 1% | 0% | 0% |
| KNORR Gravy Classics Mixes—CPC | | | | | |
| ★ Au Jus | 1/5 pkg | 15 | 0% | 0% | 0% |
| ★ Classic Brown & Onion Lyonnaise | 1/5 pkg | 20 | 1% | 0% | 0% |
| ★ Classic Brown | 1/6 pkg | 20 | 1% | 0% | 0% |
| ★ Hunter Mushroom | 1/5 pkg | 25 | 1% | 0% | 0% |
| ★ Roasted Chicken | 1/5 pkg | 30 | 2% | 0% | 1% |
| ★ Roasted Turkey | 1/5 pkg | 25 | 1% | 0% | 1% |
| LIBBY'S Gravy—NESTLÉ | | | | | |
| ❖ Country Chicken | 1/4 cup | 60 | 6% | 3% | 2% |
| ❖ Country Sausage | 1/4 cup | 90 | 11% | 8% | 2% |
| LOMA LINDA *Gravy Quik*— | | | | | |
| WORTHINGTON FOODS | | | | | |
| ★ Brown | 1 tbsp | 20 | 0% | 0% | 0% |
| ★ Chicken Style | 1 tbsp | 20 | 0% | 0% | 0% |
| ★ Country Style | 1 tbsp | 25 | 1% | 0% | 0% |
| ★ Mushroom | 1 tbsp | 15 | 0% | 0% | 0% |
| ★ Onion | 1 tbsp | 20 | 0% | 0% | 0% |
| McCORMICK/SCHILLING Gravy Mixes | | | | | |
| ★ Au Jus | 1/12 pkg | 5 | 0% | 0% | 0% |

| FOOD | Serving Size | Calories | Tot Fat | Sat Fat | Chol |
|------|-------------|----------|---------|---------|------|
| ★ Brown | 1/4 pkg | 20 | 1% | 0% | 0% |
| ★ Chicken | 1/4 pkg | 20 | 0% | 0% | 0% |
| ★ Country, Regular | 1/8 pkg | 45 | 3% | 0% | 1% |
| ★ Country, Sausage | 1/8 pkg | 40 | 2% | 0% | 0% |
| ★ Herb | 1/4 pkg | 20 | 1% | 0% | 0% |
| ★ Homestyle | 1/4 pkg | 25 | 2% | 0% | 0% |
| ★ Mushroom | 1/4 pkg | 20 | 1% | 0% | 0% |
| ★ Onion | 1/4 pkg | 20 | 1% | 0% | 0% |
| ★ Pork | 1/4 pkg | 25 | 0% | 0% | 0% |
| ★ Turkey | 1/4 pkg | 20 | 0% | 0% | 0% |
| ❖ NATURAL TOUCH Stroganoff Mix—WORTHINGTON FOODS | 4 tbsp mix | 90 | 5% | 10% | 3% |
| PEPPERIDGE FARM Gravies— CAMPBELL'S | | | | | |
| ★ Cream of Chicken | 1/4 cup | 30 | 2% | 3% | 1% |
| ★ Golden Chicken w/ Pieces of Chicken | 1/4 cup | 25 | 2% | 0% | 1% |
| ★ Hearty Beef w/Pieces of Beef | 1/4 cup | 25 | 2% | 0% | 1% |
| ★ Mushroom & Wine w/Mushroom | 1/4 cup | 30 | 2% | 3% | 1% |
| ★ Onion & Garlic | 1/4 cup | 30 | 2% | 3% | 1% |
| ★ Seasoned Turkey w/Pieces of Turkey | 1/4 cup | 30 | 2% | 0% | 1% |
| ★ Stroganoff w/Sliced Mushrooms | 1/4 cup | 30 | 2% | 3% | 1% |
| PILLSBURY Gravy Mixes (prep as dir) | | | | | |
| ★ Brown | 2 tbsp | 10 | 0% | 0% | 0% |
| ★ Chicken Style | 2 tbsp | 10 | 0% | 0% | 0% |
| ★ Homestyle | 2 tbsp | 10 | 0% | 0% | 0% |

## MEXICAN SAUCES

### Generic Foods

| FOOD | Serving Size | Calories | Tot Fat | Sat Fat | Chol |
|------|-------------|----------|---------|---------|------|
| ★ Chili Sauce | 1 tbsp | 15 | 0% | 0% | 0% |
| ★ Hot Chili Pepper Sauce | 1 tsp | 0 | 0% | 0% | 0% |
| ★ Picante Sauce | 1 tbsp | 10 | 1% | 0% | 0% |
| ★ Taco Sauce | 1 tbsp | 10 | 1% | 0% | 0% |

### Brand Name Foods

| FOOD | Serving Size | Calories | Tot Fat | Sat Fat | Chol |
|------|-------------|----------|---------|---------|------|
| ★ DEL MONTE Chili Sauce | 1 tbsp | 20 | 0% | 0% | 0% |
| GEBHARDT Sauces—HUNT WESSON | | | | | |
| ❖ Chili Hot Dog | 1/4 cup | 60 | 5% | 7% | 1% |
| ★ Enchilada | 1/4 cup | 35 | 3% | 5% | 0% |
| ★ Hot | 1 tsp | 0 | 0% | 0% | 0% |

★ Foods with this symbol have less than or equal to 5% *Daily Value* for <u>all</u> three nutrients (5% Rule).
❖ Foods with this symbol have <u>at least one</u> of the three nutrients greater than 5% *Daily Value* but less than or equal to 20% *Daily Value*.
⊘ Foods with this symbol have <u>at least one</u> of the three nutrients greater than 20% *Daily Value* (20% Rule).

| FOOD | Serving Size | Calories | Tot Fat | Sat Fat | Chol |
|---|---|---|---|---|---|
| HUNT'S Homestyle Sauces— HUNT WESSON | | | | | |
| ★ Pepper Sauce | 1 tsp | 0 | 0% | 0% | 0% |
| ★ Picante Sauce (mild or medium) | 2 tbsp | 10 | 0% | 0% | 0% |
| ★ Chunky Mexican | 1/4 cup | 20 | 0% | 0% | 0% |
| ★ KNORR Fresh Gourmet Stir 'n Sauce Mexican—CPC | 1/2 pouch | 60 | 4% | 2% | 0% |
| LA VICTORIA | | | | | |
| ★ Enchilada Sauce | 1/4 cup | 20 | 1% | 0% | 0% |
| ★ Green Taco Sauce | 1 tbsp | 0 | 0% | 0% | 0% |
| ★ Red Taco Sauce | 1 tbsp | 5 | 0% | 0% | 0% |
| LAS PALMAS Enchilada Sauce—PET | | | | | |
| ★ Green Chile | 1/4 cup | 25 | 2% | 0% | 0% |
| ★ Original or Hot | 1/4 cup | 15 | 1% | 0% | 0% |
| ★ LAS PALMAS Red Chile Sauce—PET | 1/4 cup | 15 | 1% | 0% | 0% |
| ★ McCORMICK/SCHILLING Seasoning & Sauce Mixes: Fajitas Marinade | 1/6 pkg | 15 | 0% | 0% | 0% |
| ★ NATURAL TOUCH Taco Mix— WORTHINGTON FOODS | 3 tbsp dry mix | 60 | 2% | 0% | 0% |
| OLD EL PASO Enchilada Sauce—PET | | | | | |
| ★ Green Chili | 1/4 cup | 30 | 2% | 0% | 0% |
| ★ Mild or hot | 1/4 cup | 30 | 2% | 0% | 0% |
| ★ PACE Picante Sauce | 2 tbsp | 10 | 0% | 0% | 0% |
| ★ RO-TEL Pourable Diced Tomatoes & Green Chili Sauce—AMERICAN HOME FOODS | 2 tbsp | 5 | 0% | 0% | 0% |
| ROSARITA Sauces—HUNT WESSON | | | | | |
| ★ Enchilada: Mild | 1/4 cup | 23 | 2% | 1% | 0% |
| ★ Taco Sauce | 2 tbsp | 10 | 0% | 0% | 0% |
| ★ Zesty Jalapeno Picante: Mild, medium, or hot | 2 tbsp | 10 | 0% | 0% | 0% |
| ★ Zesty Tomato Mexicali | 1/2 cup | 80 | 2% | 3% | 0% |
| ★ HEINZ Chili Sauce | 1 tbsp | 15 | 0% | 0% | 0% |
| OLD EL PASO Taco Sauces—PET | | | | | |
| ★ Extra Chunky Taco Sauce: Mild or medium | 1 tbsp | 5 | 0% | 0% | 0% |
| ★ Taco Sauce: Mild, medium, or hot | 1 tbsp | 5 | 0% | 0% | 0% |
| ★ PANCHO VILLA Taco Sauce, Mild—PET | 2 tbsp | 15 | 0% | 0% | 0% |

## ORIENTAL SAUCES

**Brand Name Foods**

| FOOD | Serving Size | Calories | Tot Fat | Sat Fat | Chol |
|---|---|---|---|---|---|
| ★ BETTY CROCKER Recipe Sauces Sweet & Sour—GENERAL MILLS | 1/2 cup | 160 | 0% | 0% | 0% |
| ★ CONTADINA Sweet 'N Sour Sauce—NESTLÉ | 2 tbsp | 40 | 1% | 0% | 0% |

| FOOD | Serving Size | Calories | Tot Fat | Sat Fat | Chol |
|---|---|---|---|---|---|
| GOLDEN DIPT Marinades— | | | | | |
| MCCORMICK | | | | | |
| ★ Ginger Teriyaki | 1 tbsp | 60 | 5% | 0% | 0% |
| ★ Honey Soy Marinade, Fat Free | 1 tbsp | 30 | 0% | 0% | 0% |
| KIKKOMAN | | | | | |
| ★ Naturally Brewed Soy Sauce: | | | | | |
| Regular or Lite | 1 tbsp | 10 | 0% | 0% | 0% |
| ★ Stir-Fry Sauce | 1 tbsp | 15 | 0% | 0% | 0% |
| ★ Sweet & Sour Sauce | 2 tbsp | 35 | 0% | 0% | 0% |
| ★ Teriyaki Baste & Glaze | 2 tbsp | 50 | 0% | 0% | 0% |
| ★ Teriyaki Baste & Glaze w/Honey & Pineapple | 2 tbsp | 80 | 0% | 0% | 0% |
| ★ Teriyaki Marinade & Sauce: | | | | | |
| Regular or Lite | 1 tbsp | 15 | 0% | 0% | 0% |
| ★ KNORR Fresh Gourmet *Stir 'n Sauce* Szechwan—CPC | 1/2 pouch | 45 | 1% | 0% | 0% |
| ★ KRAFT Sweet 'n Sour Sauce | 2 tbsp | 80 | 1% | 0% | 0% |
| LA CHOY Sauces—HUNT WESSON | | | | | |
| ★ Bead Molasses | 1 tbsp | 50 | 0% | 0% | 0% |
| ★ Brown Gravy Sauce | 1/4 cup | 280 | 0% | 0% | 0% |
| ★ Chun King Hot Teriyaki Sauce | 1 tbsp | 15 | 1% | 0% | 0% |
| ★ Plum Sauce | 1 tbsp | 25 | 0% | 0% | 0% |
| ★ Soy Sauce | 1 tbsp | 10 | 0% | 0% | 0% |
| ★ Soy Sauce, Lite | 1 tbsp | 15 | 0% | 0% | 0% |
| ★ Sweet & Sour Duck Sauce | 2 tbsp | 60 | 0% | 0% | 0% |
| ★ Sweet & Sour Sauce | 2 tbsp | 60 | 0% | 0% | 0% |
| ★ Teriyaki Sauce | 1 tbsp | 15 | 0% | 0% | 0% |
| ★ Teriyaki Sauce, Lite | 1 tbsp | 20 | 0% | 0% | 0% |
| LA CHOY Stir Fry Sauces— | | | | | |
| HUNT WESSON | | | | | |
| ★ Mandarin Soy Sauce | 1/2 cup | 70 | 0% | 0% | 0% |
| ★ Spicy Sweet & Sour | 1/2 cup | 140 | 0% | 0% | 0% |
| ★ Spicy Szechwan | 1/2 cup | 80 | 0% | 0% | 0% |
| ★ Teriyaki Sauce | 1/2 cup | 90 | 0% | 0% | 0% |
| LAWRY'S Weekday Gourmet Sauces | | | | | |
| ★ Chicken Teriyaki | 1 tbsp | 25 | 0% | 0% | 0% |
| ❖ Oriental Chicken Salad | 2 tbsp | 60 | 6% | 3% | 0% |
| McCORMICK/SCHILLING | | | | | |
| Seasoning & Sauce Mixes | | | | | |
| ★ Sweet & Sour | 1/6 pkg | 30 | 0% | 0% | 0% |
| ★ Teriyaki | 1/8 pkg | 15 | 0% | 0% | 0% |
| McCORMICK/SCHILLING Sauce Blends for Chicken | | | | | |
| ★ Sweet & Sour Chicken | 1/6 pkg | 35 | 0% | 0% | 0% |

★ Foods with this symbol have less than or equal to 5% *Daily Value* for <u>all</u> three nutrients (5% Rule).

❖ Foods with this symbol have <u>at least one</u> of the three nutrients greater than 5% *Daily Value* but less than or equal to 20% *Daily Value*.

Ⓐ Foods with this symbol have <u>at least one</u> of the three nutrients greater than 20% *Daily Value* (20% Rule).

| FOOD | Serving Size | Calories | Tot Fat | Sat Fat | Chol |
|---|---|---|---|---|---|
| ★ Teriyaki Chicken | 1/4 pkg | 40 | 2% | 0% | 0% |
| RAGU Sweet & Sour Sauces— | | | | | |
| VAN DEN BERGH | | | | | |
| ★ *Chicken Tonight* Cooking Sauce | 1/2 cup | 120 | 0% | 0% | 0% |
| ★ *Chicken Tonight* Simmer Sauce | 1/2 cup | 80 | 0% | 0% | 0% |
| S & W Cooking Sauces | | | | | |
| ★ Oriental | 1 tbsp | 20 | 0% | 0% | 0% |
| ★ Teriyaki: Regular or Lite | 1 tbsp | 25 | 0% | 0% | 0% |
| ★ SAUCEWORKS Sweet 'n Sour— | | | | | |
| KRAFT | 2 tbsp | 60 | 0% | 0% | 0% |
| ★ SIMMER CHEF Cooking Sauce: | | | | | |
| Oriental Sweet & Sour— | | | | | |
| CAMPBELL'S | 1/2 cup | 110 | 2% | 0% | 0% |
| SUN LUCK | | | | | |
| ★ Black Bean Garlic Sauce | 1 tbsp | 25 | 2% | 0% | 0% |
| ★ Char Siu BBQ Sauce | 1 tbsp | 60 | 0% | 0% | 0% |
| ★ Hoisin Sauce, Traditional | 1 tbsp | 20 | 0% | 0% | 0% |
| ★ Mirin (Sweet Rice Wine) | 1 tbsp | 20 | 0% | 0% | 0% |
| ★ Oyster Sauce, Cantonese | 1 tbsp | 25 | 0% | 0% | 0% |
| ★ Plum Sauce | 2 tbsp | 85 | 0% | 0% | 0% |
| ★ Soy Sauce: All varieties | 1 tbsp | 10 | 0% | 0% | 0% |
| ★ Stir Fry Sauce, Cantonese | 1 tbsp | 15 | 0% | 0% | 0% |
| ★ Sweet & Sour Chinese Sauce | 1 tbsp | 25 | 0% | 0% | 0% |
| SUN LUCK Chili Sauces | | | | | |
| ★ Chili Garlic Sauce, Hot | 1 tsp | 5 | 0% | 0% | 0% |
| ❖ Chili Oil, Layu | 1 tsp | 45 | 8% | 0% | 0% |
| ★ Chili Sauce, Hot | 1 tsp | 5 | 0% | 0% | 0% |

## PASTA SAUCES

**Brand Name Foods**

| FOOD | Serving Size | Calories | Tot Fat | Sat Fat | Chol |
|---|---|---|---|---|---|
| CAMPBELL'S Canned Spaghetti Sauce | | | | | |
| ★ Extra Garlic & Onion | 1/2 cup | 60 | 2% | 0% | 0% |
| ★ Flavored w/Ground Beef | 1/2 cup | 100 | 2% | 0% | 0% |
| ★ Italian Style | 1/2 cup | 120 | 2% | 0% | 0% |
| ★ Marinara | 1/2 cup | 90 | 2% | 0% | 0% |
| ★ Mushroom | 1/2 cup | 100 | 2% | 0% | 0% |
| ★ Mushroom & Garlic | 1/2 cup | 90 | 2% | 0% | 0% |
| ★ Traditional | 1/2 cup | 120 | 2% | 0% | 0% |
| CHEF BOYARDEE Spaghetti Sauce | | | | | |
| —AMERICAN HOME FOODS | | | | | |
| ★ w/Meat | 1/2 cup | 90 | 4% | 5% | 3% |
| ★ w/Mushrooms | 1/2 cup | 60 | 0% | 0% | 0% |
| CLASSICO—BORDEN | | | | | |
| ❖ D'Abruzzi (Beef & Pork) | 1/2 cup | 90 | 8% | 5% | 3% |
| ❖ Di Capri (Sun-Dried Tomato) | 1/2 cup | 80 | 7% | 5% | 0% |
| ❖ Di Genoa (Tomato & Pesto) | 1/2 cup | 110 | 9% | 8% | 1% |

| FOOD | Serving Size | Calories | Tot Fat | Sat Fat | Chol |
|---|---|---|---|---|---|
| ★ Di Napoli (Tomato & Basil) | 1/2 cup | 60 | 2% | 0% | 0% |
| ❖ Di Parma (Four Cheese) | 1/2 cup | 70 | 6% | 5% | 1% |
| ★ Di Roma Arrabbiata (Spicy Red Pepper) | 1/2 cup | 60 | 4% | 3% | 0% |
| ❖ Di Salerno (Sweet Peppers & Onions) | 1/2 cup | 70 | 6% | 3% | 0% |
| ★ Di Sicilia (Mushrooms & Ripe Olives) | 1/2 cup | 50 | 2% | 3% | 0% |
| ❖ Di Sorrento (Onion & Garlic) | 1/2 cup | 80 | 6% | 3% | 0% |
| CONTADINA *Pasta Ready* Sauces —NESTLÉ | | | | | |
| ★ Tomatoes | 1/2 cup | 40 | 3% | 0% | 0% |
| ★ Tomatoes Primavera | 1/2 cup | 50 | 2% | 0% | 0% |
| ★ Tomatoes w/Crushed Red Pepper | 1/2 cup | 60 | 5% | 2% | 0% |
| ★ Tomatoes w/Mushrooms | 1/2 cup | 50 | 2% | 0% | 0% |
| ★ Tomatoes w/Olives | 1/2 cup | 60 | 5% | 2% | 0% |
| ❖ Tomatoes w/Three Cheeses | 1/2 cup | 70 | 6% | 0% | 1% |
| DEL MONTE Chunky Spaghetti Sauces | | | | | |
| ★ Garden Style | 1/2 cup | 60 | 2% | 0% | 0% |
| ★ Garlic & Herb | 1/2 cup | 60 | 2% | 0% | 0% |
| ★ Italian Herb | 1/2 cup | 60 | 2% | 0% | 0% |
| ★ Tomato Basil | 1/2 cup | 60 | 2% | 0% | 0% |
| DEL MONTE Spaghetti Sauces | | | | | |
| ★ Traditional | 1/2 cup | 80 | 2% | 0% | 0% |
| ★ w/Garlic & Onion | 1/2 cup | 70 | 1% | 0% | 0% |
| ★ w/Green Peppers & Mushrooms | 1/2 cup | 70 | 1% | 0% | 0% |
| ★ w/Meat | 1/2 cup | 70 | 3% | 0% | 0% |
| ★ w/Mushrooms | 1/2 cup | 80 | 2% | 0% | 0% |
| DI GIORNO *Light Varieties* Sauces —KRAFT | | | | | |
| ⊛ Alfredo, Reduced Fat | 1/4 cup | 170 | 15% | 30% | 10% |
| ★ Chunky Tomato w/Basil | 1/2 cup | 70 | 0% | 0% | 0% |
| DI GIORNO Sauces—KRAFT | | | | | |
| ⊛ Alfredo | 1/4 cup | 230 | 34% | 50% | 15% |
| ⊛ Four Cheese | 1/4 cup | 200 | 29% | 55% | 15% |
| ❖ Marinara | 1/2 cup | 100 | 7% | 5% | 1% |
| ⊛ Olive Oil & Garlic w/Grated Cheeses | 1/4 cup | 370 | 55% | 40% | 7% |
| ⊛ Pesto | 1/4 cup | 320 | 48% | 35% | 5% |
| ★ Plum Tomato & Mushroom | 1/2 cup | 70 | 0% | 0% | 0% |
| ❖ Traditional Meat | 1/2 cup | 120 | 9% | 10% | 5% |
| HEALTHY CHOICE Pasta Sauces —CONAGRA | | | | | |
| ★ Extra Chunky Garlic & Onions | 1/2 cup | 50 | 1% | 0% | 0% |

★ Foods with this symbol have less than or equal to 5% *Daily Value* for all three nutrients (5% Rule).
❖ Foods with this symbol have at least one of the three nutrients greater than 5% *Daily Value* but less than or equal to 20% *Daily Value*.
⊛ Foods with this symbol have at least one of the three nutrients greater than 20% *Daily Value* (20% Rule).

| FOOD | Serving Size | Calories | Tot Fat | Sat Fat | Chol |
|------|------|------|------|------|------|
| ★ Extra Chunky Italian Style Vegetable | 1/2 cup | 50 | 1% | 0% | 0% |
| ★ Extra Chunky Mushrooms | 1/2 cup | 50 | 1% | 0% | 0% |
| ★ Original Flavored w/Meat | 1/2 cup | 50 | 2% | 0% | 0% |
| ★ Original Garlic & Herbs | 1/2 cup | 50 | 1% | 0% | 0% |
| ★ Original Mushrooms | 1/2 cup | 50 | 1% | 0% | 0% |
| ★ Original Traditional | 1/2 cup | 50 | 1% | 0% | 0% |
| ★ Super Chunky Mushrooms & Sweet Peppers | 1/2 cup | 50 | 1% | 0% | 0% |
| ★ Super Chunky Vegetable Primavera | 1/2 cup | 50 | 1% | 0% | 0% |
| HUNT'S Old Country Spaghetti Sauce—HUNT WESSON | | | | | |
| ★ Flavored w/Meat | 1/2 cup | 60 | 4% | 3% | 0% |
| ★ Traditional | 1/2 cup | 50 | 4% | 2% | 0% |
| ★ w/Garlic & Herbs | 1/2 cup | 60 | 4% | 2% | 0% |
| ★ w/Italian Style Vegetables | 1/2 cup | 60 | 4% | 2% | 0% |
| ★ w/Mushroom | 1/2 cup | 50 | 4% | 2% | 0% |
| KNORR Pasta Sauce Mixes—CPC | | | | | |
| ★ Alfredo | 1/6 pkg | 35 | 2% | 0% | 0% |
| ★ Carbonara | 1/6 pkg | 30 | 3% | 3% | 1% |
| ★ Creamy Pesto | 1/5 pkg | 30 | 2% | 0% | 0% |
| ★ Four Cheese | 1/6 pkg | 30 | 3% | 4% | 0% |
| ★ Garlic Herb | 1/6 pkg | 35 | 3% | 3% | 0% |
| ★ Parma Rosa | 1/5 pkg | 30 | 2% | 0% | 0% |
| ★ Pesto | 1/3 pkg | 15 | 1% | 0% | 0% |
| LAWRY'S Spaghetti Sauces | | | | | |
| ★ Extra Rich & Thick (prep as dir) | 1/2 cup | 35 | 2% | 0% | 0% |
| ★ Original Style (prep as dir) | 1/2 cup | 30 | 0% | 0% | 0% |
| McCORMICK/SCHILLING Seasoning & Sauce Mixes | | | | | |
| ★ American | 1/5 pkg | 25 | 0% | 0% | 0% |
| ★ Italian | 1/5 pkg | 25 | 0% | 0% | 0% |
| ★ Spaghetti | 1/5 pkg | 25 | 0% | 0% | 0% |
| ★ Thick & Zesty | 1/5 pkg | 25 | 0% | 0% | 0% |
| ❖ NEWMAN'S OWN Bombolina Sauce | 1/2 cup | 100 | 8% | 5% | 0% |
| NEWMAN'S OWN Spaghetti Sauces | | | | | |
| ★ Marinara | 1/2 cup | 60 | 3% | 0% | 0% |
| ★ Marinara w/Mushrooms | 1/2 cup | 60 | 3% | 0% | 0% |
| ★ Sockarooni | 1/2 cup | 60 | 3% | 0% | 0% |
| PASTA PRIMA Sauce Mixes— MCCORMICK | | | | | |
| ❖ Alfredo | 1/4 pkg | 40 | 4% | 8% | 3% |
| ★ Herb & Garlic | 1/4 pkg | 15 | 0% | 0% | 0% |
| ★ Parmesan | 1/5 pkg | 35 | 3% | 5% | 0% |
| ★ Vinaigrette | 1/6 pkg | 10 | 0% | 0% | 0% |

| FOOD | Serving Size | Calories | Tot Fat | Sat Fat | Chol |
|---|---|---|---|---|---|
| PREGO Extra Chunky Spaghetti Sauce—CAMPBELL'S | | | | | |
| ★ Garden Combination | 1/2 cup | 90 | 2% | 3% | 0% |
| ★ Garlic & Cheese | 1/2 cup | 130 | 5% | 5% | 0% |
| ❖ Mushroom and Diced Onion | 1/2 cup | 120 | 9% | 8% | 0% |
| ❖ Mushroom and Diced Tomato | 1/2 cup | 110 | 6% | 5% | 0% |
| ❖ Mushroom and Green Pepper | 1/2 cup | 100 | 6% | 5% | 0% |
| ❖ Mushroom Supreme | 1/2 cup | 130 | 7% | 3% | 2% |
| ❖ Mushroom w/Extra Spice | 1/2 cup | 120 | 6% | 0% | 0% |
| ❖ Sausage and Pepper | 1/2 cup | 180 | 14% | 13% | 3% |
| ❖ Tomato Onion and Garlic | 1/2 cup | 120 | 9% | 8% | 0% |
| ★ Vegetable Supreme | 1/2 cup | 90 | 5% | 3% | 2% |
| ❖ Zesty Basil | 1/2 cup | 130 | 5% | 8% | 0% |
| ★ Zesty Oregano | 1/2 cup | 140 | 5% | 5% | 0% |
| ❖ PREGO Marinara Sauce—CAMPBELL'S | 1/2 cup | 110 | 9% | 8% | 0% |
| PREGO Spaghetti Sauce—CAMPBELL'S | | | | | |
| ❖ Diced Onion and Garlic | 1/2 cup | 120 | 8% | 5% | 0% |
| ❖ Flavored w/Meat | 1/2 cup | 160 | 9% | 8% | 2% |
| ★ Three Cheese | 1/2 cup | 100 | 3% | 3% | 0% |
| ❖ Made w/Mushrooms | 1/2 cup | 150 | 8% | 8% | 0% |
| ★ Tomato and Basil | 1/2 cup | 110 | 5% | 3% | 0% |
| ❖ Traditional | 1/2 cup | 150 | 9% | 10% | 0% |
| PROGRESSO Pasta Sauces—PET | | | | | |
| Ⓐ Alfredo (Authentic) | 1/2 cup | 310 | 42% | 77% | 25% |
| ❖ Creamy Clam | 1/2 cup | 100 | 9% | 6% | 3% |
| ❖ Marinara | 1/2 cup | 90 | 7% | 4% | 1% |
| ❖ Marinara (Authentic) | 1/2 cup | 100 | 8% | 7% | 1% |
| ❖ Meat Flavored | 1/2 cup | 100 | 7% | 5% | 2% |
| ❖ Mushroom Spaghetti | 1/2 cup | 100 | 7% | 4% | 1% |
| ★ Pizza | 1/2 cup | 35 | 2% | 0% | 0% |
| ★ Red Clam | 1/2 cup | 80 | 5% | 3% | 2% |
| ❖ Rock Lobster | 1/2 cup | 100 | 11% | 5% | 2% |
| ❖ Spaghetti | 1/2 cup | 100 | 7% | 4% | 1% |
| ❖ White Clam | 1/2 cup | 120 | 14% | 7% | 5% |
| ❖ White Clam (Authentic) | 1/2 cup | 90 | 11% | 7% | 4% |
| RAGU Chunky Garden Style Pasta Sauce—VAN DEN BERGH | | | | | |
| ❖ Chunky Mushroom and Green Pepper | 1/2 cup | 120 | 7% | 2% | 0% |
| ❖ Chunky Tomato Garlic and Onion | 1/2 cup | 120 | 7% | 2% | 0% |
| ❖ Super Mushroom | 1/2 cup | 120 | 7% | 2% | 0% |
| ❖ Super Vegetable Primavera | 1/2 cup | 110 | 7% | 2% | 0% |

★ Foods with this symbol have less than or equal to 5% *Daily Value* for <u>all</u> three nutrients (5% Rule).
❖ Foods with this symbol have <u>at least one</u> of the three nutrients greater than 5% *Daily Value* but less than or equal to 20% *Daily Value*.
Ⓐ Foods with this symbol have <u>at least one</u> of the three nutrients greater than 20% *Daily Value* (20% Rule).

| FOOD | Serving Size | Calories | Tot Fat | Sat Fat | Chol |
|------|--------------|----------|---------|---------|------|
| RAGU Hearty Pasta Sauce—VAN DEN BERGH | | | | | |
| ❖ Parmesan | 1/2 cup | 120 | 6% | 5% | 1% |
| ❖ Sauteed Onion and Mushroom | 1/2 cup | 110 | 6% | 3% | 0% |
| RAGU Light Pasta Sauce—VAN DEN BERGH | | | | | |
| ★ No Sugar Added Tomato & Herb | 1/2 cup | 60 | 2% | 0% | 0% |
| ★ Tomato and Herb | 1/2 cup | 50 | 0% | 0% | 0% |
| RAGU *Old World Style* Spaghetti Sauces—VAN DEN BERGH | | | | | |
| ★ Mushroom | 1/2 cup | 80 | 5% | 3% | 0% |
| ★ Traditional | 1/2 cup | 80 | 5% | 3% | 0% |
| S & W *Simply Wonderful* California Pasta Sauces | | | | | |
| ★ Fishermen's Wharf Recipe, Chunky Tomato Marinara | 1/2 cup | 50 | 0% | 0% | 0% |
| ★ Mendocino Coast Recipe, Chunky Garden Primavera | 1/2 cup | 60 | 0% | 0% | 0% |
| ★ Wine Country Recipe, Chunky Tomato Mushroom | 1/2 cup | 45 | 0% | 0% | 0% |
| ★ SMART OPTIONS Pasta Sauce w/Mushrooms—WEIGHT WATCHERS | 1/2 cup | 60 | 0% | 0% | 0% |
| ★ WEIGHT WATCHERS Pasta Sauce w/Mushrooms | 1/2 cup | 60 | 0% | 0% | 0% |

## PIZZA SAUCES

**Brand Name Foods**

| FOOD | Serving Size | Calories | Tot Fat | Sat Fat | Chol |
|------|--------------|----------|---------|---------|------|
| CONTADINA Chunky Pizza Sauce —NESTLÉ | | | | | |
| ★ 3 Cheese | 1/4 cup | 35 | 1% | 0% | 0% |
| ★ Basic | 1/4 cup | 30 | 0% | 0% | 0% |
| ★ Mushroom | 1/4 cup | 30 | 0% | 0% | 0% |
| CONTADINA Pizza Sauces—NESTLÉ | | | | | |
| ★ Pizza Sauce | 1/4 cup | 35 | 2% | 0% | 0% |
| ★ Pizza Sauce Flavored w/ Pepperoni | 1/4 cup | 40 | 3% | 2% | 0% |
| ★ Pizza Sauce w/Italian Cheeses | 1/4 cup | 40 | 2% | 0% | 0% |
| ★ Pizza Squeeze | 1/4 cup | 35 | 2% | 0% | 0% |
| ★ Pizza Squeeze w/Italian Cheeses | 1/4 cup | 40 | 2% | 0% | 0% |
| ★ HUNT'S Angela Mia Pizza Sauce —CONAGRA | 1/4 cup | 35 | 0% | 0% | 0% |
| PREGO Pizza Sauce—CAMPBELL'S | | | | | |
| ★ Traditional | 1/4 cup | 40 | 3% | 0% | 0% |
| ★ w/Pepperoni Chunks | 1/4 cup | 70 | 5% | 5% | 3% |
| RAGU Pizza Sauce—VAN DEN BERGH | | | | | |
| ★ *Pizza Quick* Sauce | 1/4 cup | 40 | 2% | 0% | 0% |
| ★ Pizza Sauce | 1/4 cup | 30 | 1% | 0% | 0% |

| FOOD | Serving Size | Calories | Tot Fat | Sat Fat | Chol |
|------|------|------|------|------|------|

## SAUCES

**Brand Name Foods**

| FOOD | Serving Size | Calories | Tot Fat | Sat Fat | Chol |
|------|------|------|------|------|------|
| BETTY CROCKER *Hamburger Helper* Sloppy Joes Sauce— GENERAL MILLS | | | | | |
| ★  BBQ | 1/4 cup | 80 | 0% | 0% | 0% |
| ★  Pepperoni Pizza | 1/4 cup | 45 | 1% | 0% | 0% |
| ★  Sloppy Joes | 1/4 cup | 50 | 0% | 0% | 0% |
| ★  Taco | 1/4 cup | 45 | 0% | 0% | 0% |
| DEL MONTE Sloppy Joe Sauces | | | | | |
| ★  Hickory Flavor | 1/4 cup | 70 | 0% | 0% | 0% |
| ★  Italian Style | 1/4 cup | 70 | 0% | 0% | 0% |
| ★  Original Recipe | 1/4 cup | 70 | 0% | 0% | 0% |
| ★ GREEN GIANT Sloppy Joe Sandwich Sauce—PILLSBURY | 1/4 cup | 50 | 0% | 0% | 0% |
| ★ HORMEL Not-So-Sloppy-Joe Sauce | 1/4 cup | 70 | 0% | 0% | 0% |
| HUNT'S MANWICH—HUNT WESSON | | | | | |
| ★  Barbecue | 1/4 cup | 60 | 0% | 1% | 0% |
| ★  Bold | 1/4 cup | 60 | 2% | 0% | 0% |
| ★  Burrito | 1/4 cup | 25 | 0% | 0% | 0% |
| ★  Mexican | 1/4 cup | 25 | 0% | 0% | 0% |
| ★  Original | 1/4 cup | 30 | 1% | 0% | 0% |
| ★  Taco | 1/4 cup | 30 | 0% | 0% | 0% |
| ★  Thick & Chunky | 1/4 cup | 45 | 1% | 0% | 0% |
| KNORR *Classic Sauce* Mixes—CPC | | | | | |
| ★  Bearnaise | 1/5 pkg | 20 | 1% | 0% | 0% |
| ★  Demi-Glace Mix | 1/5 pkg | 30 | 1% | 0% | 0% |
| ★  Hollandaise | 1/5 pkg | 20 | 1% | 2% | 0% |
| ★  Peppercorn | 1/5 pkg | 25 | 1% | 0% | 0% |
| ★  White | 1/9 pkg | 25 | 2% | 2% | 0% |
| KNORR Sauces Mixes—CPC | | | | | |
| ★  Curry | 1/5 pkg | 30 | 2% | 0% | 0% |
| ★  Mushroom | 1/5 pkg | 20 | 1% | 0% | 0% |
| ★  Mustard Herb | 1/4 pkg | 40 | 2% | 0% | 0% |
| ★  Newburg | 1/5 pkg | 20 | 1% | 0% | 0% |
| ❖ LAWRY'S Weekday Gourmet Sauces:  Chicken Dijon | 1/4 cup | 80 | 5% | 3% | 7% |
| ★ LIBBY'S Sloppy Joe Sauce—NESTLÉ | 1/3 cup | 45 | 0% | 0% | 0% |
| McCORMICK Collection Sauce Mixes | | | | | |
| ★  Bearnaise | 1/10 pkg | 10 | 0% | 0% | 0% |
| ★  Green Peppercorn | 1/6 pkg | 20 | 0% | 0% | 0% |
| ★  Hollandaise | 1/10 pkg | 15 | 0% | 0% | 5% |
| ★  Hunter | 1/5 pkg | 30 | 0% | 0% | 0% |

★  Foods with this symbol have less than or equal to 5% *Daily Value* for <u>all</u> three nutrients (5% Rule).

❖  Foods with this symbol have <u>at least one</u> of the three nutrients greater than 5% *Daily Value* but less than or equal to 20% *Daily Value.*

Ⓐ  Foods with this symbol have <u>at least one</u> of the three nutrients greater than 20% *Daily Value* (20% Rule).

| FOOD | Serving Size | Calories | Tot Fat | Sat Fat | Chol |
|---|---|---|---|---|---|
| ★ Spring Vegetable | 1/8 env | 10 | 0% | 0% | 0% |
| ★ Toasted Onion | 1/16 env | 5 | 0% | 0% | 0% |
| ★ White | 1/6 pkg | 20 | 0% | 0% | 0% |
| McCORMICK/SCHILLING Seasoning & Sauce Mixes | | | | | |
| ★ Beef Stroganoff | 1/8 pkg | 15 | 0% | 0% | 0% |
| ★ Sloppy Joes | 1/8 pkg | 15 | 0% | 0% | 0% |

### TOMATO SAUCE AND PASTE

**Brand Name Foods**

| FOOD | Serving Size | Calories | Tot Fat | Sat Fat | Chol |
|---|---|---|---|---|---|
| CONTADINA—NESTLÉ | | | | | |
| ★ Italian Tomato Paste | 2 tbsp | 40 | 1% | 0% | 0% |
| ★ Italian Tomato Sauce | 1/4 cup | 15 | 0% | 0% | 0% |
| ★ Thick and Zesty Tomato Sauce | 1/4 cup | 15 | 0% | 0% | 0% |
| ★ Tomato Paste | 2 tbsp | 30 | 0% | 0% | 0% |
| ★ Tomato Puree | 1/4 cup | 20 | 0% | 0% | 0% |
| ★ Tomato Sauce | 1/4 cup | 20 | 0% | 0% | 0% |
| DEL MONTE | | | | | |
| ★ Tomato Paste | 2 tbsp | 30 | 0% | 0% | 0% |
| ★ Tomato Sauce | 1/4 cup | 20 | 0% | 0% | 0% |
| HUNT'S—HUNT WESSON | | | | | |
| ★ Tomato Paste | 2 tbsp | 30 | 1% | 0% | 0% |
| ★ Tomato Puree | 1/4 cup | 25 | 1% | 0% | 0% |
| ★ Tomato Sauce | 1/4 cup | 35 | 0% | 0% | 0% |
| ★ Tomato Sauce Italian | 1/4 cup | 30 | 2% | 0% | 0% |
| ★ Tomato Sauce w/Herb | 1/4 cup | 30 | 2% | 0% | 0% |
| ★ S & W Tomato Sauce | 1/4 cup | 20 | 0% | 0% | 0% |

# Ingredients

### BAKING MIXES

**Brand Name Foods**

| FOOD | Serving Size | Calories | Tot Fat | Sat Fat | Chol |
|---|---|---|---|---|---|
| BISQUICK—GENERAL MILLS | | | | | |
| ❖ Baking Mix | 1/3 cup | 170 | 9% | 8% | 0% |
| ★ Baking Mix, Reduced Fat | 1/3 cup | 150 | 4% | 4% | 0% |
| ENER-G Gluten Free Baking Mixes | | | | | |
| ★ Barley | 1/3 cup | 130 | 1% | 0% | 0% |
| ★ Basic | 1/3 cup | 120 | 1% | 0% | 0% |
| ★ Corn | 1/3 cup | 150 | 1% | 0% | 0% |
| ★ Oat | 1/3 cup | 110 | 4% | 2% | 0% |
| ★ Potato | 1/3 cup | 210 | 2% | 0% | 0% |
| ★ Rice | 1/3 cup | 180 | 1% | 0% | 0% |
| ❖ GOLD MEDAL Biscuit | 1/3 cup | 180 | 10% | 11% | 0% |

| FOOD | Serving Size | Calories | Tot Fat | Sat Fat | Chol |
|------|------|------|------|------|------|
| ❖ KRUSTEAZ Baking Mix (2" biscuits) | | | | | |
| —CONTINENTAL MILLS | 2 biscuits | 180 | 9% | 8% | 0% |

## BAKING: CONFECTION CHIPS AND BAKING BARS

**Generic Foods**

| | | | | | |
|------|------|------|------|------|------|
| ⊛ Baking Chocolate | 1 tbsp | 70 | 12% | 22% | 0% |
| ❖ Carob Chips | 1 tbsp | 80 | 7% | 19% | 0% |
| ❖ Chocolate Chips | 1 tbsp | 70 | 6% | 11% | 0% |

**Brand Name Foods**

| | | | | | |
|------|------|------|------|------|------|
| BAKER'S Chocolate Chips—KRAFT | | | | | |
| ❖ Real Milk Chocolate | 1/2 oz (~27 chips) | 70 | 6% | 11% | 0% |
| ❖ Semi-Sweet Chocolate | 1/2 oz (~27 chips) | 60 | 6% | 11% | 0% |
| ❖ Semi-Sweet Flavored Chocolate | 1/2 oz (~27 chips) | 70 | 5% | 14% | 0% |
| BAKER'S Baking Bars—KRAFT | | | | | |
| ❖ *German's* Sweet Chocolate | 2 squares | 60 | 6% | 11% | 0% |
| ⊛ Semi-Sweet Chocolate Bar | 1 square | 130 | 13% | 27% | 0% |
| ⊛ Unsweetened Chocolate Bar | 1 square | 140 | 22% | 43% | 0% |
| ⊛ White Chocolate Bar | 1 square | 160 | 14% | 28% | 2% |
| GHIRARDELLI Baking Bars | | | | | |
| ⊛ Bittersweet | 3 sections | 210 | 23% | 45% | 0% |
| ⊛ Classic White Confection | 3 sections | 240 | 23% | 44% | 2% |
| ⊛ Milk Chocolate | 3 sections | 220 | 21% | 41% | 3% |
| ⊛ Semi-Sweet | 3 sections | 210 | 22% | 43% | 1% |
| ⊛ Sweet Dark | 3 sections | 210 | 22% | 43% | 0% |
| ⊛ Unsweetened Chocolate | 3 sections | 210 | 35% | 69% | 0% |
| GHIRARDELLI Chips | | | | | |
| ❖ Classic White | 2 tbsp | 80 | 6% | 16% | 0% |
| ❖ Flickettes | 2 tbsp | 70 | 6% | 18% | 0% |
| ❖ Milk Chocolate | 2 tbsp | 70 | 6% | 11% | 0% |
| ❖ Semi-Sweet Chocolate | 2 tbsp | 70 | 7% | 12% | 0% |
| HERSHEY's Bake Shoppe | | | | | |
| ❖ Butterscotch Chips | 1 tbsp | 80 | 6% | 20% | 1% |
| ❖ Holiday Bits for Baking | 1 tbsp | 70 | 5% | 10% | 0% |
| ❖ Milk Chocolate Chips | 1 tbsp | 80 | 6% | 13% | 0% |
| ❖ Mint Chocolate Chips | 1 tbsp | 80 | 6% | 13% | 0% |
| ❖ Raspberry Chips | 1 tbsp | 80 | 6% | 13% | 0% |
| ❖ *Reese's* Bits for Baking | 1 tbsp | 70 | 5% | 8% | 0% |

★ Foods with this symbol have less than or equal to 5% *Daily Value* for <u>all</u> three nutrients (5% Rule).

❖ Foods with this symbol have <u>at least one</u> of the three nutrients greater than 5% *Daily Value* but less than or equal to 20% *Daily Value*.

⊛ Foods with this symbol have <u>at least one</u> of the three nutrients greater than 20% *Daily Value* (20% Rule).

| FOOD | Serving Size | Calories | Tot Fat | Sat Fat | Chol |
|------|------|------|------|------|------|
| ❖ *Reese's* Peanut Butter Chips | 1 tbsp | 80 | 6% | 20% | 0% |
| ❖ Semi-Sweet Chocolate Chips | 1 tbsp | 80 | 6% | 13% | 0% |
| ❖ Semi-Sweet Chunks | 5 pcs | 80 | 6% | 13% | 0% |
| ❖ *Skor* English Toffee Bits for Baking | 1 tbsp | 60 | 6% | 13% | 3% |
| ❖ Vanilla Milk Chips | 1 tbsp | 80 | 6% | 15% | 0% |
| HERSHEY's Bake Shoppe Baking Bars | | | | | |
| ❖ Bittersweet Baking Bar | 1/2 bar | 80 | 7% | 15% | 0% |
| ❖ Semi-Sweet Baking Bar | 1/2 bar | 80 | 6% | 13% | 0% |
| ❀ Unsweetened Baking Bar | 1/2 bar | 90 | 11% | 23% | 0% |
| M&M's Baking Bits | | | | | |
| ❖ Chocolate | 1/2 oz | 70 | 5% | 10% | 1% |
| ❖ Semi-Sweet | 1/2 oz | 70 | 6% | 11% | 0% |
| ❀ NESTLÉ Choco Bake | 1/2 oz | 80 | 12% | 23% | 0% |
| TOLLHOUSE Baking Bars— NESTLÉ | | | | | |
| ❖ Premier White | 1/2 oz | 80 | 8% | 17% | 1% |
| ❖ Semi-Sweet Chocolate | 1/2 oz | 70 | 6% | 12% | 0% |
| ❖ Unsweetened Chocolate | 1/2 oz | 80 | 11% | 9% | 0% |
| TOLLHOUSE Morsels—NESTLÉ | | | | | |
| ❖ Butterscotch | 1 tbsp | 80 | 6% | 19% | 0% |
| ❖ Milk Chocolate | 1 tbsp | 70 | 6% | 11% | 0% |
| ❖ Mint Chocolate | 1 tbsp | 70 | 6% | 11% | 0% |
| ❖ Premier White | 1 tbsp | 80 | 6% | 19% | 0% |
| ❖ Rainbow | 1 tbsp | 70 | 4% | 8% | 0% |
| ❖ Semi-Sweet | 1 tbsp | 70 | 6% | 12% | 0% |
| ❖ Semi-Sweet Mini | 1 tbsp | 70 | 6% | 12% | 0% |

## BAKING: OTHER

**Generic Foods**

| FOOD | Serving Size | Calories | Tot Fat | Sat Fat | Chol |
|------|------|------|------|------|------|
| ❀ Coconut: dried, flaked, canned | 2 tbsp | 70 | 7% | 21% | 0% |
| ❀ Coconut: raw, shredded | 2 tbsp | 50 | 8% | 22% | 0% |
| ★ Cornstarch | 1 tbsp | 30 | 0% | 0% | 0% |
| ★ Potato Starch | 1 tbsp | 40 | 0% | 0% | 0% |
| ★ Tapioca: Pearl (dry) | 1/3 cup | 170 | 0% | 0% | 0% |
| ★ Tapioca Starch | 1 tbsp | 10 | 0% | 0% | 0% |

**Brand Name Foods**

| FOOD | Serving Size | Calories | Tot Fat | Sat Fat | Chol |
|------|------|------|------|------|------|
| BAKER'S Coconut—KRAFT | | | | | |
| ❀ *Angel Flake* (bag) | 2 tbsp | 70 | 7% | 21% | 0% |
| ❀ *Angel Flake* (can) | 2 tbsp | 70 | 8% | 24% | 0% |
| ❖ Premium Shred | 2 tbsp | 60 | 6% | 19% | 0% |
| ❖ HERSHEY's Bake Shoppe *Mounds* Baking Coconut | 2 tbsp | 70 | 7% | 18% | 0% |
| ★ SURE-JELL Fruit Pectin—KRAFT | 1/4 tsp | 5 | 0% | 0% | 0% |

| FOOD | Serving Size | Calories | Tot Fat | Sat Fat | Chol |
|---|---|---|---|---|---|

## BATTER MIXES AND COATINGS

**Brand Name Foods**

GOLDEN DIPT Mixes—MCCORMICK

| FOOD | Serving Size | Calories | Tot Fat | Sat Fat | Chol |
|---|---|---|---|---|---|
| ★ All Purpose Batter | 1/4 cup mix | 120 | 0% | 0% | 0% |
| ★ All Purpose Bread Crumb | 1/4 cup mix | 120 | 1% | 0% | 0% |
| ★ All Purpose Cracker Meal | 1/4 cup mix | 140 | 1% | 0% | 0% |
| ★ Beer Batter | 1/4 cup mix | 120 | 0% | 0% | 0% |
| ★ Corn Dog Batter | 1/4 cup mix | 120 | 0% | 0% | 0% |
| ★ Fish & Chips Batter | 1/4 cup mix | 120 | 0% | 0% | 0% |
| ★ Onion Ring Batter | 1/4 cup mix | 120 | 0% | 0% | 0% |
| ★ Tempura Batter | 1/4 cup mix | 120 | 0% | 0% | 0% |

GOLDEN DIPT Fry Mixes—MCCORMICK

| FOOD | Serving Size | Calories | Tot Fat | Sat Fat | Chol |
|---|---|---|---|---|---|
| ★ Extra Crispy Chicken Seasoned Mix | ~1 1/2 tbsp mix | 60 | 0% | 0% | 0% |
| ★ Fisherman's Choice Fish Mix: All flavors | ~1 1/3 tbsp mix | 40 | 0% | 0% | 0% |
| ★ Herbs & Spices Chicken Seasoned Mix | ~2 tbsp mix | 60 | 0% | 0% | 0% |
| ★ Hot 'n Spicy Chicken Seasoned Mix | ~2 tbsp mix | 60 | 0% | 0% | 0% |
| ★ Original Homestyle Chicken Seasoned Mix | ~2 tbsp mix | 50 | 0% | 0% | 0% |
| ★ Seafood Mix | ~1 2/3 tbsp mix | 60 | 0% | 0% | 0% |

GOLDEN DIPT *Oven Easy* Coating Mixes—MCCORMICK

| FOOD | Serving Size | Calories | Tot Fat | Sat Fat | Chol |
|---|---|---|---|---|---|
| ❖ Cajun Style | 1/4 cup mix | 90 | 5% | 6% | 0% |
| ★ Lemon & Pepper | 1/4 cup mix | 80 | 2% | 0% | 0% |
| ★ Shrimp & Seafood | 2 tbsp mix | 70 | 3% | 0% | 0% |

KRUSTEAZ—CONTINENTAL MILLS

| FOOD | Serving Size | Calories | Tot Fat | Sat Fat | Chol |
|---|---|---|---|---|---|
| ★ Bake 'N Fry Mix | 1/4 cup mix | 100 | 2% | 0% | 1% |
| ★ Tempura Mix | 1/4 cup mix | 110 | 1% | 0% | 0% |

OVEN FRY Coating Mix—KRAFT

| FOOD | Serving Size | Calories | Tot Fat | Sat Fat | Chol |
|---|---|---|---|---|---|
| ★ Extra Crispy Recipe for Chicken | 1/8 packet | 60 | 2% | 0% | 0% |
| ★ Extra Crispy Recipe for Pork | 1/8 packet | 60 | 2% | 0% | 0% |
| ★ Home Style Flour Recipe for Chicken | 1/8 packet | 40 | 2% | 0% | 0% |

SHAKE 'N BAKE Seasoning & Coating Mixture—KRAFT

| FOOD | Serving Size | Calories | Tot Fat | Sat Fat | Chol |
|---|---|---|---|---|---|
| ★ Country Mild Recipe | 1/8 packet | 35 | 3% | 4% | 0% |
| ★ Hot and Spicy Chicken | 1/8 packet | 40 | 1% | 0% | 0% |
| ★ Hot and Spicy Pork | 1/8 packet | 45 | 1% | 0% | 0% |
| ★ Italian Herb Recipe | 1/8 packet | 40 | 1% | 0% | 0% |

★ Foods with this symbol have less than or equal to 5% *Daily Value* for <u>all</u> three nutrients (5% Rule).
❖ Foods with this symbol have <u>at least one</u> of the three nutrients greater than 5% *Daily Value* but less than or equal to 20% *Daily Value.*
Ⓐ Foods with this symbol have <u>at least one</u> of the three nutrients greater than 20% *Daily Value* (20% Rule).

| FOOD | Serving Size | Calories | Tot Fat | Sat Fat | Chol |
|------|-------------|----------|---------|---------|------|
| ★ Original Recipe for Chicken | 1/8 packet | 40 | 1% | 0% | 0% |
| ★ Original Recipe for Fish | 1/4 packet | 70 | 2% | 0% | 0% |
| ★ Original Recipe for Pork | 1/8 packet | 40 | 0% | 0% | 0% |
| SHAKE 'N BAKE Seasoning & Coating Mixture Glaze—KRAFT | | | | | |
| ★ Barbecue Chicken | 1/8 packet | 45 | 2% | 0% | 0% |
| ★ Barbecue Pork | 1/8 packet | 35 | 0% | 0% | 0% |
| ★ Honey Mustard | 1/8 packet | 45 | 2% | 0% | 0% |
| ★ Tangy Honey | 1/8 packet | 45 | 1% | 0% | 0% |

## BREAD AND CRACKER CRUMBS

**Generic Foods**

| | | | | | |
|------|-------------|----------|---------|---------|------|
| ★ Bread Crumbs | 1/3 cup | 120 | 2% | 2% | 0% |
| ★ Cracker Meal | 1/4 cup | 120 | 1% | 0% | 0% |

**Brand Name Foods**

| | | | | | |
|------|-------------|----------|---------|---------|------|
| ★ CONTADINA Bread Crumbs—NESTLÉ | 1/3 cup | 100 | 2% | 0% | 0% |
| ★ KELLOGG'S Corn Flake Crumbs | 2 tbsp | 40 | 0% | 0% | 0% |
| ★ PREMIUM Fat Free Cracker Crumbs—NABISCO | 1/4 cup | 100 | 0% | 0% | 0% |
| PROGRESSO Bread Crumbs—PET | | | | | |
| ★ Italian Style | 1/4 cup | 110 | 2% | 0% | 0% |
| ★ Lemon Herb | 1/4 cup | 100 | 1% | 0% | 0% |
| ★ Plain | 1/4 cup | 100 | 2% | 0% | 0% |
| ★ Tomato Basil | 1/4 cup | 120 | 2% | 0% | 0% |
| ❖ RITZ Cracker Crumbs—NABISCO | 1/3 cup | 140 | 11% | 6% | 0% |
| ★ SUN LUCK Panko Breading | 1/2 cup | 110 | 2% | 0% | 0% |

## COOKIE CRUMBS

**Brand Name Foods**

| | | | | | |
|------|-------------|----------|---------|---------|------|
| ❖ HONEY MAID Graham Cracker Crumbs—NABISCO | To make 1/8 of 9" pie | 70 | 2% | 10% | 0% |
| ★ NILLA Cookie Crumbs—NABISCO | 2 tbsp | 70 | 4% | 2% | 1% |
| ★ OREO Cookie Crumbs—NABISCO | 2 tbsp | 80 | 4% | 3% | 0% |
| ★ SUNSHINE Graham Cracker Crumbs | 3 tbsp | 80 | 3% | 3% | 0% |

## FLOURS AND MEALS

**Generic Foods**

| | | | | | |
|------|-------------|----------|---------|---------|------|
| ★ Arrowroot Flour | 1/4 cup | 110 | 0% | 0% | 0% |
| ★ Barley Flour | 1/4 cup | 100 | 1% | 0% | 0% |

| FOOD | Serving Size | Calories | Tot Fat | Sat Fat | Chol |
|------|--------------|----------|---------|---------|------|
| ★ Buckwheat Groats | 1/4 cup | 100 | 1% | 1% | 0% |
| ★ Cake/Pastry | 1/4 cup | 100 | 0% | 0% | 0% |
| ★ Carob | 1/4 cup | 100 | 0% | 0% | 0% |
| ★ Corn Masa | 1/4 cup | 100 | 2% | 1% | 0% |
| ★ Corn: Whole Grain | 1/4 cup | 110 | 2% | 1% | 0% |
| ★ Cornmeal, degermed | 1/4 cup | 130 | 1% | 0% | 0% |
| ★ Durum Wheat | 1/4 cup | 130 | 2% | 1% | 0% |
| ★ Rice | 1/4 cup | 150 | 1% | 1% | 0% |
| ★ Rye Flour: Light, medium, or dark | 1/4 cup | 70 | 1% | 0% | 0% |
| ★ Soy Flour: defatted | 1/3 cup | 120 | 1% | 0% | 0% |
| ❖ Soy Flour: full fat | 1/3 cup | 170 | 9% | 4% | 0% |
| ★ Soy Flour: lowfat | 1/3 cup | 130 | 3% | 1% | 0% |
| ★ Wheat: self-rising | 1/4 cup | 110 | 0% | 0% | 0% |
| ★ Wheat Gluten | 1/4 cup | 130 | 1% | 0% | 0% |
| ★ Wheat/White: All Purpose | 1/4 cup | 110 | 0% | 0% | 0% |
| ★ Wheat/White: Bread Flour | 1/4 cup | 120 | 1% | 0% | 0% |
| ★ Wheat/White: Cake Flour | 1/4 cup | 100 | 0% | 0% | 0% |
| ★ Whole Wheat | 1/4 cup | 100 | 1% | 0% | 0% |
| **Brand Name Foods** | | | | | |
| ★ ALBERS Cornmeal: Yellow or White—NESTLÉ | 3 tbsp | 110 | 0% | 0% | 0% |
| ★ ARROWHEAD MILLS Amaranth Flour | 1/4 cup | 110 | 2% | 0% | 0% |
| ★ AUNT JEMIMA White Corn Meal (enriched)—QUAKER | 3 tbsp | 90 | 1% | 0% | 0% |
| ★ BALLARD All-Purpose Flour—PILLSBURY | 1 cup | 400 | 2% | 0% | 0% |
| ENER-G Breadmaker Flours | | | | | |
| ★ Bleached | 1/4 cup | 120 | 1% | 0% | 0% |
| ★ Dark Rye | 1/4 cup | 110 | 1% | 2% | 0% |
| ❖ Rice Bran | 1/4 cup | 120 | 9% | 5% | 0% |
| ❖ Soy | 1/4 cup | 100 | 7% | 3% | 0% |
| ★ Wheat Bran | 1/4 cup | 30 | 1% | 0% | 0% |
| ★ Wheat, cracked | 1/3 cup | 120 | 1% | 2% | 0% |
| ★ ENER-G Gluten Free Brown Rice Flour | 1/4 cup | 120 | 2% | 2% | 0% |
| PILLSBURY BEST Flour | 1 cup | 400 | 2% | 0% | 0% |
| ★ All varieties except Whole Wheat | 1/4 cup | 100 | 0% | 0% | 0% |
| ★ Whole Wheat | 1/4 cup | 120 | 2% | 0% | 0% |

★ Foods with this symbol have less than or equal to 5% *Daily Value* for <u>all</u> three nutrients (5% Rule).

❖ Foods with this symbol have <u>at least one</u> of the three nutrients greater than 5% *Daily Value* but less than or equal to 20% *Daily Value.*

Ⓑ Foods with this symbol have <u>at least one</u> of the three nutrients greater than 20% *Daily Value* (20% Rule).

| FOOD | Serving Size | Calories | Tot Fat | Sat Fat | Chol |
|------|------|------|------|------|------|
| | | | | | |

SEASONINGS

**Brand Name Foods**

| FOOD | Serving Size | Calories | Tot Fat | Sat Fat | Chol |
|------|------|------|------|------|------|
| ★ AC'CENT Flavor Enhancer—PET | 1/8 tsp | 0 | 0% | 0% | 0% |
| CHICKEN BLENDS Seasoning Mixes—MCCORMICK | | | | | |
| ★ L'Orange | 1/4 pkg | 40 | 0% | 0% | 0% |
| ★ Parmesan | 1/6 pkg | 40 | 2% | 3% | 1% |
| ★ Piccata | 1/4 pkg | 25 | 0% | 0% | 0% |
| ★ Stir Fry | 1/6 pkg | 20 | 0% | 0% | 0% |
| ★ GOLDEN DIPT Salt Seasonings: All flavors—MCCORMICK | 1/4–1/2 tsp | 0 | 0% | 0% | 0% |
| ★ HAIN Taco Seasoning Mix | 2 tsp dry mix | 15 | 0% | 0% | 0% |
| LAWRY'S Spices & Seasonings for: | | | | | |
| ★ Burrito | 1 tbsp | 35 | 1% | 0% | 0% |
| ★ Chicken Taco | 2 tsp | 20 | 0% | 0% | 0% |
| ★ Enchilada Sauce | 2 tsp | 20 | 0% | 0% | 0% |
| ★ Fajitas | 2 tsp | 15 | 0% | 0% | 0% |
| ★ Guacamole | 1/2 tsp | 5 | 0% | 0% | 0% |
| ★ Taco | 1 tbsp | 25 | 0% | 0% | 0% |
| McCORMICK/SCHILLING Seasoning & Sauce Mixes | | | | | |
| ★ Beef Stew | 1/8 pkg | 15 | 0% | 0% | 0% |
| ★ Burrito | 1/6 pkg | 25 | 0% | 0% | 0% |
| ★ Chili | 1/8 pkg | 30 | 0% | 0% | 0% |
| ★ Enchilada | 1/8 pkg | 15 | 0% | 0% | 0% |
| ★ Fried Rice | 1/4 pkg | 20 | 0% | 0% | 0% |
| ★ Hamburger | 1/6 pkg | 15 | 0% | 0% | 0% |
| ★ Meat Loaf | 1/10 pkg | 15 | 0% | 0% | 0% |
| ★ Season 'n Fry | 1/8 pkg | 35 | 0% | 0% | 0% |
| ★ Stir Fry | 1/6 pkg | 20 | 0% | 0% | 0% |
| ★ Swedish Meatballs | 1/6 pkg | 45 | 2% | 0% | 0% |
| ★ Swiss Steak | 1/6 pkg | 10 | 0% | 0% | 0% |
| ★ Taco Mix | 1/6 pkg | 20 | 0% | 0% | 0% |
| McCORMICK/SCHILLING Bag 'n Season | | | | | |
| ★ Beef Stew | 1/8 pkg | 10 | 0% | 0% | 0% |
| ★ Chicken | 1/6 pkg | 20 | 0% | 0% | 0% |
| ★ Country Chicken | 1/6 pkg | 25 | 2% | 0% | 0% |
| ★ Hot & Spicy Wings | 1/4 pkg | 35 | 0% | 0% | 0% |
| ★ Meat Loaf | 1/8 pkg | 15 | 0% | 0% | 0% |
| ★ Oriental Style | 1/6 pkg | 25 | 0% | 0% | 0% |
| ★ Pork Chops | 1/6 pkg | 15 | 0% | 0% | 0% |
| ★ Pot Roast | 1/8 pkg | 10 | 0% | 0% | 0% |
| ★ Roast Turkey | 1/12 pkg | 15 | 0% | 0% | 1% |
| ★ Spareribs | 1/6 pkg | 30 | 0% | 0% | 0% |
| ★ Swiss Steak | 1/6 pkg | 15 | 0% | 0% | 0% |

| FOOD | Serving Size | Calories | Tot Fat | Sat Fat | Chol |
|------|------|------|------|------|------|
| OLD BAY *Classic*—MCCORMICK | | | | | |
| ❖ Crab Cake | 1/6 pkg | 30 | 2% | 0% | 10% |
| ❖ Salmon | 1/5 pkg | 40 | 2% | 0% | 18% |
| ❖ Tuna | 1/5 pkg | 30 | 2% | 0% | 13% |
| OLD BAY *Seas'n Easy*—MCCORMICK | | | | | |
| ★ Creole | 1/5 pkg | 25 | 1% | 0% | 0% |
| ★ Garlic & Herb | 1/4 pkg | 30 | 0% | 0% | 0% |
| ★ Honey Mustard | 1/8 pkg | 35 | 2% | 0% | 0% |
| ★ Lemon Dill | 1/5 pkg | 30 | 0% | 0% | 0% |
| ★ Seafood Marinara | 1/4 pkg | 25 | 0% | 0% | 0% |
| OLD EL PASO Seasoning Mix—PET | | | | | |
| ★ Burrito | 2 tsp | 20 | 0% | 0% | 0% |
| ★ Chili | 1 tbsp | 25 | 1% | 0% | 0% |
| ★ Enchilada Sauce | 2 tsp | 10 | 0% | 0% | 0% |
| ★ Taco | 2 tsp | 20 | 0% | 0% | 0% |
| ★ PANCHO VILLA Taco Seasoning Mix—PET | 2 tsp | 20 | 0% | 0% | 0% |

# Jams, Jellies, Sugars, and Syrups

## FRUIT BUTTERS, HONEY, JAMS, JELLIES, AND PRESERVES

**Generic Foods**

| FOOD | Serving Size | Calories | Tot Fat | Sat Fat | Chol |
|------|------|------|------|------|------|
| ★ Apple Butter | 1 tbsp | 40 | 0% | 0% | 0% |
| ★ Green Pepper Jelly | 1 tbsp | 50 | 0% | 0% | 0% |
| ★ Honey | 1 tbsp | 70 | 0% | 0% | 0% |
| ★ Jam/Preserves, Low Calorie | 1 tbsp | 25 | 0% | 0% | 0% |
| ★ Jam/Preserves: All varieties | 1 tbsp | 60 | 0% | 0% | 0% |
| ★ Jelly: All varieties | 1 tbsp | 50 | 0% | 0% | 0% |
| ★ Marmalade | 1 tbsp | 50 | 0% | 0% | 0% |

**Brand Name Foods**

| FOOD | Serving Size | Calories | Tot Fat | Sat Fat | Chol |
|------|------|------|------|------|------|
| ★ ESTEE Spreads: All varieties | 1 tbsp | 10 | 0% | 0% | 0% |
| ★ FEATHERWEIGHT Fruit Spreads: All varieties | 1 tbsp | 15 | 0% | 0% | 0% |
| KRAFT Jams | | | | | |
| ★ Grape | 1 tbsp | 60 | 0% | 0% | 0% |
| ★ Red Plum | 1 tbsp | 60 | 0% | 0% | 0% |
| ★ Strawberry | 1 tbsp | 50 | 0% | 0% | 0% |

★ Foods with this symbol have less than or equal to 5% *Daily Value* for <u>all</u> three nutrients (5% Rule).

❖ Foods with this symbol have <u>at least one</u> of the three nutrients greater than 5% *Daily Value* but less than or equal to 20% *Daily Value*.

Ⓐ Foods with this symbol have <u>at least one</u> of the three nutrients greater than 20% *Daily Value* (20% Rule).

| FOOD | Serving Size | Calories | Tot Fat | Sat Fat | Chol |
|---|---|---|---|---|---|
| KRAFT Jellies | | | | | |
| ★ Apple | 1 tbsp | 60 | 0% | 0% | 0% |
| ★ Apple-Strawberry | 1 tbsp | 50 | 0% | 0% | 0% |
| ★ Blackberry | 1 tbsp | 50 | 0% | 0% | 0% |
| ★ Grape | 1 tbsp | 50 | 0% | 0% | 0% |
| ★ Guava | 1 tbsp | 50 | 0% | 0% | 0% |
| ★ Red Currant | 1 tbsp | 50 | 0% | 0% | 0% |
| ★ Strawberry | 1 tbsp | 60 | 0% | 0% | 0% |
| ★ KRAFT Preserves: All varieties | 1 tbsp | 50 | 0% | 0% | 0% |
| ★ KRAFT Reduced Calorie Fruit Spreads: All varieties | 1 tbsp | 20 | 0% | 0% | 0% |
| ★ MARY ELLEN Dutch Girl Apple Butter—SMUCKER'S | 1 tbsp | 35 | 0% | 0% | 0% |
| POLANER—AMERICAN HOME FOODS | | | | | |
| ★ All Fruit Spreadable Fruit: All varieties | 1 tbsp | 40 | 0% | 0% | 0% |
| ★ Reduced Sugar Fruit Spreads: All varieties | 1 tbsp | 25 | 0% | 0% | 0% |
| ★ Jellies | 1 tbsp | 60 | 0% | 0% | 0% |
| POLANER Fancy Fruit Preserves —AMERICAN HOME FOODS | | | | | |
| ★ Apricot | 1 tbsp | 60 | 0% | 0% | 0% |
| ★ Blueberry | 1 tbsp | 50 | 0% | 0% | 0% |
| ★ Cherry | 1 tbsp | 60 | 0% | 0% | 0% |
| ★ Red Raspberry | 1 tbsp | 60 | 0% | 0% | 0% |
| ★ Seedless Blackberry | 1 tbsp | 50 | 0% | 0% | 0% |
| ★ Strawberry | 1 tbsp | 50 | 0% | 0% | 0% |
| POLANER Fruit Butters— AMERICAN HOME FOODS | | | | | |
| ★ Apple Butter | 1 tbsp | 35 | 0% | 0% | 0% |
| ★ Pumpkin Butter | 1 tbsp | 35 | 0% | 0% | 0% |
| POLANER Marmalades— AMERICAN HOME FOODS | | | | | |
| ★ California Navel Sweet Orange | 1 tbsp | 45 | 0% | 0% | 0% |
| ★ Orange Fancy Fruit | 1 tbsp | 60 | 0% | 0% | 0% |
| POLANER Preserves— AMERICAN HOME FOODS | | | | | |
| ★ Apricot | 1 tbsp | 50 | 0% | 0% | 0% |
| ★ Chunky Pineapple | 1 tbsp | 60 | 0% | 0% | 0% |
| ★ Damson Plum | 1 tbsp | 50 | 0% | 0% | 0% |
| ★ Natural Strawberry | 1 tbsp | 60 | 0% | 0% | 0% |
| ★ Peach | 1 tbsp | 40 | 0% | 0% | 0% |
| ★ Red Raspberry | 1 tbsp | 60 | 0% | 0% | 0% |
| ★ Seedless Blackberry | 1 tbsp | 50 | 0% | 0% | 0% |
| ★ Selected Blueberry | 1 tbsp | 60 | 0% | 0% | 0% |
| ★ Strawberry | 1 tbsp | 50 | 0% | 0% | 0% |
| SMUCKER'S | | | | | |
| ★ Fruit Butters | 1 tbsp | 45 | 0% | 0% | 0% |
| ★ Homestyle Fruit Spread | 1 tbsp | 45 | 0% | 0% | 0% |

| FOOD | Serving Size | Calories | Tot Fat | Sat Fat | Chol |
|---|---|---|---|---|---|
| ★ Jams and Jellies | 1 tbsp | 50 | 0% | 0% | 0% |
| ★ *Light* Fruit Preserves | 1 tbsp | 20 | 0% | 0% | 0% |
| ★ Marmalades | 1 tbsp | 50 | 0% | 0% | 0% |
| ★ Preserves | 1 tbsp | 50 | 0% | 0% | 0% |
| ★ Preserves: Reduced Sugar | 1 tbsp | 25 | 0% | 0% | 0% |
| ★ *Simply Fruit* Spreadable Fruit | 1 tbsp | 50 | 0% | 0% | 0% |
| ★ *Slenderella* Reduced Calorie Fruit Spread | 1 tbsp | 20 | 0% | 0% | 0% |

% DAILY VALUE

## FRUIT DIPS

**Brand Name Foods**

| FOOD | Serving Size | Calories | Tot Fat | Sat Fat | Chol |
|---|---|---|---|---|---|
| ❖ MARIE'S Caramel Dip—CAMPBELL'S | 2 tbsp | 150 | 8% | 20% | 2% |
| MARIE'S Creamy Glaze—CAMPBELL'S | | | | | |
| ★ For Bananas | 2 tbsp | 40 | 0% | 0% | 0% |
| ★ For Blueberries | 2 tbsp | 40 | 0% | 0% | 0% |
| ★ For Peaches | 2 tbsp | 40 | 0% | 0% | 0% |
| ★ For Strawberries | 2 tbsp | 40 | 0% | 0% | 0% |
| SMUCKER'S Fat Free Fruit Dip | | | | | |
| ★ Caramel | 2 tbsp | 130 | 0% | 0% | 0% |
| ★ Chocolate | 2 tbsp | 130 | 1% | 0% | 0% |

## SUGAR

**Generic Foods**

| FOOD | Serving Size | Calories | Tot Fat | Sat Fat | Chol |
|---|---|---|---|---|---|
| ★ Sugar, Brown | 1 tsp | 20 | 0% | 0% | 0% |
| ★ Sugar, Powdered | 1 tsp | 10 | 0% | 0% | 0% |
| ★ Sugar, White | 1 tsp | 20 | 0% | 0% | 0% |

## SYRUPS

**Brand Name Foods**

| FOOD | Serving Size | Calories | Tot Fat | Sat Fat | Chol |
|---|---|---|---|---|---|
| AUNT JEMIMA—QUAKER | | | | | |
| ★ Butter Rich | 1/4 cup | 210 | 0% | 0% | 0% |
| ★ Butterlite | 1/4 cup | 100 | 0% | 0% | 0% |
| ★ Pancake & Waffle Syrup | 1/4 cup | 210 | 0% | 0% | 0% |
| ESTEE Syrups | | | | | |
| ★ Blueberry | 1/4 cup | 80 | 0% | 0% | 0% |
| ★ Maple | 1/4 cup | 80 | 0% | 0% | 0% |
| FEATHERWEIGHT Lite Syrups | | | | | |
| ★ Blueberry | 1/4 cup | 80 | 0% | 0% | 0% |

★ Foods with this symbol have less than or equal to 5% *Daily Value* for all three nutrients (5% Rule).
❖ Foods with this symbol have at least one of the three nutrients greater than 5% *Daily Value* but less than or equal to 20% *Daily Value*.
Ⓐ Foods with this symbol have at least one of the three nutrients greater than 20% *Daily Value* (20% Rule).

| FOOD | Serving Size | Calories | Tot Fat | Sat Fat | Chol |
|---|---|---|---|---|---|
| ★ Maple | 1/4 cup | 80 | 0% | 0% | 0% |
| ★ GOLDEN GRIDDLE Syrup—CPC | 1 tbsp | 50 | 0% | 0% | 0% |
| GRANDMA'S Molasses— | | | | | |
| CADBURY BEVERAGES | | | | | |
| ★ 4 Star | 1 tbsp | 50 | 0% | 0% | 0% |
| ★ Gold | 1 tbsp | 50 | 0% | 0% | 0% |
| ★ Green Label | 1 tbsp | 50 | 0% | 0% | 0% |
| HUNGRY JACK Microwave Syrup | | | | | |
| —PILLSBURY | | | | | |
| ★ Butter Maple | 1/4 cup | 210 | 0% | 0% | 0% |
| ★ Lite Butter Maple | 1/4 cup | 100 | 0% | 0% | 0% |
| KARO—CPC | | | | | |
| ★ Dark or Light Corn Syrup | 1 tbsp | 60 | 0% | 0% | 0% |
| ★ Pancake Syrup | 1 tbsp | 60 | 0% | 0% | 0% |
| LOG CABIN Syrup—KRAFT | | | | | |
| ★ Lite Reduced Calorie | 1/4 cup | 100 | 0% | 0% | 0% |
| ★ Original | 1/4 cup | 200 | 0% | 0% | 0% |
| LOG CABIN Country Kitchen | | | | | |
| Syrups—KRAFT | | | | | |
| ★ Butter Flavored | 1/4 cup | 200 | 0% | 0% | 0% |
| ★ Lite Reduced Calorie | 1/4 cup | 100 | 0% | 0% | 0% |
| ★ Original | 1/4 cup | 200 | 0% | 0% | 0% |
| MRS. BUTTERWORTH'S Syrups | | | | | |
| —VAN DEN BERGH | | | | | |
| ★ Lite Reduced Calorie | 1/4 cup | 100 | 0% | 0% | 0% |
| ★ Original | 1/4 cup | 230 | 0% | 0% | 0% |
| MRS. RICHARDSON'S Syrups— | | | | | |
| QUAKER | | | | | |
| ★ Lite | 1/4 cup | 100 | 0% | 0% | 0% |
| ★ Original | 1/4 cup | 210 | 0% | 0% | 0% |
| POLANER Pourable All Fruit— | | | | | |
| AMERICAN HOME FOODS | | | | | |
| ★ Apricot | 1/4 cup | 110 | 0% | 0% | 0% |
| ★ Black Cherry | 1/4 cup | 110 | 0% | 0% | 0% |
| ★ Blueberry | 1/4 cup | 120 | 0% | 0% | 0% |
| ★ Seedless Red Raspberry | 1/4 cup | 120 | 0% | 0% | 0% |
| ★ Strawberry | 1/4 cup | 110 | 0% | 0% | 0% |
| POLANER Syrups—AMERICAN | | | | | |
| HOME FOODS | | | | | |
| ★ Blueberry w/Whole Blueberries | 1/4 cup | 150 | 0% | 0% | 0% |
| ★ Red Raspberry | 1/4 cup | 150 | 0% | 0% | 0% |
| ★ Strawberry | 1/4 cup | 160 | 0% | 0% | 0% |
| SMUCKER'S Syrups | | | | | |
| ★ Light Fruit | 1/4 cup | 130 | 0% | 0% | 0% |
| ★ Natural Fruit | 1/4 cup | 210 | 0% | 0% | 0% |

| FOOD | Serving Size | Calories | Tot Fat | Sat Fat | Chol |
|------|-------------|----------|---------|---------|------|

# Main Dishes, Entrées, and Dinners: Canned and Shelf-Stable

## CHICKEN

**Brand Name Foods**

SWANSON—CAMPBELL'S
| | | | | | |
|------|-------------|----------|---------|---------|------|
| ⊛ Chicken & Dumplings | 1 cup | 260 | 20% | 25% | 22% |
| ⊛ Chicken à la King | 1 cup | 320 | 32% | 35% | 20% |
| ❖ Mixin' Chicken in Broth | 1/4 cup | 110 | 11% | 15% | 15% |

## CHILI

**Generic Foods**

| | | | | | |
|------|-------------|----------|---------|---------|------|
| ⊛ Chili Con Carne w/Beans | 1 cup | 340 | 25% | 38% | 13% |
| ⊛ Chili w/Beans | 1 cup | 290 | 22% | 30% | 14% |

**Brand Name Foods**

BEARITOS Vegetarian Chili—
LITTLE BEAR ORGANIC FOODS
| | | | | | |
|------|-------------|----------|---------|---------|------|
| ★ Black Bean | 1 cup | 150 | 2% | 1% | 0% |
| ★ Original | 1 cup | 190 | 2% | 1% | 0% |
| ★ Spicy | 1 cup | 190 | 2% | 1% | 0% |

CHEF BOYARDEE Chili—
AMERICAN HOME FOODS
| | | | | | |
|------|-------------|----------|---------|---------|------|
| ⊛ Chili Con Carne w/Beans | 1 can | 310 | 28% | 35% | 13% |
| ⊛ Hot Chili Con Carne w/Beans | 1 can | 330 | 31% | 40% | 13% |

DENNISON'S Chili—AMERICAN
HOME FOODS
| | | | | | |
|------|-------------|----------|---------|---------|------|
| ★ Chili Beans in Chili Gravy | 1/2 cup | 110 | 0% | 0% | 0% |
| ⊛ Chunky Chili Con Carne w/Beans | 1 cup | 340 | 25% | 35% | 13% |
| ⊛ Deluxe Chili Con Carne w/Beans | 1 cup | 360 | 26% | 30% | 15% |
| ⊛ Hot Chili Con Carne, No Beans | 1 cup | 350 | 34% | 50% | 23% |
| ⊛ Hot Chili Con Carne w/Beans | 1 cup | 370 | 28% | 40% | 15% |
| ❖ Lite Chili w/Beans | 1 cup | 200 | 6% | 8% | 13% |
| ❖ Reduced Fat Chili Con Carne w/Beans | 1 cup | 290 | 11% | 13% | 12% |
| ❖ Select Chili w/Beans, Caliente: Hot & Spicy | 1 cup | 240 | 9% | 10% | 12% |
| ❖ Select Chili w/Beans, Homestyle: Mild w/Kidney Beans | 1 cup | 250 | 11% | 15% | 12% |

★ Foods with this symbol have less than or equal to 5% *Daily Value* for <u>all</u> three nutrients (5% Rule).
❖ Foods with this symbol have <u>at least one</u> of the three nutrients greater than 5% *Daily Value* but less than or equal to 20% *Daily Value*.
⊛ Foods with this symbol have <u>at least one</u> of the three nutrients greater than 20% *Daily Value* (20% Rule).

| FOOD | Serving Size | Calories | Tot Fat | Sat Fat | Chol |
|------|--------------|----------|---------|---------|------|
| HEALTH VALLEY Fat Free Vegetarian Chili | | | | | |
| ★ Mild w/3 beans | 1/2 cup | 80 | 0% | 0% | 0% |
| ★ Mild w/Black Beans | 1/2 cup | 80 | 0% | 0% | 0% |
| ★ Spicy w/Black Beans | 1/2 cup | 80 | 0% | 0% | 0% |
| ★ HUNT'S Homestyle Separates Chili Fixings—HUNT WESSON | 1/2 cup | 80 | 2% | 1% | 0% |
| KNORR Chili—CPC | | | | | |
| ★ Four Bean | 1 pkg | 230 | 2% | 0% | 0% |
| ★ Italian Beans | 1 pkg | 230 | 3% | 0% | 0% |
| LIBBY'S Chili—NESTLÉ | | | | | |
| ✲ Chili No Beans | 1 cup | 480 | 57% | 86% | 24% |
| ✲ Chili w/Beans | 1 cup | 420 | 42% | 63% | 17% |
| ✲ *Diner* Chili w/Beans | 1 container | 320 | 34% | 40% | 14% |
| ❖ NATURAL TOUCH Vegetarian Chili—WORTHINGTON FOODS | 1 cup | 270 | 18% | 10% | 0% |
| STAGG Chili w/Beans | | | | | |
| ✲ *Chunkero* | 1 cup | 330 | 24% | 27% | 13% |
| ✲ *Classic* | 1 cup | 330 | 23% | 31% | 10% |
| ✲ *Country* | 1 cup | 330 | 25% | 31% | 13% |
| ✲ *Dynamite Hot* | 1 cup | 330 | 23% | 31% | 10% |
| ✲ *Laredo* | 1 cup | 300 | 19% | 26% | 13% |
| ❖ *Ranch House* Chicken | 1 cup | 270 | 9% | 9% | 17% |
| ✲ *Steak House* Straight | 1 cup | 360 | 34% | 47% | 20% |
| ❖ *Turkey Ranchero* | 1 cup | 280 | 14% | 15% | 7% |
| ✲ WORTHINGTON Meatless Chili | 1 cup | 290 | 23% | 13% | 0% |

## HASH

**Brand Name Foods**

| FOOD | Serving Size | Calories | Tot Fat | Sat Fat | Chol |
|------|--------------|----------|---------|---------|------|
| LIBBY'S Hash—NESTLÉ | | | | | |
| ✲ Corned Beef | 1 cup | 490 | 55% | 84% | 32% |
| ✲ Roast Beef | 1 cup | 460 | 51% | 63% | 27% |
| MORNING CLASSICS Hash—NESTLÉ | | | | | |
| ✲ Original | 1 cup | 240 | 20% | 31% | 6% |
| ✲ Sausage | 1 cup | 240 | 20% | 31% | 6% |
| ✲ Smoke | 1 cup | 240 | 20% | 31% | 6% |

## MEXICAN

**Brand Name Foods**

| FOOD | Serving Size | Calories | Tot Fat | Sat Fat | Chol |
|------|--------------|----------|---------|---------|------|
| ✲ OLD EL PASO Tamales—PET | 3 tamales | 330 | 30% | 36% | 9% |
| OLD EL PASO Dinner Kits (prep as dir)—PET | | | | | |
| ✲ Burrito | 1 burrito | 280 | 11% | 14% | 22% |
| ✲ Soft Taco | 2 tacos | 380 | 16% | 22% | 21% |
| ✲ Taco | 2 tacos | 270 | 20% | 24% | 20% |

| FOOD | Serving Size | Calories | Tot Fat | Sat Fat | Chol |
|------|--------------|----------|---------|---------|------|

ORIENTAL

**Brand Name Foods**

*Beef*

LA CHOY Dinners—HUNT WESSON

| | | | | | |
|------|--------------|----------|---------|---------|------|
| ★ Beef Chow Mein | 1 cup | 110 | 3% | 4% | 4% |
| ❖ Beef Pepper Oriental | 1 cup | 100 | 4% | 6% | 7% |
| ★ *Dinner Classics* Pepper Steak | 1/5 pkg | 35 | 0% | 0% | 0% |
| ★ Noodles w/Beef | 1 cup | 150 | 2% | 3% | 4% |
| ❖ Noodles w/Vegetables & Beef | 1 cup | 160 | 5% | 7% | 2% |

*Chicken*

LA CHOY Chicken Dinners—
HUNT WESSON

| | | | | | |
|------|--------------|----------|---------|---------|------|
| ❖ Chicken Chow Mein | 1 cup | 110 | 7% | 6% | 3% |
| ❖ Chicken Sweet & Sour | 1 cup | 160 | 4% | 4% | 8% |
| ❖ Chicken Teriyaki | 1 cup | 110 | 5% | 6% | 9% |
| ❖ Noodles w/Chicken | 1 cup | 160 | 6% | 5% | 4% |
| ❖ Noodles w/Vegetables & Chicken | 1 cup | 160 | 5% | 7% | 6% |
| ❖ Spicy Chicken, Szechwan | 1 cup | 100 | 4% | 5% | 6% |
| ❖ Sweet & Sour Noodles w/Chicken | 1 cup | 260 | 5% | 7% | 3% |

*Pork and Other*

| | | | | | |
|------|--------------|----------|---------|---------|------|
| ★ LA CHOY Pork Chow Mein—HUNT WESSON | 1 cup | 80 | 3% | 5% | 3% |
| LA CHOY Dinners—HUNT WESSON | | | | | |
| ★ Noodles w/Vegetables • | 1 cup | 130 | 2% | 3% | 0% |
| ★ Shrimp Chow Mein | 1 cup | 50 | 1% | 2% | 3% |

STEW

**Brand Name Foods**

| | | | | | |
|------|--------------|----------|---------|---------|------|
| ★ CASBAH Morrocan Stew | 1 cup | 180 | 0% | 0% | 0% |
| ⊛ CHEF BOYARDEE Beef Stew—AMERICAN HOME FOODS | 1 can | 210 | 18% | 25% | 12% |
| ❖ HUNT'S Homestyle Separates: Beef Stew—HUNT WESSON | 1 cup | 160 | 7% | 10% | 7% |
| ★ KNORR Vegetable Stew Mix—CPC | 1 pkg mix | 160 | 3% | 0% | 0% |
| ⊛ LIBBY'S *Diner* Beef Stew—NESTLÉ | 1 container | 290 | 30% | 25% | 12% |
| ⊛ LUCK'S Brunswick Stew | 1 cup | 150 | 15% | 48% | 0% |

★ Foods with this symbol have less than or equal to 5% *Daily Value* for <u>all</u> three nutrients (5% Rule).
❖ Foods with this symbol have <u>at least one</u> of the three nutrients greater than 5% *Daily Value* but less than or equal to 20% *Daily Value*.
⊛ Foods with this symbol have <u>at least one</u> of the three nutrients greater than 20% *Daily Value* (20% Rule).

| FOOD | Serving Size | Calories | Tot Fat | Sat Fat | Chol |
|------|--------------|----------|---------|---------|------|
| ❖ SWANSON Chicken Stew—CAMPBELL'S | 1 cup | 180 | 12% | 15% | 12% |
| ❖ WORTHINGTON Meatless Country Stew | 1 cup | 210 | 14% | 8% | 0% |

<u>TURKEY</u>

**Brand Name Foods**

| | | | | | |
|------|--------------|----------|---------|---------|------|
| ❖ LIBBY'S *Diner* Gravy w/Turkey & Dressing—NESTLÉ | 1 container | 180 | 11% | 8% | 11% |

# Main Dishes, Entrées, and Dinners: Frozen and Refrigerated

<u>BEEF</u>

**Brand Name Foods**

| FOOD | Serving Size | Calories | Tot Fat | Sat Fat | Chol |
|------|--------------|----------|---------|---------|------|
| ARMOUR CLASSICS—CONAGRA | | | | | |
| ❖ Lite Beef Pepper Steak | 1 meal | 210 | 6% | 8% | 20% |
| ❖ Lite Salisbury Steak | 1 meal | 260 | 11% | 20% | 18% |
| ⊛ Meatloaf | 1 meal | 300 | 15% | 25% | 22% |
| ⊛ Salisbury Steak | 1 meal | 330 | 28% | 40% | 17% |
| ⊛ Swedish Meatballs | 1 meal | 300 | 26% | 35% | 13% |
| BANQUET *Extra Helping* Dinners —CONAGRA | | | | | |
| ⊛ Chicken Fried Steak | 1 meal | 800 | 68% | 70% | 18% |
| ⊛ Meatloaf | 1 meal | 650 | 58% | 80% | 28% |
| ⊛ Salisbury Steak | 1 meal | 740 | 71% | 95% | 25% |
| BANQUET Dinners—CONAGRA | | | | | |
| ⊛ Beef | 1 meal | 240 | 11% | 15% | 23% |
| ⊛ Gravy w/Beef Patty | 1 meal | 300 | 31% | 40% | 12% |
| ⊛ Meatloaf | 1 meal | 280 | 26% | 35% | 13% |
| ⊛ Salisbury Steak | 1 meal | 310 | 25% | 35% | 12% |
| BANQUET *Extra Helping* Family Entrees—CONAGRA | | | | | |
| ❖ Beef Stew | 1 cup | 160 | 6% | 10% | 8% |
| ❖ Gravy and Sliced Beef | 2 slcs w/ gravy | 100 | 5% | 8% | 13% |
| ⊛ Gravy w/Charbroiled Beef | 1 pattie w/ gravy | 180 | 20% | 30% | 8% |
| ❖ Noodles and Beef | 1 cup | 140 | 6% | 10% | 12% |
| ⊛ Onion Gravy w/Beef | 1 patty w/ gravy | 180 | 22% | 30% | 7% |
| ⊛ Salisbury Steak | 1 pattie w/ gravy | 200 | 22% | 30% | 8% |

| FOOD | Serving Size | Calories | Tot Fat | Sat Fat | Chol |
|---|---|---|---|---|---|
| BUDGET GOURMET *Light & Healthy Dinners*—ALL AMERICAN GOURMET | | | | | |
| ❖ Beef Sirloin Meatballs and Gravy | 11 oz | 310 | 12% | 15% | 12% |
| ❖ Beef Sirloin Salisbury Steak w/ Red Skinned Potatoes | 11 oz | 260 | 12% | 15% | 12% |
| ❖ Sirloin of Beef in Wine Sauce | 11 oz | 270 | 9% | 10% | 13% |
| ❖ Special Recipe Sirloin of Beef | 11 oz | 310 | 11% | 15% | 8% |
| ❖ Yankee Pot Roast | 10.5 oz | 270 | 11% | 13% | 10% |
| BUDGET GOURMET *Light & Healthy Entrées*—ALL AMERICAN GOURMET | | | | | |
| ❖ Beef Sirloin Salisbury Steak | 9 oz | 240 | 8% | 10% | 13% |
| ❖ Beef Stroganoff | 8.75 oz | 290 | 11% | 20% | 12% |
| ❖ Sirloin of Beef in Herb Sauce | 9.5 oz | 260 | 11% | 20% | 10% |
| BUDGET GOURMET *Original Entrées*—ALL AMERICAN GOURMET | | | | | |
| Ⓐ Open Faced Roast Beef w/ Mashed Potatoes & Gravy | 9 oz | 340 | 26% | 30% | 13% |
| ❖ Pepper Steak w/Rice | 10 oz | 290 | 12% | 15% | 13% |
| Ⓐ Roast Sirloin Supreme | 9 oz | 300 | 20% | 35% | 22% |
| Ⓐ Sirloin Cheddar Melt | 9.4 oz | 370 | 32% | 50% | 28% |
| Ⓐ Sirloin Tips w/Country Style Vegetables | 10 oz | 250 | 20% | 30% | 13% |
| Ⓐ Swedish Meatballs | 10 oz | 550 | 52% | 80% | 50% |
| HEALTHY CHOICE Classics— CONAGRA | | | | | |
| ❖ Mesquite Beef Barbecue | 1 meal | 310 | 6% | 8% | 15% |
| ❖ Salisbury Steak | 1 meal | 260 | 9% | 13% | 10% |
| Ⓐ Traditional Swedish Meatballs | 1 meal | 320 | 14% | 15% | 22% |
| HEALTHY CHOICE Dinners— CONAGRA | | | | | |
| ❖ Beef Tips w/Sauce | 1 meal | 290 | 9% | 12% | 14% |
| ❖ Traditional Beef Tips | 1 meal | 260 | 8% | 10% | 14% |
| ❖ Traditional Meatloaf | 1 meal | 320 | 12% | 20% | 12% |
| ❖ Traditional Salisbury Steak | 1 meal | 320 | 9% | 15% | 15% |
| ❖ Yankee Pot Roast | 1 meal | 280 | 8% | 10% | 15% |
| HEALTHY CHOICE Entrees— CONAGRA | | | | | |
| ★ Beef Macaroni Casserole | 1 meal | 200 | 2% | 3% | 5% |
| ❖ *Beef Tips Francais* | 1 meal | 280 | 8% | 8% | 10% |
| MARIE CALLENDER'S—CONAGRA | | | | | |
| ❖ Old Fashioned Beef Pot Roast & Gravy | 1 cup | 180 | 8% | 5% | 12% |

★ Foods with this symbol have less than or equal to 5% *Daily Value* for <u>all</u> three nutrients (5% Rule).

❖ Foods with this symbol have <u>at least one</u> of the three nutrients greater than 5% *Daily Value* but less than or equal to 20% *Daily Value*.

Ⓐ Foods with this symbol have <u>at least one</u> of the three nutrients greater than 20% *Daily Value* (20% Rule).

| FOOD | Serving Size | Calories | Tot Fat | Sat Fat | Chol |
|---|---|---|---|---|---|
| ⊛ Meatloaf & Gravy w/Mashed Potatoes | 1 dinner | 540 | 46% | 55% | 27% |
| ⊛ Beef Stroganoff & Noodles | 1 cup | 440 | 42% | 55% | 13% |
| STOUFFER'S *Lean Cuisine* Entrées —NESTLÉ | | | | | |
| ❖ Beef Pot Roast & Whipped Potatoes | 1 pkg | 210 | 11% | 8% | 13% |
| ❖ Cafe Classics Sirloin Beef Peppercorn | 1 pkg | 210 | 11% | 8% | 8% |
| ❖ Meatloaf & Whipped Potatoes | 1 pkg | 250 | 11% | 10% | 15% |
| ❖ Salisbury Steak w/Macaroni & Cheese | 1 pkg | 280 | 14% | 18% | 20% |
| ❖ Stuffed Cabbage w/Whipped Potatoes | 1 pkg | 220 | 11% | 8% | 8% |
| ❖ Swedish Meatballs w/Pasta | 1 pkg | 290 | 12% | 15% | 18% |
| ⊛ STOUFFER'S *Lunch Express* Swedish Meatballs w/Pasta —NESTLÉ | 1 pkg | 530 | 49% | 55% | 22% |
| STOUFFER'S Entrées—NESTLÉ | | | | | |
| ❖ Creamed Chipped Beef | 1 pkg | 150 | 17% | 15% | 13% |
| ⊛ Creamed Chipped Beef over Country Biscuit | 1 pkg | 510 | 45% | 40% | 13% |
| ❖ Green Pepper Steak | 1 pkg | 330 | 14% | 15% | 12% |
| ⊛ Swedish Meatballs | 1 pkg | 440 | 35% | 40% | 28% |
| STOUFFER'S Homestyle Entrées —NESTLÉ | | | | | |
| ❖ Beef Pot Roast & Browned Potatoes | 1 pkg | 270 | 15% | 15% | 13% |
| ⊛ Meatloaf & Whipped Potatoes | 1 pkg | 380 | 37% | 40% | 27% |
| ⊛ Salisbury Steak & Gravy & Macaroni & Cheese | 1 pkg | 370 | 29% | 30% | 17% |
| ⊛ SWANSON *Budget Meals* Meatloaf —CAMPBELL'S | 1 pkg | 350 | 32% | 50% | 8% |
| SWANSON *Hungry Man* Dinners —CAMPBELL'S | | | | | |
| ⊛ Meatloaf | 1 pkg | 620 | 48% | 80% | 20% |
| ⊛ Salisbury Steak | 1 pkg | 610 | 52% | 85% | 27% |
| ⊛ Sirloin Beef Tips | 1 pkg | 450 | 25% | 30% | 40% |
| ❖ Yankee Pot Roast | 1 pkg | 400 | 17% | 15% | 15% |
| SWANSON Complete Dinners —CAMPBELL'S | | | | | |
| ❖ Beef & Broccoli | 1 pkg | 340 | 15% | 20% | 8% |
| ⊛ Beef & Gravy | 1 pkg | 330 | 14% | 25% | 13% |
| ⊛ Chopped Sirloin Beef w/Gravy | 1 pkg | 350 | 26% | 55% | 20% |
| ⊛ Meatloaf | 1 pkg | 410 | 28% | 45% | 12% |
| ⊛ Salisbury Steak | 1 pkg | 390 | 28% | 35% | 17% |
| ⊛ Sirloin Beef Tips w/Noodles & Beef Gravy | 1 pkg | 290 | 17% | 25% | 17% |

| FOOD | Serving Size | Calories | Tot Fat | Sat Fat | Chol |
|------|-------------|----------|---------|---------|------|
| ❖ Smothered Hot Roast Beef Sandwich | 1 pkg | 380 | 20% | 20% | 10% |
| ❖ Yankee Pot Roast | 1 pkg | 270 | 11% | 20% | 17% |
| SWANSON Homestyle Entrées —CAMPBELL'S | | | | | |
| Ⓐ Salisbury Steak in Gravy w/ Mashed Potatoes | 1 pkg | 350 | 31% | 55% | 12% |
| Ⓐ Sirloin Beef Tips & Noodles w/Gravy | 1 pkg | 410 | 34% | 40% | 15% |
| Ⓐ TYSON Premium Dinners: Beef Champignon | 1 pkg | 330 | 22% | 30% | 22% |
| WEIGHT WATCHERS Frozen Entrees | | | | | |
| ❖ Grilled Salisbury Steak | 1 entrée | 250 | 14% | 15% | 10% |
| ❖ Swedish Meatballs | 1 entrée | 280 | 12% | 15% | 10% |

## CHICKEN

**Brand Name Foods**

| FOOD | Serving Size | Calories | Tot Fat | Sat Fat | Chol |
|------|-------------|----------|---------|---------|------|
| ARMOUR CLASSICS—CONAGRA | | | | | |
| Ⓐ Chicken & Noodles | 1 meal | 280 | 14% | 25% | 20% |
| Ⓐ Chicken Mesquite | 1 meal | 280 | 20% | 20% | 22% |
| Ⓐ Chicken w/Wine & Mushrooms | 1 meal | 260 | 17% | 25% | 17% |
| Ⓐ Glazed Chicken | 1 meal | 280 | 22% | 20% | 18% |
| ❖ Lite Chicken Burgundy | 1 meal | 210 | 8% | 8% | 15% |
| ❖ Lite Sweet & Sour Chicken | 1 meal | 220 | 2% | 0% | 10% |
| BANQUET Extra Helping Dinners —CONAGRA | | | | | |
| Ⓐ All White Meat Chicken | 1 meal | 820 | 63% | 45% | 32% |
| Ⓐ Fried Chicken | 1 meal | 790 | 60% | 45% | 37% |
| Ⓐ Southern Fried Chicken | 1 meal | 750 | 57% | 45% | 40% |
| BANQUET Dinners—CONAGRA | | | | | |
| ❖ Barbecue Style Chicken | 1 meal | 320 | 18% | 13% | 20% |
| ❖ Chicken & Dumpling | 1 meal | 260 | 12% | 13% | 12% |
| Ⓐ Chicken Nuggets | 1 meal | 410 | 32% | 25% | 15% |
| Ⓐ Fried Chicken Meal | 1 meal | 470 | 42% | 45% | 35% |
| Ⓐ Southern Fried Meal | 1 meal | 530 | 46% | 40% | 28% |
| Ⓐ White Meat Meal | 1 meal | 470 | 43% | 55% | 33% |
| BANQUET Extra Helping Family Entrées—CONAGRA | | | | | |
| Ⓐ Chicken & Dumplings | 1 cup | 290 | 22% | 25% | 13% |
| ❖ Noodle and Chicken | 1 cup | 210 | 14% | 15% | 13% |

★ Foods with this symbol have less than or equal to 5% *Daily Value* for all three nutrients (5% Rule).
❖ Foods with this symbol have at least one of the three nutrients greater than 5% *Daily Value* but less than or equal to 20% *Daily Value*.
Ⓐ Foods with this symbol have at least one of the three nutrients greater than 20% *Daily Value* (20% Rule).

| FOOD | Serving Size | Calories | Tot Fat | Sat Fat | Chol |
|------|------|------|------|------|------|
| BUDGET GOURMET *Light & Healthy* Dinners—ALL AMERICAN GOURMET | | | | | |
| ❖ Chicken in Mesquite Barbecue Sauce | 11 oz | 280 | 9% | 10% | 13% |
| ✇ Herbed Chicken Breast w/ Fettucini | 11 oz | 300 | 12% | 15% | 22% |
| ❖ Honey Mustard Chicken Breast | 11 oz | 310 | 9% | 8% | 17% |
| ❖ Roast Chicken Breast w/ Herb Gravy | 11 oz | 240 | 11% | 10% | 12% |
| BUDGET GOURMET *Light & Healthy* Entrées—ALL AMERICAN GOURMET | | | | | |
| ✇ Chicken Au Gratin | 9.1 oz | 250 | 12% | 25% | 15% |
| ❖ French Recipe Chicken | 10 oz | 200 | 12% | 15% | 10% |
| ❖ Orange Glazed Chicken Breast | 9 oz | 300 | 3% | 5% | 10% |
| BUDGET GOURMET *Original* Entrées—ALL AMERICAN GOURMET | | | | | |
| ✇ Chicken and Egg Noodles | 10 oz | 410 | 35% | 60% | 37% |
| ✇ Chicken Marsala | 9 oz | 270 | 11% | 20% | 27% |
| ✇ Chicken w/Fettucini | 10 oz | 380 | 29% | 50% | 28% |
| ❖ HEALTHY CHOICE Classics Chicken Francesca—CONAGRA | 1 meal | 360 | 8% | 11% | 10% |
| HEALTHY CHOICE Dinners— CONAGRA | | | | | |
| ❖ Chicken Dijon | 1 meal | 280 | 6% | 8% | 11% |
| ❖ Country Herb Chicken | 1 meal | 270 | 6% | 8% | 12% |
| ❖ Mesquite Chicken BBQ | 1 meal | 320 | 3% | 3% | 12% |
| ❖ Smoky Chicken Barbecue | 1 meal | 380 | 8% | 8% | 17% |
| ❖ Southwestern Glazed Chicken | 1 meal | 300 | 5% | 5% | 15% |
| HEALTHY CHOICE Entrées— CONAGRA | | | | | |
| ❖ Chicken Imperial | 1 meal | 230 | 6% | 5% | 13% |
| ❖ Country Glazed Chicken | 1 meal | 200 | 2% | 3% | 10% |
| ❖ Country Roast Turkey w/ Mushroom | 1 meal | 220 | 6% | 6% | 9% |
| ❖ Honey Mustard Chicken | 1 meal | 260 | 3% | 0% | 10% |
| LUCK'S | | | | | |
| ❖ Chicken & Dumplings | 1 cup | 170 | 3% | 3% | 8% |
| ❖ Chicken & Potatoes | 1 cup | 190 | 6% | 5% | 7% |
| MARIE CALLENDER'S—CONAGRA | | | | | |
| ✇ Escalloped Noodles & Chicken | 1 cup | 270 | 25% | 30% | 7% |
| ✇ Pasta Primavera w/Chicken | 1 cup | 310 | 29% | 40% | 8% |
| ✇ Country Fried Chicken & Gravy | 1 dinner | 610 | 42% | 40% | 18% |
| ✇ Chicken Fried Steak & Gravy | 1 dinner | 650 | 48% | 50% | 17% |
| ✇ Herb Roasted Chicken & Mashed Potatoes | 1 dinner | 670 | 65% | 75% | 68% |

| FOOD | Serving Size | Calories | Tot Fat | Sat Fat | Chol |
|------|--------------|----------|---------|---------|------|
| **SMART ONES**—WEIGHT WATCHERS | | | | | |
| ❖ Honey Mustard Chicken | 1 entrée | 200 | 3% | 3% | 10% |
| ❖ Lemon Herb Chicken Piccata | 1 entrée | 190 | 3% | 3% | 8% |
| STOUFFER'S *Lean Cuisine* Entrees—NESTLÉ | | | | | |
| ❖ Baked Chicken & Whipped Potatoes & Stuffing | 1 pkg | 240 | 8% | 3% | 12% |
| ❖ Chicken & Vegetables | 1 pkg | 240 | 8% | 5% | 12% |
| ❖ Chicken a L'Orange | 1 pkg | 260 | 4% | 3% | 13% |
| ❖ Chicken in Honey Barbecue Sauce | 1 pkg | 250 | 7% | 5% | 17% |
| ❖ Chicken in Peanut Sauce | 1 pkg | 280 | 9% | 5% | 15% |
| ❖ Fiesta Chicken w/Rice & Vegetables | 1 pkg | 240 | 8% | 5% | 15% |
| ❖ Glazed Chicken w/Vegetable Rice | 1 pkg | 240 | 9% | 5% | 20% |
| ❖ Honey Mustard Chicken w/ Vegetable Rice | 1 pkg | 250 | 7% | 5% | 17% |
| ❖ *Lunch Express* Chicken Fettucini w/Broccoli | 1 pkg | 290 | 12% | 18% | 13% |
| STOUFFER'S *Lean Cuisine* Cafe Classics Entrees—NESTLÉ | | | | | |
| ❖ Calypso Chicken | 1 pkg | 280 | 9% | 10% | 13% |
| ❖ Chicken Mediterranean | 1 pkg | 250 | 6% | 5% | 10% |
| ❖ Herb Roasted Chicken | 1 pkg | 210 | 8% | 5% | 13% |
| STOUFFER'S *Lunch Express*— NESTLÉ | | | | | |
| ❖ Chicken w/Garden Vegetables & Rice | 1 pkg | 340 | 17% | 15% | 10% |
| ❖ Chicken w/Linguini | 1 pkg | 300 | 17% | 10% | 13% |
| ❖ Grilled Chicken & Angel Hair Pasta | 1 pkg | 340 | 20% | 15% | 17% |
| STOUFFER'S Entrées—NESTLÉ | | | | | |
| ❖ Chicken a la King | 1 pkg | 320 | 15% | 15% | 18% |
| Ⓐ Creamed Chicken | 1 pkg | 280 | 31% | 35% | 27% |
| Ⓐ Creamy Chicken & Broccoli | 1 pkg | 320 | 23% | 25% | 20% |
| Ⓐ Escalloped Chicken & Noodles | 1 pkg | 440 | 45% | 30% | 27% |
| STOUFFER'S Homestyle Entrées —NESTLÉ | | | | | |
| Ⓐ Baked Chicken & Gravy & Whipped Potatoes | 1 pkg | 270 | 18% | 15% | 25% |
| Ⓐ Breaded Chicken Filets & Potato Rounds | 1 pkg | 380 | 28% | 15% | 17% |
| Ⓐ Chicken & Noodles | 1 pkg | 310 | 22% | 25% | 27% |

★ Foods with this symbol have less than or equal to 5% *Daily Value* for all three nutrients (5% Rule).

❖ Foods with this symbol have at least one of the three nutrients greater than 5% *Daily Value* but less than or equal to 20% *Daily Value*.

Ⓐ Foods with this symbol have at least one of the three nutrients greater than 20% *Daily Value* (20% Rule).

| FOOD | Serving Size | Calories | Tot Fat | Sat Fat | Chol |
|---|---|---|---|---|---|
| ⊛ Fried Chicken & Whipped Potatoes | 1 pkg | 330 | 25% | 20% | 18% |
| ⊛ SWANSON *Budget Meals* Fried Chicken (dark portion)— CAMPBELL'S | 1 pkg | 420 | 34% | 40% | 33% |
| SWANSON *Hungry Man* Dinners —CAMPBELL'S | | | | | |
| ⊛ Boneless Chicken | 1 pkg | 700 | 43% | 55% | 35% |
| ⊛ Fried Chicken (dark portions) | 1 pkg | 810 | 63% | 70% | 40% |
| ⊛ Fried Chicken (mostly white meat) | 1 pkg | 810 | 62% | 70% | 40% |
| ⊛ Grilled Chicken Patties | 1 pkg | 580 | 29% | 40% | 30% |
| SWANSON Complete Dinners —CAMPBELL'S | | | | | |
| ⊛ Chicken Nuggets | 1 pkg | 450 | 32% | 35% | 12% |
| ❖ Chicken Tenders Platter | 1 pkg | 320 | 18% | 15% | 8% |
| ⊛ Fried Chicken (dark portion) | 1 pkg | 560 | 43% | 55% | 20% |
| ⊛ Fried Chicken (white portion) | 1 pkg | 550 | 40% | 55% | 20% |
| ❖ Grilled Chicken White Meat in Garlic Sauce | 1 pkg | 270 | 11% | 15% | 10% |
| SWANSON Homestyle Entrées— CAMPBELL'S | | | | | |
| ⊛ Chicken & Noodles w/ Vegetables in Cream Sauce | 1 pkg | 320 | 23% | 40% | 17% |
| ⊛ Chicken Nibbles | 1 pkg | 340 | 31% | 45% | 30% |
| ⊛ Deluxe Chicken Pie | 1 pkg | 410 | 34% | 40% | 15% |
| ⊛ Fried Chicken & Whipped Potatoes | 1 pkg | 400 | 32% | 40% | 27% |
| TAJ Entrees | | | | | |
| ⊛ Chicken Curry w/Brown Rice | 1 pkg | 330 | 14% | 10% | 30% |
| ⊛ Chicken Masala w/Brown Rice | 1 pkg | 330 | 14% | 14% | 32% |
| TYSON | | | | | |
| ❖ Grilled Mesquite Chicken Breast | 1 patty | 110 | 9% | 5% | 13% |
| ⊛ Stuffed Chicken Cordon Bleu | 1 pc | 390 | 28% | 30% | 30% |
| TYSON *Healthy Portion* Meals | | | | | |
| ❖ BBQ Chicken | 1 pkg | 420 | 14% | 13% | 18% |
| ❖ Herb Chicken | 1 pkg | 450 | 5% | 5% | 20% |
| ❖ Honey Mustard Chicken | 1 pkg | 400 | 5% | 5% | 18% |
| ❖ Mesquite Chicken | 1 pkg | 430 | 15% | 10% | 20% |
| TYSON Premium Dinners | | | | | |
| ❖ Blackened Chicken | 1 pkg | 270 | 8% | 5% | 15% |
| ❖ Chicken Francais | 1 pkg | 260 | 15% | 15% | 15% |
| ❖ Chicken Mesquite | 1 pkg | 310 | 12% | 15% | 20% |
| ❖ Chicken Supreme | 1 pkg | 260 | 14% | 13% | 17% |
| ❖ Chicken w/Broccoli & Cheese | 1 pkg | 230 | 9% | 10% | 13% |
| ❖ Glazed Chicken Tenders w/ Rice Pilaf | 1 pkg | 270 | 9% | 5% | 18% |
| ❖ Grilled Chicken | 1 pkg | 220 | 5% | 5% | 17% |
| ❖ Honey Roasted Chicken | 1 pkg | 220 | 6% | 5% | 18% |

| FOOD | Serving Size | Calories | Tot Fat | Sat Fat | Chol |
|------|--------------|----------|---------|---------|------|
| **WEIGHT WATCHERS** | | | | | |
| ❖ Barbecue Glazed Chicken | 1 entrée | 190 | 5% | 5% | 7% |
| ❖ Chicken Cordon Bleu | 1 entrée | 220 | 9% | 10% | 7% |
| ❖ Roast Glazed Chicken | 1 entrée | 200 | 8% | 13% | 5% |
| Ⓐ Southern Fried Chicken | 1 entrée | 280 | 17% | 23% | 22% |

## CHILI

**Brand Name Foods**

| | | | | | |
|------|--------------|----------|---------|---------|------|
| MARIE CALLENDER'S—CONAGRA | | | | | |
| Ⓐ Chili & Cornbread | 1 cup + 1/2 oz bread | 350 | 20% | 30% | 10% |
| ❖ Chili w/Beans | 1 pkg | 270 | 15% | 20% | 12% |
| ❖ *Lean Cuisine* Three Bean Chili w/Rice | 1 pkg | 210 | 9% | 10% | 3% |

## FISH AND SEAFOOD

**Brand Name Foods**

| | | | | | |
|------|--------------|----------|---------|---------|------|
| ❖ ARMOUR CLASSICS Lite Shrimp Creole—CONAGRA | 1 meal | 220 | 1% | 0% | 7% |
| ❖ BUDGET GOURMET *Light & Healthy* Dinners Shrimp Mariner—ALL AMERICAN GOURMET | 11 oz | 260 | 9% | 10% | 20% |
| HEALTHY CHOICE—CONAGRA | | | | | |
| ❖ Classics Shrimp and Vegetables Maria | 1 meal | 270 | 5% | 5% | 12% |
| ❖ Lemon Pepper Fish | 1 meal | 290 | 7% | 6% | 9% |
| ❖ MARIE CALLENDER'S Breaded Shrimp over Angel Hair Pasta | 1 cup | 300 | 18% | 10% | 10% |
| Ⓐ PEPPERIDGE FARM *Meal Kits* Shrimp Newburg—CAMPBELL'S | 1 filled | 340 | 31% | 35% | 20% |
| ❖ SMART ONES Shrimp Marinara —WEIGHT WATCHERS | 1 entrée | 190 | 3% | 3% | 13% |
| STOUFFER'S *Lean Cuisine* Entrées—NESTLÉ | | | | | |
| Ⓐ Fish Divan | 1 pkg | 210 | 9% | 5% | 22% |
| ❖ *Lunch Express* Pasta & Tuna Casserole | 1 pkg | 280 | 9% | 10% | 7% |
| STOUFFER'S Entrées—NESTLÉ | | | | | |
| Ⓐ Homestyle Fish Fillet w/ Macaroni & Cheese | 1 pkg | 430 | 32% | 25% | 23% |

★ Foods with this symbol have less than or equal to 5% *Daily Value* for <u>all</u> three nutrients (5% Rule).

❖ Foods with this symbol have <u>at least one</u> of the three nutrients greater than 5% *Daily Value* but less than or equal to 20% *Daily Value*.

Ⓐ Foods with this symbol have <u>at least one</u> of the three nutrients greater than 20% *Daily Value* (20% Rule).

| FOOD | Serving Size | Calories | Tot Fat | Sat Fat | Chol |
|------|--------------|----------|---------|---------|------|
| ✺ Tuna Noodle Casserole | 1 pkg | 330 | 22% | 10% | 13% |
| SWANSON—CAMPBELL'S | | | | | |
| ✺ *Budget Meals* Breaded Fish Sticks | 1 pkg | 370 | 20% | 30% | 8% |
| ✺ Complete Dinners:  Fish 'n Chips | 1 pkg | 480 | 31% | 20% | 15% |
| ✺ Homestyle Entrée:  Fish 'n Chips | 1 pkg | 310 | 18% | 25% | 12% |
| ❖ TYSON Crab Delights Stir Fry Kit | 1 cup | 240 | 11% | 10% | 5% |
| ❖ WEIGHT WATCHERS Frozen Entrées:  Fried Fillet of Fish | 1 entrée | 230 | 12% | 13% | 8% |

## HAM AND PORK

**Brand Name Foods**

| FOOD | Serving Size | Calories | Tot Fat | Sat Fat | Chol |
|------|--------------|----------|---------|---------|------|
| ✺ BUDGET GOURMET *Light & Healthy* Entrées:  Ham and Asparagus Au Gratin—ALL AMERICAN GOURMET | 8.7 oz | 290 | 20% | 25% | 17% |
| ✺ STOUFFER'S Entrées:  Ham & Asparagus Bake—NESTLÉ | 1 pkg | 520 | 55% | 70% | 25% |
| SWANSON—CAMPBELL'S | | | | | |
| ✺ Complete Dinners:  Rib Shaped Pork Patty | 1 pkg | 510 | 35% | 40% | 17% |
| ✺ Homestyle Entrée:  Scalloped Potatoes & Ham | 1 pkg | 290 | 18% | 40% | 15% |

## ITALIAN

*Beef*
**Brand Name Foods**

| FOOD | Serving Size | Calories | Tot Fat | Sat Fat | Chol |
|------|--------------|----------|---------|---------|------|
| ✺ ARMOUR CLASSICS Veal Parmigiana—CONAGRA | 1 meal | 400 | 34% | 55% | 22% |
| BANQUET—CONAGRA | | | | | |
| ✺ Dinners:  Veal Parmigiana | 1 meal | 320 | 22% | 25% | 8% |
| ✺ *Extra Helping* Family Entrées:  Veal Parmigiana | 1 patty w/ sauce | 230 | 22% | 20% | 7% |
| ❖ MORTON Dinners:  Veal Parmesan —CONAGRA | 1 meal | 280 | 20% | 20% | 7% |
| ✺ STOUFFER'S Entrées:  Homestyle Veal Parmigiana w/Spaghetti —NESTLÉ | 1 pkg | 420 | 29% | 20% | 25% |
| SWANSON—CAMPBELL'S | | | | | |
| ✺ Complete Dinners:  Veal Parmigiana | 1 pkg | 400 | 28% | 40% | 28% |
| ✺ Homestyle Entrée:  Veal Parmigiana | 1 pkg | 310 | 18% | 25% | 20% |
| ✺ *Hungry Man* Dinners:  Veal Parmigiana | 1 pkg | 590 | 38% | 70% | 32% |

| FOOD | Serving Size | Calories | Tot Fat | Sat Fat | Chol |
|------|-------------|----------|---------|---------|------|

### Chicken
### Brand Name Foods

ARMOUR CLASSICS—CONAGRA

| FOOD | Serving Size | Calories | Tot Fat | Sat Fat | Chol |
|------|-------------|----------|---------|---------|------|
| ❖ Chicken Fettucini | 1 meal | 230 | 12% | 20% | 8% |
| ⊛ Chicken Parmigiana | 1 meal | 360 | 28% | 30% | 15% |
| BANQUET—CONAGRA | | | | | |
| ⊛ Dinners: Chicken Parmigiana | 1 meal | 290 | 23% | 20% | 17% |
| ⊛ *Extra Helping* Dinners: Chicken Parmesan | 1 meal | 650 | 51% | 40% | 22% |
| ⊛ *Extra Helping* Family Entrées: Chicken Parmesan | 1 patty w/ gravy | 240 | 20% | 25% | 7% |
| BUDGET GOURMET— ALL AMERICAN GOURMET | | | | | |
| ❖ *Light & Healthy* Dinners: Chicken Parmigiana | 11 oz | 300 | 15% | 15% | 15% |
| ❖ *Light & Healthy Special Selections:* Italian Style Vegetables & Chicken | 10 oz | 280 | 11% | 10% | 8% |
| ❖ HEALTHY CHOICE Classics: Cacciatore Chicken—CONAGRA | 1 meal | 260 | 4% | 3% | 8% |
| HEALTHY CHOICE Dinners —CONAGRA | | | | | |
| ❖ Chicken Broccoli Alfredo | 1 meal | 370 | 12% | 15% | 15% |
| ❖ Chicken Parmigiana | 1 meal | 300 | 6% | 10% | 12% |
| HEALTHY CHOICE Entrées— CONAGRA | | | | | |
| ❖ Chicken and Vegetables Marsala | 1 meal | 220 | 2% | 0% | 10% |
| ❖ Chicken Fettuccini Alfredo | 1 meal | 260 | 7% | 10% | 13% |
| ❖ Garlic Chicken Milano | 1 meal | 240 | 6% | 10% | 12% |
| ⊛ MARIE CALLENDER'S Breaded Chicken Parmigiana | 1 dinner | 620 | 42% | 40% | 17% |
| SMART ONES—WEIGHT WATCHERS | | | | | |
| ❖ Chicken Marsala | 1 entrée | 150 | 3% | 3% | 8% |
| ❖ Chicken Mirabella | 1 entrée | 170 | 3% | 3% | 7% |
| STOUFFER'S *Lean Cuisine* Entrées—NESTLÉ | | | | | |
| ❖ Chicken Italiano w/Fettucini & Vegetables | 1 pkg | 270 | 9% | 8% | 13% |
| ❖ Chicken Marsala & Vegetables | 1 pkg | 180 | 6% | 5% | 20% |
| ❖ *Lunch Express* Pasta & Chicken Marinara | 1 pkg | 270 | 9% | 8% | 7% |

★ Foods with this symbol have less than or equal to 5% *Daily Value* for <u>all</u> three nutrients (5% Rule).
❖ Foods with this symbol have <u>at least one</u> of the three nutrients greater than 5% *Daily Value* but less than or equal to 20% *Daily Value.*
⊛ Foods with this symbol have <u>at least one</u> of the three nutrients greater than 20% *Daily Value* (20% Rule).

| FOOD | Serving Size | Calories | Tot Fat | Sat Fat | Chol |
|------|-------------|----------|---------|---------|------|
| STOUFFER'S *Lean Cuisine* Cafe Classics Entrées—NESTLÉ | | | | | |
| ❖ Cheese Lasagna w/Chicken Scaloppini | 1 pkg | 290 | 12% | 13% | 13% |
| ❖ Chicken Carbonara | 1 pkg | 290 | 12% | 10% | 13% |
| ❖ Chicken Piccata | 1 pkg | 290 | 9% | 8% | 10% |
| STOUFFER'S Entrées—NESTLÉ | | | | | |
| Ⓐ Homestyle Chicken Parmigiana w/Spaghetti | 1 pkg | 320 | 15% | 10% | 25% |
| Ⓐ *Lunch Express* Chicken Alfredo | 1 pkg | 360 | 26% | 30% | 20% |
| SWANSON—CAMPBELL'S | | | | | |
| Ⓐ *Budget Meals* Chicken Parmigiana | 1 pkg | 340 | 28% | 40% | 13% |
| Ⓐ Complete Dinners: Chicken Parmigiana | 1 pkg | 400 | 29% | 35% | 12% |
| TYSON *Healthy Portion* Meals | | | | | |
| Ⓐ Chicken Marinara | 1 pkg | 420 | 8% | 5% | 23% |
| ❖ Italian Style Chicken | 1 pkg | 385 | 6% | 5% | 18% |
| TYSON Premium Dinners | | | | | |
| ❖ Chicken Marsala | 1 pkg | 180 | 6% | 5% | 15% |
| ❖ Chicken Parmigiana | 1 pkg | 290 | 17% | 10% | 7% |
| ❖ Chicken Picatta | 1 pkg | 190 | 5% | 5% | 17% |
| ❖ Grilled Italian Chicken w/ Herb Glaze | 1 pkg | 190 | 5% | 5% | 15% |
| ❖ WEIGHT WATCHERS Chicken Parmigiana | 1 entrée | 230 | 9% | 15% | 17% |

## Other
### Brand Name Foods

| FOOD | Serving Size | Calories | Tot Fat | Sat Fat | Chol |
|------|-------------|----------|---------|---------|------|
| Ⓐ BUDGET GOURMET *Original Entrées* Linguini w/Bay Shrimp & Clams Marinara—ALL AMERICAN GOURMET | 10 oz | 300 | 17% | 30% | 18% |
| HEALTHY CHOICE Dinners | | | | | |
| ❖ Classics Turkey Fettuccine alla Crema | 1 meal | 350 | 6% | 8% | 10% |
| ❖ Shrimp Marinara | 1 meal | 220 | 1% | 0% | 17% |

## MEXICAN

### Generic Foods

| FOOD | Serving Size | Calories | Tot Fat | Sat Fat | Chol |
|------|-------------|----------|---------|---------|------|
| Ⓐ Taco | 1 taco | 370 | 32% | 57% | 19% |
| Ⓐ Tostada w/Guacamole | 1 tostada | 180 | 18% | 25% | 7% |

### Brand Name Foods

| FOOD | Serving Size | Calories | Tot Fat | Sat Fat | Chol |
|------|-------------|----------|---------|---------|------|
| BANQUET Dinners—CONAGRA | | | | | |
| Ⓐ Chimichanga Meal | 1 meal | 470 | 35% | 35% | 5% |

| FOOD | Serving Size | Calories | Tot Fat | Sat Fat | Chol |
|---|---|---|---|---|---|
| ⊛ *Extra Helpin'* Mexican Style | 1 meal | 820 | 52% | 70% | 17% |
| ⊛ Mexican Combo Meal | 1 meal | 380 | 17% | 25% | 5% |
| ⊛ Mexican Style Meal | 1 meal | 400 | 20% | 25% | 5% |
| GEBHARDT Tamales—HUNT WESSON | | | | | |
| ⊛ Jumbo Tamales | 2 tamales | 330 | 39% | 58% | 11% |
| ⊛ Tamales | 2 tamales | 270 | 32% | 48% | 9% |
| ❖ HAIN Vegetarian Classics: | | | | | |
| Mexican Style Taco | 1 pkg | 420 | 14% | 5% | 0% |
| ❖ MORTON Dinners: Mexican— | | | | | |
| CONAGRA | 1 meal | 260 | 11% | 15% | 2% |
| PATIO Dinners—CONAGRA | | | | | |
| ❖ Fiesta | 1 meal | 340 | 14% | 20% | 5% |
| ⊛ Mexican | 1 meal | 440 | 23% | 30% | 7% |
| ⊛ Ranchera | 1 meal | 410 | 23% | 30% | 8% |
| SWANSON—CAMPBELL'S | | | | | |
| ⊛ *Budget Meals* Mexican Style | 1 pkg | 400 | 25% | 35% | 7% |
| ⊛ Complete Dinners: Mexican | | | | | |
| Style Combination | 1 pkg | 480 | 29% | 65% | 10% |
| ⊛ *Hungry Man* Dinners: Mexican | | | | | |
| Style | 1 pkg | 780 | 55% | 80% | 20% |

### *Beef*

### Generic Foods

| | | | | | |
|---|---|---|---|---|---|
| ⊛ Beef Chimichanga | 1 chimichanga | 430 | 30% | 43% | 3% |
| ❖ Beef Fajita | 1 cup | 240 | 16% | 19% | 9% |

### Brand Name Foods

| | | | | | |
|---|---|---|---|---|---|
| ⊛ OLD EL PASO Beef Chimichanga | | | | | |
| —PET | 1 each | 370 | 31% | 27% | 3% |
| ⊛ PATIO Dinners: Salisbury Con | | | | | |
| Queso—CONAGRA | 1 meal | 390 | 3% | 55% | 13% |
| ❖ TYSON Complete Kits: Beef | | | | | |
| Fajita Kit | 1 fajita | 150 | 6% | 5% | 7% |

### *Burritos*

### Generic Foods

| | | | | | |
|---|---|---|---|---|---|
| ⊛ Beans & Cheese Burrito | 2 burritos | 380 | 18% | 34% | 9% |
| ⊛ Beef, Cheese, & Bean Enchirito | 1 enchirito | 340 | 25% | 40% | 16% |

★ Foods with this symbol have less than or equal to 5% *Daily Value* for <u>all</u> three nutrients (5% Rule).
❖ Foods with this symbol have <u>at least one</u> of the three nutrients greater than 5% *Daily Value* but less than or equal to 20% *Daily Value*.
⊛ Foods with this symbol have <u>at least one</u> of the three nutrients greater than 20% *Daily Value* (20% Rule).

| FOOD | Serving Size | Calories | Tot Fat | Sat Fat | Chol |
|---|---|---|---|---|---|
| **Brand Name Foods** | | | | | |
| HEALTHY CHOICE Beef Burrito Ranchero Entrées—CONAGRA | | | | | |
| ❖ Medium Spice | 1 burrito | 290 | 11% | 12% | 5% |
| ❖ Mild Spice | 1 burrito | 300 | 11% | 12% | 4% |
| OLD EL PASO Burritos—PET | | | | | |
| ◑ Bean & Cheese Burrito | 1 burrito | 290 | 13% | 22% | 5% |
| ❖ Beef & Bean Burrito: Hot | 1 burrito | 320 | 15% | 20% | 4% |
| ❖ Beef & Bean Burrito: Medium | 1 burrito | 320 | 16% | 20% | 6% |
| ❖ Beef & Bean Burrito: Mild | 1 burrito | 330 | 14% | 17% | 5% |
| ❖ Pizza Burrito: Cheese | 1 burrito | 320 | 14% | 20% | 6% |
| ◑ Pizza Burrito: Pepperoni | 1 burrito | 260 | 16% | 24% | 7% |
| ❖ Pizza Burrito: Sausage | 1 burrito | 260 | 14% | 18% | 5% |
| PATIO *Britos*—CONAGRA | | | | | |
| ◑ Beef & Bean | 10 britos | 420 | 29% | 35% | 7% |
| ◑ Nacho Beef | 10 britos | 410 | 28% | 90% | 7% |
| ❖ Nacho Cheese | 10 britos | 360 | 20% | 20% | 5% |
| ◑ Spicy Chicken | 10 britos | 400 | 25% | 20% | 8% |
| PATIO Burritos—CONAGRA | | | | | |
| ❖ Beef & Bean | 1 burrito | 280 | 11% | 15% | 5% |
| ❖ Beef & Bean Cheese | 1 burrito | 270 | 8% | 13% | 2% |
| ❖ Beef & Bean Green Chili | 1 burrito | 260 | 8% | 8% | 3% |
| ❖ Beef & Bean Red Chili | 1 burrito | 260 | 8% | 10% | 3% |
| ❖ Chicken | 1 burrito | 260 | 6% | 8% | 5% |
| ❖ Red Chili | 1 burrito | 270 | 9% | 10% | 3% |
| SWANSON Burritos—CAMPBELL'S | | | | | |
| ❖ Ham & Cheese | 1 pkg | 210 | 9% | 10% | 20% |
| ❖ Hot & Spicy | 1 pkg | 220 | 11% | 15% | 18% |
| ❖ Pizza w/Cheese & Pepperoni | 1 pkg | 240 | 14% | 15% | 20% |
| ***Chicken*** | | | | | |
| **Generic Foods** | | | | | |
| ★ Chicken Fajita | 1 cup | 170 | 4% | 4% | 4% |
| **Brand Name Foods** | | | | | |
| ❖ HEALTHY CHOICE Dinners: Chicken Picante—CONAGRA | 1 meal | 220 | 3% | 7% | 11% |
| HEALTHY CHOICE Entrées —CONAGRA | | | | | |
| ❖ Chicken Con Queso Burrito | 1 burrito | 280 | 10% | 9% | 4% |
| ❖ Fiesta Chicken Fajitas | 1 meal | 260 | 6% | 6% | 11% |
| ◑ OLD EL PASO Chicken Chimichanga—PET | 1 chimichanga | 350 | 25% | 21% | 7% |
| ❖ SMART ONES Fiesta Chicken— WEIGHT WATCHERS | 1 entrée | 220 | 3% | 3% | 8% |

| FOOD | Serving Size | Calories | Tot Fat | Sat Fat | Chol |
|---|---|---|---|---|---|
| STOUFFER'S Entrées—NESTLÉ | | | | | |
| ⊛   Homestyle Chicken Monterey w/Mexican-Style Rice | 1 pkg | 410 | 31% | 45% | 25% |
| ❖   *Lunch Express* Mexican-Style Chicken & Rice | 1 pkg | 280 | 12% | 5% | 13% |
| STOUFFER'S *Lean Cuisine* Entrées—NESTLÉ | | | | | |
| ❖   Cafe Classics Grilled Chicken Salsa | 1 pkg | 240 | 9% | 8% | 13% |
| ❖   *Lunch Express* Mexican-Style Rice w/Chicken | 1 pkg | 270 | 12% | 8% | 7% |
| ❖ TYSON Complete Kits: Chicken Fajita Kit | 1 fajita | 150 | 6% | 5% | 7% |
| ❖ WEIGHT WATCHERS Tex-Mex Chicken | 1 entrée | 260 | 6% | 8% | 12% |

### *Enchiladas*
### Generic Foods

| | | | | | |
|---|---|---|---|---|---|
| ⊛ Cheese Enchilada | 1 enchilada | 320 | 29% | 53% | 15% |

### Brand Name Foods

| | | | | | |
|---|---|---|---|---|---|
| BANQUET Dinners—CONAGRA | | | | | |
| ⊛   Beef Enchilada | 1 meal | 380 | 18% | 25% | 5% |
| ❖   Cheese Enchilada | 1 meal | 340 | 9% | 13% | 5% |
| ❖   Chicken Enchilada | 1 meal | 360 | 15% | 15% | 7% |
| ❖ BANQUET *Extra Helping* Family Entrées: Beef Enchilada w/ Cheese—CONAGRA | 1 enchilada w/cheese | 130 | 6% | 8% | 2% |
| ⊛ GEBHARDT Enchiladas— HUNT WESSON | 2 enchiladas | 260 | 29% | 45% | 8% |
| HEALTHY CHOICE Dinners— CONAGRA | | | | | |
| ❖   Beef Enchiladas Rio Grande | 1 meal | 410 | 13% | 17% | 5% |
| ⊛   Chicken Enchilada Suprema | 1 meal | 390 | 14% | 23% | 10% |
| ❖ HEALTHY CHOICE Chicken Enchiladas Suiza Entrée— CONAGRA | 1 meal | 270 | 7% | 10% | 8% |
| PATIO Dinners—CONAGRA | | | | | |
| ❖   Beef Enchilada | 1 meal | 350 | 15% | 20% | 5% |
| ❖   Cheese Enchilada | 1 meal | 330 | 12% | 15% | 5% |
| ❖   Chicken Enchilada | 1 meal | 380 | 14% | 15% | 8% |

★   Foods with this symbol have less than or equal to 5% *Daily Value* for all three nutrients (5% Rule).

❖   Foods with this symbol have at least one of the three nutrients greater than 5% *Daily Value* but less than or equal to 20% *Daily Value*.

⊛   Foods with this symbol have at least one of the three nutrients greater than 20% *Daily Value* (20% Rule).

| FOOD | Serving Size | Calories | Tot Fat | Sat Fat | Chol |
|------|--------------|----------|---------|---------|------|
| PATIO Family Entrées—CONAGRA | | | | | |
| ❖ Beef & Cheese Enchilada (15.5 oz) | 2 enchiladas w/sauce | 250 | 9% | 13% | 7% |
| ❖ Beef Enchilada (15.5 oz) | 2 enchiladas w/sauce | 200 | 9% | 15% | 5% |
| ❖ Cheese Enchilada (6 oz) | 2 enchiladas w/sauce | 170 | 6% | 10% | 3% |
| STOUFFER'S Entrées—NESTLÉ | | | | | |
| Ⓐ Cheese Enchilada & Mexican-Style Rice | 1 pkg | 370 | 22% | 25% | 8% |
| ❖ *Lean Cuisine* Chicken Enchilada Suiza w/Mexican-Style Rice | 1 pkg | 290 | 8% | 10% | 8% |
| Ⓐ SWANSON Complete Dinners: Beef Enchilada—CAMPBELL'S | 1 pkg | 480 | 32% | 60% | 13% |
| WEIGHT WATCHERS | | | | | |
| ❖ Chicken Enchiladas Suiza | 1 entrée | 250 | 12% | 15% | 8% |
| ❖ Nacho Grande Chicken Enchiladas | 1 entrée | 290 | 12% | 13% | 7% |

ORIENTAL

**Brand Name Foods**

| FOOD | Serving Size | Calories | Tot Fat | Sat Fat | Chol |
|------|--------------|----------|---------|---------|------|
| CREATE A MEAL! Vegetables (prep w/lean meat and oil as dir)—GREEN GIANT | | | | | |
| ❖ Broccoli Stir Fry | 1 1/3 cups | 290 | 20% | 15% | 20% |
| Ⓐ LoMein Stir Fry | 1 1/3 cups | 320 | 11% | 5% | 22% |
| ❖ Sweet & Sour Stir Fry | 1 1/4 cups | 290 | 11% | 5% | 20% |
| Ⓐ Szechuan Stir Fry | 1 1/4 cups | 320 | 22% | 15% | 20% |
| ❖ Teriyaki Stir Fry | 1 1/4 cups | 240 | 9% | 5% | 18% |
| Ⓐ Vegetable Almond Stir Fry | 1 1/3 cups | 320 | 17% | 8% | 22% |
| ❖ STOUFFER'S *Lean Cuisine Lunch Express* Teriyaki Stir-Fry—NESTLÉ | 1 pkg | 260 | 8% | 5% | 10% |

*Beef*
**Brand Name Foods**

| FOOD | Serving Size | Calories | Tot Fat | Sat Fat | Chol |
|------|--------------|----------|---------|---------|------|
| BUDGET GOURMET *Light & Healthy Dinners*—ALL AMERICAN GOURMET | | | | | |
| ❖ Oriental Beef | 1 pkg | 270 | 12% | 20% | 12% |
| ❖ Teriyaki Beef | 1 pkg | 310 | 9% | 10% | 15% |
| ❖ BUDGET GOURMET *Original Entrées* Beef Cantonese—ALL AMERICAN GOURMET | 1 pkg | 280 | 12% | 15% | 10% |

| FOOD | Serving Size | Calories | Tot Fat | Sat Fat | Chol |
|------|------|------|------|------|------|
| ❖ CHUN KING MEALS Beef Pepper Steak—CONAGRA | 1 meal | 300 | 6% | 5% | 3% |
| HEALTHY CHOICE | | | | | |
| ❖ Classics: Beef Broccoli Beijing | 1 meal | 330 | 5% | 4% | 6% |
| ❖ Dinners: Beef & Peppers Cantonese | 1 meal | 270 | 8% | 11% | 12% |
| ❖ Entrées: Beef Pepper Steak Oriental | 1 meal | 250 | 6% | 7% | 11% |
| ❖ STOUFFER'S *Lean Cuisine* Entrées: Oriental Beef—NESTLÉ | 1 pkg | 250 | 12% | 15% | 10% |
| ❖ STOUFFER'S *Lunch Express* Oriental Beef—NESTLÉ | 1 pkg | 260 | 12% | 8% | 7% |
| ❖ TYSON Complete Kits: Beef Stir Fry Kit—TYSON FOODS | 1 cup | 150 | 5% | 5% | 10% |

## *Chicken*
## Brand Name Foods

| FOOD | Serving Size | Calories | Tot Fat | Sat Fat | Chol |
|------|------|------|------|------|------|
| BANQUET Dinners—CONAGRA | | | | | |
| ❖ Chicken Chow Mein | 1 meal | 210 | 11% | 10% | 10% |
| ❖ Oriental Style Chicken | 1 meal | 260 | 14% | 13% | 13% |
| BUDGET GOURMET *Light & Healthy*—ALL AMERICAN GOURMET | | | | | |
| ❖ Dinners: Teriyaki Chicken Breast w/Oriental Style Vegetables | 1 pkg | 290 | 9% | 5% | 12% |
| ❖ Entrées: Chicken Oriental | 1 pkg | 300 | 9% | 10% | 7% |
| ❖ Entrées: Mandarin Chicken | 1 pkg | 250 | 8% | 5% | 15% |
| ❖ *Special Selections:* Chinese Style Vegetables & Chicken | 1 pkg | 290 | 14% | 8% | 5% |
| BUDGET GOURMET *Original*—ALL AMERICAN GOURMET | | | | | |
| ❖ Entrées: Sweet and Sour Chicken | 1 pkg | 330 | 8% | 5% | 13% |
| ❖ *Special Selections* Spicy Szechwan Style Vegetables & Chicken | 1 pkg | 300 | 14% | 8% | 3% |
| CHUN KING MEALS—CONAGRA | | | | | |
| Ⓐ Chix Chow Mein | 1 meal | 370 | 22% | 25% | 15% |
| ❖ Fried Rice w/Chicken | 1 meal | 270 | 9% | 8% | 8% |
| ❖ Imperial Chicken | 1 meal | 460 | 15% | 15% | 8% |
| Ⓐ Walnut Chicken | 1 meal | 460 | 29% | 25% | 12% |

★ Foods with this symbol have less than or equal to 5% *Daily Value* for all three nutrients (5% Rule).
❖ Foods with this symbol have at least one of the three nutrients greater than 5% *Daily Value* but less than or equal to 20% *Daily Value*.
Ⓐ Foods with this symbol have at least one of the three nutrients greater than 20% *Daily Value* (20% Rule).

| FOOD | Serving Size | Calories | Tot Fat | Sat Fat | Chol |
|---|---|---|---|---|---|
| HEALTHY CHOICE Classics—CONAGRA | | | | | |
| ❖ Ginger Chicken Hunan | 1 meal | 350 | 4% | 3% | 8% |
| ❖ Sesame Chicken Shanghai | 1 meal | 310 | 8% | 5% | 10% |
| HEALTHY CHOICE Dinners—CONAGRA | | | | | |
| ❖ Chicken Cantonese | 1 meal | 210 | 1% | 0% | 10% |
| ❖ Chicken Teriyaki | 1 meal | 270 | 3% | 3% | 13% |
| ❖ Sweet & Sour Chicken | 1 meal | 310 | 8% | 5% | 17% |
| HEALTHY CHOICE Entrées—CONAGRA | | | | | |
| ❖ Chicken Bangkok | 1 meal | 270 | 6% | 3% | 15% |
| ❖ Mandarin Chicken | 1 meal | 280 | 4% | 2% | 8% |
| ❖ Sesame Chicken | 1 meal | 240 | 5% | 3% | 10% |
| ❖ SMART ONES Chicken Chow Mein—WEIGHT WATCHERS | 1 entrée | 200 | 3% | 3% | 8% |
| STOUFFER'S Lean Cuisine Entrées—NESTLÉ | | | | | |
| ❖ Chicken Chow Mein w/Rice | 1 pkg | 210 | 8% | 5% | 12% |
| ❖ Chicken Oriental w/Vegetables & Vermicelli | 1 pkg | 260 | 9% | 5% | 15% |
| ❖ Lunch Express Mandarin Chicken | 1 pkg | 270 | 9% | 5% | 10% |
| ❖ Lunch Express Rice & Chicken Stir-Fry | 1 pkg | 280 | 14% | 5% | 5% |
| ❖ Sweet & Sour Chicken w/ Vegetables & Rice | 1 pkg | 260 | 4% | 5% | 15% |
| STOUFFER'S Lunch Express —NESTLÉ | | | | | |
| ❖ Chicken Chow Mein w/Rice | 1 pkg | 260 | 6% | 5% | 10% |
| ❖ Chicken Oriental | 1 pkg | 320 | 14% | 8% | 13% |
| TYSON Complete Kits | | | | | |
| ❖ Chicken Stir Fry Kit | 1 cup | 150 | 3% | 3% | 10% |
| ❖ Sweet & Sour Chicken | 1 cup | 200 | 6% | 5% | 15% |
| ⊛ TYSON Premium Dinners: Chicken Sweet & Sour | 1 pkg | 350 | 23% | 15% | 17% |

### Egg Rolls

### Brand Name Foods

| | | | | | |
|---|---|---|---|---|---|
| CHUN KING Mini Egg Rolls—CONAGRA | | | | | |
| ❖ Chicken | 6 egg rolls | 210 | 11% | 8% | 3% |
| ❖ Pork & Shrimp | 6 egg rolls | 220 | 12% | 10% | 3% |
| ❖ Shrimp | 6 egg rolls | 190 | 9% | 5% | 3% |
| CHUN KING Restaurant Style Egg Rolls—CONAGRA | | | | | |
| ❖ Chicken | 1 egg roll | 170 | 8% | 13% | 3% |
| ❖ Pork | 1 egg roll | 170 | 9% | 8% | 2% |

| FOOD | Serving Size | Calories | Tot Fat | Sat Fat | Chol |
|---|---|---|---|---|---|
| ❖ Shrimp | 1 egg roll | 150 | 6% | 3% | 3% |
| LACHOY Egg Rolls—CONAGRA | | | | | |
| ❖ Lobster | 7 egg rolls | 210 | 9% | 5% | 0% |
| ❖ Meat & Shrimp | 15 pcs | 240 | 14% | 10% | 3% |
| ❖ Mini Egg Rolls: Chicken | 7 egg rolls | 220 | 9% | 8% | 2% |
| ❖ Mini Egg Rolls: Pork & Shrimp | 7 egg rolls | 220 | 9% | 8% | 3% |
| ❖ Mini Egg Rolls: Shrimp | 7 egg rolls | 210 | 6% | 5% | 2% |
| LA CHOY Restaurant Style Egg Rolls—CONAGRA | | | | | |
| ❖ Chicken | 1 egg roll | 170 | 8% | 13% | 3% |
| ❖ Moo Shu Pork | 1 egg roll | 190 | 11% | 8% | 5% |
| ❖ Pork | 1 egg roll | 170 | 9% | 8% | 2% |
| ❖ Shrimp | 1 egg roll | 150 | 6% | 3% | 3% |
| ❖ Sweet & Sour | 1 egg roll | 180 | 6% | 5% | 2% |
| ❖ WORTHINGTON Vegetarian Egg Rolls | 1 egg roll | 180 | 12% | 8% | 0% |

### *Ham and Pork*

**Brand Name Foods**

| | | | | | |
|---|---|---|---|---|---|
| CHUN KING Meals—CONAGRA | | | | | |
| ❖ Fried Rice w/Pork | 1 meal | 290 | 9% | 10% | 8% |
| ❖ Sweet & Sour Pork | 1 meal | 450 | 9% | 13% | 7% |

### PIZZA

**Generic Foods**

| | | | | | |
|---|---|---|---|---|---|
| ❖ Cheese Pizza | 1 slc | 280 | 10% | 15% | 6% |
| ❖ Cheese, Meat, and Vegetable Pizza | 1 slc | 370 | 17% | 15% | 14% |
| ❖ Pepperoni Pizza | 1 slc | 180 | 11% | 11% | 5% |

**Brand Name Foods**

| | | | | | |
|---|---|---|---|---|---|
| Ⓐ ACT II Pizza Pocket—GOLDEN VALLEY | 1 pocket | 410 | 31% | 45% | 8% |
| HEALTHY CHOICE French Bread Pizza Entrees—CONAGRA | | | | | |
| ❖ Cheese | 1 pizza | 310 | 6% | 9% | 4% |
| ❖ Pepperoni | 1 pizza | 360 | 14% | 20% | 8% |
| ❖ Sausage | 1 pizza | 330 | 6% | 8% | 6% |
| ❖ Supreme | 1 pizza | 340 | 9% | 11% | 8% |
| JENO'S *Crisp 'N Tasty*—PILLSBURY | | | | | |
| Ⓐ Canadian Style Bacon | 1 pkg | 430 | 28% | 18% | 3% |
| Ⓐ Cheese | 1 pkg | 450 | 29% | 30% | 7% |
| Ⓐ Combination | 1 pkg | 520 | 43% | 35% | 8% |

★ Foods with this symbol have less than or equal to 5% *Daily Value* for <u>all</u> three nutrients (5% Rule).
❖ Foods with this symbol have <u>at least one</u> of the three nutrients greater than 5% *Daily Value* but less than or equal to 20% *Daily Value.*
Ⓐ Foods with this symbol have <u>at least one</u> of the three nutrients greater than 20% *Daily Value* (20% Rule).

| FOOD | Serving Size | Calories | Tot Fat | Sat Fat | Chol |
|------|------|------|------|------|------|
| ✿ Hamburger | 1 pkg | 480 | 35% | 25% | 8% |
| ✿ Pepperoni | 1 pkg | 500 | 40% | 30% | 8% |
| ✿ Sausage | 1 pkg | 510 | 42% | 30% | 7% |
| ✿ Supreme | 1 pkg | 520 | 43% | 35% | 8% |
| ✿ Three Meat | 1 pkg | 500 | 40% | 30% | 8% |
| JENO'S Microwave Pizza For One—PILLSBURY | | | | | |
| ❖ Cheese | 1 pkg | 240 | 17% | 18% | 5% |
| ✿ Combination | 1 pkg | 310 | 28% | 23% | 5% |
| ✿ Pepperoni | 1 pkg | 280 | 25% | 18% | 5% |
| ✿ Sausage | 1 pkg | 280 | 25% | 20% | 3% |
| MARIE CALLENDER'S Pizza— CONAGRA | | | | | |
| ✿ Chicken & Broccoli | 1/2 pizza | 350 | 23% | 35% | 8% |
| ✿ Classic 5 Meat Combo | 1/2 pizza | 330 | 22% | 35% | 7% |
| ✿ Deluxe | 1/2 pizza | 380 | 35% | 25% | 10% |
| ✿ Extra Cheese | 1/2 pizza | 410 | 38% | 50% | 7% |
| ✿ Pepperoni | 1/2 pizza | 440 | 45% | 55% | 8% |
| ✿ Primavera | 1/2 pizza | 350 | 23% | 30% | 7% |
| ✿ Sausage & Pepperoni | 1/2 pizza | 430 | 43% | 55% | 12% |
| ✿ Sliced Tomato & Mozzarella | 1/2 pizza | 350 | 23% | 30% | 10% |
| PAPPALO'S Deep Dish—PILLSBURY | | | | | |
| ✿ Pepperoni | 1/5 pizza | 340 | 22% | 30% | 10% |
| ✿ Sausage | 1/5 pizza | 330 | 20% | 40% | 8% |
| ✿ Sausage & Pepperoni | 1/5 pizza | 330 | 22% | 40% | 8% |
| ✿ Supreme | 1/5 pizza | 340 | 22% | 40% | 8% |
| ✿ Three Cheese | 1/4 pizza | 370 | 18% | 30% | 8% |
| PAPPALO'S For One—PILLSBURY | | | | | |
| ✿ Pepperoni | 1 pkg | 570 | 42% | 65% | 20% |
| ✿ Sausage & Pepperoni | 1 pkg | 570 | 42% | 80% | 18% |
| ✿ Supreme | 1 pkg | 560 | 42% | 80% | 18% |
| ✿ Three Cheese | 1 pkg | 500 | 31% | 50% | 15% |
| PAPPALO'S Pizzeria Style Crust (12")—PILLSBURY | | | | | |
| ✿ Pepperoni | 1/4 pizza | 380 | 26% | 40% | 13% |
| ✿ Sausage | 1/4 pizza | 370 | 25% | 50% | 10% |
| ✿ Sausage & Pepperoni | 1/4 pizza | 380 | 26% | 45% | 12% |
| ✿ Supreme | 1/4 pizza | 380 | 25% | 45% | 10% |
| ✿ Three Cheese | 1/4 pizza | 340 | 18% | 30% | 10% |
| PEPPERIDGE FARM Croissant Crust Pizza—CAMPBELL'S | | | | | |
| ✿ Cheese | 1 pizza | 390 | 31% | 35% | 30% |
| ✿ Deluxe | 1 pizza | 450 | 42% | 50% | 28% |
| ✿ Pepperoni | 1 pizza | 420 | 35% | 45% | 30% |
| RED BARON—SCHWAN'S SALES | | | | | |
| ✿ 4-Cheese | 1/5 pizza | 350 | 26% | 40% | 10% |
| ✿ Canadian Style Bacon | 1/5 pizza | 310 | 20% | 25% | 8% |
| ✿ Pepperoni | 1/5 pizza | 360 | 29% | 35% | 10% |
| ✿ Sausage & Pepperoni | 1/5 pizza | 380 | 31% | 40% | 10% |

| FOOD | Serving Size | Calories | Tot Fat | Sat Fat | Chol |
|---|---|---|---|---|---|
| ⊛ Special Deluxe | 1/5 pizza | 340 | 28% | 35% | 8% |
| ⊛ Supreme | 1/5 pizza | 360 | 29% | 35% | 8% |
| STOUFFER'S French Bread Pizzas—NESTLÉ | | | | | |
| ⊛ Bacon Cheddar | 1/2 pkg | 440 | 34% | 35% | 10% |
| ⊛ Cheese | 1/2 pkg | 350 | 22% | 25% | 5% |
| ⊛ Cheeseburger | 1/2 pkg | 440 | 40% | 45% | 18% |
| ⊛ Deluxe | 1/2 pkg | 440 | 34% | 35% | 12% |
| ⊛ Double Cheese | 1/2 pkg | 420 | 29% | 35% | 10% |
| ⊛ Garden Vegetable | 1/2 pkg | 370 | 22% | 25% | 5% |
| ⊛ Pepperoni | 1/2 pkg | 420 | 31% | 30% | 12% |
| ⊛ Pepperoni & Mushroom | 1/2 pkg | 430 | 32% | 30% | 10% |
| ⊛ Sausage | 1/2 pkg | 420 | 31% | 25% | 12% |
| ⊛ Sausage & Pepperoni | 1/2 pkg | 490 | 38% | 35% | 13% |
| ⊛ Vegetable Deluxe | 1/2 pkg | 380 | 26% | 30% | 8% |
| ⊛ White | 1/2 pkg | 490 | 43% | 40% | 8% |
| STOUFFER'S Lean Cuisine French Bread Pizzas—NESTLÉ | | | | | |
| ❖ Cheese | 1 pkg | 350 | 12% | 20% | 7% |
| ❖ Deluxe | 1 pkg | 330 | 9% | 13% | 10% |
| ❖ Pepperoni | 1 pkg | 330 | 11% | 15% | 8% |
| STOUFFER'S Lunch Express —NESTLÉ | | | | | |
| ⊛ Deluxe Pizza | 1 pkg | 470 | 38% | 40% | 15% |
| ⊛ Pepperoni Pizza | 1 pkg | 440 | 35% | 40% | 13% |
| TOMBSTONE Double Top Pizza —KRAFT | | | | | |
| ⊛ Pepperoni w/Double Cheese | 1/6 pizza | 350 | 31% | 50% | 15% |
| ⊛ Sausage & Pepperoni w/Double Cheese | 1/6 pizza | 360 | 31% | 50% | 15% |
| ⊛ Sausage w/Double Cheese | 1/6 pizza | 350 | 29% | 50% | 13% |
| TOMBSTONE For One 1/2 Less Fat Pizza—KRAFT | | | | | |
| ⊛ Cheese | 1 pizza | 360 | 15% | 23% | 5% |
| ⊛ Pepperoni | 1 pizza | 400 | 20% | 25% | 12% |
| ⊛ Supreme | 1 pizza | 400 | 20% | 25% | 12% |
| ❖ Vegetable | 1 pizza | 360 | 15% | 20% | 5% |
| TOMBSTONE For One Pizza —KRAFT | | | | | |
| ⊛ Cheese & Pepperoni | 1 pizza | 580 | 54% | 75% | 17% |
| ⊛ Extra Cheese | 1 pizza | 540 | 46% | 70% | 15% |
| ⊛ Italian Sausage | 1 pizza | 560 | 51% | 70% | 18% |
| ⊛ Sausage & Pepperoni | 1 pizza | 590 | 57% | 75% | 18% |
| ⊛ Supreme | 1 pizza | 570 | 52% | 70% | 17% |

★ Foods with this symbol have less than or equal to 5% *Daily Value* for all three nutrients (5% Rule).
❖ Foods with this symbol have at least one of the three nutrients greater than 5% *Daily Value* but less than or equal to 20% *Daily Value*.
⊛ Foods with this symbol have at least one of the three nutrients greater than 20% *Daily Value* (20% Rule).

| FOOD | Serving Size | Calories | Tot Fat | Sat Fat | Chol |
|------|------|------|------|------|------|
| TOMBSTONE *Light* Pizza—KRAFT | | | | | |
| ❖ Supreme | 1/5 pizza | 270 | 14% | 18% | 7% |
| ❖ Vegetable | 1/5 pizza | 240 | 11% | 13% | 3% |
| TOMBSTONE Original Pizza (12")—KRAFT | | | | | |
| ☻ Canadian Style Bacon | 1/4 pizza | 360 | 23% | 35% | 13% |
| ☻ Cheese & Hamburger | 1/5 pizza | 320 | 25% | 40% | 10% |
| ☻ Cheese & Pepperoni | 1/5 pizza | 340 | 28% | 40% | 12% |
| ☻ Cheese & Sausage | 1/5 pizza | 320 | 25% | 40% | 10% |
| ☻ Cheese, Sausage & Mushroom | 1/5 pizza | 320 | 25% | 35% | 10% |
| ☻ Deluxe | 1/5 pizza | 320 | 25% | 35% | 10% |
| ☻ Extra Cheese | 1/4 pizza | 370 | 26% | 45% | 10% |
| ☻ Sausage & Pepperoni | 1/5 pizza | 340 | 28% | 40% | 12% |
| ☻ Supreme | 1/5 pizza | 330 | 26% | 40% | 12% |
| TOMBSTONE *Special Order* Pizza (12")—KRAFT | | | | | |
| ☻ Four Cheese | 1/5 pizza | 400 | 29% | 50% | 13% |
| ☻ Four Meats | 1/6 pizza | 350 | 28% | 40% | 13% |
| ☻ Pepperoni | 1/6 pizza | 360 | 29% | 45% | 13% |
| ☻ Super Supreme | 1/6 pizza | 350 | 28% | 45% | 13% |
| ☻ Three Sausage | 1/6 pizza | 340 | 26% | 40% | 12% |
| TOMBSTONE *ThinCrust* Pizza, Italian Style—KRAFT | | | | | |
| ☻ Four Meat Combo | 1/4 pizza | 410 | 38% | 60% | 17% |
| ☻ Italian Sausage | 1/4 pizza | 400 | 37% | 55% | 17% |
| ☻ Pepperoni | 1/4 pizza | 420 | 42% | 65% | 18% |
| ☻ Supreme | 1/4 pizza | 400 | 37% | 55% | 15% |
| ☻ Three Cheese | 1/4 pizza | 380 | 34% | 60% | 15% |
| ☻ TOMBSTONE *ThinCrust* Pizza, Mexican Style Supreme Taco —KRAFT | 1/4 pizza | 380 | 35% | 55% | 17% |
| TONY'S—SCHWAN'S SALES | | | | | |
| ☻ Canadian Style Bacon | 1/3 pizza | 370 | 29% | 34% | 8% |
| ☻ Pepperoni | 1/3 pizza | 420 | 37% | 44% | 10% |
| ☻ Sausage & Pepperoni | 1/3 pizza | 440 | 39% | 46% | 10% |
| TONY'S *Pizza D'Primo*— SCHWAN'S SALES | | | | | |
| ☻ 4-Cheese | 1/3 pizza | 380 | 22% | 25% | 7% |
| ☻ Sausage & Pepperoni | 1/3 pizza | 430 | 29% | 30% | 9% |
| TOTINO'S *Party* Pizza—PILLSBURY | | | | | |
| ☻ Bacon Burger | 1/2 pizza | 370 | 31% | 23% | 5% |
| ☻ Canadian Style Bacon | 1/2 pizza | 320 | 23% | 13% | 3% |
| ☻ Cheese | 1/2 pizza | 320 | 22% | 25% | 7% |
| ☻ Combination | 1/2 pizza | 390 | 32% | 23% | 7% |
| ☻ Hamburger | 1/2 pizza | 350 | 28% | 20% | 7% |
| ☻ Pepperoni | 1/2 pizza | 380 | 32% | 25% | 7% |
| ☻ Sausage | 1/2 pizza | 380 | 31% | 23% | 5% |
| ☻ Supreme | 1/2 pizza | 380 | 31% | 23% | 7% |
| ☻ Three Meat | 1/2 pizza | 360 | 29% | 20% | 5% |

| FOOD | Serving Size | Calories | Tot Fat | Sat Fat | Chol |
|------|--------------|----------|---------|---------|------|
| ✇ Zesty Italiano | 1/2 pizza | 390 | 32% | 23% | 7% |
| ✇ Zesty Mexican Style | 1/2 pizza | 370 | 29% | 23% | 5% |
| TOTINO'S *Pizza Pops*—PILLSBURY | | | | | |
| ✇ Italian Sausage | 1 pop | 310 | 23% | 30% | 7% |
| ✇ Italian Sausage & Pepperoni | 1 pop | 320 | 26% | 30% | 7% |
| ✇ Pepperoni | 1 pop | 320 | 25% | 30% | 8% |
| ✇ Supreme | 1 pop | 300 | 23% | 25% | 7% |
| TOTINO'S *Pizza Rolls*—PILLSBURY | | | | | |
| ✇ Combination | 10 rolls | 370 | 26% | 25% | 13% |
| ✇ Hamburger & Cheese | 10 rolls | 350 | 22% | 23% | 12% |
| ✇ Nacho Cheese & Beef | 10 rolls | 340 | 25% | 30% | 13% |
| ✇ Pepperoni & Cheese | 10 rolls | 360 | 26% | 25% | 12% |
| ✇ Sausage & Cheese | 10 rolls | 350 | 23% | 20% | 10% |
| ✇ Sausage & Mushroom | 10 rolls | 330 | 22% | 20% | 10% |
| ✇ Spicy Italian Style | 10 rolls | 370 | 28% | 25% | 13% |
| ✇ Three Cheese | 10 rolls | 360 | 23% | 30% | 12% |
| ✇ Three Meat | 10 rolls | 340 | 23% | 23% | 12% |
| TOTINO'S Microwave Pizza for One—PILLSBURY | | | | | |
| ❖ Cheese | 1 pizza | 240 | 17% | 18% | 5% |
| ✇ Combination | 1 pizza | 310 | 28% | 23% | 5% |
| ✇ Pepperoni | 1 pizza | 280 | 25% | 18% | 5% |
| ✇ Sausage | 1 pizza | 280 | 25% | 20% | 3% |
| ✇ Supreme | 1 pizza | 290 | 26% | 20% | 5% |
| ✇ Zesty Mexican Style | 1 pizza | 280 | 25% | 20% | 5% |
| ❖ TOTINO'S Pizza Crusts—PILLSBURY | 1/4 crust | 180 | 11% | 5% | 0% |
| TOTINO'S Select Pizza—PILLSBURY | | | | | |
| ✇ Sausage & Pepperoni | 1/3 pizza | 360 | 29% | 35% | 10% |
| ✇ Supreme | 1/3 pizza | 340 | 28% | 35% | 10% |
| ✇ Three Cheese | 1/3 pizza | 300 | 22% | 30% | 7% |
| ✇ Two Cheese and Canadian Style Bacon | 1/3 pizza | 310 | 22% | 25% | 8% |
| ✇ Two Cheese and Pepperoni | 1/3 pizza | 360 | 31% | 40% | 12% |
| ✇ Two Cheese and Sausage | 1/3 pizza | 360 | 29% | 35% | 10% |
| WEIGHT WATCHERS Pizza | | | | | |
| ❖ Deluxe Combo | 1 entrée | 380 | 17% | 18% | 13% |
| ❖ Extra Cheese | 1 entrée | 390 | 18% | 20% | 12% |
| ❖ Pepperoni | 1 entrée | 390 | 18% | 20% | 15% |

## POTPIES, MEAT-FILLED PASTRIES, AND POCKETS

**Generic Foods**

| | | | | | |
|------|--------------|----------|---------|---------|------|
| ✇ Beef Potpie | 1 slc | 520 | 46% | 40% | 15% |
| ✇ Chicken Potpie | 1 slc | 550 | 48% | 55% | 24% |

---

★ Foods with this symbol have less than or equal to 5% *Daily Value* for <u>all</u> three nutrients (5% Rule).

❖ Foods with this symbol have <u>at least one</u> of the three nutrients greater than 5% *Daily Value* but less than or equal to 20% *Daily Value*.

✇ Foods with this symbol have <u>at least one</u> of the three nutrients greater than 20% *Daily Value* (20% Rule).

| FOOD | Serving Size | Calories | Tot Fat | Sat Fat | Chol |
|------|--------------|----------|---------|---------|------|
| ✦ Turkey Potpie | 1 cup | 470 | 38% | 42% | 7% |

**Brand Name Foods**

BANQUET *Extra Helping* Family
Entrées—CONAGRA

| | | | | | |
|------|--------------|----------|---------|---------|------|
| ✦ Beef Pie | ~ 1/3 pie | 450 | 38% | 55% | 10% |
| ✦ Chicken Pie | ~ 1/3 pie | 450 | 46% | 60% | 12% |

BANQUET Pot Pies—CONAGRA

| | | | | | |
|------|--------------|----------|---------|---------|------|
| ✦ Beef | 1 pie | 330 | 23% | 35% | 8% |
| ✦ Chicken | 1 pie | 350 | 28% | 35% | 13% |
| ✦ Supreme Beef | 1 pie | 270 | 18% | 25% | 10% |
| ✦ Supreme Chicken | 1 pie | 330 | 23% | 25% | 10% |
| ✦ Supreme Turkey | 1 pie | 330 | 20% | 25% | 8% |
| ✦ Turkey | 1 pie | 370 | 31% | 40% | 15% |
| ✦ Vegetable & Cheese | 1 pie | 390 | 28% | 40% | 5% |

MARIE CALLENDER'S POT PIES
—CONAGRA

| | | | | | |
|------|--------------|----------|---------|---------|------|
| ✦ Chicken | 1 pie | 680 | 68% | 45% | 10% |
| ✦ Chicken & Broccoli | 1 pie | 780 | 71% | 78% | 7% |
| ✦ Chicken Au Gratin | 1 pie | 720 | 71% | 65% | 8% |
| ✦ Turkey | 1 pie | 710 | 71% | 50% | 7% |
| ✦ Yankee | 1 pie | 690 | 68% | 50% | 8% |

MORTON Vegetable Pot Pies
—CONAGRA

| | | | | | |
|------|--------------|----------|---------|---------|------|
| ✦ w/Beef | 1 pie | 310 | 26% | 40% | 5% |
| ✦ w/Chicken | 1 pie | 320 | 28% | 35% | 8% |
| ✦ w/Turkey | 1 pie | 300 | 28% | 45% | 8% |

MRS. PATERSON'S AUSSIE PIE
Meat Filled Pastries—
HORMEL FOODS

| | | | | | |
|------|--------------|----------|---------|---------|------|
| ✦ Chicken | 1 pie | 460 | 38% | 40% | 30% |
| ✦ Pizza Supreme | 1 pie | 466 | 40% | 45% | 24% |
| ✦ Steak & Mushroom | 1 pie | 405 | 31% | 30% | 24% |
| ✦ Turkey w/Broccoli | 1 pie | 470 | 40% | 50% | 32% |

RED BARON *Premium Pockets*
—SCHWAN'S SALES

| | | | | | |
|------|--------------|----------|---------|---------|------|
| ✦ Chicken, Broccoli, & Cheddar | 1 pocket | 290 | 20% | 25% | 10% |
| ✦ Ham & Cheese | 1 pocket | 320 | 23% | 41% | 13% |
| ✦ Philly Steak & Cheese | 1 pocket | 280 | 18% | 28% | 11% |
| ❖ Turkey Swiss, Lean | 1 pocket | 250 | 14% | 20% | 9% |
| ✦ Turkey, Cheddar & Bacon | 1 pocket | 330 | 25% | 35% | 13% |

STOUFFER'S Entrées—NESTLÉ

| | | | | | |
|------|--------------|----------|---------|---------|------|
| ✦ Beef Pie | 1 pkg | 450 | 40% | 45% | 22% |
| ✦ Chicken Pie (10 oz) | 1 pkg | 520 | 51% | 40% | 23% |
| ✦ Turkey Pie (10 oz) | 1 pkg | 530 | 51% | 45% | 22% |

| FOOD | Serving Size | Calories | Tot Fat | Sat Fat | Chol |
|---|---|---|---|---|---|
| **STOUFFER'S** *Lean Cuisine* Entrées—NESTLÉ | | | | | |
| ❖ Chicken Pie | 1 pkg | 320 | 15% | 13% | 12% |
| ❖ Turkey Pie | 1 pkg | 300 | 14% | 10% | 17% |
| **SWANSON** *Hungry Man* Pot Pies —CAMPBELL'S | | | | | |
| Ⓐ Beef | 1 pkg | 620 | 45% | 70% | 18% |
| Ⓐ Chicken | 1 pkg | 650 | 54% | 70% | 22% |
| Ⓐ Turkey | 1 pkg | 650 | 52% | 65% | 15% |
| **SWANSON** Pot Pies—CAMPBELL'S | | | | | |
| Ⓐ Chicken | 1 pkg | 410 | 34% | 40% | 10% |
| Ⓐ Turkey | 1 pkg | 440 | 37% | 45% | 7% |
| **TONY'S** *Personal Pizza Pockets* —SCHWAN'S SALES | | | | | |
| Ⓐ Pepperoni | 1 pocket | 350 | 26% | 35% | 10% |
| Ⓐ Supreme | 1 pocket | 310 | 22% | 28% | 7% |
| **TYSON** Pot Pies | | | | | |
| Ⓐ Chicken Pie (white meat & vegetables) | 1 cup | 550 | 52% | 35% | 15% |
| Ⓐ Meat Lover's Recipe Chicken Pie (all white meat) | 1 cup | 620 | 54% | 40% | 18% |
| Ⓐ Turkey Pie (white meat & vegetables) | 1 cup | 540 | 49% | 30% | 10% |
| **VEGGIE POCKETS**—IMAGINE FOODS | | | | | |
| ❖ Bar B Que Style | 1 pocket | 290 | 13% | 3% | 0% |
| ❖ Broccoli & Cheddar Style | 1 pocket | 250 | 13% | 0% | 0% |
| ❖ Greek Style | 1 pocket | 250 | 13% | 0% | 0% |
| ❖ Indian Style | 1 pocket | 260 | 13% | 3% | 0% |
| ❖ Oriental Style | 1 pocket | 250 | 15% | 4% | 0% |
| ❖ Pizza Style | 1 pocket | 270 | 13% | 3% | 0% |
| ❖ Tex Mex Style | 1 pocket | 280 | 13% | 3% | 0% |
| **WORTHINGTON** Vegetarian Pie | | | | | |
| Ⓐ Beef Style | 1 pie | 410 | 37% | 20% | 0% |
| Ⓐ Chicken Style | 1 pie | 450 | 42% | 30% | 0% |

## TURKEY

### Brand Name Foods

| FOOD | Serving Size | Calories | Tot Fat | Sat Fat | Chol |
|---|---|---|---|---|---|
| ❖ **ARMOUR CLASSICS** Turkey & Dressing—CONAGRA | 1 meal | 270 | 11% | 20% | 20% |
| **BANQUET**—CONAGRA | | | | | |
| ❖ Dinners: Turkey | 1 meal | 270 | 15% | 15% | 15% |
| Ⓐ *Extra Helping* Dinners: Turkey | 1 meal | 560 | 31% | 25% | 25% |

★ Foods with this symbol have less than or equal to 5% *Daily Value* for <u>all</u> three nutrients (5% Rule).
❖ Foods with this symbol have <u>at least one</u> of the three nutrients greater than 5% *Daily Value* but less than or equal to 20% *Daily Value*.
Ⓐ Foods with this symbol have <u>at least one</u> of the three nutrients greater than 20% *Daily Value* (20% Rule).

| FOOD | Serving Size | Calories | Tot Fat | Sat Fat | Chol |
|------|-------------|----------|---------|---------|------|
| ❖ *Extra Helping* Family Entrées: Gravy & Sliced Turkey | 2 slcs w/gravy | 120 | 12% | 15% | 12% |
| BUDGET GOURMET *Light & Healthy*—ALL AMERICAN GOURMET | | | | | |
| ❖ Dinners: Stuffed Turkey Breast | 1 pkg | 260 | 9% | 10% | 12% |
| ❖ Entrées: Glazed Turkey | 1 pkg | 250 | 6% | 10% | 10% |
| ✆ BUDGET GOURMET *Original Entrées* Open Faced Turkey & Gravy w/Mashed Potatoes— ALL AMERICAN GOURMET | 1 pkg | 330 | 23% | 20% | 13% |
| HEALTHY CHOICE Dinners —CONAGRA | | | | | |
| ❖ Classics Country Inn Roast Turkey | 1 meal | 250 | 5% | 5% | 10% |
| ❖ Country Turkey and Pasta | 1 meal | 300 | 7% | 10% | 12% |
| ❖ Traditional Breast of Turkey | 1 meal | 280 | 5% | 6% | 16% |
| HEALTHY CHOICE Entrées— CONAGRA | | | | | |
| ❖ Country Roast Turkey w/ Mushrooms | 1 meal | 220 | 6% | 6% | 9% |
| ❖ Homestyle Turkey w/Vegetables Entrée | 1 meal | 260 | 3% | 3% | 12% |
| ✆ MARIE CALLENDER'S Turkey w/Gravy & Dressing—CONAGRA | 1 dinner | 530 | 26% | 35% | 28% |
| ❖ MORTON Dinners: Turkey Meal —CONAGRA | 1 meal | 230 | 12% | 15% | 12% |
| ❖ SMART ONES Roast Turkey Medallions—WEIGHT WATCHERS | 1 entrée | 190 | 3% | 3% | 7% |
| STOUFFER'S *Lean Cuisine* Entrées—NESTLÉ | | | | | |
| ❖ Homestyle Turkey | 1 pkg | 230 | 9% | 8% | 17% |
| ❖ *Lunch Express* Pasta & Turkey Dijon | 1 pkg | 270 | 9% | 8% | 10% |
| ❖ Roasted Turkey Breast & Stuffing & Cinnamon Apples | 1 pkg | 290 | 6% | 5% | 8% |
| STOUFFER'S Entrées—NESTLÉ | | | | | |
| ❖ Homestyle Roast Turkey & Homestyle Stuffing | 1 pkg | 280 | 17% | 13% | 13% |
| ✆ Turkey Tetrazzini | 1 pkg | 360 | 29% | 15% | 13% |
| ✆ SWANSON *Hungry Man* Dinner: Turkey (mostly white meat)— CAMPBELL'S | 1 pkg | 490 | 20% | 40% | 15% |
| SWANSON Complete Dinners— CAMPBELL'S | | | | | |
| ✆ Turkey (mostly white meat) in Gravy w/Dressing | 1 pkg | 280 | 15% | 25% | 13% |
| ❖ Turkey Breast Meat w/Pasta | 1 pkg | 290 | 12% | 20% | 12% |
| ❖ Turkey Dinner (mostly white meat) | 1 pkg | 310 | 11% | 10% | 12% |
| ❖ TYSON Premium Dinners: Turkey w/Dressing | 1 pkg | 320 | 18% | 10% | 12% |

| FOOD | Serving Size | Calories | Tot Fat | Sat Fat | Chol |
|---|---|---|---|---|---|
| ❖ WEIGHT WATCHERS Stuffed Turkey Breast | 1 entrée | 240 | 12% | 15% | 7% |

VEGETARIAN

**Brand Name Foods**

| FOOD | Serving Size | Calories | Tot Fat | Sat Fat | Chol |
|---|---|---|---|---|---|
| HAIN Vegetarian Classics | | | | | |
| ❖ Hawaiian Nuggets | 1 pkg | 310 | 8% | 3% | 0% |
| ❖ Pepper Steak | 1 pkg | 310 | 9% | 5% | 0% |
| NATURAL TOUCH Loaf— WORTHINGTON FOODS | | | | | |
| ❖ Lentil Rice | 1" slc | 170 | 14% | 13% | 0% |
| ❖ Nine Bean | 1" slc | 160 | 12% | 8% | 1% |
| ⊛ PEPPERIDGE FARM Broccoli w/ Cheese in Pastry—CAMPBELL'S | 1 pastry | 240 | 22% | 23% | 17% |
| TAJ Vegetarian Entrées | | | | | |
| ❖ Bean Masala | 12 oz | 390 | 17% | 5% | 0% |
| ❖ Channa Masala | 12 oz | 360 | 16% | 5% | 0% |
| ❖ Dal Bahaar | 12 oz | 385 | 20% | 5% | 0% |
| ⊛ Palak Paneer | 12 oz | 370 | 26% | 12% | 2% |
| ❖ Raj Mah | 12 oz | 370 | 17% | 5% | 0% |
| ⊛ Shahi Paneer | 12 oz | 410 | 37% | 48% | 15% |
| ⊛ Vegetable Korma | 12 oz | 370 | 21% | 5% | 0% |

# Main Dishes, Entrées, and Dinners: The Makings

BEEF DISHES

**Brand Name Foods**

| FOOD | Serving Size | Calories | Tot Fat | Sat Fat | Chol |
|---|---|---|---|---|---|
| BETTY CROCKER *Hamburger Helper* (prep as dir)— GENERAL MILLS | | | | | |
| ⊛ Beef Noodle | 1 cup | 260 | 15% | 18% | 25% |
| ❖ Beef Romanoff | 1 cup | 290 | 16% | 20% | 17% |
| ❖ Beef Taco | 1 cup | 300 | 17% | 20% | 17% |
| ❖ Beef Teriyaki | 1 cup | 320 | 16% | 20% | 18% |
| ❖ Beef Vegetable Soup | 1 cup | 190 | 12% | 15% | 17% |
| ⊛ Cheddar 'n Bacon | 1 cup | 350 | 24% | 29% | 22% |
| ⊛ Cheeseburger Macaroni | 1 cup | 320 | 21% | 24% | 19% |
| ⊛ Cheesy Italian | 1 cup | 330 | 21% | 8% | 21% |
| ⊛ Cheesy Shells | 1 cup | 340 | 24% | 28% | 20% |
| ❖ Chili Macaroni | 1 cup | 290 | 16% | 19% | 18% |

★ Foods with this symbol have less than or equal to 5% *Daily Value* for all three nutrients (5% Rule).

❖ Foods with this symbol have at least one of the three nutrients greater than 5% *Daily Value* but less than or equal to 20% *Daily Value*.

⊛ Foods with this symbol have at least one of the three nutrients greater than 20% *Daily Value* (20% Rule).

| FOOD | Serving Size | Calories | Tot Fat | Sat Fat | Chol |
|------|------|------|------|------|------|
| ✆ Fettuccini Alfredo | 1 cup | 310 | 21% | 31% | 21% |
| ❖ Hamburger Stew | 1 cup | 250 | 16% | 20% | 18% |
| ✆ Meat Loaf | 1 cup | 280 | 23% | 30% | 37% |
| ✆ Mushroom & Wild Rice | 1 cup | 350 | 20% | 25% | 20% |
| ✆ Nacho Cheese | 1 cup | 340 | 21% | 27% | 20% |
| ✆ Potato Stroganoff | 1 cup | 270 | 18% | 22% | 18% |
| ✆ Potatoes Au Gratin | 1 cup | 290 | 21% | 24% | 18% |
| ❖ Rice Oriental | 1 cup | 310 | 16% | 19% | 18% |
| ✆ Stroganoff | 1 cup | 350 | 21% | 26% | 21% |
| ✆ Three Cheese | 1 cup | 350 | 24% | 29% | 20% |
| ❖ Zesty Italian | 1 cup | 320 | 16% | 19% | 18% |
| ❖ Beef Stew | 1 cup | 250 | 15% | 18% | 17% |
| ❖ Italian Rigatoni | 1 cup | 290 | 15% | 19% | 17% |
| ❖ Salisbury | 1 cup | 280 | 15% | 19% | 17% |
| ✆ Swedish Meatballs | 1 cup | 320 | 25% | 28% | 37% |
| ★ BIRDS EYE *Easy Recipe* For Beef: Oriental Beef (as packaged)—DEAN FOODS | 2/3 cup | 70 | 2% | 0% | 0% |
| ✆ BIRDS EYE *Easy Recipe* Meal Starter: Oriental Stir Fry (prep as dir)—DEAN FOODS | 2 1/4 cups | 310 | 15% | 10% | 27% |
| KNORR—CPC | | | | | |
| ★ Bourguignonne Beef Stew w/ Wine Recipe Mix | 1/6 pkg | 40 | 1% | 2% | 0% |
| ★ Goulash Beef Stew Recipe Mix | 1/6 pkg | 40 | 2% | 3% | 1% |
| ★ Sauerbraten Beef Pot Roast Recipe Mix | 1/6 pkg | 35 | 2% | 3% | 0% |

## CHICKEN DISHES

**Brand Name Foods**

| FOOD | Serving Size | Calories | Tot Fat | Sat Fat | Chol |
|------|------|------|------|------|------|
| ❖ BETTY CROCKER *Dinner Sensations* Sweet & Sour Chicken (prep as dir)—GENERAL MILLS | 1 cup | 330 | 6% | 5% | 11% |
| ✆ BETTY CROCKER *Skillet Chicken Helper* Stir-Fried Chicken (prep as dir)—GENERAL MILLS | 1 cup | 270 | 14% | 10% | 36% |
| BIRDS EYE *Easy Recipe* For Chicken (as packaged)—DEAN FOODS | | | | | |
| ❖ Chicken Alfredo | 2/3 cup | 180 | 12% | 18% | 5% |
| ❖ Chicken Primavera | 3/4 cup | 140 | 6% | 3% | 0% |
| ★ Chicken Teriyaki | 1/2 cup | 100 | 2% | 0% | 0% |
| ★ Orange Glazed Chicken | 2/3 cup | 90 | 1% | 0% | 0% |
| ✆ BIRDS EYE *Easy Recipe* Meal Starter: Cacciatore (prep as dir)—DEAN FOODS | 2 cups | 280 | 14% | 8% | 31% |

| FOOD | Serving Size | Calories | Tot Fat | Sat Fat | Chol |
|------|------|------|------|------|------|

## FISH DISHES

**Brand Name Foods**

BETTY CROCKER *Tuna Helper*
(prep as dir)—GENERAL MILLS

| FOOD | Serving Size | Calories | Tot Fat | Sat Fat | Chol |
|------|------|------|------|------|------|
| ❖ Au Gratin | 1 cup | 300 | 18% | 15% | 6% |
| ❖ Cheesy Noodles | 1 cup | 290 | 19% | 14% | 17% |
| ❖ Creamy Broccoli | 1 cup | 310 | 19% | 16% | 6% |
| Ⓐ Creamy Noodles | 1 cup | 310 | 22% | 18% | 17% |
| Ⓐ Fettuccine Alfredo | 1 cup | 340 | 24% | 22% | 9% |
| ❖ Garden Cheddar | 1 cup | 310 | 19% | 15% | 7% |
| Ⓐ Pasta Salad | 1 cup | 380 | 41% | 15% | 3% |
| ❖ Tetrazzini | 1 cup | 310 | 18% | 16% | 8% |
| Ⓐ Tuna Pot Pie | 1 cup | 440 | 37% | 33% | 36% |
| ❖ Tuna Romanoff | 1 cup | 280 | 12% | 8% | 6% |

## PIZZA

**Brand Name Foods**

| FOOD | Serving Size | Calories | Tot Fat | Sat Fat | Chol |
|------|------|------|------|------|------|
| ❖ BETTY CROCKER *Hamburger Helper* Pizzabake (prep as dir) —GENERAL MILLS | 1 cup | 270 | 15% | 18% | 15% |
| CHEF BOYARDEE *Complete* Pizza Kits—AMERICAN HOME FOODS | | | | | |
| ❖ Cheese | 1/3 pkg | 320 | 12% | 13% | 5% |
| ❖ Pepperoni | 1/4 pkg | 260 | 12% | 15% | 7% |
| ❖ Sausage | 1/4 pkg | 260 | 11% | 13% | 7% |

## VEGETARIAN DISHES

**Brand Name Foods**

| FOOD | Serving Size | Calories | Tot Fat | Sat Fat | Chol |
|------|------|------|------|------|------|
| FANTASTIC FOODS *Tofu Classics* | | | | | |
| ❖ Chow Mein w/Tofu | 1 cup | 330 | 8% | 5% | 0% |
| Ⓐ Stroganoff w/Tofu | 1 cup | 430 | 18% | 30% | 3% |
| LOMA LINDA Meatless Products —WORTHINGTON FOODS | | | | | |
| ★ Chicken Supreme | 1/3 cup dry mix | 90 | 2% | 0% | 0% |
| ★ Patty Mix | 1/3 cup dry mix | 90 | 2% | 0% | 0% |

★ Foods with this symbol have less than or equal to 5% *Daily Value* for all three nutrients (5% Rule).
❖ Foods with this symbol have at least one of the three nutrients greater than 5% *Daily Value* but less than or equal to 20% *Daily Value*.
Ⓐ Foods with this symbol have at least one of the three nutrients greater than 20% *Daily Value* (20% Rule).

| FOOD | Serving Size | Calories | Tot Fat | Sat Fat | Chol |
|------|-------------|----------|---------|---------|------|
| ★ Savory Dinner Loaf | 1/3 cup dry mix | 90 | 2% | 0% | 0% |
| MANISCHEWITZ | | | | | |
| ★ Spinach Quiche Mix | 1/5 cup mix | 120 | 2% | 3% | 0% |
| ★ Tomato & Basil Quiche Mix | 1/3 cup mix | 130 | 2% | 3% | 0% |
| ★ NATURAL TOUCH Loaf Mix— | | | | | |
| WORTHINGTON FOODS | 4 tbsp dry mix | 100 | 1% | 0% | 0% |

# Meal Replacements

BARS

**Brand Name Foods**

| FOOD | Serving Size | Calories | Tot Fat | Sat Fat | Chol |
|------|-------------|----------|---------|---------|------|
| FIGURINES 100 Diet Bars— PILLSBURY | | | | | |
| ❖ Chocolate | 2 bars | 220 | 17% | 13% | 1% |
| ❖ Chocolate Caramel | 2 bars | 220 | 17% | 13% | 1% |
| ❖ Chocolate Peanut Butter | 2 bars | 220 | 17% | 15% | 1% |
| ❖ S'Mores | 2 bars | 220 | 17% | 13% | 1% |
| ❖ Vanilla | 2 bars | 220 | 17% | 13% | 1% |
| SWEET SUCCESS Bars—NESTLÉ | | | | | |
| ❖ Chewy Chocolate Brownie | 1 bar | 120 | 6% | 9% | 1% |
| ❖ Chewy Chocolate Chip | 1 bar | 120 | 6% | 8% | 1% |
| ❖ Chewy Oatmeal Raisin | 1 bar | 120 | 6% | 8% | 1% |
| ❖ Chewy Chocolate Raspberry | 1 bar | 120 | 6% | 8% | 1% |
| ❖ Chewy Chocolate Peanut Butter | 1 bar | 120 | 6% | 8% | 1% |
| SLIM-FAST Breakfast & Lunch Bars | | | | | |
| ❖ Dutch Chocolate | 1 bar | 140 | 8% | 10% | 1% |
| ❖ Peanut Butter | 1 bar | 150 | 8% | 15% | 1% |
| ULTRA SLIM-FAST Nutrition Bars | | | | | |
| ❖ Chewy Caramel Crunch | 1 bar | 120 | 5% | 10% | 1% |
| ❖ Chocolate Chip Crunch | 1 bar | 120 | 6% | 10% | 0% |
| ❖ Cocoa Almond Crunch | 1 bar | 120 | 6% | 10% | 0% |
| ❖ Peanut Butter Crunch | 1 bar | 120 | 6% | 10% | 0% |
| ❖ Peanut Caramel Crunch | 1 bar | 120 | 6% | 10% | 1% |
| ❖ Vanilla Almond Crunch | 1 bar | 120 | 6% | 10% | 0% |

CANNED DRINKS

**Brand Name Foods**

| FOOD | Serving Size | Calories | Tot Fat | Sat Fat | Chol |
|------|-------------|----------|---------|---------|------|
| SWEET SUCCESS Drink (10 fl oz) —NESTLÉ | | | | | |
| ★ Rich Chocolate Almond | 1 can | 200 | 5% | 5% | 1% |
| ★ Dark Chocolate Fudge | 1 can | 200 | 5% | 5% | 1% |

| FOOD | Serving Size | Calories | Tot Fat | Sat Fat | Chol |
|------|--------------|----------|---------|---------|------|
| ★ Chocolate Mocha Supreme | 1 can | 200 | 5% | 5% | 1% |
| ★ Creamy Milk Chocolate | 1 can | 200 | 5% | 5% | 1% |
| ★ Chocolate Raspberry Truffle | 1 can | 200 | 5% | 5% | 1% |
| ★ Smooth Vanilla Creme | 1 can | 200 | 5% | 5% | 1% |
| SEGO Liquid Diet Meal (10 fl oz) —PET | | | | | |
| ★ *Very* Chocolate | 1 can | 240 | 2% | 0% | 2% |
| ★ *Very* Chocolate Malt | 1 can | 240 | 2% | 0% | 2% |
| ❖ *Very* Strawberry | 1 can | 240 | 7% | 4% | 2% |
| ❖ *Very* Vanilla | 1 can | 240 | 7% | 4% | 2% |
| SEGO Lite Liquid Diet Meal (10 fl oz)—PET | | | | | |
| ★ Chocolate | 1 can | 150 | 5% | 0% | 2% |
| ★ Dutch Chocolate | 1 can | 150 | 5% | 0% | 2% |
| ❖ French Vanilla | 1 can | 150 | 6% | 0% | 2% |
| ❖ Strawberry | 1 can | 150 | 6% | 0% | 2% |
| ❖ Vanilla | 1 can | 150 | 6% | 0% | 2% |
| ULTRA SLIM-FAST Ready-to-Drink Meal | | | | | |
| ★ Apple-Cranberry-Raspberry (11.5 fl oz) | 1 can | 220 | 2% | 3% | 3% |
| ★ Chocolate Fudge (11 fl oz) | 1 can | 220 | 5% | 5% | 3% |
| ★ Chocolate Royale (11 fl oz) | 1 can | 220 | 5% | 5% | 2% |
| ★ Coffee (11 fl oz) | 1 can | 220 | 5% | 3% | 2% |
| ★ French Vanilla (11 fl oz) | 1 can | 220 | 5% | 3% | 2% |
| ★ Golden Apple (11.5 fl oz) | 1 can | 220 | 2% | 3% | 3% |
| ★ Milk Chocolate (11 fl oz) | 1 can | 230 | 5% | 5% | 2% |
| ★ Orange-Pineapple (11.5 fl oz) | 1 can | 220 | 2% | 3% | 3% |
| ★ Orange-Strawberry-Banana (11.5 fl oz) | 1 can | 220 | 2% | 3% | 3% |
| ★ Strawberry Supreme (11 fl oz) | 1 can | 230 | 5% | 3% | 2% |

## DRINK MIXES

**Brand Name Foods**

| FOOD | Serving Size | Calories | Tot Fat | Sat Fat | Chol |
|------|--------------|----------|---------|---------|------|
| SWEET SUCCESS (prep w/skim milk)—NESTLÉ | | | | | |
| ★ Chocolate Mocha Supreme | 9 fl oz | 180 | 2% | 5% | 2% |
| ★ Chocolate Raspberry Truffle | 9 fl oz | 180 | 3% | 5% | 2% |
| ❖ Classic Chocolate Chip | 9 fl oz | 180 | 4% | 8% | 2% |
| ★ Creamy Milk Chocolate | 9 fl oz | 180 | 3% | 5% | 2% |
| ★ Creamy Vanilla Delight | 9 fl oz | 180 | 1% | 3% | 2% |
| ★ Dark Chocolate Fudge | 9 fl oz | 180 | 3% | 5% | 2% |
| ★ Rich Chocolate Almond | 9 fl oz | 180 | 2% | 5% | 2% |

★ Foods with this symbol have less than or equal to 5% *Daily Value* for <u>all</u> three nutrients (5% Rule).
❖ Foods with this symbol have <u>at least one</u> of the three nutrients greater than 5% *Daily Value* but less than or equal to 20% *Daily Value*.
Ⓐ Foods with this symbol have <u>at least one</u> of the three nutrients greater than 20% *Daily Value* (20% Rule).

| FOOD | Serving Size | Calories | Tot Fat | Sat Fat | Chol |
|------|------|------|------|------|------|
| SLIM-FAST Instant Nutritional Meal (prep w/3 tbsp in 8 oz skim milk) | | | | | |
| ★ Cafe Mocha | 8 fl oz | 200 | 2% | 4% | 3% |
| ★ Chocolate | 8 fl oz | 190 | 2% | 4% | 3% |
| ❖ Chocolate Fudge | 8 fl oz | 200 | 4% | 6% | 3% |
| ★ Chocolate Malt | 8 fl oz | 190 | 2% | 4% | 3% |
| ★ Chocolate Royale | 8 fl oz | 200 | 2% | 4% | 3% |
| ★ French Vanilla | 8 fl oz | 200 | 1% | 3% | 3% |
| ★ Strawberry | 8 fl oz | 190 | 1% | 3% | 3% |
| ★ Strawberry Supreme | 8 fl oz | 200 | 1% | 3% | 3% |
| ★ Vanilla | 8 fl oz | 190 | 1% | 3% | 3% |
| ★ ULTRA SLIM-FAST Instant Nutritional Meal (prep w/5 tbsp in 8 oz orange juice) | 8 fl oz | 220 | 1% | 0% | 3% |

# Meat and Meat Substitutes

## BACON

**Generic Foods**

| FOOD | Serving Size | Calories | Tot Fat | Sat Fat | Chol |
|------|------|------|------|------|------|
| ❖ Bacon, Pork | 2 slcs | 90 | 11% | 13% | 4% |
| ★ Bacon Bits | 1 tbsp | 30 | 2% | 1% | 0% |
| ★ Canadian Bacon (grilled) | 1 slc | 30 | 2% | 2% | 3% |

**Brand Name Foods**

| FOOD | Serving Size | Calories | Tot Fat | Sat Fat | Chol |
|------|------|------|------|------|------|
| ❖ HORMEL Canadian Style Bacon | 2 oz | 70 | 5% | 8% | 10% |
| ★ JENNIE-O *Extra Lean* Turkey Bacon | 1 slc | 20 | 1% | 0% | 4% |
| ★ LOUIS RICH Turkey Bacon— OSCAR MAYER | 1 slc | 30 | 4% | 3% | 3% |
| ❖ MORNINGSTAR FARMS Meatless Breakfast Strips—WORTHINGTON FOODS | 2 strips | 60 | 7% | 3% | 0% |
| ❖ OLD SMOKEHOUSE Bacon (cooked)—HORMEL FOODS | 2 slcs | 80 | 11% | 13% | 5% |
| OSCAR MAYER Bacon (cooked) | | | | | |
| ❖ 1/8" Thick Cut | 1 slc | 60 | 8% | 8% | 3% |
| ❖ Bacon | 2 slcs | 60 | 8% | 8% | 3% |
| ❖ Canadian-Style Bacon | 2 slcs | 50 | 3% | 5% | 8% |
| ❖ Center Cut | 3 slcs | 90 | 11% | 13% | 7% |
| ❖ Lower Sodium | 2 slcs | 60 | 6% | 8% | 3% |
| ❖ RED LABEL Bacon (cooked)— HORMEL FOODS | 2 slcs | 80 | 11% | 13% | 5% |

| FOOD | Serving Size | Calories | Tot Fat | Sat Fat | Chol |
|------|--------------|----------|---------|---------|------|
| ❖ WORTHINGTON Stripples (frozen meatless bacon)—WORTHINGTON FOODS | 2 strips | 60 | 8% | 3% | 0% |

### BEEF: CANNED AND DRIED

**Brand Name Foods**

HORMEL

| | | | | | |
|------|--------------|----------|---------|---------|------|
| ❖ Corned Beef | 2 oz | 120 | 11% | 15% | 17% |
| ❖ Roast Beef with Gravy | 2 oz | 60 | 3% | 5% | 10% |
| ❖ Sliced Dried Beef | 10 slcs | 50 | 2% | 3% | 8% |
| LIBBY'S—NESTLÉ | | | | | |
| ⊛ Deviled Meat | 1 can | 160 | 20% | 26% | 29% |
| ⊛ Potted Meat | 1 can | 160 | 20% | 26% | 29% |
| ⊛ Roast Beef w/Gravy | 2/3 cup | 140 | 5% | 8% | 24% |

### BEEF: FRESH

**Generic Foods**

| | | | | | |
|------|--------------|----------|---------|---------|------|
| ❖ Beefalo: All cuts (roasted) | 3 oz | 160 | 8% | 11% | 16% |
| Bottom Round, Steak | | | | | |
| ⊛ Trimmed of visible fat (broiled) | 3 oz | 150 | 6% | 5% | 23% |
| ⊛ Trimmed to 1/8" fat (broiled) | 3 oz | 180 | 11% | 15% | 23% |
| ⊛ Brain | 3 oz | 140 | 16% | 12% | 582% |
| ⊛ Brisket, Corned | 3 oz | 210 | 25% | 27% | 28% |
| Brisket, Flat Half | | | | | |
| ⊛ Trimmed of visible fat (braised) | 3 oz | 160 | 8% | 9% | 27% |
| ⊛ Trimmed to 1/4" fat (braised) | 3 oz | 190 | 13% | 14% | 27% |
| Brisket, Point Half | | | | | |
| ⊛ Trimmed of visible fat (braised) | 3 oz | 250 | 26% | 32% | 26% |
| ⊛ Trimmed to 1/4" fat (braised) | 3 oz | 330 | 41% | 53% | 22% |
| Brisket, Whole | | | | | |
| ⊛ Trimmed of visible fat (braised) | 3 oz | 210 | 17% | 20% | 27% |
| ⊛ Trimmed to 1/8" fat (braised) | 3 oz | 290 | 32% | 40% | 27% |
| Chuck Arm Pot Roast | | | | | |
| ⊛ Trimmed to 1/8" fat (braised) | 3 oz | 260 | 28% | 35% | 28% |
| ⊛ Trimmed of visible fat (braised) | 3 oz | 180 | 11% | 15% | 28% |
| Chuck Blade Roast | | | | | |
| ⊛ Trimmed of visible fat (braised) | 3 oz | 210 | 17% | 20% | 30% |
| ⊛ Trimmed to 1/8" fat (braised) | 3 oz | 290 | 32% | 45% | 30% |
| Eye Round, Roast | | | | | |
| ❖ Trimmed of visible fat (roasted) | 3 oz | 140 | 6% | 10% | 20% |
| ❖ Trimmed to 1/8" fat (roasted) | 3 oz | 170 | 11% | 15% | 20% |

★ Foods with this symbol have less than or equal to 5% *Daily Value* for <u>all</u> three nutrients (5% Rule).
❖ Foods with this symbol have <u>at least one</u> of the three nutrients greater than 5% *Daily Value* but less than or equal to 20% *Daily Value*.
⊛ Foods with this symbol have <u>at least one</u> of the three nutrients greater than 20% *Daily Value* (20% Rule).

| FOOD | Serving Size | Calories | Tot Fat | Sat Fat | Chol |
|------|------|------|------|------|------|
| ❖ Flank Steak (Choice): | | | | | |
| Trimmed of visible fat (broiled) | 3 oz | 180 | 13% | 19% | 19% |
| Ground (broiled, well done) | | | | | |
| ☻ 10% fat (before cooking) | 3 oz | 210 | 17% | 20% | 28% |
| ☻ 17% fat (before cooking) | 3 oz | 230 | 20% | 25% | 28% |
| ☻ 27% fat (before cooking) | 3 oz | 250 | 26% | 30% | 28% |
| ☻ Heart | 3 oz | 150 | 7% | 7% | 55% |
| ☻ Kidneys | 3 oz | 120 | 4% | 5% | 110% |
| ☻ Liver | 3 oz | 140 | 6% | 8% | 110% |
| Loin, Sirloin Steak | | | | | |
| ☻ Trimmed of visible fat (broiled) | 3 oz | 170 | 9% | 10% | 25% |
| ☻ Trimmed to 1/8" fat (broiled) | 3 oz | 210 | 18% | 25% | 25% |
| Loin, Tenderloin Steak | | | | | |
| ☻ Trimmed of visible fat (broiled) | 3 oz | 180 | 14% | 15% | 23% |
| ☻ Trimmed to 1/8" fat (broiled) | 3 oz | 240 | 25% | 30% | 23% |
| ☻ Porterhouse (Choice, broiled) | 3 oz | 190 | 14% | 18% | 23% |
| Rib Roast, Large End | | | | | |
| ☻ Trimmed of visible fat (roasted) | 3 oz | 200 | 17% | 20% | 23% |
| ☻ Trimmed to 1/8" fat (roasted) | 3 oz | 300 | 37% | 50% | 23% |
| Rib Steak, Small End | | | | | |
| ☻ Trimmed of visible fat (broiled) | 3 oz | 190 | 15% | 20% | 23% |
| ☻ Trimmed to 1/8" fat (broiled) | 3 oz | 280 | 32% | 45% | 23% |
| Round, Tip Roast | | | | | |
| ☻ Trimmed of visible fat (roasted) | 3 oz | 160 | 9% | 10% | 23% |
| ☻ Trimmed to 1/8" fat (roasted) | 3 oz | 190 | 15% | 20% | 23% |
| ☻ Shank (Choice, simmered) | 3 oz | 170 | 8% | 10% | 22% |
| ☻ Rib, Short Ribs (Choice, braised) | 3 oz | 250 | 24% | 33% | 26% |
| ❖ Steak, T-Bone: Trimmed to 1/4" fat (broiled) | 3 oz | 190 | 14% | 18% | 18% |
| Stew | | | | | |
| ☻ Trimmed of visible fat (simmered) | 3 oz | 170 | 8% | 10% | 23% |
| ☻ Trimmed to 1/4" fat (simmered) | 3 oz | 190 | 12% | 14% | 23% |
| ☻ Tongue (simmered) | 3 oz | 240 | 27% | 38% | 30% |
| Top Loin, Steak | | | | | |
| ☻ Trimmed of visible fat (broiled) | 3 oz | 70 | 12% | 15% | 22% |
| ☻ Trimmed to 1/8" fat (broiled) | 3 oz | 130 | 23% | 30% | 22% |
| Top Round, Steak | | | | | |
| ☻ Trimmed of visible fat (broiled) | 3 oz | 150 | 6% | 5% | 23% |
| ☻ Trimmed to 1/8" fat (broiled) | 3 oz | 180 | 11% | 15% | 23% |
| ❖ Tripe, pickled | 3 oz | 300 | 0% | 1% | 19% |

### FRANKS

**Generic Foods**

| FOOD | Serving Size | Calories | Tot Fat | Sat Fat | Chol |
|------|------|------|------|------|------|
| ❖ Chicken Frankfurter | 1 frank | 140 | 16% | 15% | 18% |
| ☻ Corn Dog | 1 dog | 460 | 29% | 26% | 26% |

| FOOD | Serving Size | Calories | Tot Fat | Sat Fat | Chol |
|---|---|---|---|---|---|
| ⊛ Bratwurst, Pork | 1 link (2 oz) | 170 | 22% | 26% | 11% |
| ⊛ Frankfurter, Beef (10 per pound) | 1 frank | 140 | 20% | 27% | 9% |
| ⊛ Knockwurst, Pork & Beef | 1 link (2 oz) | 170 | 24% | 28% | 11% |

### Brand Name Foods

| FOOD | Serving Size | Calories | Tot Fat | Sat Fat | Chol |
|---|---|---|---|---|---|
| ❖ BUTTERBALL Turkey Frankfurters | 1 frank | 140 | 16% | 17% | 13% |
| ❖ GRILLMASTER Chicken Franks | 1 frank | 130 | 16% | 15% | 20% |
| HEALTHY CHOICE Franks— CONAGRA | | | | | |
| ❖ Beef Frank | 1 frank | 60 | 2% | 3% | 7% |
| ❖ Bunsize Frank | 1 frank | 70 | 2% | 3% | 7% |
| ❖ Franks | 1 frank | 50 | 2% | 3% | 7% |
| ❖ Jumbo Frank | 1 frank | 70 | 2% | 3% | 10% |
| ❖ Deli Beef Franks | 1 frank | 100 | 5% | 5% | 8% |
| ❖ Deli Meat Franks | 1 frank | 100 | 5% | 5% | 10% |
| HORMEL Franks | | | | | |
| ⊛ Cocktail Smokies | 5 Smokies | 180 | 25% | 35% | 13% |
| ❖ Corn Dogs | 2.75 oz | 220 | 17% | 15% | 15% |
| ⊛ Meat Franks | 1 frank | 140 | 20% | 30% | 12% |
| ⊛ Wieners | 5 wieners | 160 | 22% | 35% | 13% |
| ❖ JENNIE-O *Extra Lean* Premium Turkey Franks | 1 frank | 45 | 3% | 3% | 10% |
| ★ LIGHT & LEAN 97 Beef Franks— HORMEL FOODS | 1 frank | 45 | 2% | 3% | 3% |
| LOMA LINDA Meatless Hot Dogs—WORTHINGTON FOODS | | | | | |
| ❖ Big Franks | 1 frank | 110 | 11% | 5% | 0% |
| ❖ Corn Dogs | 1 pc | 200 | 14% | 8% | 0% |
| ❖ Linketts | 1 frank | 70 | 7% | 3% | 0% |
| LOUIS RICH Franks made w/ Turkey & Chicken—OSCAR MAYER | | | | | |
| ❖ *Bun-Length* (8–16 oz pkg) | 1 frank | 110 | 12% | 13% | 17% |
| ❖ Cheese Franks (10–16 oz pkg) | 1 frank | 90 | 11% | 13% | 13% |
| ❖ Franks (10–16 oz pkg) | 1 frank | 90 | 11% | 10% | 13% |
| ❖ MORNINGSTAR FARMS Meatless Deli Franks— WORTHINGTON FOODS | 1 frank | 110 | 11% | 5% | 0% |
| MR. TURKEY Franks | | | | | |
| ⊛ Chicken Cheese Franks | 1 frank | 140 | 18% | 22% | 12% |
| ❖ Turkey Franks | 1 frank | 130 | 17% | 16% | 13% |
| ❖ NATURAL TOUCH Vege Frank | 1 link | 100 | 9% | 5% | 0% |
| OSCAR MAYER *Big & Juicy* Franks | | | | | |
| ⊛ Deli Style Beef Franks | 1 link | 230 | 34% | 50% | 17% |
| ⊛ Hot 'N Spicy Wieners | 1 link | 220 | 31% | 40% | 15% |

★  Foods with this symbol have less than or equal to 5% *Daily Value* for <u>all</u> three nutrients (5% Rule).

❖  Foods with this symbol have <u>at least one</u> of the three nutrients greater than 5% *Daily Value* but less than or equal to 20% *Daily Value*.

⊛  Foods with this symbol have <u>at least one</u> of the three nutrients greater than 20% *Daily Value* (20% Rule).

| FOOD | Serving Size | Calories | Tot Fat | Sat Fat | Chol |
|------|------|------|------|------|------|
| ⊛ Original Beef Franks | 1 link | 240 | 34% | 45% | 15% |
| ⊛ Original Wieners | 1 link | 240 | 34% | 45% | 15% |
| ⊛ Quarter Pound Beef Franks | 1 link | 350 | 51% | 65% | 22% |
| ⊛ Smokie Links Wieners | 1 link | 220 | 29% | 35% | 17% |
| ★ OSCAR MAYER Fat Free Hot Dogs made w/Turkey & Beef | 1 frank | 40 | 0% | 0% | 5% |
| OSCAR MAYER Franks | | | | | |
| ⊛ Beef | 1 link | 140 | 20% | 30% | 8% |
| ⊛ Beef *Bun-Length* | 1 link | 190 | 26% | 35% | 12% |
| ❖ Beef Light | 1 link | 110 | 14% | 18% | 8% |
| ⊛ Cheese Hot Dogs made w/ Pork, Turkey & Beef | 1 link | 140 | 20% | 25% | 12% |
| OSCAR MAYER Wieners | | | | | |
| ⊛ *Bun-Length* made w/Pork & Turkey | 1 link | 190 | 26% | 30% | 12% |
| ❖ Light made w/Pork, Turkey & Beef | 1 link | 110 | 14% | 15% | 12% |
| ⊛ Little | 6 links | 180 | 26% | 30% | 10% |
| ⊛ Made w/Pork & Turkey | 1 link | 150 | 20% | 23% | 10% |
| WORTHINGTON Meatless Franks | | | | | |
| ❖ Super Link (canned) | 1 link | 110 | 12% | 5% | 0% |
| ★ Veja-Links (canned) | 1 link | 50 | 5% | 3% | 0% |
| WRANGLERS Franks—HORMEL FOODS | | | | | |
| ⊛ Beef or Smoked Franks | 1 frank | 170 | 23% | 30% | 13% |
| ⊛ Cheese Franks | 1 frank | 170 | 23% | 35% | 13% |

## GAME

**Generic Foods**

| | | | | | |
|------|------|------|------|------|------|
| ⊛ Deer (roasted) | 3 oz | 130 | 4% | 5% | 32% |
| ⊛ Elk (roasted) | 3 oz | 120 | 2% | 3% | 21% |
| ⊛ Rabbit, Domestic: All cuts (roasted) | 3 oz | 170 | 11% | 10% | 23% |
| ⊛ Venison (roasted) | 3 oz | 120 | 3% | 4% | 23% |

## HAM

**Generic Foods**

| | | | | | |
|------|------|------|------|------|------|
| ❖ Ham (roasted) | 3 oz | 130 | 7% | 8% | 16% |
| Ham (cured) | | | | | |
| ❖ Steak, Extra lean (cooked) | 3 oz | 100 | 6% | 6% | 13% |
| ❖ Whole, Lean (roasted) | 3 oz | 130 | 7% | 8% | 16% |
| Ham, Cured and canned | | | | | |
| ❖ Lean (roasted) | 3 oz | 120 | 6% | 7% | 9% |
| ⊛ Medium fat (roasted) | 3 oz | 190 | 20% | 21% | 18% |

| FOOD | Serving Size | Calories | Tot Fat | Sat Fat | Chol |
|---|---|---|---|---|---|
| **Brand Name Foods** | | | | | |
| ❖ BLACK LABEL Canned Ham— | | | | | |
| HORMEL FOODS | 3 oz | 100 | 8% | 10% | 13% |
| ❖ CURE 81 Ham—HORMEL FOODS | 3 oz | 100 | 8% | 8% | 15% |
| ❖ CUREMASTER Ham—HORMEL FOODS | 3 oz | 80 | 5% | 5% | 13% |
| ❖ HEALTHY CHOICE Boneless | | | | | |
| Honey Ham—CONAGRA | 3 oz | 100 | 4% | 5% | 13% |
| HORMEL | | | | | |
| ⊛ Ham & Cheese Patties | 1 patty | 190 | 26% | 30% | 15% |
| ⊛ Ham Patties | 1 patty | 180 | 26% | 30% | 12% |
| JENNIE-O Turkey Ham | | | | | |
| ❖ Honey Cured | 2 oz | 80 | 5% | 5% | 10% |
| ❖ Lean Turkey Ham | 2 oz | 70 | 5% | 5% | 13% |
| ❖ Turkey Ham (Water & | | | | | |
| Carrageenan Product) | 2 oz | 50 | 3% | 3% | 10% |
| ❖ LIGHT & LEAN 97 Ham— | | | | | |
| HORMEL FOODS | 3 oz | 90 | 4% | 5% | 12% |
| OSCAR MAYER Dinner Ham | | | | | |
| ❖ Slice | 3 oz | 80 | 5% | 5% | 13% |
| ❖ Steak | 1 steak | 60 | 3% | 3% | 10% |
| ⊛ OSCAR MAYER *Sweet Morsel* | | | | | |
| Smoked Boneless Pork | | | | | |
| Shoulder Butt | 3 oz | 180 | 23% | 25% | 17% |
| ❖ PRIMISSIMO Proscuitti Ham— | | | | | |
| HORMEL FOODS | 1 oz | 70 | 7% | 8% | 8% |

LAMB

| FOOD | Serving Size | Calories | Tot Fat | Sat Fat | Chol |
|---|---|---|---|---|---|
| **Generic Foods** | | | | | |
| ⊛ Ground (broiled) | 3 oz | 240 | 26% | 35% | 27% |
| Leg, Whole | | | | | |
| ⊛ Trimmed of visible fat (roasted) | 3 oz | 160 | 11% | 10% | 25% |
| ⊛ Trimmed to 1/8" fat (roasted) | 3 oz | 210 | 18% | 25% | 27% |
| Loin Chop | | | | | |
| ⊛ Trimmed of visible fat (broiled) | 3 oz | 180 | 12% | 15% | 27% |
| ⊛ Trimmed to 1/8" fat (broiled) | 3 oz | 250 | 28% | 35% | 28% |
| Rib Roast | | | | | |
| ⊛ Trimmed of visible fat (roasted) | 3 oz | 200 | 17% | 20% | 25% |
| ⊛ Trimmed to 1/8" fat (roasted) | 3 oz | 290 | 35% | 50% | 27% |
| Shank | | | | | |
| ⊛ Trimmed of visible fat (braised) | 3 oz | 160 | 8% | 10% | 30% |
| ⊛ Trimmed to 1/8" fat (braised) | 3 oz | 210 | 17% | 25% | 30% |

★ Foods with this symbol have less than or equal to 5% *Daily Value* for <u>all</u> three nutrients (5% Rule).

❖ Foods with this symbol have <u>at least one</u> of the three nutrients greater than 5% *Daily Value* but less than or equal to 20% *Daily Value*.

⊛ Foods with this symbol have <u>at least one</u> of the three nutrients greater than 20% *Daily Value* (20% Rule).

| FOOD | Serving Size | Calories | Tot Fat | Sat Fat | Chol |
|------|--------------|----------|---------|---------|------|
| Shoulder, Arm Chop | | | | | |
| ⊛ Trimmed of visible fat (broiled) | 3 oz | 170 | 12% | 15% | 27% |
| ⊛ Trimmed to 1/8" fat (broiled) | 3 oz | 230 | 23% | 35% | 27% |
| Shoulder, Blade Chop | | | | | |
| ⊛ Trimmed of visible fat (broiled) | 3 oz | 180 | 15% | 15% | 27% |
| ⊛ Trimmed to 1/8" fat (broiled) | 3 oz | 230 | 25% | 30% | 27% |

## MEAT SUBSTITUTES

**Brand Name Foods**

| FOOD | Serving Size | Calories | Tot Fat | Sat Fat | Chol |
|------|--------------|----------|---------|---------|------|
| ❖ FANTASTIC FOODS Falafel Mix (prep as dir) | 1 cup | 250 | 6% | 3% | 0% |
| HARVEST BURGERS—GREEN GIANT | | | | | |
| ❖ Italian Style | 1 burger | 140 | 7% | 8% | 0% |
| ❖ Original Flavor | 1 burger | 140 | 6% | 8% | 0% |
| ❖ Southwestern Style | 1 burger | 140 | 6% | 8% | 0% |
| ⊛ LOMA LINDA *Nuteena*— | | | | | |
| WORTHINGTON FOODS | 3/8" slc | 160 | 20% | 25% | 0% |
| LOMA LINDA Meatless Products —WORTHINGTON FOODS | | | | | |
| ⊛ Chik-Nuggets | 5 pcs | 240 | 25% | 13% | 0% |
| ★ Dinner Cuts | 1 slc | 80 | 2% | 3% | 0% |
| ⊛ Fried Chik'n | 1 pc | 180 | 23% | 10% | 0% |
| ⊛ Fried Chik'n w/Gravy | 2 pcs | 390 | 48% | 23% | 2% |
| ❖ Griddle Steaks | 1 pc | 130 | 11% | 5% | 0% |
| ❖ Redi-Burger | 5/8" slc | 170 | 15% | 8% | 0% |
| ❖ Sizzle Burger | 1 patty | 200 | 18% | 8% | 1% |
| ❖ Swiss Steak w/Gravy | 1 pc | 120 | 9% | 5% | 0% |
| ❖ Tender Bits | 6 avg pcs | 110 | 7% | 3% | 0% |
| ❖ Tender Rounds w/Gravy | 6 pcs | 120 | 8% | 5% | 0% |
| ★ Vege-Burger | 1/4 cup | 70 | 2% | 3% | 0% |
| ★ Vita-Burger Chunks | 1/4 cup | 70 | 2% | 0% | 0% |
| ★ Vita-Burger Granules | 3 tbsp | 70 | 2% | 0% | 0% |
| MORNINGSTAR FARMS Meatless Products—WORTHINGTON FOODS | | | | | |
| ★ Better 'N Burgers | 1 patty | 70 | 0% | 0% | 0% |
| ❖ Chik Patties | 1 patty | 170 | 15% | 8% | 0% |
| ❖ Garden Vege-Patties | 1 patty | 110 | 6% | 3% | 0% |
| ❖ Grillers | 1 patty | 140 | 11% | 8% | 0% |
| ❖ Prime Patties | 1 patty | 130 | 8% | 8% | 0% |
| NATURAL TOUCH Meatless Products—WORTHINGTON FOODS | | | | | |
| ❖ Garden Grain Patties | 1 patty | 160 | 11% | 5% | 0% |
| ❖ Garden Vege Patties | 1 patty | 10 | 6% | 5% | 0% |
| ❖ Okara Patties | 1 patty | 110 | 8% | 5% | 0% |
| ★ Vegan Burger | 1 patty | 70 | 0% | 0% | 0% |
| ❖ Vege Burger | 1 patty | 140 | 9% | 5% | 0% |

| FOOD | Serving Size | Calories | Tot Fat | Sat Fat | Chol |
|------|------|------|------|------|------|
| WORTHINGTON Meatless Cold Cuts | | | | | |
| ★ Bolono (frozen slices) | 3 slcs | 80 | 5% | 5% | 0% |
| ❖ Protose (3/8") | 1 slc | 130 | 11% | 5% | 0% |
| ❖ Salami (3/8") | 1 slc | 120 | 12% | 5% | 0% |
| ❖ Wham | 2 slcs | 80 | 8% | 5% | 0% |
| WORTHINGTON Meatless Products | | | | | |
| ❖ Beef Style (frozen roll) (3/8") | 1 slc | 110 | 11% | 5% | 0% |
| ❖ Chic-Ketts (3/8") | 2 slcs | 120 | 11% | 5% | 0% |
| ❖ Chicken | 2 slcs | 80 | 7% | 5% | 0% |
| ❖ Chicken (frozen roll) (3/8") | 1 slc | 80 | 7% | 5% | 0% |
| ❖ Chik Stiks | 1 pc | 110 | 11% | 5% | 0% |
| ★ Choplets | 2 slcs | 90 | 2% | 5% | 0% |
| ❖ Corned Beef (frozen slices) | 4 slcs | 140 | 14% | 10% | 0% |
| ❖ Crispy Chik Patties | 1 patty | 170 | 14% | 8% | 0% |
| ★ Diced Chik (canned) | 1/4 cup (drained) | 60 | 5% | 3% | 0% |
| ❖ Dinner Roast (3/4") | 1 slc | 180 | 18% | 10% | 1% |
| ❖ Frichik (canned) | 2 pcs | 120 | 12% | 5% | 0% |
| ❖ Golden Croquettes | 4 pcs | 210 | 15% | 8% | 0% |
| ★ Granburger (dry) | 3 tbsp | 60 | 1% | 0% | 0% |
| ★ Multigrain Cutlets | 1 slc | 80 | 2% | 3% | 0% |
| ❖ Numete (3/8") | 1 slc | 130 | 15% | 13% | 0% |
| ❖ Prime Stakes | 1 pc | 140 | 14% | 8% | 0% |
| ❖ Savory Slices | 3 slcs | 150 | 14% | 18% | 0% |
| ❖ Sliced Chik (canned) | 3 slcs | 90 | 9% | 5% | 0% |
| ❖ Smoked Beef (frozen slices) | 6 slcs | 120 | 9% | 5% | 0% |
| ❖ Smoked Turkey | 3 slcs | 140 | 15% | 10% | 0% |
| ❖ Stakelets | 1 pc | 140 | 12% | 8% | 0% |
| ❖ Tuno (frozen) | 1/2 cup | 80 | 9% | 5% | 0% |
| Ⓐ Turkee Slices (canned) | 3 slcs | 190 | 22% | 13% | 0% |
| ❖ Veelets (frozen) | 1 patty | 180 | 14% | 8% | 0% |
| ★ Vegetable Skallops | 1 cup | 90 | 2% | 3% | 0% |
| ★ Vegetable Steaks | 2 slcs | 80 | 2% | 3% | 0% |
| ★ Vegetarian Burger | 1/4 cup | 60 | 3% | 0% | 0% |
| ★ Vegetarian Cutlets | 1 slc | 70 | 2% | 0% | 0% |

## PORK

**Generic Foods**

| FOOD | Serving Size | Calories | Tot Fat | Sat Fat | Chol |
|------|------|------|------|------|------|
| ❖ Chitterlings, Pork | 1 oz | 90 | 13% | 14% | 14% |
| ❖ Feet, Pork (Pickled) | 1 oz | 60 | 7% | 8% | 9% |
| Ⓐ Ground (broiled) | 3 oz | 250 | 28% | 35% | 27% |

---

★ Foods with this symbol have less than or equal to 5% *Daily Value* for <u>all</u> three nutrients (5% Rule).

❖ Foods with this symbol have <u>at least one</u> of the three nutrients greater than 5% *Daily Value* but less than or equal to 20% *Daily Value*.

Ⓐ Foods with this symbol have <u>at least one</u> of the three nutrients greater than 20% *Daily Value* (20% Rule).

| FOOD | Serving Size | Calories | Tot Fat | Sat Fat | Chol |
|------|--------------|----------|---------|---------|------|
| Loin, Country Style Ribs | | | | | |
| ⊛ Trimmed of visible fat (roasted) | 3 oz | 210 | 20% | 25% | 27% |
| ⊛ Trimmed to 1/8" fat (roasted) | 3 oz | 280 | 34% | 40% | 27% |
| Loin, Center Chop | | | | | |
| ⊛ Trimmed of visible fat (broiled) | 3 oz | 170 | 11% | 15% | 23% |
| ⊛ Trimmed to 1/8" fat (broiled) | 3 oz | 200 | 17% | 20% | 23% |
| Loin, Rib Chop | | | | | |
| ⊛ Trimmed of visible fat (broiled) | 3 oz | 190 | 12% | 15% | 23% |
| ⊛ Trimmed to 1/8" fat (broiled) | 3 oz | 220 | 20% | 25% | 23% |
| Loin, Sirloin Roast | | | | | |
| ⊛ Trimmed of visible fat (roasted) | 3 oz | 180 | 14% | 15% | 25% |
| ⊛ Trimmed to 1/8" fat (roasted) | 3 oz | 220 | 22% | 25% | 25% |
| Loin, Tenderloin Roast | | | | | |
| ⊛ Trimmed of visible fat (roasted) | 3 oz | 140 | 6% | 5% | 22% |
| ⊛ Trimmed to 1/8" fat (roasted) | 3 oz | 150 | 8% | 10% | 22% |
| Shoulder, Blade Steak | | | | | |
| ⊛ Trimmed of visible fat (broiled) | 3 oz | 190 | 17% | 20% | 27% |
| ⊛ Trimmed to 1/8" fat (broiled) | 3 oz | 220 | 22% | 25% | 27% |
| Spareribs | | | | | |
| ⊛ Trimmed to 1/8" fat (braised) | 3 oz | 340 | 40% | 45% | 35% |
| Top Loin, Chop (boneless) | | | | | |
| ⊛ Trimmed of visible fat (broiled) | 3 oz | 170 | 11% | 10% | 23% |
| ⊛ Trimmed to 1/8" fat (broiled) | 3 oz | 200 | 15% | 15% | 23% |
| Top Loin, Roast (boneless) | | | | | |
| ⊛ Trimmed of visible fat (roasted) | 3 oz | 170 | 9% | 10% | 22% |
| ⊛ Trimmed to 1/8" fat (roasted) | 3 oz | 190 | 15% | 20% | 22% |

**Brand Name Foods**

| | | | | | |
|------|--------------|----------|---------|---------|------|
| HORMEL Pickled Products | | | | | |
| ❖ Pickled Pigs Feet | 2 oz | 80 | 9% | 10% | 15% |
| ❖ Pickled Pork Hocks | 2 oz | 110 | 12% | 15% | 15% |

SAUSAGES

**Generic Foods**

| | | | | | |
|------|--------------|----------|---------|---------|------|
| ⊛ Kielbasa, Pork and Beef | 1 link (2 oz) | 170 | 23% | 27% | 12% |
| ⊛ Polish Sausage | 2 oz | 180 | 24% | 28% | 13% |
| ⊛ Sausage (smoked and cured) | 2 oz | 170 | 23% | 31% | 12% |
| ❖ Sausage, Meatless | 2 oz | 140 | 15% | 8% | 0% |
| ⊛ Sausage, Pork | 4 links | 200 | 26% | 30% | 16% |
| ⊛ Sausage Patty, Pork | 2 patties | 200 | 26% | 30% | 15% |
| ⊛ Vienna Sausage, Pork and Beef | 2 oz | 150 | 21% | 25% | 10% |

**Brand Name Foods**

| | | | | | |
|------|--------------|----------|---------|---------|------|
| GREEN GIANT Sausage Substitutes —PILLSBURY | | | | | |
| ❖ Breakfast Links | 3 links | 110 | 8% | 3% | 0% |
| ❖ Breakfast Patties | 2 patties | 100 | 6% | 3% | 0% |

| FOOD | Serving Size | Calories | Tot Fat | Sat Fat | Chol |
|------|------|------|------|------|------|
| ★ HEALTHY CHOICE Breakfast Sausage: Links or Patties—CONAGRA | 2 links/patties | 50 | 2% | 3% | 5% |
| HEALTHY CHOICE Low Fat Link Line—CONAGRA | | | | | |
| ❖ Polska Kielbasa | 1 link | 100 | 5% | 5% | 12% |
| ❖ Smoked Sausage | 1 link | 100 | 5% | 5% | 12% |
| HEALTHY CHOICE Low-Fat Smoked Sausage—CONAGRA | | | | | |
| ❖ Polska Kielbasa | 2 oz | 70 | 2% | 3% | 8% |
| ❖ Smoked Sausage | 2 oz | 70 | 2% | 3% | 8% |
| Ⓐ HORMEL Kielbasa Skinless Sausage | 2 oz | 150 | 20% | 25% | 13% |
| Ⓐ HORMEL Pickled Smoked or Hot Sausage | 6 links | 140 | 17% | 25% | 13% |
| HORMEL Sausage | | | | | |
| ❖ Chicken Vienna Sausage | 2 oz | 110 | 15% | 15% | 18% |
| ❖ Vienna Sausage | 2 oz | 140 | 20% | 20% | 15% |
| JENNIE-O *Extra Lean* Sausages | | | | | |
| ❖ Smoked Turkey Sausage | 2 oz | 70 | 4% | 3% | 12% |
| ❖ Turkey Kielbasa | 2 oz | 70 | 4% | 4% | 12% |
| ❖ JENNIE-O Turkey Sausage | 2 links | 130 | 17% | 15% | 16% |
| LIBBY'S Vienna Sausage—NESTLÉ | | | | | |
| ❖ Chicken Vienna Sausage | 3 links | 100 | 12% | 13% | 17% |
| ❖ Vienna Sausage | 3 links | 130 | 18% | 12% | 16% |
| ❖ Vienna Sausage in BBQ Sauce | 3 links w/ sauce | 130 | 18% | 12% | 16% |
| LITTLE SIZZLERS—HORMEL FOODS | | | | | |
| Ⓐ Brown 'N Serve Sausage Link | 3 links | 230 | 34% | 40% | 15% |
| Ⓐ Brown 'N Serve Sausage Patties | 2 patties | 190 | 28% | 30% | 13% |
| Ⓐ Sausage Link (cooked) | 3 links | 210 | 31% | 35% | 15% |
| Ⓐ Sausage Patties (cooked) | 2 patties | 250 | 35% | 40% | 17% |
| ❖ LOMA LINDA Little Links—WORTHINGTON FOODS | 2 links | 90 | 9% | 5% | 0% |
| LOUIS RICH Turkey Sausage—OSCAR MAYER | | | | | |
| ❖ Polska Kielbasa | 2 oz | 80 | 7% | 8% | 12% |
| ❖ Sausage Links | 2 links | 90 | 9% | 8% | 15% |
| ❖ Smoked | 2 oz | 90 | 8% | 8% | 12% |
| ❖ Smoked w/cheddar | 2 oz | 90 | 8% | 10% | 12% |
| MORNINGSTAR FARMS Meatless Sausages—WORTHINGTON FOODS | | | | | |
| ❖ Breakfast Links | 2 links | 90 | 8% | 5% | 0% |
| ❖ Breakfast Patties | 1 patty | 90 | 8% | 8% | 0% |

★ Foods with this symbol have less than or equal to 5% *Daily Value* for <u>all</u> three nutrients (5% Rule).

❖ Foods with this symbol have <u>at least one</u> of the three nutrients greater than 5% *Daily Value* but less than or equal to 20% *Daily Value*.

Ⓐ Foods with this symbol have <u>at least one</u> of the three nutrients greater than 20% *Daily Value* (20% Rule).

| FOOD | Serving Size | Calories | Tot Fat | Sat Fat | Chol |
|---|---|---|---|---|---|
| MR. TURKEY Sausage | | | | | |
| ❖ Breakfast | 3 links | 110 | 13% | 8% | 10% |
| ❖ Smoked | 3 links | 100 | 10% | 12% | 12% |
| ❖ OLD SMOKEHOUSE Smoked Summer Sausage—HORMEL FOODS | 1 oz | 110 | 15% | 20% | 10% |
| ❖ OSCAR MAYER Braunschweiger (Liver Sausage) | 1 slc | 100 | 14% | 15% | 17% |
| Ⓐ OSCAR MAYER Pork Sausage Link | 2 links | 170 | 23% | 25% | 13% |
| OSCAR MAYER Smokies | | | | | |
| Ⓐ Beef | 1 link | 120 | 17% | 25% | 10% |
| Ⓐ Cheese | 1 link | 130 | 18% | 23% | 10% |
| ❖ Links Sausage | 1 link | 130 | 18% | 20% | 8% |
| Ⓐ Little Cheese | 6 links | 180 | 25% | 30% | 12% |
| Ⓐ Little Sausage | 6 links | 170 | 25% | 30% | 12% |
| SPECIAL RECIPE Sausage— HORMEL FOODS | | | | | |
| ❖ Sausage Link | 2 links | 108 | 15% | 20% | 6% |
| ❖ Sausage Patty | 1 patty | 108 | 15% | 20% | 6% |
| TURKEY STORE Turkey Sausage | | | | | |
| ❖ Breakfast | 2 links | 140 | 16% | 17% | 13% |
| ❖ Italian | 2 links | 130 | 15% | 8% | 15% |
| WORTHINGTON Meatless Sausage | | | | | |
| ❖ Leanies Links (frozen) | 1 link | 110 | 12% | 8% | 0% |
| ❖ Prosage Links (frozen) | 2 links | 120 | 14% | 8% | 0% |
| ❖ Prosage Patties (frozen) | 1 patty | 100 | 11% | 10% | 0% |
| ❖ Saucettes | 1 link | 90 | 9% | 5% | 0% |

### VEAL

**Generic Foods**

| FOOD | Serving Size | Calories | Tot Fat | Sat Fat | Chol |
|---|---|---|---|---|---|
| Cutlets | | | | | |
| ❖ Trimmed of visible fat (roasted) | 3 oz | 130 | 5% | 5% | 20% |
| ❖ Trimmed to 1/8" fat (roasted) | 3 oz | 140 | 6% | 10% | 20% |
| Ⓐ Ground (broiled) | 3 oz | 150 | 10% | 13% | 29% |
| Loin Chop | | | | | |
| Ⓐ Trimmed of visible fat (roasted) | 3 oz | 150 | 9% | 10% | 27% |
| Ⓐ Trimmed to 1/8" fat (roasted) | 3 oz | 180 | 15% | 20% | 27% |
| Rib Roast | | | | | |
| Ⓐ Trimmed of visible fat (roasted) | 3 oz | 150 | 9% | 10% | 27% |
| Ⓐ Trimmed to 1/8" fat (roasted) | 3 oz | 190 | 18% | 25% | 27% |

| FOOD | Serving Size | Calories | Tot Fat | Sat Fat | Chol |
|------|--------------|----------|---------|---------|------|
| Shoulder, Arm Steak | | | | | |
| ⊛   Trimmed of visible fat (braised) | 3 oz | 170 | 8% | 5% | 25% |
| ⊛   Trimmed to 1/8" fat (braised) | 3 oz | 200 | 14% | 15% | 25% |
| Shoulder, Blade Steak | | | | | |
| ⊛   Trimmed of visible fat (braised) | 3 oz | 170 | 9% | 10% | 28% |
| ⊛   Trimmed to 1/8" fat (braised) | 3 oz | 190 | 14% | 15% | 28% |

# Nuts and Seeds

### BUTTERS

**Generic Foods**

| FOOD | Serving Size | Calories | Tot Fat | Sat Fat | Chol |
|------|--------------|----------|---------|---------|------|
| ⊛ Almond Butter | 2 tbsp | 200 | 29% | 9% | 0% |
| ⊛ Cashew Butter | 2 tbsp | 190 | 24% | 16% | 0% |
| ⊛ Peanut Butter: Chunky or Smooth Style | 2 tbsp | 190 | 25% | 15% | 0% |
| ⊛ Sesame Butter (Tahini) | 2 tbsp | 170 | 23% | 11% | 0% |

**Brand Name Foods**

| FOOD | Serving Size | Calories | Tot Fat | Sat Fat | Chol |
|------|--------------|----------|---------|---------|------|
| ⊛ ESTEE Peanut Butter | 2 tbsp | 190 | 23% | 15% | 0% |
| ⊛ FEATHERWEIGHT Peanut Butter | 2 tbsp | 190 | 23% | 15% | 0% |
| ❖ GOOBER Peanut Butter & Jelly—SMUCKER'S | 3 tbsp | 230 | 20% | 10% | 0% |
| JIF Peanut Butter—PROCTER & GAMBLE | | | | | |
| ⊛   Creamy or Extra Crunchy | 2 tbsp | 190 | 25% | 15% | 0% |
| ❖   Reduced Fat JIF: Creamy or Crunchy | 2 tbsp | 190 | 18% | 12% | 0% |
| ⊛   *Simply* JIF: Creamy or Crunchy | 2 tbsp | 190 | 25% | 15% | 0% |
| PETER PAN Peanut Butter—HUNT WESSON | | | | | |
| ⊛   Creamy | 2 tbsp | 190 | 25% | 17% | 0% |
| ⊛   Crunchy | 2 tbsp | 190 | 24% | 16% | 0% |
| ⊛   Very Low Sodium Creamy | 2 tbsp | 200 | 27% | 12% | 0% |
| ⊛   Very Low Sodium Crunchy | 2 tbsp | 200 | 27% | 12% | 0% |
| ❖   Whipped Creamy | 2 tbsp | 150 | 19% | 13% | 0% |
| ❖   Whipped Crunchy | 2 tbsp | 150 | 19% | 12% | 0% |

★  Foods with this symbol have less than or equal to 5% *Daily Value* for <u>all</u> three nutrients (5% Rule).

❖  Foods with this symbol have <u>at least one</u> of the three nutrients greater than 5% *Daily Value* but less than or equal to 20% *Daily Value*.

⊛  Foods with this symbol have <u>at least one</u> of the three nutrients greater than 20% *Daily Value* (20% Rule).

| FOOD | Serving Size | Calories | Tot Fat | Sat Fat | Chol |
|---|---|---|---|---|---|
| ❖ PETER PAN *Smart Choice* Reduced Fat Peanut Butter Spread | 2 tbsp | 190 | 18% | 10% | 0% |
| ❖   Creamy | 2 tbsp | 180 | 17% | 11% | 0% |
| ❖   Crunchy | 2 tbsp | 200 | 18% | 8% | 0% |
| POLANER Peanut Butter— AMERICAN HOME FOODS | | | | | |
| ❖   Grape Jelly & Peanut Butter | 2 tbsp | 120 | 8% | 5% | 0% |
| ⊛   Natural Crunchy | 2 tbsp | 190 | 22% | 10% | 0% |
| ⊛   Natural Smooth: Regular or No Salt | 2 tbsp | 190 | 22% | 10% | 0% |
| ⊛ REESE'S Peanut Butter: Creamy or Crunchy—HERSHEY FOODS | 2 tbsp | 200 | 25% | 15% | 0% |
| SKIPPY Peanut Butter—CPC | | | | | |
| ⊛   Creamy or Super Chunk | 2 tbsp | 190 | 26% | 17% | 0% |
| ❖   Creamy or Super Chunk, Reduced Fat | 2 tbsp | 190 | 19% | 13% | 0% |
| SMUCKER'S | | | | | |
| ⊛   Natural Peanut Butter | 2 tbsp | 200 | 25% | 10% | 0% |
| ⊛   Peanut Butter | 2 tbsp | 190 | 23% | 15% | 0% |

## NUTS

**Generic Foods**

| FOOD | Serving Size | Calories | Tot Fat | Sat Fat | Chol |
|---|---|---|---|---|---|
| ⊛ Almonds (dry roasted) | 1 oz | 170 | 23% | 7% | 0% |
| ⊛ Almonds (honey roasted) | 1 oz | 170 | 22% | 7% | 0% |
| ⊛ Almonds (oil roasted) | 1 oz | 180 | 25% | 8% | 0% |
| ⊛ Beechnuts (dried) | 1 oz | 170 | 22% | 8% | 0% |
| ⊛ Brazil Nuts (dried and shelled) | 1 oz | 190 | 29% | 23% | 0% |
| ⊛ Butternuts (dried) | 1 oz | 170 | 25% | 2% | 0% |
| ❖ Cashews (dry roasted) | 1 oz | 160 | 20% | 13% | 0% |
| ⊛ Cashews (oil roasted) | 1 oz | 160 | 21% | 14% | 0% |
| ★ Chinese Chestnuts (raw) | 1 oz | 60 | 0% | 0% | 0% |
| ⊛ Coconut flesh | 1 oz | 100 | 15% | 42% | 0% |
| ★ European Chestnuts (roasted) | 1 oz | 70 | 1% | 1% | 0% |
| ⊛ Filberts (dry roasted) | 1 oz | 190 | 29% | 7% | 0% |
| ⊛ Hazelnuts (dry roasted) | 1 oz | 190 | 29% | 7% | 0% |
| ⊛ Hickory Nuts (dried) | 1 oz | 200 | 30% | 11% | 0% |
| ⊛ Macadamia Nuts (oil roasted) | 1 oz | 200 | 34% | 16% | 0% |
| ⊛ Mixed Nuts (dry roasted) | 1 oz | 170 | 22% | 10% | 0% |
| ⊛ Mixed Nuts (oil roasted) | 1 oz | 180 | 25% | 12% | 0% |
| ⊛ Peanuts: All types (dry roasted) | 1 oz | 170 | 22% | 10% | 0% |
| ⊛ Pecans (dry roasted) | 1 oz | 190 | 28% | 7% | 0% |
| ⊛ Pecans (oil roasted) | 1 oz | 200 | 31% | 8% | 0% |
| ⊛ Pine Nuts/Pignolia | 1 oz | 150 | 22% | 11% | 0% |
| ⊛ Pistachio (dry roasted) | 1 oz | 170 | 23% | 9% | 0% |
| ⊛ Walnuts (dried) | 1 oz | 180 | 23% | 7% | 0% |

| FOOD | Serving Size | Calories | Tot Fat | Sat Fat | Chol |
|------|--------------|----------|---------|---------|------|

**Brand Name Foods**

BLUE DIAMOND Almonds

| FOOD | Serving Size | Calories | Tot Fat | Sat Fat | Chol |
|------|--------------|----------|---------|---------|------|
| ⊛ Blanched Sliced | 1/3 cup | 200 | 26% | 8% | 0% |
| ❖ Blanched Almond Paste | 2 tbsp | 150 | 15% | 5% | 0% |
| ⊛ Blanched Slivered | 1/4 cup | 190 | 25% | 5% | 0% |
| ⊛ Blanched Whole | 3 tbsp | 190 | 25% | 5% | 0% |
| ⊛ Chopped Natural | 1/4 cup | 200 | 26% | 5% | 0% |
| ⊛ Dry Roasted, No Salt | 3 tbsp | 190 | 25% | 8% | 0% |
| ⊛ Dry Roasted, Salted | 3 tbsp | 200 | 25% | 5% | 0% |
| ⊛ Honey Roasted | 3 tbsp | 170 | 22% | 5% | 0% |
| ⊛ Oil Roasted Whole | 3 tbsp | 200 | 26% | 5% | 0% |
| ⊛ Roasted, Salted | 3 tbsp | 180 | 26% | 5% | 0% |
| ⊛ Sliced Natural | 1/3 cup | 200 | 26% | 5% | 0% |
| ⊛ Smokehouse | 3 tbsp | 180 | 25% | 5% | 0% |
| ⊛ Whole Natural | 3 tbsp | 180 | 23% | 5% | 0% |
| EAGLE Nuts—ANHEUSER BUSCH | | | | | |
| ⊛ Ballpark Peanuts | 1 oz (28 nuts) | 180 | 23% | 15% | 0% |
| ⊛ Deluxe Mixed Nuts w/o Peanuts | 1 oz (1/4 cup) | 200 | 26% | 15% | 0% |
| ⊛ Honey Roast Cashew & Peanut Mix | 1 oz (1/4 cup) | 180 | 22% | 15% | 0% |
| ⊛ Honey Roast Cashews | 1 oz (18 nuts) | 180 | 22% | 15% | 0% |
| ❖ Honey Roast Peanuts | 1 oz (35 nuts) | 170 | 20% | 15% | 0% |
| ⊛ Lightly Salted Cashews | 1 oz (19 nuts) | 190 | 23% | 15% | 0% |
| ⊛ Lightly Salted Mixed Nuts | 1 oz (1/4 cup) | 200 | 26% | 15% | 0% |
| ⊛ Lightly Salted Peanuts | 1 oz (29 nuts) | 180 | 23% | 15% | 0% |
| ⊛ Mixed Nuts | 1 oz (1/4 cup) | 200 | 26% | 15% | 0% |
| ⊛ Roasted Peanuts | 1 oz (28 nuts) | 180 | 23% | 10% | 0% |
| FISHER FAVORITES Glazed Nut Mix & Cashews—PROCTER & GAMBLE | | | | | |
| ❖ Honey | 1 oz | 170 | 19% | 10% | 0% |
| ❖ Praline | 1 oz | 170 | 18% | 10% | 0% |
| ❖ Toffee | 1 oz | 170 | 17% | 9% | 0% |
| FISHER Golden Roast Crunchy Nuts—PROCTER & GAMBLE | | | | | |
| ❖ Baked Honey Peanuts | 1 oz | 150 | 14% | 8% | 0% |

★ Foods with this symbol have less than or equal to 5% *Daily Value* for all three nutrients (5% Rule).

❖ Foods with this symbol have at least one of the three nutrients greater than 5% *Daily Value* but less than or equal to 20% *Daily Value*.

⊛ Foods with this symbol have at least one of the three nutrients greater than 20% *Daily Value* (20% Rule).

| FOOD | Serving Size | Calories | Tot Fat | Sat Fat | Chol |
|---|---|---|---|---|---|
| ❖ BBQ Peanuts | 1 oz | 160 | 18% | 9% | 0% |
| ❖ Peanuts | 1 oz | 160 | 18% | 9% | 0% |
| FISHER Nuts—PROCTER & GAMBLE | | | | | |
| ⊛ Cashew Halves | 1 oz | 170 | 23% | 13% | 0% |
| ❖ Honey Dry Roasted Peanuts | 1 oz | 170 | 20% | 12% | 0% |
| ⊛ Honey Roasted Peanuts | 1 oz | 160 | 21% | 12% | 0% |
| ❖ Honey Roasted Peanuts & Cashews | 1 oz | 170 | 20% | 9% | 0% |
| ⊛ Jumbo Cashews | 1 oz | 170 | 23% | 13% | 0% |
| ⊛ Mixed Nuts: Plain or Lightly Salted | 1 oz | 180 | 25% | 13% | 0% |
| ⊛ Oil Roast Peanuts | 1 oz | 170 | 23% | 13% | 0% |
| ⊛ Oil Roasted Cashews | 1 oz | 170 | 23% | 13% | 0% |
| ⊛ Red Pistachios | 1 bag | 170 | 23% | 12% | 0% |
| ⊛ Salted In-shell Peanuts | 1 oz (shelled) | 170 | 21% | 8% | 0% |
| ⊛ Spanish Peanuts | 1 oz | 180 | 25% | 12% | 0% |
| ⊛ LITTLE DEBBIE Individual Snacks: Salted Peanuts—MCKEE FOODS | 1/2 pkg (1 oz) | 160 | 22% | 10% | 0% |
| ⊛ PROGRESSO Pignoli (Pine) Nuts—PET | 1 oz | 170 | 21% | 6% | 0% |

SEEDS

**Generic Foods**

| FOOD | Serving Size | Calories | Tot Fat | Sat Fat | Chol |
|---|---|---|---|---|---|
| ❖ Pumpkin Seeds (roasted) | 1 oz | 130 | 8% | 5% | 0% |
| ⊛ Sesame Seeds (dried) | 2 tbsp | 160 | 22% | 10% | 0% |
| ⊛ Sunflower Kernels (dry roasted) | 1 oz | 170 | 22% | 7% | 0% |
| ⊛ Sunflower Kernels (oil roasted) | 1 oz | 180 | 25% | 9% | 0% |

**Brand Name Foods**

| FOOD | Serving Size | Calories | Tot Fat | Sat Fat | Chol |
|---|---|---|---|---|---|
| ARROWHEAD MILLS Seeds | | | | | |
| ⊛ Sesame, hulled | 1/4 cup | 210 | 31% | 13% | 0% |
| ⊛ Sesame, whole brown | 1/4 cup | 200 | 31% | 13% | 0% |
| ⊛ Sunflower, hulled | 1/4 cup | 180 | 23% | 8% | 0% |
| FISHER Seeds—PROCTER & GAMBLE | | | | | |
| ⊛ Salted In-shell Sunflower Seeds | 1 oz (shelled) | 170 | 23% | 7% | 0% |
| ⊛ Sunflower Nuts | 1 oz | 170 | 23% | 7% | 0% |

| FOOD | Serving Size | Calories | Tot Fat | Sat Fat | Chol |
|------|------|------|------|------|------|

# Pasta, Rice, and Other Grains

*Note: Values are for cooked pasta, rice, and other grains unless otherwise noted.*

### ORIENTAL NOODLES

**Generic Foods**

| FOOD | Serving Size | Calories | Tot Fat | Sat Fat | Chol |
|------|------|------|------|------|------|
| ★ Cellophane Rice Noodles | 1/2 cup | 250 | 0% | 0% | 0% |
| ⊛ Fried Chow Mein Noodles | 1 cup | 240 | 21% | 10% | 0% |
| ★ Japanese Soba | 1 cup | 110 | 0% | 0% | 0% |
| ★ Japanese Somen | 1 cup | 230 | 0% | 0% | 0% |
| ★ Mung Bean Noodles | 1/2 cup | 190 | 0% | 0% | 0% |
| ❖ Ramen | 2/3 cup | 140 | 9% | 1% | 8% |
| ★ Rice Cellophane | 1/2 cup | 70 | 0% | 0% | 0% |
| ★ Rice Sticks | 1/2 cup | 70 | 5% | 2% | 0% |
| ❖ Rice Sticks (fried) | 1/2 cup | 100 | 8% | 3% | 5% |
| ★ Somen, Wheat (uncooked) | 1/2 cup | 200 | 1% | 0% | 0% |
| ★ Soybean Noodles | 1/2 cup | 190 | 0% | 0% | 0% |
| ★ Sweet Potato Noodles | 1/2 cup | 190 | 0% | 0% | 0% |
| ★ Udon | 1/2 cup | 190 | 2% | 0% | 0% |
| ★ Wonton Wrappers | 6 wrappers | 140 | 1% | 1% | 2% |

**Brand Name Foods**

| FOOD | Serving Size | Calories | Tot Fat | Sat Fat | Chol |
|------|------|------|------|------|------|
| ❖ KNORR Oriental Noodles—CPC | 1 pkg | 210 | 4% | 2% | 6% |
| LA CHOY Noodles & Rice— HUNT WESSON | | | | | |
| ❖ Chow Mein Noodles | 1/2 cup | 140 | 9% | 6% | 0% |
| ❖ Crispy Wide Noodles | 1/2 cup | 150 | 13% | 8% | 0% |
| ★ Rice Noodles | 1/2 cup | 120 | 5% | 3% | 0% |
| SUN LUCK Noodles | | | | | |
| ★ Bean Threads Saifun (uncooked) | 2 oz | 190 | 0% | 0% | 0% |
| ★ Chow Mein Chuka Soba | 1 1/2 cups | 200 | 1% | 0% | 0% |
| ★ Maifun (rice sticks, uncooked) | 2 oz | 200 | 1% | 1% | 0% |
| ★ Somen Tomoshiraga | 1 bundle | 320 | 4% | 0% | 0% |
| ★ Steamed Stir-Fry Noodles | 1 cup | 400 | 3% | 0% | 0% |
| ★ Udon Noodles | 1 cup | 400 | 3% | 0% | 0% |
| ★ Yakisoba Noodles | 1 cup | 400 | 0% | 0% | 0% |

---

★ Foods with this symbol have less than or equal to 5% *Daily Value* for <u>all</u> three nutrients (5% Rule).

❖ Foods with this symbol have <u>at least one</u> of the three nutrients greater than 5% *Daily Value* but less than or equal to 20% *Daily Value*.

⊛ Foods with this symbol have <u>at least one</u> of the three nutrients greater than 20% *Daily Value* (20% Rule).

| FOOD | Serving Size | Calories | Tot Fat | Sat Fat | Chol |
|------|--------------|----------|---------|---------|------|

PASTA: DRY

**Generic Foods**

| | | | | | |
|------|--------------|----------|---------|---------|------|
| ★ Macaroni | 1 cup | 220 | 1% | 1% | 0% |
| ★ Macaroni (uncooked) | 1/2 cup (2 oz) | 190 | 1% | 1% | 0% |
| ★ Macaroni, Vegetable | 1 cup | 170 | 0% | 0% | 0% |
| ★ Macaroni, Vegetable (uncooked) | 1/2 cup (2 oz) | 150 | 1% | 0% | 0% |
| ★ Pasta: All shapes (uncooked) | 1/2 cup (2 oz) | 200 | 2% | 1% | 0% |
| Spaghetti | | | | | |
| ★ Cooked Al Dente | 1 cup | 190 | 2% | 0% | 0% |
| ★ Cooked Tender | 1 cup | 160 | 2% | 0% | 0% |
| ★ Spinach | 1 cup | 180 | 1% | 1% | 0% |
| ★ Uncooked | 2 oz | 200 | 1% | 1% | 0% |
| ★ Whole Wheat | 1 cup | 170 | 1% | 1% | 0% |

**Brand Name Foods**

| | | | | | |
|------|--------------|----------|---------|---------|------|
| ★ ENER-G Gluten Free Rice Macaroni (uncooked) | 2 oz | 200 | 0% | 0% | 0% |
| ENER-G Gluten Free Noodles | | | | | |
| ★ Brown Rice Shells (uncooked) | 2 oz | 210 | 0% | 0% | 0% |
| ★ Rice Spaghetti | 1/2 cup | 210 | 0% | 0% | 0% |
| ★ Rice Tagliatelle | 1/2 cup | 210 | 0% | 0% | 0% |
| ★ Rice Vermicelli | 1/2 cup | 210 | 0% | 0% | 0% |
| ★ Spaghetti | 1/2 cup | 180 | 1% | 0% | 0% |
| ★ Spiral Noodle (uncooked) | 2 oz | 180 | 1% | 0% | 0% |
| ⊛ MANISCHEWITZ Egg Noodles | 1 1/4 cups | 220 | 4% | 4% | 22% |
| MUELLER'S Pasta (uncooked)—CPC | | | | | |
| ❖ Egg Noodles | 2 oz | 220 | 5% | 0% | 18% |
| ★ Pasta | 2 oz | 210 | 2% | 0% | 0% |
| ★ Yolk Free Cholesterol Free Noodles | 2 oz | 210 | 2% | 0% | 0% |
| WESTBRAE Pasta (uncooked) | | | | | |
| ★ Spinach Lasagna | 2 pcs | 180 | 3% | 0% | 0% |
| ★ Whole Wheat Lasagna | 2 pcs | 180 | 2% | 0% | 0% |

PASTA: FROZEN AND REFRIGERATED

**Brand Name Foods**

| | | | | | |
|------|--------------|----------|---------|---------|------|
| BUDGET GOURMET *Original Entrées*—ALL AMERICAN GOURMET | | | | | |
| ⊛ Cheese Manicotti w/Meat Sauce | 1 pkg | 420 | 34% | 55% | 28% |
| ⊛ Italian Sausage Lasagna | 1 pkg | 430 | 32% | 45% | 20% |
| CONTADINA Pasta—NESTLÉ | | | | | |
| ⊛ Angel's Hair | 1 1/4 cups | 240 | 5% | 4% | 30% |
| ⊛ Beef & Garlic Ravioli | 1 1/4 cups | 350 | 21% | 24% | 36% |

| | FOOD | Serving Size | Calories | Tot Fat | Sat Fat | Chol |
|---|---|---|---|---|---|---|
| ▲ | Cheese & Basil Tortelloni | 1 cup | 360 | 16% | 20% | 21% |
| ▲ | Cheese Ravioli | 1 cup | 280 | 18% | 31% | 27% |
| ❖ | Cheese Tortelloni | 3/4 cup | 260 | 9% | 13% | 14% |
| ▲ | Chicken & Prosciutto Tortelloni | 1 cup | 360 | 20% | 19% | 23% |
| ▲ | Chicken & Rosemary Ravioli | 1 1/4 cups | 330 | 19% | 16% | 27% |
| ❖ | Chicken & Vegetable Tortelloni | 3/4 cup | 260 | 10% | 8% | 14% |
| ▲ | Fettuccine | 1 1/4 cups | 250 | 5% | 4% | 31% |
| ★ | Fettuccine, Cholesterol Free | 1 cup | 240 | 3% | 2% | 0% |
| ❖ | Light Cheese Ravioli | 1 cup | 240 | 7% | 10% | 18% |
| ▲ | Light Garden Vegetable Ravioli | 1 1/4 cups | 290 | 9% | 15% | 21% |
| ❖ | Light Garlic & Cheese Tortelloni | 1 cup | 280 | 8% | 11% | 17% |
| ▲ | Linguine | 1 1/4 cups | 260 | 5% | 4% | 32% |
| ★ | Linguine, Cholesterol Free | 1 1/4 cups | 250 | 4% | 2% | 0% |
| ★ | Plain Pasta: All varieties | 1/4 pkg | 210 | 2% | 1% | 0% |
| ▲ | Spicy Italian Sausage & Bell Pepper Tortelloni | 1 cup | 330 | 15% | 19% | 29% |
| ★ | Spinach Linguine | 1/4 pkg | 210 | 2% | 1% | 0% |
| ▲ | Spinach Tagliatelle (Fettuccine) | 1 1/4 cups | 270 | 6% | 5% | 34% |
| ❖ | Spinach Three Cheese Tortelloni | 3/4 cup | 260 | 9% | 14% | 18% |
| ★ | Tricolor Rotelle | 1/6 pkg | 210 | 2% | 1% | 0% |
| | DI GIORNO *Light Varieties* Ravioli —KRAFT | | | | | |
| ★ | Cheese & Garlic | 1 cup | 270 | 3% | 5% | 2% |
| ❖ | Tomato & Cheese | 1 cup | 280 | 5% | 8% | 3% |
| | DI GIORNO Pastas (uncooked)— KRAFT | | | | | |
| ★ | Angels Hair | 2 oz | 160 | 2% | 0% | 0% |
| ★ | Fettuccini | 2 1/2 oz | 190 | 2% | 0% | 0% |
| ★ | Herb Linguine | 2 1/2 oz | 190 | 2% | 0% | 0% |
| ★ | Linguine | 2 1/2 oz | 190 | 2% | 0% | 0% |
| ★ | Spinach Fettuccini | 2 1/2 oz | 190 | 2% | 0% | 0% |
| ❖ | Egg Noodles (cooked) | 1 cup | 210 | 3% | 2% | 13% |
| ❖ | Egg Spinach Noodles (cooked) | 1 cup | 230 | 3% | 3% | 19% |
| | DI GIORNO Stuffed Ravioli—KRAFT | 1 cup | 350 | 20% | 40% | 15% |
| ▲ | Italian Herb Cheese | 1 cup | 350 | 20% | 40% | 15% |
| ▲ | w/Italian Sausage | 3/4 cup | 340 | 18% | 25% | 17% |
| | DI GIORNO Stuffed Tortelloni— KRAFT | | | | | |
| ❖ | Cheese | 3/4 cup | 260 | 9% | 18% | 10% |
| ▲ | Hot Red Pepper Cheese | 1 cup | 310 | 14% | 25% | 13% |
| ▲ | Mozzarella Garlic | 1 cup | 300 | 14% | 25% | 15% |
| ▲ | Mushroom | 1 cup | 290 | 11% | 23% | 10% |
| ❖ | w/Chicken & Herbs | 1 cup | 260 | 8% | 13% | 12% |
| ▲ | w/Meat | 3/4 cup | 290 | 14% | 23% | 13% |

★ Foods with this symbol have less than or equal to 5% *Daily Value* for <u>all</u> three nutrients (5% Rule).

❖ Foods with this symbol have <u>at least one</u> of the three nutrients greater than 5% *Daily Value* but less than or equal to 20% *Daily Value*.

▲ Foods with this symbol have <u>at least one</u> of the three nutrients greater than 20% *Daily Value* (20% Rule).

| FOOD | Serving Size | Calories | Tot Fat | Sat Fat | Chol |
|------|--------------|----------|---------|---------|------|

## PASTA DISHES: CANNED AND SHELF-STABLE

**Brand Name Foods**

CHEF BOYARDEE—AMERICAN
HOME FOODS

| FOOD | Serving Size | Calories | Tot Fat | Sat Fat | Chol |
|------|--------------|----------|---------|---------|------|
| ❖ Beefogetti (Pasta w/Mini Meatballs in Tomato Sauce) | 1 cup | 250 | 11% | 15% | 8% |
| ❖ Cannelloni (Beef Filled Macaroni in Meat Sauce) | 1 cup | 260 | 14% | 15% | 8% |
| ★ Cheese Tortelloni in Hearty Tomato Sauce | 1 cup | 230 | 2% | 0% | 5% |
| Ⓐ Chili Mac (Macaroni w/Beef in Chili Gravy) | 1 cup | 260 | 17% | 25% | 10% |
| ❖ Fettuccini in Hearty Meat Sauce | 1 cup | 230 | 9% | 13% | 7% |
| Ⓐ Mini Bites (Cheese Ravioli & Meatballs in Tomato Sauce) | 1 cup | 270 | 17% | 25% | 8% |
| ❖ Mini Cannelloni (Beef Filled Pasta in Meat Sauce) | 1 cup | 260 | 14% | 15% | 8% |
| ❖ Mini Ravioli (Beef Ravioli in Tomato & Meat Sauce) | 1 cup | 240 | 11% | 13% | 7% |
| ❖ Rigatoni (Macaroni in Tomato & Meat Sauce) | 1 cup | 250 | 11% | 13% | 8% |
| ❖ Roller Coasters (Pasta w/Mini Meatballs in Tomato Sauce) | 1 cup | 250 | 11% | 15% | 8% |
| ★ Sharks (Pasta Shapes in Tomato & Cheese Flavored Sauce) | 1 cup | 180 | 0% | 0% | 1% |
| ❖ Sir Chomps-A-Lot (Bite Size Lasagna) | 1 cup | 210 | 5% | 8% | 5% |
| ❖ Sir Chomps-A-Lot (Bite Size O-Rings w/Mini Meatballs in Tomato Sauce) | 1 cup | 260 | 15% | 20% | 8% |

CHEF BOYARDEE Individual
Serving Cans (7 oz)—AMERICAN
HOME FOODS

| FOOD | Serving Size | Calories | Tot Fat | Sat Fat | Chol |
|------|--------------|----------|---------|---------|------|
| ★ ABC's & 123's (Pasta Shapes in Tomato & Cheese Flavored Sauce) | 1 can | 150 | 0% | 0% | 0% |
| ❖ ABC's & 123's (Pasta Shapes w/Mini Meatballs in Tomato Sauce) | 1 can | 210 | 12% | 15% | 7% |
| ❖ Beef Ravioli in Tomato & Meat Sauce | 1 can | 170 | 6% | 10% | 5% |
| ❖ Beefaroni (Macaroni w/Beef in Tomato Sauce) | 1 can | 190 | 8% | 10% | 5% |
| ❖ Beefogetti (Pasta w/Mini Meatballs in Tomato Sauce) | 1 can | 200 | 12% | 15% | 7% |
| ★ Dinosaurs (Pasta Shapes in Tomato and Cheese Sauce) | 1 can | 170 | 0% | 0% | 1% |
| ❖ Lasagna (Pasta & Beef in Sauce) | 1 can | 190 | 9% | 13% | 7% |

| FOOD | Serving Size | Calories | Tot Fat | Sat Fat | Chol |
|---|---|---|---|---|---|
| ❖ Roller Coasters (Pasta & Mini Meatballs in Tomato Sauce) | 1 can | 220 | 13% | 17% | 7% |
| ★ Sir Chomps-A-Lot (Bite Size Cheese Ravioli in Tomato & Cheese Flavored Sauce) | 1 can | 150 | 0% | 0% | 1% |
| ★ Sir Chomps-A-Lot (Bite Size Beef Ravioli in Tomato & Meat Sauce) | 1 can | 150 | 2% | 3% | 3% |
| ❖ Spaghetti & Meat Balls in Tomato Sauce | 1 can | 210 | 12% | 15% | 7% |
| CHEF BOYARDEE *Main Meals* Microwave Bowls—AMERICAN HOME FOODS | | | | | |
| ❖ Beef Ravioli Suprema | 1 bowl | 270 | 8% | 10% | 7% |
| ❖ Cheese Ravioli Suprema | 1 bowl | 280 | 8% | 10% | 7% |
| ❖ Classic Noodles & Chicken w/ Vegetables | 1 bowl | 170 | 2% | 0% | 12% |
| ❖ Fettuccine in Meat Sauce | 1 bowl | 320 | 14% | 18% | 9% |
| ❖ Hearty Lasagna | 1 bowl | 300 | 17% | 20% | 12% |
| ❖ Meat Tortellini | 1 bowl | 300 | 6% | 9% | 10% |
| ❖ Spaghetti Suprema | 1 bowl | 230 | 9% | 15% | 8% |
| ★ Ziti in Tomato Sauce | 1 bowl | 240 | 0% | 0% | 0% |
| CHEF BOYARDEE Microwave Bowl—AMERICAN HOME FOODS | | | | | |
| ❖ ABC's & 123's (Pasta w/Mini Meatballs in Tomato Sauce) | 1 bowl | 230 | 14% | 20% | 7% |
| ❖ Beef Ravioli in Tomato & Meat Sauce | 1 bowl | 180 | 5% | 8% | 3% |
| ★ Beefaroni (Macaroni w/Beef in Tomato Sauce) | 1 bowl | 190 | 5% | 5% | 5% |
| ❖ Cheese Ravioli in Tomato & Meat Sauce | 1 bowl | 190 | 5% | 8% | 5% |
| ❖ Dinosaurs (Pasta Shapes w/Mini Meatballs in Tomato Sauce) | 1 bowl | 230 | 12% | 15% | 7% |
| ❖ Lasagna (Pasta & Beef in Sauce) | 1 bowl | 230 | 12% | 15% | 7% |
| ❖ Macaroni & Cheese | 1 bowl | 180 | 8% | 13% | 7% |
| ★ Meat Tortellini | 1 bowl | 210 | 4% | 5% | 5% |
| ★ Sir Chomps-A-Lot (Bite Size Beef Ravioli in Tomato & Meat Sauce) | 1 bowl | 180 | 3% | 5% | 3% |
| ❖ Spaghetti & Meat Balls in Tomato Sauce | 1 bowl | 200 | 9% | 13% | 7% |
| ❖ Spaghetti Rings & Meat Balls in Tomato Sauce | 1 bowl | 240 | 12% | 18% | 7% |
| FRANCO-AMERICAN—CAMPBELL'S | | | | | |
| ❖ Beef Ravioli in Meat Sauce | 1 cup | 300 | 15% | 20% | 8% |
| ❖ Beef Raviolios in Meat Sauce | 1 can | 250 | 11% | 20% | 5% |

★ Foods with this symbol have less than or equal to 5% *Daily Value* for <u>all</u> three nutrients (5% Rule).

❖ Foods with this symbol have <u>at least one</u> of the three nutrients greater than 5% *Daily Value* but less than or equal to 20% *Daily Value*.

Ⓐ Foods with this symbol have <u>at least one</u> of the three nutrients greater than 20% *Daily Value* (20% Rule).

| FOOD | Serving Size | Calories | Tot Fat | Sat Fat | Chol |
|------|--------------|----------|---------|---------|------|
| ❖ Beefy Mac | 1 can | 230 | 12% | 18% | 3% |
| Ⓐ Circusos Pasta w/Meatballs in Tomato Sauce | 1 cup | 260 | 17% | 25% | 7% |
| ❖ Elbow Macaroni & Cheese | 1 can | 190 | 9% | 13% | 2% |
| ❖ Hearty Twists Pasta w/Meat Sauce | 1 cup | 250 | 8% | 10% | 3% |
| ❖ Macaroni & Cheese | 1 cup | 200 | 11% | 15% | 3% |
| ❖ Spaghetti 'n Beef in Tomato | 1 can | 230 | 14% | 20% | 7% |
| ★ Spaghetti in Tomato Sauce w/ Cheese | 1 cup | 180 | 3% | 3% | 2% |
| ★ Spaghetti Pasta in Tomato & Cheese Sauce | 1 cup | 210 | 3% | 5% | 2% |
| Ⓐ Spaghetti w/Meatballs in Tomato Sauce | 1 cup | 270 | 15% | 25% | 10% |
| ★ Spaghettios Garfield Pizzos | 1 cup | 210 | 4% | 5% | 2% |
| Ⓐ Spaghettios Garfield Pizzos w/Beef | 1 cup | 260 | 15% | 25% | 5% |
| ★ Spaghettios Pasta in Tomato & Cheese | 1 cup | 190 | 3% | 3% | 2% |
| Ⓐ Spaghettios Pasta w/Sliced Franks in Tomato Sauce | 1 cup | 250 | 17% | 25% | 8% |
| Ⓐ Spaghettios w/Meatballs | 1 cup | 260 | 17% | 25% | 7% |
| HEALTH VALLEY Fat Free Pasta Vegetarian Cuisine | | | | | |
| ★ Linguini Primavera | 1 cup | 110 | 0% | 0% | 0% |
| ★ Pasta Gaioli | 1 cup | 120 | 0% | 0% | 0% |
| ★ Spicy Rotini | 1 cup | 100 | 0% | 0% | 0% |
| HUNT'S Homestyle Separates— HUNT WESSON | | | | | |
| ❖ Beef Ravioli | 1 cup | 220 | 12% | 14% | 4% |
| ❖ Noodles & Beef | 1 cup | 150 | 6% | 9% | 6% |
| ❖ Noodles & Chicken | 1 cup | 180 | 9% | 10% | 12% |
| ❖ Noodles & Chicken Cacciatore | 1 cup | 180 | 9% | 10% | 12% |
| ❖ Noodles & Chicken w/Mushroom | 1 cup | 200 | 7% | 10% | 8% |
| ❖ Rigatoni w/Italian Garden Style Sauce | 1 cup | 170 | 8% | 7% | 0% |
| KRAFT Deluxe Original | | | | | |
| Ⓐ Deluxe Original | ~ 1 cup | 320 | 15% | 30% | 8% |
| Ⓐ *Thick 'N Creamy* | ~ 1 cup | 320 | 16% | 30% | 8% |
| KRAFT Dinners (prep as dir) | | | | | |
| Ⓐ Cheddar Cheese Egg Noodle | ~ 1 cup | 430 | 32% | 30% | 23% |
| ❖ Chicken Egg Noodle | ~ 1 cup | 330 | 18% | 18% | 20% |
| ❖ Mild American Spaghetti | ~ 1 cup | 270 | 7% | 5% | 1% |
| ❖ Spaghetti with Meat Sauce | ~ 1 cup | 330 | 17% | 20% | 5% |
| ❖ Tangy Italian Spaghetti | ~ 1 cup | 270 | 7% | 5% | 1% |
| KRAFT Macaroni & Cheese Dinners (prep as dir) | | | | | |
| Ⓐ *Dinosaurs* | ~ 1 cup | 390 | 26% | 23% | 3% |
| Ⓐ Mild White Cheddar | ~ 1 cup | 390 | 26% | 20% | 3% |
| Ⓐ Original | ~ 1 cup | 390 | 26% | 20% | 3% |
| Ⓐ Spirals | ~ 1 cup | 390 | 26% | 23% | 3% |
| Ⓐ *Super Mario Bros.* | ~ 1 cup | 390 | 26% | 23% | 3% |

| FOOD | Serving Size | Calories | Tot Fat | Sat Fat | Chol |
|------|--------------|----------|---------|---------|------|
| ⊛ Teddy Bears | ~ 1 cup | 390 | 26% | 23% | 3% |
| ⊛ *The Flintstones* | ~ 1 cup | 390 | 26% | 23% | 3% |
| VELVEETA—KRAFT | | | | | |
| ⊛ Rotini & Cheese, Broccoli | ~ 1 cup | 400 | 25% | 50% | 15% |
| ⊛ Shells & Cheese, Bacon | ~ 1 cup | 360 | 22% | 40% | 13% |
| ⊛ Shells & Cheese, Original | ~ 1 cup | 360 | 20% | 40% | 13% |
| ⊛ Shells & Cheese, Salsa | ~ 1 cup | 380 | 22% | 45% | 13% |
| LIBBY'S *Diner*—NESTLÉ | | | | | |
| ❖ Beef Ravioli | 1 container | 230 | 13% | 18% | 4% |
| ❖ Lasagna | 1 container | 200 | 11% | 17% | 5% |
| ❖ Macaroni & Beef | 1 container | 220 | 14% | 20% | 6% |
| ⊛ Macaroni & Cheese | 1 container | 320 | 31% | 34% | 11% |
| ❖ Pasta Spirals & Chicken | 1 container | 130 | 7% | 4% | 4% |
| ❖ Spaghetti & Meatballs | 1 container | 190 | 8% | 10% | 6% |
| PROGRESSO Pasta—PET | | | | | |
| ❖ Beef Ravioli | 1 cup | 260 | 8% | 10% | 2% |
| ★ Cheese Ravioli | 1 cup | 220 | 3% | 5% | 1% |

## PASTA DISHES: FROZEN AND REFRIGERATED

**Brand Name Foods**

| FOOD | Serving Size | Calories | Tot Fat | Sat Fat | Chol |
|------|--------------|----------|---------|---------|------|
| BANQUET *Extra Helping* Family Entrées—CONAGRA | | | | | |
| ❖ Lasagna w/Meat Sauce | 1 cup | 230 | 12% | 20% | 12% |
| ❖ Mac & Cheese | 1 cup | 210 | 8% | 10% | 3% |
| ❖ Macaroni & Beef | 1 cup | 230 | 11% | 15% | 8% |
| ⊛ Macaroni & Cheese | 1 cup | 300 | 15% | 25% | 8% |
| ❖ BANQUET Macaroni & Cheese—CONAGRA | 1 container | 200 | 5% | 8% | 3% |
| BUDGET GOURMET *Light & Healthy* Entrées—ALL AMERICAN GOURMET | | | | | |
| ⊛ Cheese Ravioli | 1 pkg | 310 | 20% | 45% | 15% |
| ❖ Lasagna w/Meat Sauce | 1 pkg | 250 | 11% | 15% | 10% |
| ⊛ Linguini w/Shrimp & Clams | 1 pkg | 280 | 12% | 25% | 23% |
| ⊛ Vegetable Lasagna | 1 pkg | 290 | 15% | 25% | 7% |
| BUDGET GOURMET *Light & Healthy Special Selections*—ALL AMERICAN GOURMET | | | | | |
| ⊛ Macaroni & Cheese w/Cheddar & Parmesan | 1 pkg | 340 | 12% | 25% | 8% |
| ❖ Penne Pasta w/Chunky Tomato Sauce & Italian Sausage | 1 pkg | 330 | 15% | 13% | 3% |
| ❖ Rigatoni in Cream Sauce w/ Broccoli & Chicken | 1 pkg | 310 | 9% | 13% | 5% |

★ Foods with this symbol have less than or equal to 5% *Daily Value* for <u>all</u> three nutrients (5% Rule).

❖ Foods with this symbol have <u>at least one</u> of the three nutrients greater than 5% *Daily Value* but less than or equal to 20% *Daily Value*.

⊛ Foods with this symbol have <u>at least one</u> of the three nutrients greater than 20% *Daily Value* (20% Rule).

| FOOD | Serving Size | Calories | Tot Fat | Sat Fat | Chol |
|---|---|---|---|---|---|
| ❖ Spaghetti w/Chunky Tomato & Meat Sauce | 1 pkg | 320 | 11% | 13% | 2% |
| Ⓐ Three Cheese Lasagna | 1 pkg | 370 | 25% | 50% | 20% |
| BUDGET GOURMET *Original Special Selections*—ALL AMERICAN GOURMET | | | | | |
| Ⓐ Escalloped Noodles & Turkey | 1 pkg | 440 | 31% | 50% | 38% |
| Ⓐ Fettucini Alfredo w/Four Cheeses | 1 pkg | 480 | 37% | 65% | 18% |
| Ⓐ Homestyle Macaroni & Cheese | 1 pkg | 400 | 31% | 60% | 15% |
| Ⓐ Linguini w/Tomato Sauce & Italian Sausage | 1 pkg | 360 | 22% | 20% | 8% |
| Ⓐ Wide Ribbon Pasta w/Ricotta & Chunky Tomato Sauce | 1 pkg | 420 | 34% | 40% | 22% |
| BUDGET GOURMET *Side Dishes* —ALL AMERICAN GOURMET | | | | | |
| ❖ Cheese Tortellini | 1 pkg | 190 | 12% | 10% | 4% |
| Ⓐ Macaroni & Cheese | 1 pkg | 270 | 20% | 38% | 13% |
| Ⓐ Pasta Alfredo w/Broccoli | 1 pkg | 230 | 16% | 35% | 11% |
| ❖ Ziti in Marinara Sauce | 1 pkg | 220 | 15% | 20% | 4% |
| ★ HAIN Vegetarian Classics: Radiatore Bolognese | 1 pkg | 290 | 4% | 0% | 0% |
| HEALTHY CHOICE Entrées— CONAGRA | | | | | |
| ❖ Cheese Ravioli Parmigiana | 1 meal | 250 | 6% | 1% | 7% |
| ❖ Classics Pasta Shells Marinara | 1 meal | 370 | 6% | 10% | 8% |
| ❖ Fettucini Alfredo | 1 meal | 250 | 8% | 10% | 5% |
| ❖ Lasagna Roma | 1 meal | 390 | 8% | 9% | 5% |
| ❖ Macaroni & Cheese | 1 meal | 290 | 8% | 11% | 5% |
| ★ Spaghetti Bolognese | 1 meal | 260 | 4% | 5% | 5% |
| Ⓐ Three Cheese Manicotti | 1 meal | 310 | 14% | 24% | 7% |
| ★ Vegetable Pasta Italiano | 1 meal | 240 | 2% | 1% | 0% |
| ★ Zucchini Lasagna | 1 meal | 330 | 3% | 5% | 3% |
| MARIE CALLENDER'S Pasta— CONAGRA | | | | | |
| Ⓐ Angel Hair Pasta w/Sausage & Breadstick | 1 cup + 1 oz bread | 370 | 23% | 20% | 3% |
| Ⓐ Callender's Deluxe Pasta | 1 cup | 350 | 35% | 45% | 10% |
| Ⓐ Cheese Ravioli in Marinara Sauce w/Spirals & Garlic Bread | 1 cup + 1 oz bread | 370 | 22% | 25% | 12% |
| Ⓐ Extra Cheese Lasagna | 1 cup | 330 | 25% | 40% | 11% |
| Ⓐ Family Size Escalloped Noodles & Chicken | 1 cup | 270 | 25% | 30% | 7% |
| Ⓐ Family Size Lasagna w/Meat | 1 cup | 350 | 25% | 40% | 17% |
| Ⓐ Family Size Rigatoni Parmigiana | 1 cup | 320 | 22% | 35% | 8% |
| Ⓐ Fettucini Alfredo | 1 cup | 350 | 32% | 45% | 15% |
| Ⓐ Fettucini Primavera w/Tortellini | 1 cup | 310 | 29% | 40% | 17% |
| Ⓐ Fettucini w/Broccoli & Chicken | 1 cup | 420 | 40% | 55% | 18% |
| Ⓐ Lasagna w/Meat Sauce | 1 cup | 370 | 28% | 45% | 12% |

| FOOD | Serving Size | Calories | Tot Fat | Sat Fat | Chol |
|---|---|---|---|---|---|
| ❖ Macaroni & Beef w/Tomatoes & Soft Breadstick | 1 cup + 1 oz bread | 310 | 17% | 20% | 5% |
| ⊛ Marie's Special Macaroni & Cheese | 1 cup | 420 | 26% | 45% | 13% |
| ⊛ Rigatoni Parmigiana w/Soft Breadstick | 1 cup + 1 oz bread | 300 | 22% | 30% | 8% |
| ❖ Spaghetti & Meat Sauce w/Garlic Bread | 1 cup + 1 oz bread | 260 | 15% | 15% | 2% |
| ❖ Spaghetti Marinara w/Cheese Garlic Bread | 1 cup + 1 3/8 oz bread | 270 | 15% | 15% | 3% |
| ★ MORTON Dinners: Spaghetti—CONAGRA | 1 meal | 170 | 5% | 5% | 1% |
| ❖ MORTON Macaroni & Cheese—CONAGRA | 1 cup | 230 | 6% | 10% | 2% |
| ❖ MORTON Mac & Cheese—CONAGRA | 1 container | 200 | 5% | 8% | 3% |
| PASTA ACCENTS—GREEN GIANT | | | | | |
| ❖ Alfredo | 2 cups | 210 | 12% | 13% | 5% |
| ❖ Creamy Cheddar | 2 1/3 cups | 250 | 12% | 15% | 5% |
| ❖ Florentine | 2 cups | 310 | 14% | 15% | 7% |
| ❖ Garden Herb Seasoning | 2 cups | 230 | 11% | 20% | 5% |
| ⊛ Garlic Seasoning | 2 cups | 260 | 15% | 25% | 5% |
| ⊛ Primavera | 2 1/4 cups | 320 | 18% | 25% | 7% |
| ❖ White Cheddar Sauce | 1 3/4 cups | 300 | 18% | 18% | 7% |
| SMART ONES—WEIGHT WATCHERS | | | | | |
| ★ Angel Hair Pasta | 1 entrée | 180 | 3% | 3% | 0% |
| ★ Lasagna Curls w/Italian Vegetables | 1 entrée | 170 | 3% | 3% | 2% |
| ★ Lasagna Florentine | 1 entrée | 210 | 3% | 3% | 3% |
| ★ Ravioli Florentine | 1 entrée | 200 | 3% | 3% | 2% |
| STOUFFER'S Entrées—NESTLÉ | | | | | |
| ⊛ Beef Ravioli | 1 pkg | 370 | 22% | 20% | 27% |
| ⊛ Beef Stroganoff | 1 pkg | 380 | 31% | 35% | 28% |
| ⊛ Cheese Manicotti (9 oz) | 1 pkg | 340 | 25% | 35% | 17% |
| ⊛ Cheese Ravioli w/Tomato Sauce | 1 pkg | 360 | 22% | 25% | 28% |
| ⊛ Cheese Shells w/Tomato Sauce | 1 pkg | 340 | 25% | 35% | 17% |
| ⊛ Cheese Tortellini w/Alfredo Sauce | 1 pkg | 550 | 51% | 90% | 53% |
| ⊛ Cheese Tortellini w/Tomato Sauce | 1 pkg | 290 | 9% | 25% | 35% |
| ⊛ Fettucini Alfredo | 1 pkg | 580 | 60% | 105% | 40% |
| ⊛ Four Cheese Lasagna | 1 pkg | 410 | 29% | 50% | 18% |
| ⊛ Homestyle Chicken Fettucini | 1 pkg | 380 | 23% | 20% | 22% |
| ⊛ Lasagna w/Meat Sauce (10.5 oz) | 1 pkg | 360 | 20% | 25% | 17% |
| ⊛ Macaroni & Beef | 1 pkg | 340 | 18% | 25% | 17% |
| ⊛ Macaroni & Cheese | 1 cup | 310 | 25% | 30% | 10% |
| ⊛ Noodles Romanoff | 1 pkg | 460 | 38% | 30% | 20% |
| ⊛ Spaghetti w/Meatballs | 1 pkg | 420 | 23% | 20% | 15% |
| ⊛ Vegetable Lasagna (10.5 oz) | 1 pkg | 370 | 29% | 25% | 12% |

★  Foods with this symbol have less than or equal to 5% *Daily Value* for all three nutrients (5% Rule).
❖  Foods with this symbol have at least one of the three nutrients greater than 5% *Daily Value* but less than or equal to 20% *Daily Value*.
⊛  Foods with this symbol have at least one of the three nutrients greater than 20% *Daily Value* (20% Rule).

| FOOD | Serving Size | Calories | Tot Fat | Sat Fat | Chol |
|---|---|---|---|---|---|
| STOUFFER'S *Lean Cuisine* Entrées —NESTLÉ | | | | | |
| ❖ Angel Hair Pasta | 1 pkg | 210 | 6% | 5% | 0% |
| ❖ Cafe Classics Bow Tie Pasta & Chicken | 1 pkg | 270 | 9% | 8% | 20% |
| ❖ Cheddar Bake w/Pasta | 1 pkg | 220 | 9% | 10% | 7% |
| ❖ Cheese Cannelloni | 1 pkg | 270 | 12% | 18% | 10% |
| ❖ Cheese Ravioli | 1 pkg | 240 | 11% | 15% | 17% |
| ❖ Chicken Fettucini | 1 pkg | 270 | 9% | 13% | 15% |
| ❖ Chicken Parmesan & Pasta | 1 pkg | 220 | 8% | 8% | 17% |
| ❖ Classic Cheese Lasagna | 1 pkg | 290 | 9% | 15% | 10% |
| ❖ Fettucini Alfredo | 1 pkg | 270 | 11% | 15% | 5% |
| ❖ Fettucini Primavera | 1 pkg | 260 | 12% | 13% | 12% |
| ❖ Lasagna w/Meat Sauce | 1 pkg | 270 | 9% | 13% | 8% |
| ❖ Macaroni & Beef | 1 pkg | 280 | 12% | 10% | 8% |
| ❖ Macaroni & Cheese | 1 pkg | 270 | 11% | 18% | 7% |
| ❖ Rigatoni | 1 pkg | 180 | 6% | 8% | 7% |
| ❖ Spaghetti w/Meatballs | 1 pkg | 290 | 11% | 10% | 10% |
| ❖ Spaghetti w/Meat Sauce | 1 pkg | 290 | 9% | 8% | 7% |
| ❖ Zucchini Lasagna | 1 pkg | 240 | 6% | 8% | 5% |
| STOUFFER'S *Lean Cuisine Lunch Express*—NESTLÉ | | | | | |
| ❖ Cheese Lasagna Casserole | 1 pkg | 270 | 11% | 13% | 5% |
| ❖ Macaroni & Cheese & Broccoli | 1 pkg | 240 | 9% | 15% | 5% |
| STOUFFER'S *Lunch Express*— NESTLÉ | | | | | |
| ⊛ Cheese Ravioli | 1 pkg | 360 | 22% | 25% | 20% |
| ⊛ Fettucini Primavera | 1 pkg | 420 | 38% | 60% | 32% |
| ⊛ Lasagna w/Meat Sauce | 1 pkg | 330 | 15% | 25% | 13% |
| ⊛ Macaroni & Cheese w/Broccoli | 1 pkg | 360 | 29% | 25% | 10% |
| ❖ Spaghetti w/Meat Sauce | 1 pkg | 320 | 15% | 18% | 10% |
| SWANSON—CAMPBELL'S | | | | | |
| ❖ *Mac and More* Classic Macaroni 'n Cheese | 1 pkg | 180 | 8% | 15% | 5% |
| ❖ Macaroni & Cheese | 1 pkg | 240 | 14% | 20% | 7% |
| SWANSON *Budget Meals*— CAMPBELL'S | | | | | |
| ⊛ Macaroni & Cheese | 1 pkg | 320 | 17% | 35% | 7% |
| ⊛ Spaghetti & Meatballs | 1 pkg | 300 | 20% | 30% | 7% |
| SWANSON Homestyle Entrées— CAMPBELL'S | | | | | |
| ⊛ Lasagna w/Meat Sauce | 1 pkg | 410 | 23% | 35% | 22% |
| ⊛ Macaroni & Cheese | 1 pkg | 280 | 15% | 25% | 7% |
| WEIGHT WATCHERS Pasta Dishes | | | | | |
| ❖ Cheese Manicotti | 1 entrée | 290 | 14% | 18% | 7% |
| ❖ Chicken Fettucini | 1 entrée | 280 | 14% | 15% | 13% |
| ❖ Fettucini Alfredo w/Broccoli | 1 entrée | 220 | 9% | 13% | 5% |
| ❖ Garden Lasagna | 1 entrée | 230 | 8% | 5% | 2% |
| ❖ Italian Cheese Lasagna | 1 entrée | 300 | 12% | 15% | 8% |

| FOOD | Serving Size | Calories | Tot Fat | Sat Fat | Chol |
|------|------|------|------|------|------|
| ❖ Lasagna w/Meat Sauce | 1 entrée | 290 | 11% | 13% | 5% |
| ❖ Macaroni & Beef | 1 entrée | 220 | 7% | 8% | 3% |
| ❖ Macaroni & Cheese | 1 entrée | 260 | 9% | 10% | 7% |
| ❖ Penne Pasta w/Sun-Dried Tomatoes | 1 entrée | 290 | 14% | 13% | 5% |
| ❖ Spaghetti w/Meat Sauce | 1 entrée | 250 | 9% | 10% | 3% |
| ❖ Tuna Noodle Casserole | 1 entrée | 240 | 11% | 13% | 5% |

<u>PASTA DISHES: MIXES</u>

**Brand Name Foods**

| FOOD | Serving Size | Calories | Tot Fat | Sat Fat | Chol |
|------|------|------|------|------|------|
| BETTY CROCKER *Hamburger Helper* (prep as dir)—GENERAL MILLS | | | | | |
| ❖ Lasagne | 1 cup | 280 | 15% | 19% | 17% |
| ❖ Pizza Pasta w/Cheese Topping | 1 cup | 290 | 17% | 20% | 16% |
| ❖ Spaghetti | 1 cup | 300 | 16% | 20% | 18% |
| CHEF BOYARDEE *Complete* Dinners—AMERICAN HOME FOODS | | | | | |
| ❖ Italian Sausage Lasagna | 1/4 pkg | 260 | 8% | 8% | 7% |
| ❖ Lasagna | 1/4 pkg | 290 | 11% | 15% | 7% |
| ★ Spaghetti w/Meat Sauce | ~1/3 pkg | 260 | 5% | 5% | 3% |
| GOLDEN SAUTE (prep as dir)—LIPTON | | | | | |
| ❖ Angel Hair Parmesan | 1 cup | 290 | 15% | 16% | 3% |
| ❖ Savory Herb & Garlic Penne | 1 cup | 280 | 13% | 13% | 1% |
| NOODLES & SAUCE (prep as dir)—LIPTON | | | | | |
| ➂ Alfredo | 1 cup | 250 | 11% | 18% | 24% |
| ➂ Alfredo Broccoli | 1 cup | 260 | 11% | 18% | 24% |
| ➂ Alfredo Carbonara | 1 cup | 260 | 11% | 16% | 29% |
| ❖ Beef | 1 cup | 220 | 5% | 5% | 20% |
| ➂ Butter | 1 cup | 260 | 13% | 17% | 22% |
| ➂ Butter & Herb | 1 cup | 250 | 10% | 13% | 22% |
| ➂ Cheddar Bacon | 1 cup | 230 | 7% | 9% | 21% |
| ➂ Cheese | 1 cup | 250 | 7% | 11% | 22% |
| ➂ Chicken Broccoli | 1 cup | 220 | 6% | 7% | 21% |
| ➂ Chicken Flavor | 1 cup | 230 | 7% | 8% | 21% |
| ➂ Chicken Tetrazinni | 1 cup | 220 | 7% | 10% | 22% |
| ➂ Creamy Chicken | 1 cup | 230 | 9% | 12% | 22% |
| ➂ Parmesan | 1 cup | 250 | 12% | 19% | 23% |
| ➂ Romanoff | 1 cup | 260 | 11% | 16% | 23% |
| ➂ Sour Cream & Chives | 1 cup | 260 | 13% | 18% | 24% |
| ➂ Stroganoff | 1 cup | 210 | 6% | 10% | 22% |

★ Foods with this symbol have less than or equal to 5% *Daily Value* for <u>all</u> three nutrients (5% Rule).

❖ Foods with this symbol have <u>at least one</u> of the three nutrients greater than 5% *Daily Value* but less than or equal to 20% *Daily Value*.

➂ Foods with this symbol have <u>at least one</u> of the three nutrients greater than 20% *Daily Value* (20% Rule).

| FOOD | Serving Size | Calories | Tot Fat | Sat Fat | Chol |
|---|---|---|---|---|---|
| RICE-A-RONI *Noodle Roni*— | | | | | |
| GOLDEN GRAIN | | | | | |
| ⊛ Angel Hair Pasta w/Herbs | 1 cup | 320 | 22% | 13% | 2% |
| ⊛ Angel Hair Pasta w/Parmesan Cheese | 1 cup | 320 | 22% | 15% | 2% |
| ⊛ Corkscrew Pasta w/Creamy Garlic Sauce | 1 cup | 420 | 38% | 25% | 2% |
| ⊛ Corkscrew Pasta w/Four Cheese Sauce | 1 cup | 410 | 28% | 25% | 3% |
| ⊛ Fettuccine Pasta w/Alfredo Sauce | 1 cup | 470 | 38% | 30% | 3% |
| ❖ Fettuccine Pasta w/Broccoli au Gratin | 1 cup | 290 | 15% | 18% | 3% |
| ⊛ Fettuccine Pasta w/Chicken Sauce | 1 cup | 320 | 21% | 13% | 2% |
| ❖ Fettuccine Pasta w/Mild Cheddar Sauce | 1 cup | 300 | 16% | 18% | 3% |
| ⊛ Fettuccine Pasta w/Romanoff Sauce | 1 cup | 410 | 29% | 28% | 3% |
| ⊛ Fettuccine Pasta w/Stroganoff Sauce | 1 cup | 370 | 22% | 18% | 3% |
| ⊛ Linguine Pasta w/Chicken & Broccoli | 1 cup | 370 | 25% | 20% | 2% |
| ⊛ Linguine Pasta w/Creamy Chicken Parmesan | 1 cup | 410 | 28% | 23% | 2% |
| ❖ Oriental Style Pasta w/Stir Fry Sauce | 1 cup | 290 | 18% | 5% | 0% |
| ⊛ Pasta Shells w/White Cheddar Sauce | 1 cup | 390 | 25% | 23% | 5% |
| ⊛ Penne Pasta w/Herb & Butter Sauce | 1 cup | 430 | 38% | 28% | 0% |
| ❖ Rigatoni Pasta w/Tomato Basic | 1 cup | 240 | 14% | 5% | 0% |
| ⊛ Rigatoni Pasta w/White Cheddar & Broccoli Sauce | 1 cup | 400 | 29% | 25% | 3% |
| ⊛ Tenderthin Pasta w/Broccoli & Mushroom | 1 cup | 460 | 37% | 25% | 2% |
| ⊛ Tenderthin Pasta w/Parmesano Sauce | 1 cup | 400 | 26% | 23% | 3% |
| ⊛ Vermicelli Pasta w/Garlic & Olive Oil Sauce | 1 cup | 360 | 24% | 13% | 0% |

RICE

**Generic Foods**

| FOOD | Serving Size | Calories | Tot Fat | Sat Fat | Chol |
|---|---|---|---|---|---|
| ★ Brown Rice (long grain) | 1 cup | 220 | 3% | 2% | 0% |
| ★ Brown Rice (long grain, uncooked) | 1/4 cup | 170 | 2% | 1% | 0% |
| ★ Parboiled | 1 cup | 200 | 1% | 1% | 0% |
| ★ Parboiled (uncooked) | 1/4 cup | 170 | 0% | 0% | 0% |
| ★ White Glutinous Rice | 1/2 cup | 120 | 0% | 0% | 0% |
| ★ White Glutinous Rice (uncooked) | 1/4 cup | 170 | 0% | 0% | 0% |

| FOOD | Serving Size | Calories | Tot Fat | Sat Fat | Chol |
|---|---|---|---|---|---|
| ★ White Rice | 1 cup | 160 | 0% | 0% | 0% |
| ★ White rice (long, medium, or short grain) | 1 cup | 230 | 1% | 1% | 0% |
| ★ White Rice (long, medium, or short grain; uncooked) | 1/4 cup | 180 | 0% | 0% | 0% |
| ★ Wild Rice (uncooked) | 1/4 cup | 140 | 1% | 0% | 0% |

**Brand Name Foods**

| | | | | | |
|---|---|---|---|---|---|
| ARROWHEAD MILLS Rice (uncooked) | | | | | |
| ★ Basmati Style Rice (long grain) | 1/4 cup | 150 | 2% | 0% | 0% |
| ★ Brown Rice (long grain) | 1/4 cup | 150 | 2% | 0% | 0% |
| ★ Brown Rice (medium grain) | 1/4 cup | 160 | 2% | 0% | 0% |
| ★ Brown Rice (short grain) | 1/4 cup | 170 | 2% | 0% | 0% |
| MINUTE Rice (prep w/o fat)—KRAFT | | | | | |
| ★ Boil-in-Bag | 1 cup | 190 | 0% | 0% | 0% |
| ★ Instant Whole Grain Brown Rice | 2/3 cup | 170 | 2% | 0% | 0% |
| ★ Long Grain & Wild Rice Mix | 1 cup | 230 | 1% | 0% | 0% |
| ★ Original | 3/4 cup | 170 | 0% | 0% | 0% |
| ★ Premium Long Grain | 1 cup | 170 | 0% | 0% | 0% |
| ★ NIKO NIKO Calrose Rice (uncooked) | 1/4 cup | 170 | 1% | 0% | 0% |
| ★ SUN LUCK Long Grain Rice (uncooked) | 1/4 cup | 170 | 1% | 0% | 0% |
| UNCLE BEN'S | | | | | |
| ★ Brown & Wild Mushroom Flavor Rice | 2/3 cup | 140 | 2% | 0% | 0% |
| ★ *Converted* Brand Rice | 1 cup | 170 | 0% | 0% | 0% |
| ★ Instant Brown Rice | 1 cup | 190 | 2% | 0% | 0% |
| ★ Instant Rice | 1 cup | 190 | 1% | 0% | 0% |
| UNCLE BEN'S Long Grain & Wild Rice | | | | | |
| ★ Original | 1 cup | 190 | 1% | 0% | 0% |
| ★ Vegetable & Herb | 3/4 cup | 200 | 2% | 0% | 0% |

### RICE DISHES: CANNED AND SHELF-STABLE

**Brand Name Foods**

| | | | | | |
|---|---|---|---|---|---|
| BEARITOS Beans & Rice—LITTLE BEAR ORGANIC | | | | | |
| ★ Cajun Style | 1 cup | 140 | 1% | 0% | 0% |
| ★ Cuban Style | 1 cup | 150 | 1% | 0% | 0% |
| ★ Mexican Style | 1 cup | 160 | 1% | 0% | 0% |

★ Foods with this symbol have less than or equal to 5% *Daily Value* for all three nutrients (5% Rule).

❖ Foods with this symbol have at least one of the three nutrients greater than 5% *Daily Value* but less than or equal to 20% *Daily Value*.

Ⓐ Foods with this symbol have at least one of the three nutrients greater than 20% *Daily Value* (20% Rule).

| FOOD | Serving Size | Calories | Tot Fat | Sat Fat | Chol |
|------|--------------|----------|---------|---------|------|
| **CHEF BOYARDEE Microwave** | | | | | |
| Bowls—AMERICAN HOME FOODS | | | | | |
| ❖ Rice w/Beef & Vegetables | 1 bowl | 240 | 11% | 13% | 7% |
| ★ Rice w/Chicken & Vegetables | 1 bowl | 180 | 4% | 3% | 5% |
| ★ Fried Rice | 1 cup | 240 | 2% | 1% | 0% |
| **OLD EL PASO**—PET | | | | | |
| ★ Mexican Rice | 1/2 cup | 410 | 3% | 2% | 0% |
| ★ Spanish Rice | 1 cup | 130 | 1% | 0% | 0% |

## RICE DISHES: FROZEN

**Brand Name Foods**

| FOOD | Serving Size | Calories | Tot Fat | Sat Fat | Chol |
|------|--------------|----------|---------|---------|------|
| **BIRDS EYE**—DEAN FOODS | | | | | |
| ❖ French Style Rice | 1 pkg | 310 | 10% | 17% | 5% |
| ❖ Rice & Broccoli Au Gratin | 1 pkg | 290 | 10% | 16% | 5% |
| **BUDGET GOURMET** *Side Dishes* | | | | | |
| —ALL AMERICAN GOURMET | | | | | |
| ⊕ Oriental Rice w/Vegetables | 1 pkg | 220 | 18% | 24% | 6% |
| ❖ Rice Pilaf w/Green Beans | 1 pkg | 230 | 18% | 14% | 3% |
| **GREEN GIANT Rice & Vegetable** | | | | | |
| Combinations—PILLSBURY | | | | | |
| ❖ Rice & Broccoli | 1 pkg | 320 | 18% | 18% | 5% |
| ❖ Rice Medley | 1 pkg | 240 | 5% | 8% | 2% |
| ❖ Rice Pilaf | 1 pkg | 230 | 5% | 8% | 2% |
| ❖ White & Wild Rice | 1 pkg | 250 | 8% | 3% | 0% |

## RICE DISHES: MIXES

**Brand Name Foods**

| FOOD | Serving Size | Calories | Tot Fat | Sat Fat | Chol |
|------|--------------|----------|---------|---------|------|
| **FANTASTIC FOODS** | | | | | |
| ❖ Bombay Curry Rice & Beans | 1 cup | 230 | 5% | 8% | 0% |
| ★ Cajun Rice & Beans | 1 cup | 210 | 3% | 0% | 0% |
| ★ Caribbean Rice & Beans | 1 cup | 190 | 2% | 0% | 0% |
| ★ Italian Rice & Beans | 1 cup | 210 | 2% | 0% | 0% |
| ★ Pilaf | 1 cup | 240 | 3% | 0% | 0% |
| ★ Szechuan Rice & Beans | 1 cup | 190 | 3% | 0% | 0% |
| ★ Spanish Rice & Beans | 1 cup | 210 | 2% | 0% | 0% |
| **KNORR Rice Mixes**—CPC | | | | | |
| ★ Basmati Rice Pilaf Tomato & Herbs | 1/4 pkg | 150 | 1% | 0% | 0% |
| ★ Harvest Pilaf Rice Medley & Carrots | 1/4 pkg | 90 | 1% | 0% | 0% |
| ★ Jasmine Rice Pilaf Lemon & Herbs | 1/4 pkg | 130 | 1% | 0% | 0% |
| ★ Risotto Milanese | 1/4 pkg | 130 | 1% | 0% | 0% |
| ★ Risotto Primavera | 1/4 pkg | 140 | 1% | 0% | 0% |
| ★ Risotto w/Mushrooms | 1/4 pkg | 140 | 1% | 0% | 0% |
| ★ Risotto w/Onions & Herbs | 1/4 pkg | 150 | 1% | 0% | 0% |

| FOOD | Serving Size | Calories | Tot Fat | Sat Fat | Chol |
|---|---|---|---|---|---|
| **RICE & SAUCE (prep as dir)—** | | | | | |
| LIPTON | | | | | |
| ❖ Alfredo Broccoli | 1 cup | 250 | 7% | 10% | 3% |
| ★ Beef Broccoli | 1 cup | 230 | 1% | 0% | 0% |
| ★ Beans Cajun | 1 cup | 260 | 2% | 0% | 0% |
| ★ Chicken Broccoli | 1 cup | 250 | 3% | 4% | 1% |
| ★ Chicken Risotto | 1 cup | 230 | 3% | 3% | 2% |
| ❖ Creamy Chicken | 1 cup | 260 | 7% | 5% | 0% |
| ★ Medley | 1 cup | 240 | 3% | 2% | 1% |
| ★ Oriental | 1 cup | 230 | 2% | 0% | 1% |
| ★ Pilaf | 1 cup | 230 | 1% | 0% | 0% |
| **RICE-A-RONI (prep as dir)—** | | | | | |
| GOLDEN GRAIN | | | | | |
| ❖ Beef & Mushroom | 1 cup | 290 | 9% | 5% | 0% |
| ❖ Beef Flavor | 1 cup | 320 | 15% | 5% | 0% |
| ❖ Beef Flavor, 1/3 less salt | 1 cup | 280 | 8% | 5% | 0% |
| Ⓐ Broccoli Au Gratin | 1 cup | 370 | 26% | 20% | 2% |
| ❖ Broccoli Au Gratin, 1/3 less salt | 1 cup | 320 | 17% | 13% | 2% |
| ❖ Chicken & Broccoli | 1 cup | 290 | 12% | 5% | 0% |
| Ⓐ Chicken & Mushroom | 1 cup | 360 | 22% | 13% | 0% |
| ❖ Chicken & Vegetables | 1 cup | 290 | 11% | 5% | 0% |
| ❖ Chicken Flavor | 1 cup | 320 | 15% | 5% | 0% |
| ❖ Chicken Flavor, 1/3 less salt | 1 cup | 280 | 8% | 5% | 0% |
| ❖ Fried Rice | 1 cup | 320 | 17% | 10% | 0% |
| ★ Fried Rice, 1/3 less salt | 1 cup | 260 | 5% | 3% | 0% |
| ❖ Herb & Butter | 1 cup | 310 | 14% | 8% | 2% |
| ❖ Long Grain & Wild Pilaf | 1 cup | 240 | 8% | 5% | 0% |
| ❖ Long Grain & Wild Rice Chicken with Almonds | 1 cup | 290 | 13% | 8% | 0% |
| ❖ Long Grain & Wild Rice Original | 1 cup | 290 | 13% | 8% | 0% |
| ❖ Oriental Stir Fry | 1 cup | 290 | 8% | 5% | 0% |
| ❖ Red Beans & Rice | 1 cup | 280 | 11% | 5% | 0% |
| ❖ Rice Pilaf | 1 cup | 310 | 14% | 5% | 0% |
| ❖ Spanish Rice | 1 cup | 270 | 12% | 5% | 0% |
| Ⓐ Stroganoff | 1 cup | 360 | 22% | 18% | 2% |
| Ⓐ White Cheddar & Herbs | 1 cup | 340 | 22% | 20% | 2% |
| **RICE-A-RONI Fast Cook—GOLDEN** | | | | | |
| GRAIN | | | | | |
| ❖ Broccoli Cheese | 1 cup | 300 | 18% | 13% | 2% |
| ❖ Chicken Flavor | 1 cup | 250 | 10% | 8% | 2% |
| ❖ Oriental Flavor | 1 cup | 290 | 15% | 10% | 0% |
| ❖ Spanish | 1 cup | 250 | 8% | 5% | 0% |
| **UNCLE BEN'S *Country Inn Recipes*** | | | | | |
| ❖ Broccoli & White Cheddar | 1 cup | 270 | 8% | 15% | 2% |
| ❖ Broccoli Rice Au Gratin | 1 cup | 260 | 6% | 10% | 2% |

★ Foods with this symbol have less than or equal to 5% *Daily Value* for <u>all</u> three nutrients (5% Rule).

❖ Foods with this symbol have <u>at least one</u> of the three nutrients greater than 5% *Daily Value* but less than or equal to 20% *Daily Value*.

Ⓐ Foods with this symbol have <u>at least one</u> of the three nutrients greater than 20% *Daily Value* (20% Rule).

| FOOD | Serving Size | Calories | Tot Fat | Sat Fat | Chol |
|------|------|------|------|------|------|
| ❖ Chicken & Broccoli | 1 cup | 270 | 11% | 18% | 3% |
| ★ Chicken w/Wild Rice | 1 cup | 200 | 2% | 0% | 0% |
| ❖ Creamy Mushroom & Wild Rice | 1 cup | 250 | 4% | 8% | 2% |
| ❖ Herbed Rice Au Gratin | 1 cup | 260 | 5% | 8% | 2% |
| ❖ Homestyle Chicken & Vegetable | 1 cup | 270 | 9% | 15% | 5% |
| ★ Tomato & Herb | 1 cup | 240 | 2% | 0% | 0% |
| ★ Vegetable Pilaf | 1 cup | 200 | 2% | 0% | 0% |

## OTHER GRAINS

**Generic Foods**

| FOOD | Serving Size | Calories | Tot Fat | Sat Fat | Chol |
|------|------|------|------|------|------|
| ★ Amaranth | 1/4 cup | 180 | 5% | 4% | 0% |
| ★ Barley (uncooked) | 1/4 cup | 160 | 2% | 1% | 0% |
| ★ Barley, Pearl | 1 cup | 190 | 1% | 1% | 0% |
| ★ Buckwheat Groats | 1 cup | 180 | 2% | 1% | 0% |
| ★ Bulgar Wheat | 1 cup | 150 | 1% | 0% | 0% |
| ★ Bulgar Wheat (uncooked) | 1/4 cup | 120 | 1% | 0% | 0% |
| ★ Couscous | 1 cup | 200 | 0% | 0% | 0% |
| ★ Couscous (uncooked) | 1/4 cup | 170 | 0% | 0% | 0% |
| ★ Quinoa (uncooked) | 1/4 cup | 160 | 4% | 1% | 0% |
| ★ Rye | 1/4 cup | 140 | 2% | 1% | 0% |
| ★ Triticale | 1/4 cup | 160 | 2% | 1% | 0% |

**Brand Name Foods**

| FOOD | Serving Size | Calories | Tot Fat | Sat Fat | Chol |
|------|------|------|------|------|------|
| ★ ALA (uncooked)—CONTINENTAL MILLS | 1/4 cup | 150 | 1% | 0% | 0% |
| ARROWHEAD MILLS Grains (uncooked) | | | | | |
| ★ Amaranth | 1/4 cup | 170 | 3% | 3% | 0% |
| ★ Barley, pearled | 1/4 cup | 140 | 2% | 0% | 0% |
| ★ Buckwheat Groats | 1/4 cup | 140 | 2% | 0% | 0% |
| ❖ Flax | 3 tbsp | 140 | 15% | 5% | 0% |
| ★ Millet, hulled | 1/4 cup | 150 | 2% | 0% | 0% |
| ★ Oat Groats | 1/4 cup | 160 | 5% | 3% | 0% |
| ★ Quinoa | 1/4 cup | 140 | 3% | 0% | 0% |
| ★ Rye, whole | 1/4 cup | 160 | 2% | 0% | 0% |
| ★ KNORR Spicy Couscous Raisins & Almonds—CPC | 1/4 pkg | 150 | 2% | 0% | 0% |
| ❖ MANISCHEWITZ Kasha & Gravy | 1/2 cup | 100 | 5% | 8% | 0% |

| FOOD | Serving Size | Calories | Tot Fat | Sat Fat | Chol |
|------|--------------|----------|---------|---------|------|

# Poultry

<u>CHICKEN</u>

*Canned*
**Brand Name Foods**

| | | | | | |
|------|--------------|----------|---------|---------|------|
| SWANSON Chicken—CAMPBELL'S | | | | | |
| ❖   Chunk Chicken | 1/4 cup | 90 | 5% | 5% | 12% |
| ❖   Premium Chunk Chicken in Water | 1/4 cup | 90 | 5% | 5% | 13% |
| ★   Premium Chunk White Chicken in Water | 1/4 cup | 80 | 2% | 3% | 5% |

*Coated and Fried*
**Generic Foods**

| | | | | | |
|------|--------------|----------|---------|---------|------|
| ⊛ Breast w/Skin (floured) | 3 oz | 190 | 12% | 10% | 25% |
| ⊛ Breast w/Skin (battered) | 3 oz | 220 | 17% | 15% | 24% |
| ⊛ Breast w/o Skin (fried) | 3 oz | 160 | 6% | 5% | 26% |
| ⊛ Drumstick w/Skin (battered) | 3 oz | 230 | 21% | 18% | 24% |
| ⊛ Drumstick w/Skin (floured) | 3 oz | 210 | 18% | 16% | 25% |
| ⊛ Drumstick w/o Skin (fried) | 3 oz | 170 | 11% | 9% | 27% |
| ⊛ Leg w/o Skin (fried) | 3 oz | 180 | 12% | 11% | 28% |
| ⊛ Thigh w/Skin (battered) | 3 oz | 240 | 22% | 19% | 26% |
| ⊛ Thigh w/Skin (floured) | 3 oz | 220 | 20% | 17% | 27% |
| ⊛ Thigh w/o Skin (fried) | 3 oz | 190 | 13% | 12% | 29% |
| ⊛ Wing w/Skin (battered) | 3 oz | 280 | 29% | 25% | 23% |
| ⊛ Wing w/Skin (floured) | 3 oz | 270 | 29% | 26% | 23% |
| ⊛ Wing w/o Skin (fried) | 3 oz | 180 | 12% | 11% | 24% |

**Brand Name Foods**

| | | | | | |
|------|--------------|----------|---------|---------|------|
| BANQUET Fried Bone-In Chicken—CONAGRA | | | | | |
| ⊛   Barbecue Game Time Wings | 4 pcs | 190 | 18% | 20% | 23% |
| ⊛   Country Fried Chicken | 3 oz | 270 | 28% | 25% | 22% |
| ⊛   Fried Chicken, Drums & Thighs | 3 oz | 260 | 28% | 25% | 22% |
| ⊛   Fried Chicken Breast | 1 pc | 410 | 40% | 65% | 28% |
| ⊛   Hot & Spicy Fried Chicken | 3 oz | 260 | 28% | 25% | 22% |
| ⊛   Hot & Spicy Game Time Wings | 4 pcs | 230 | 25% | 25% | 28% |
| ⊛   Original Fried Chicken | 3 oz | 270 | 28% | 25% | 22% |
| ❖   Skinless Fried Chicken | 3 oz | 210 | 20% | 15% | 18% |
| ⊛   Southern Fried Chicken | 1 pc | 270 | 28% | 25% | 22% |

★  Foods with this symbol have less than or equal to 5% *Daily Value* for <u>all</u> three nutrients (5% Rule).
❖  Foods with this symbol have <u>at least one</u> of the three nutrients greater than 5% *Daily Value* but less than or equal to 20% *Daily Value*.
⊛  Foods with this symbol have <u>at least one</u> of the three nutrients greater than 20% *Daily Value* (20% Rule).

| | FOOD | Serving Size | Calories | Tot Fat | Sat Fat | Chol |
|---|---|---|---|---|---|---|
| | BANQUET Fried Chicken (boneless)—CONAGRA | | | | | |
| ☻ | Chicken & Cheddar Nuggets | 4 chunks | 280 | 29% | 30% | 8% |
| ☻ | Hot Popcorn Chicken | 3 oz | 290 | 29% | 20% | 12% |
| ❖ | Mozzarella Nuggets | 6 pcs | 210 | 17% | 20% | 3% |
| ☻ | Nuggets | 6 nuggets | 240 | 23% | 15% | 12% |
| ❖ | Original Chicken Breast Tenders | 3 tenders | 260 | 25% | 20% | 8% |
| ☻ | Patties | 1 patty | 180 | 17% | 13% | 8% |
| ☻ | Southern Fried Nuggets | 6 nuggets | 340 | 31% | 20% | 15% |
| ❖ | Southern Fried Patties | 1 patty | 170 | 15% | 10% | 6% |
| ❖ | Southern Fried Tenders | 3 tenders | 260 | 25% | 20% | 5% |
| ☻ | Sweet & Sour Nuggets | 6 nuggets | 320 | 28% | 20% | 15% |
| ❖ | Tenders | 3 tenders | 210 | 15% | 10% | 8% |
| | COUNTRY SKILLET—CONAGRA | | | | | |
| ☻ | Chunks | 5 chunks | 270 | 26% | 15% | 7% |
| ☻ | Nuggets | 10 nuggets | 280 | 28% | 20% | 8% |
| ☻ | Patties | 1 patty | 190 | 18% | 13% | 7% |
| ☻ | Southern Fried Chunks | 5 chunks | 250 | 23% | 15% | 7% |
| ❖ | Southern Fried Patties | 1 patty | 190 | 18% | 13% | 7% |
| | TYSON Breaded Chicken | | | | | |
| ☻ | Breaded Chicken Breast Patties | 1 patty | 240 | 25% | 20% | 12% |
| ☻ | Breaded Chicken Chunks | 6 nuggets | 250 | 23% | 15% | 15% |
| ☻ | Breast Chunks | 6 chunks | 220 | 22% | 15% | 12% |
| ❖ | Breast Fillets | 2 fillets | 160 | 9% | 5% | 10% |
| ❖ | Breast Patties | 1 patty | 190 | 18% | 15% | 10% |
| ☻ | Breast Tenders | 5 tenders | 210 | 22% | 15% | 13% |
| ☻ | Chick'n Chunks | 6 chunks | 280 | 31% | 25% | 17% |
| ☻ | Southern Fried Chunks | 6 chunks | 250 | 28% | 20% | 15% |
| | TYSON *Chick'n Chippers* | | | | | |
| ☻ | Hot & Spicy | 5 chippers | 310 | 32% | 20% | 13% |
| ☻ | Original | 5 chippers | 310 | 32% | 20% | 13% |
| ☻ | Ranch | 5 chippers | 310 | 32% | 20% | 13% |
| | TYSON Wings & Drums | | | | | |
| ☻ | Barbecue Chicken Wings | 4 pcs | 220 | 23% | 20% | 43% |
| ☻ | Buffalo Style *Hot Wings* | 6 portions | 190 | 18% | 15% | 35% |
| ☻ | Hot 'n Spicy Chicken Wings | 4 pcs | 220 | 23% | 18% | 37% |
| ☻ | Hot Barbecue Drums | 1 drumstick | 90 | 6% | 5% | 23% |
| ☻ | Teriyaki Chicken Wings | 4 pcs | 190 | 18% | 15% | 40% |

**Fresh and Frozen**

**Generic Foods**

| | | | | | | |
|---|---|---|---|---|---|---|
| | Breast | | | | | |
| ☻ | Skinless, baked | 3 oz | 120 | 2% | 3% | 23% |
| ☻ | With skin, baked | 3 oz | 170 | 11% | 10% | 23% |
| | Drumstick | | | | | |
| ☻ | Skinless, baked | 3 oz | 130 | 6% | 5% | 27% |
| ☻ | With skin, baked | 3 oz | 180 | 14% | 15% | 25% |
| ☻ | Giblets, simmered | 3 oz | 130 | 6% | 6% | 111% |

| FOOD | Serving Size | Calories | Tot Fat | Sat Fat | Chol |
|------|------|------|------|------|------|
| &#9412; Liver, simmered | 3 oz | 130 | 7% | 8% | 179% |
| Thigh | | | | | |
| &#9412;   Skinless, baked | 3 oz | 150 | 11% | 10% | 25% |
| &#9412;   With skin, baked | 3 oz | 210 | 20% | 20% | 23% |
| Whole | | | | | |
| &#9412;   Skinless, baked | 3 oz | 130 | 6% | 5% | 25% |
| &#9412;   With skin, baked | 3 oz | 200 | 18% | 15% | 25% |
| Wing | | | | | |
| &#9412;   Skinless, baked | 3 oz | 150 | 9% | 8% | 23% |
| &#9412;   With skin, baked | 3 oz | 250 | 26% | 25% | 23% |

**Brand Name Foods**

CHICKEN BY GEORGE—HORMEL FOODS

| FOOD | Serving Size | Calories | Tot Fat | Sat Fat | Chol |
|------|------|------|------|------|------|
| ❖   Cajun | 1 breast | 120 | 6% | 5% | 18% |
| ❖   Caribbean Grill | 1 breast | 150 | 6% | 5% | 18% |
| ❖   Garlic & Herb | 1 breast | 120 | 5% | 5% | 17% |
| ❖   Italian Blue Cheese | 1 breast | 130 | 8% | 5% | 20% |
| ❖   Lemon Herb | 1 breast | 120 | 5% | 5% | 17% |
| ❖   Lemon Oregano | 1 breast | 130 | 6% | 5% | 17% |
| ❖   Mesquite Barbecue | 1 breast | 120 | 3% | 3% | 17% |
| &#9412;   Mustard Dill | 1 breast | 140 | 8% | 5% | 22% |
| ❖   Roasted | 1 breast | 110 | 5% | 5% | 18% |
| ❖   Teriyaki | 1 breast | 130 | 5% | 5% | 17% |
| ❖   Tomato Herb with Basil | 1 breast | 140 | 8% | 5% | 20% |
| &#9412; TYSON Rock Cornish Game Hen | 1/2 hen (7.5 oz) | 350 | 35% | 40% | 83% |

*Prepared*

**Brand Name Foods**

TYSON Roasted Chicken, Ready to Eat

| FOOD | Serving Size | Calories | Tot Fat | Sat Fat | Chol |
|------|------|------|------|------|------|
| &#9412;   Breast Halves | 1/2 breast | 250 | 20% | 20% | 37% |
| &#9412;   Drumsticks | 3 drumsticks | 330 | 28% | 25% | 75% |
| &#9412;   Thighs | 1 thigh | 260 | 29% | 30% | 45% |
| &#9412;   Whole | 3 oz | 180 | 18% | 15% | 33% |

TYSON Rotisserie Chicken, Ready to Eat

| FOOD | Serving Size | Calories | Tot Fat | Sat Fat | Chol |
|------|------|------|------|------|------|
| &#9412;   Breast Quarter w/Skin | 1 pc | 470 | 45% | 45% | 62% |
| &#9412;   Breast Quarter w/o Skin | 1 pc | 250 | 12% | 13% | 48% |
| &#9412;   Half Bird w/Skin | 3 oz | 170 | 15% | 15% | 30% |
| &#9412;   Half Bird w/o Skin | 3 oz | 140 | 11% | 13% | 28% |

★   Foods with this symbol have less than or equal to 5% *Daily Value* for <u>all</u> three nutrients (5% Rule).
❖   Foods with this symbol have <u>at least one</u> of the three nutrients greater than 5% *Daily Value* but less than or equal to 20% *Daily Value.*
&#9412;   Foods with this symbol have <u>at least one</u> of the three nutrients greater than 20% *Daily Value* (20% Rule).

| FOOD | Serving Size | Calories | Tot Fat | Sat Fat | Chol |
|------|-------------|----------|---------|---------|------|
| ⊛ Leg Quarter w/Skin | 1 pc | 480 | 49% | 50% | 85% |
| ⊛ Leg Quarter w/o Skin | 1 pc | 270 | 18% | 20% | 63% |

TURKEY

**Canned**
**Brand Name Foods**

SWANSON Premium Turkey—
CAMPBELL'S
| ❖ Chunk Turkey in Water | 1/4 cup | 100 | 6% | 5% | 17% |
| ❖ Chunk White Turkey in Water | 1/4 cup | 90 | 3% | 3% | 12% |

**Coated**
**Brand Name Foods**

LOUIS RICH Breaded Turkey—
OSCAR MAYER
| ⊛ Turkey Nuggets | 4 nuggets | 260 | 25% | 15% | 12% |
| ❖ Turkey Patties | 1 patty | 220 | 20% | 13% | 12% |
| ⊛ Turkey Sticks | 3 sticks | 230 | 23% | 15% | 12% |

**Fresh and Frozen**
**Generic Foods**

Breast
| ❖ Skinless (baked) | 3 oz | 120 | 2% | 0% | 15% |
| ❖ With skin (baked) | 3 oz | 160 | 9% | 10% | 18% |

Drumstick
| ⊛ Skinless (baked) | 3 oz | 140 | 6% | 5% | 27% |
| ⊛ With skin (baked) | 3 oz | 170 | 12% | 10% | 25% |

Thigh
| ⊛ Skinless (baked) | 3 oz | 140 | 8% | 8% | 23% |
| ⊛ With skin (baked) | 3 oz | 160 | 11% | 10% | 23% |
| ⊛ Ground (cooked) | 3 oz | 200 | 17% | 14% | 29% |

Turkey Roll
| ❖ Light meat | 3 oz | 130 | 9% | 9% | 12% |
| ❖ Light and dark meat | 3 oz | 130 | 9% | 9% | 16% |

Whole
| ❖ Skinless (roasted) | 3 oz | 130 | 5% | 5% | 20% |
| ❖ With skin (roasted) | 3 oz | 180 | 12% | 10% | 20% |

Wing
| ⊛ Skinless (baked) | 3 oz | 140 | 5% | 5% | 25% |
| ❖ With skin (baked) | 3 oz | 200 | 17% | 15% | 17% |

**Brand Name Foods**

| ❖ JENNIE-O *Extra Lean* White Turkey Roast | 4 oz roast, 2 tbsp gravy | 120 | 5% | 4% | 19% |

| FOOD | Serving Size | Calories | Tot Fat | Sat Fat | Chol |
|------|--------------|----------|---------|---------|------|

*Prepared*
**Brand Name Foods**

JENNIE-O Half Turkey Breast

| FOOD | Serving Size | Calories | Tot Fat | Sat Fat | Chol |
|------|--------------|----------|---------|---------|------|
| ❖ Dark Carameled | 2 oz | 60 | 2% | 0% | 9% |
| ❖ Oven Roasted | 2 oz | 70 | 3% | 2% | 9% |

JENNIE-O *Natural Choice* Premium

| FOOD | Serving Size | Calories | Tot Fat | Sat Fat | Chol |
|------|--------------|----------|---------|---------|------|
| ⊛ Boneless Breast of Young Turkey | 4 oz | 170 | 12% | 10% | 22% |
| ⊛ Boneless Young Turkey | 4 oz | 170 | 13% | 14% | 24% |
| ⊛ Lean Ground Turkey | 4 oz | 130 | 7% | 6% | 25% |
| ⊛ Turkey Breast | 4 oz | 170 | 12% | 11% | 23% |
| ❖ Turkey Breast Tenderloins | 4 oz | 120 | 1% | 0% | 17% |

JENNIE-O Turkey Breast

| FOOD | Serving Size | Calories | Tot Fat | Sat Fat | Chol |
|------|--------------|----------|---------|---------|------|
| ★ Festive (96% fat free) | 2 oz | 60 | 3% | 3% | 5% |
| ★ Our Blue Ribbon (99% fat free) | 2 oz | 45 | 0% | 0% | 5% |
| ❖ LIGHT & LEAN 97 Smoked Turkey Breast—HORMEL FOODS | 3 oz | 80 | 2% | 3% | 12% |

LOUIS RICH Breast of Turkey—
OSCAR MAYER

| FOOD | Serving Size | Calories | Tot Fat | Sat Fat | Chol |
|------|--------------|----------|---------|---------|------|
| ❖ Barbecued | 2 oz | 60 | 1% | 0% | 8% |
| ❖ Hickory Smoked | 2 oz | 60 | 1% | 0% | 8% |
| ❖ Honey Roasted | 2 oz | 60 | 1% | 0% | 8% |
| ❖ Oven Roasted | 2 oz | 50 | 1% | 0% | 8% |

LOUIS RICH Dinner Slices—
OSCAR MAYER

| FOOD | Serving Size | Calories | Tot Fat | Sat Fat | Chol |
|------|--------------|----------|---------|---------|------|
| ❖ Hickory Smoked Breast of Turkey | 1 slice | 80 | 2% | 0% | 12% |
| ❖ Honey Roasted Breast of Turkey | 1 slice | 80 | 2% | 3% | 12% |
| ❖ Oven Roasted Breast of Turkey | 1 slice | 70 | 2% | 0% | 12% |

### *OTHER* POULTRY

**Generic Foods**

| FOOD | Serving Size | Calories | Tot Fat | Sat Fat | Chol |
|------|--------------|----------|---------|---------|------|
| ⊛ Capon (all parts), roasted or broiled | 3 oz | 190 | 15% | 14% | 29% |
| ⊛ Duck Liver, raw | 3 oz | 120 | 6% | 6% | 146% |
| ⊛ Duck w/Skin, roasted | 3 oz | 290 | 37% | 41% | 24% |
| ⊛ Goose w/Skin, roasted | 3 oz | 260 | 29% | 29% | 26% |

★   Foods with this symbol have less than or equal to 5% *Daily Value* for <u>all</u> three nutrients (5% Rule).
❖   Foods with this symbol have <u>at least one</u> of the three nutrients greater than 5% *Daily Value* but less than or equal to 20% *Daily Value*.
⊛   Foods with this symbol have <u>at least one</u> of the three nutrients greater than 20% *Daily Value* (20% Rule).

| FOOD | Serving Size | Calories | Tot Fat | Sat Fat | Chol |
|------|--------------|----------|---------|---------|------|

# Salads, Dressings, and Toppers

## SALADS

### Generic Foods

| FOOD | Serving Size | Calories | Tot Fat | Sat Fat | Chol |
|------|--------------|----------|---------|---------|------|
| ⊛ Chef Salad w/Ham & Cheese | 2 cups | 200 | 20% | 35% | 15% |
| ⊛ Chicken Salad | 1/2 cup | 500 | 56% | 21% | 22% |
| ❖ Macaroni Salad | 1/2 cup | 200 | 18% | 4% | 1% |
| ★ Mandarin Orange Gelatin Salad | 1/2 cup | 90 | 0% | 0% | 0% |
| ⊛ Potato Salad | 1/2 cup | 180 | 16% | 9% | 29% |
| ⊛ Taco Salad | 1 cup | 280 | 23% | 34% | 15% |
| ★ Waldorf Gelatin Salad | 1/2 cup | 110 | 1% | 0% | 0% |

### Brand Name Foods

| FOOD | Serving Size | Calories | Tot Fat | Sat Fat | Chol |
|------|--------------|----------|---------|---------|------|
| BETTY CROCKER *Suddenly Salad* (prep as dir)—GENERAL MILLS | | | | | |
| ❖ Caesar | 3/4 cup | 250 | 16% | 7% | 0% |
| ❖ Classic Pasta | 3/4 cup | 220 | 11% | 5% | 0% |
| ⊛ Creamy Macaroni | 3/4 cup | 320 | 31% | 15% | 5% |
| ★ Garden Italian (98% Fat-Free) | 3/4 cup | 130 | 1% | 0% | 0% |
| ⊛ Ranch & Bacon | 3/4 cup | 320 | 30% | 17% | 5% |
| ★ FANTASTIC FOODS Tabouli Salad Mix (prep as dir) | 1 cup | 240 | 2% | 0% | 0% |
| KRAFT Pasta Salads (prep as dir) | | | | | |
| ⊛ Classic Ranch with Bacon | ~ 1 cup | 360 | 35% | 20% | 5% |
| ⊛ Creamy Caesar | ~ 1 cup | 350 | 34% | 20% | 5% |
| ❖ Garden Primavera | ~ 1 cup | 280 | 18% | 13% | 2% |
| ★ Light Italian | ~ 1 cup | 190 | 3% | 5% | 1% |
| ⊛ Parmesan Peppercorn | ~ 1 cup | 360 | 38% | 23% | 7% |

## SALAD DRESSINGS

### *Caesar Dressings*
### Brand Name Foods

| FOOD | Serving Size | Calories | Tot Fat | Sat Fat | Chol |
|------|--------------|----------|---------|---------|------|
| ⊛ GOOD SEASONS Mix: Gourmet Caesar (prep as dir)—KRAFT | 2 tbsp | 150 | 24% | 12% | 0% |
| KRAFT | | | | | |
| ⊛ Caesar | 2 tbsp | 130 | 21% | 12% | 1% |
| ❖ *Deliciously Right* Reduced Calorie Caesar | 2 tbsp | 60 | 8% | 6% | 1% |
| ❖ MARIE'S Dressing & Dip: Creamy Caesar—CAMPBELL'S | 1 pouch | 250 | 8% | 20% | 8% |
| ⊛ NEWMAN'S OWN Caesar | 2 tbsp | 150 | 25% | 8% | 1% |
| SALAD CELEBRATIONS—WEIGHT WATCHERS | | | | | |
| ★ Caesar, Fat Free | 2 tbsp | 10 | 0% | 0% | 0% |
| ★ Three Cheese Caesar | 2 tbsp | 40 | 3% | 0% | 3% |

| FOOD | Serving Size | Calories | Tot Fat | Sat Fat | Chol |
|---|---|---|---|---|---|
| SEVEN SEAS—KRAFT | | | | | |
| ☻ Creamy Caesar | 2 tbsp | 140 | 23% | 13% | 3% |
| ❖ *Viva* Caesar | 2 tbsp | 120 | 19% | 11% | 0% |
| ❖ WISH-BONE Caesar w/Olive Oil | | | | | |
| —LIPTON | 2 tbsp | 100 | 15% | 8% | 0% |
| **Cheese Dressings** | | | | | |
| **Generic Foods** | | | | | |
| ☻ Blue Cheese | 2 tbsp | 150 | 25% | 15% | 6% |
| ★ Blue Cheese, Low Calorie | 2 tbsp | 20 | 3% | 5% | 3% |
| **Brand Name Foods** | | | | | |
| ★ ESTEE Blue Cheese | 2 tbsp | 15 | 1% | 0% | 0% |
| ☻ GOOD SEASONS Mix: Cheese | | | | | |
| Garlic (prep as dir)—KRAFT | 2 tbsp | 140 | 24% | 12% | 0% |
| HIDDEN VALLEY RANCH (Bottled) | | | | | |
| ☻ Blue Cheese | 2 tbsp | 160 | 26% | 20% | 3% |
| ★ Blue Cheese, Fat Free | 2 tbsp | 20 | 0% | 0% | 0% |
| ☻ Creamy Parmesan | 2 tbsp | 140 | 23% | 15% | 3% |
| ★ Creamy Parmesan, Fat Free | 2 tbsp | 30 | 0% | 0% | 0% |
| KRAFT | | | | | |
| ★ *Free* Fat Free Blue Cheese Flavor | 2 tbsp | 50 | 0% | 0% | 0% |
| ❖ *Roka* Brand Blue Cheese | 2 tbsp | 90 | 11% | 19% | 4% |
| MARIE'S *Luscious Low Fat*— | | | | | |
| CAMPBELL'S | | | | | |
| ★ Creamy Blue Cheese | 2 tbsp | 45 | 2% | 0% | 0% |
| ★ Creamy Parmesan | 2 tbsp | 45 | 2% | 0% | 0% |
| MARIE'S *Salad Bar*—CAMPBELL'S | | | | | |
| ☻ Blue Cheese | 2 tbsp | 180 | 29% | 18% | 5% |
| ❖ Blue Cheese, Reduced Calorie | 2 tbsp | 100 | 11% | 5% | 2% |
| MARIE'S Dressing & Dip— | | | | | |
| CAMPBELL'S | | | | | |
| ☻ Chunky Blue Cheese | 2 tbsp | 180 | 29% | 18% | 5% |
| ❖ Chunky Blue Cheese, Reduced | | | | | |
| Calorie | 2 tbsp | 100 | 11% | 5% | 3% |
| ☻ Parmesan Ranch | 2 tbsp | 180 | 29% | 15% | 5% |
| ❖ SEVEN SEAS Chunky Blue | | | | | |
| Cheese—KRAFT | 2 tbsp | 90 | 11% | 19% | 4% |
| WISH-BONE—LIPTON | | | | | |
| ☻ Chunky Blue Cheese | 2 tbsp | 170 | 26% | 13% | 4% |
| ★ Chunky Blue Cheese, Fat Free | 2 tbsp | 35 | 0% | 0% | 0% |

★ Foods with this symbol have less than or equal to 5% *Daily Value* for <u>all</u> three nutrients (5% Rule).

❖ Foods with this symbol have <u>at least one</u> of the three nutrients greater than 5% *Daily Value* but less than or equal to 20% *Daily Value*.

☻ Foods with this symbol have <u>at least one</u> of the three nutrients greater than 20% *Daily Value* (20% Rule).

| FOOD | Serving Size | Calories | Tot Fat | Sat Fat | Chol |
|---|---|---|---|---|---|
| **Coleslaw Dressings** | | | | | |
| **Brand Name Foods** | | | | | |
| HIDDEN VALLEY RANCH (Bottled) | | | | | |
| ⊛   Coleslaw | 2 tbsp | 150 | 23% | 15% | 3% |
| ★   Coleslaw, Fat Free | 2 tbsp | 35 | 0% | 0% | 0% |
| ❖ KRAFT Coleslaw | 2 tbsp | 150 | 19% | 10% | 9% |
| ❖ MARIE'S Cole Slaw—CAMPBELL'S | 2 tbsp | 150 | 2% | 10% | 3% |
| **French Dressings** | | | | | |
| **Generic Foods** | | | | | |
| ❖ French | 2 tbsp | 130 | 20% | 15% | 1% |
| **Brand Name Foods** | | | | | |
| ★ ESTEE Creamy French | 2 tbsp | 10 | 0% | 0% | 0% |
| ★ FEATHERWEIGHT French | 2 tbsp | 10 | 0% | 0% | 0% |
| ★ HIDDEN VALLEY RANCH (Bottled) | | | | | |
|   Fat Free French | 2 tbsp | 35 | 0% | 0% | 0% |
| KRAFT | | | | | |
| ❖   *Catalina* French | 2 tbsp | 140 | 18% | 9% | 0% |
| ❖   *Catalina* w/Honey | 2 tbsp | 140 | 18% | 10% | 0% |
| ★   *Deliciously Right* French, | | | | | |
|     Reduced Calorie | 2 tbsp | 50 | 5% | 2% | 0% |
| ★   *Free* French Style, Fat Free | 2 tbsp | 50 | 0% | 0% | 0% |
| ❖   French | 2 tbsp | 120 | 18% | 9% | 0% |
| MARIE'S—CAMPBELL'S | | | | | |
| ❖   Dressing & Dip: Tangy French | 2 tbsp | 130 | 17% | 8% | 0% |
| ❖   *Salad Bar* French | 2 tbsp | 130 | 15% | 8% | 0% |
| ★ SALAD CELEBRATIONS Fat Free | | | | | |
|   French Style—WEIGHT WATCHERS | 2 tbsp | 40 | 0% | 0% | 0% |
| ★ WISH-BONE Fat Free Sweet & | | | | | |
|   Spicy French—LIPTON | 2 tbsp | 30 | 0% | 0% | 0% |
| **Herb Dressings** | | | | | |
| **Brand Name Foods** | | | | | |
| GOOD SEASONS Mixes | | | | | |
|   (prep as dir)—KRAFT | | | | | |
| ⊛   Garlic and Herbs | 2 tbsp | 140 | 24% | 11% | 0% |
| ★   Zesty Herb, Fat Free | 2 tbsp | 10 | 0% | 0% | 0% |
| ❖ SEVEN SEAS Herbs & Spices— | | | | | |
|   KRAFT | 2 tbsp | 120 | 19% | 10% | 0% |

| FOOD | Serving Size | Calories | Tot Fat | Sat Fat | Chol |
|---|---|---|---|---|---|
| ***Honey Mustard Dressings*** | | | | | |
| **Brand Name Foods** | | | | | |
| GOOD SEASONS Mixes (prep as dir)—KRAFT | | | | | |
| ⊛ Honey Mustard | 2 tbsp | 150 | 24% | 11% | 0% |
| ★ Honey Mustard, Fat Free | 2 tbsp | 20 | 0% | 0% | 0% |
| ❖ HAIN Natural Classics: Dijon | 2 tbsp | 130 | 20% | 10% | 0% |
| HIDDEN VALLEY RANCH (Bottled) | | | | | |
| ⊛ Honey Dijon | 2 tbsp | 140 | 23% | 10% | 2% |
| ★ Honey Dijon, Fat Free | 2 tbsp | 35 | 0% | 0% | 0% |
| KRAFT | | | | | |
| ★ *Free* Honey Dijon, Fat Free | 2 tbsp | 50 | 0% | 0% | 0% |
| ⊛ Honey Dijon | 2 tbsp | 150 | 23% | 10% | 0% |
| ⊛ MARIE'S Dressing & Dip: Honey Mustard—CAMPBELL'S | 2 tbsp | 160 | 23% | 10% | 2% |
| ★ SALAD CELEBRATIONS Fat Free Honey Dijon—WEIGHT WATCHERS | 2 tbsp | 45 | 0% | 0% | 0% |
| WISH-BONE—LIPTON | | | | | |
| ❖ Honey Dijon | 2 tbsp | 130 | 15% | 7% | 0% |
| ★ Honey Dijon, Fat Free | 2 tbsp | 45 | 0% | 0% | 0% |
| ***Italian Dressings*** | | | | | |
| **Generic Foods** | | | | | |
| ★ Creamy Italian, Fat Free | 2 tbsp | 30 | 0% | 0% | 0% |
| ⊛ Italian | 2 tbsp | 140 | 22% | 10% | 0% |
| **Brand Name Foods** | | | | | |
| ESTEE | | | | | |
| ★ Creamy Italian | 2 tbsp | 15 | 1% | 0% | 0% |
| ★ Italian | 2 tbsp | 5 | 0% | 0% | 0% |
| ★ FEATHERWEIGHT Italian | 2 tbsp | 5 | 0% | 0% | 0% |
| GOOD SEASONS Mixes (prep as dir)—KRAFT | | | | | |
| ★ Creamy Italian, Fat Free | 2 tbsp | 20 | 0% | 0% | 0% |
| ⊛ Italian | 2 tbsp | 140 | 24% | 11% | 0% |
| ★ Italian, Fat Free | 2 tbsp | 10 | 0% | 0% | 0% |
| ❖ Italian, Reduced Calorie | 2 tbsp | 50 | 8% | 5% | 0% |
| ⊛ Mild Italian | 2 tbsp | 150 | 24% | 13% | 0% |
| ❖ Zesty Italian, Reduced Calorie | 2 tbsp | 50 | 8% | 5% | 0% |
| ⊛ Zesty Italian | 2 tbsp | 140 | 24% | 11% | 0% |

★ Foods with this symbol have less than or equal to 5% *Daily Value* for <u>all</u> three nutrients (5% Rule).

❖ Foods with this symbol have <u>at least one</u> of the three nutrients greater than 5% *Daily Value* but less than or equal to 20% *Daily Value*.

⊛ Foods with this symbol have <u>at least one</u> of the three nutrients greater than 20% *Daily Value* (20% Rule).

| | | % DAILY VALUE | | |

| FOOD | Serving Size | Calories | Tot Fat | Sat Fat | Chol |
|---|---|---|---|---|---|
| **HAIN** | | | | | |
| ★ Italian, Fat Free | 2 tbsp | 35 | 0% | 0% | 0% |
| ☻ *Natural Classics* Creamy Italian | 2 tbsp | 180 | 25% | 12% | 0% |
| **HIDDEN VALLEY RANCH (Bottled)** | | | | | |
| ❖ Creamy Herb Italian | 2 tbsp | 140 | 20% | 10% | 3% |
| ★ Italian Parmesan, Fat Free | 2 tbsp | 20 | 0% | 0% | 0% |
| **KRAFT** | | | | | |
| ❖ Creamy Italian | 2 tbsp | 110 | 17% | 18% | 0% |
| ❖ *Deliciously Right* Creamy Italian, Reduced Calorie | 2 tbsp | 50 | 7% | 5% | 0% |
| ❖ *Deliciously Right* Italian, Reduced Calorie | 2 tbsp | 70 | 11% | 5% | 0% |
| ★ *Free* Italian, Fat Free | 2 tbsp | 10 | 0% | 0% | 0% |
| ❖ House Italian | 2 tbsp | 120 | 19% | 10% | 1% |
| ★ Oil-Free Italian, Fat Free | 2 tbsp | 5 | 0% | 0% | 0% |
| ☻ Presto Italian | 2 tbsp | 140 | 23% | 11% | 0% |
| ❖ Zesty Italian | 2 tbsp | 110 | 16% | 8% | 0% |
| ☻ LAWRY'S Italian w/Aged Parmesan Cheese—LIPTON | 2 tbsp | 140 | 22% | 13% | 2% |
| ★ MARIE'S *Luscious Low Fat* Creamy Italian Herb—CAMPBELL'S | 2 tbsp | 40 | 3% | 0% | 0% |
| **MARIE'S Dressing & Dip—CAMPBELL'S** | | | | | |
| ☻ Creamy Italian Garlic | 2 tbsp | 180 | 29% | 15% | 5% |
| ❖ Creamy Italian Garlic, Reduced Calorie | 2 tbsp | 90 | 11% | 3% | 2% |
| ★ NEWMAN'S OWN Light Italian, Reduced Calorie | 2 tbsp | 20 | 1% | 0% | 0% |
| **SALAD CELEBRATIONS Fat Free —WEIGHT WATCHERS** | | | | | |
| ★ Creamy Italian | 2 tbsp | 30 | 0% | 0% | 0% |
| ★ Italian | 2 tbsp | 10 | 0% | 0% | 0% |
| **SEVEN SEAS Dressing—KRAFT** | | | | | |
| ❖ Creamy Italian | 2 tbsp | 110 | 18% | 9% | 0% |
| ❖ Creamy Italian, Reduced Calorie | 2 tbsp | 60 | 8% | 4% | 0% |
| ★ *Free* Italian, Fat Free | 2 tbsp | 10 | 0% | 0% | 0% |
| ❖ Italian w/Olive Oil, Reduced Calorie | 2 tbsp | 50 | 7% | 4% | 0% |
| ❖ Two Cheese Italian | 2 tbsp | 70 | 11% | 5% | 0% |
| ❖ *Viva* Italian | 2 tbsp | 110 | 17% | 8% | 0% |
| ❖ *Viva* Italian, Reduced Calorie | 2 tbsp | 45 | 6% | 3% | 0% |
| **WISH-BONE—LIPTON** | | | | | |
| ☻ Classic House Italian | 2 tbsp | 140 | 22% | 11% | 1% |
| ❖ Classic Olive Oil Italian | 2 tbsp | 70 | 10% | 5% | 0% |
| ❖ Creamy Italian | 2 tbsp | 100 | 15% | 8% | 0% |
| ❖ Italian | 2 tbsp | 100 | 14% | 7% | 0% |
| ★ Italian, Fat Free | 2 tbsp | 15 | 0% | 0% | 0% |
| ❖ Robusto Italian | 2 tbsp | 100 | 15% | 7% | 0% |

| FOOD | Serving Size | Calories | Tot Fat | Sat Fat | Chol |
|---|---|---|---|---|---|
| **Ranch Dressings** | | | | | |
| **Generic Foods** | | | | | |
| ❖ Ranch Style | 2 tbsp | 110 | 18% | 7% | 3% |
| **Brand Name Foods** | | | | | |
| GOOD SEASONS Mixes (prep as dir)—KRAFT | | | | | |
| ❖  Buttermilk Farm Style | 2 tbsp | 120 | 18% | 10% | 3% |
| ❖  Ranch | 2 tbsp | 120 | 18% | 10% | 3% |
| ❖  Ranch, Reduced Calorie | 2 tbsp | 60 | 7% | 6% | 2% |
| HAIN Natural Classics | | | | | |
| ⊛  Old Fashioned Buttermilk | 2 tbsp | 130 | 21% | 11% | 1% |
| ⊛  Poppyseed Rancher's | 2 tbsp | 140 | 21% | 10% | 2% |
| KRAFT | | | | | |
| ⊛  Buttermilk Ranch | 2 tbsp | 150 | 24% | 14% | 2% |
| ⊛  Caesar Ranch | 2 tbsp | 140 | 23% | 13% | 3% |
| ⊛  Cucumber Ranch | 2 tbsp | 150 | 23% | 12% | 0% |
| ❖  *Deliciously Right* Ranch, Reduced Calorie | 2 tbsp | 110 | 17% | 9% | 3% |
| ★  *Free* Peppercorn Ranch, Fat Free | 2 tbsp | 50 | 0% | 0% | 0% |
| ★  *Free* Ranch, Fat Free | 2 tbsp | 50 | 0% | 0% | 0% |
| ⊛  Peppercorn Ranch | 2 tbsp | 170 | 28% | 14% | 3% |
| ⊛  Ranch | 2 tbsp | 170 | 28% | 15% | 2% |
| ★ MARIE'S *Luscious Low Fat* Zesty Ranch—CAMPBELL'S | 2 tbsp | 45 | 2% | 0% | 0% |
| MARIE'S *Salad Bar*—CAMPBELL'S | | | | | |
| ❖  Ranch | 2 tbsp | 130 | 15% | 8% | 0% |
| ❖  Ranch, Reduced Calorie | 2 tbsp | 90 | 11% | 5% | 2% |
| MARIE'S Dressing & Dip— CAMPBELL'S | | | | | |
| ⊛  Buttermilk Spice Ranch Style | 2 tbsp | 180 | 28% | 15% | 5% |
| ⊛  Creamy Ranch | 2 tbsp | 190 | 31% | 15% | 5% |
| ❖  Reduced Calorie Creamy Ranch | 2 tbsp | 100 | 11% | 3% | 2% |
| ⊛ NEWMAN'S OWN Ranch | 2 tbsp | 180 | 29% | 15% | 2% |
| ★ SALAD CELEBRATIONS Fat Free Ranch—WEIGHT WATCHERS | 2 tbsp | 35 | 0% | 0% | 0% |
| SEVEN SEAS Dressing—KRAFT | | | | | |
| ⊛  Ranch | 2 tbsp | 150 | 24% | 12% | 2% |
| ★  *Free* Ranch, Fat Free | 2 tbsp | 50 | 0% | 0% | 0% |
| ❖  Ranch, Reduced Calorie | 2 tbsp | 100 | 14% | 8% | 0% |
| WISH-BONE—LIPTON | | | | | |
| ⊛  Ranch | 2 tbsp | 160 | 25% | 13% | 4% |
| ★  Ranch, Fat Free | 2 tbsp | 40 | 0% | 0% | 0% |

★  Foods with this symbol have less than or equal to 5% *Daily Value* for all three nutrients (5% Rule).

❖  Foods with this symbol have at least one of the three nutrients greater than 5% *Daily Value* but less than or equal to 20% *Daily Value*.

⊛  Foods with this symbol have at least one of the three nutrients greater than 20% *Daily Value* (20% Rule).

| FOOD | Serving Size | Calories | Tot Fat | Sat Fat | Chol |
|------|------|------|------|------|------|
| ***Thousand Island Dressings*** | | | | | |
| **Generic Foods** | | | | | |
| ❖ Thousand Island | 2 tbsp | 120 | 17% | 9% | 3% |
| ★ Thousand Island, Low Calorie | 2 tbsp | 50 | 5% | 2% | 1% |
| **Brand Name Foods** | | | | | |
| ★ ESTEE Thousand Island | 2 tbsp | 10 | 0% | 0% | 0% |
| ❖ HAIN Natural Classics: 1000 Island | 2 tbsp | 110 | 14% | 8% | 1% |
| KRAFT | | | | | |
| ❖ *Deliciously Right* Thousand Island, Reduced Calorie | 2 tbsp | 70 | 6% | 4% | 2% |
| ★ *Free* Thousand Island, Fat Free | 2 tbsp | 45 | 0% | 0% | 0% |
| ❖ Thousand Island | 2 tbsp | 110 | 16% | 8% | 3% |
| ❖ Thousand Island w/Bacon | 2 tbsp | 120 | 18% | 9% | 0% |
| MARIE'S—CAMPBELL'S | | | | | |
| ☻ *Salad Bar* Thousand Island | 2 tbsp | 170 | 25% | 13% | 3% |
| ☻ Dressing & Dip: Thousand Island | 2 tbsp | 240 | 35% | 20% | 7% |
| ★ SALAD CELEBRATIONS Thousand Island—WEIGHT WATCHERS | 2 tbsp | 45 | 2% | 0% | 3% |
| WISH-BONE—LIPTON | | | | | |
| ❖ Thousand Island | 2 tbsp | 130 | 18% | 9% | 4% |
| ★ Thousand Island, Fat Free | 2 tbsp | 35 | 0% | 0% | 0% |
| ***Vinaigrette Dressings*** | | | | | |
| **Brand Name Foods** | | | | | |
| HAIN Fat Free Dressings | | | | | |
| ★ Raspberry Vinaigrette | 2 tbsp | 25 | 0% | 0% | 0% |
| ★ White Wine Vinaigrette | 2 tbsp | 25 | 0% | 0% | 0% |
| KRAFT | | | | | |
| ★ *Free* Red Wine Vinegar, Fat Free | 2 tbsp | 15 | 0% | 0% | 0% |
| ❖ *Herb* Garden Tomato Basil & Oregano | 2 tbsp | 80 | 9% | 5% | 0% |
| ❖ *Herb* Red Wine Vinegar & Thyme | 2 tbsp | 90 | 14% | 8% | 0% |
| ❖ LAWRY'S Red Wine Vinaigrette —LIPTON | 2 tbsp | 90 | 11% | 5% | 0% |
| MARIE'S Zesty Fat Free Vinaigrette—CAMPBELL'S | | | | | |
| ★ Classic Herb | 2 tbsp | 30 | 0% | 0% | 0% |
| ★ Honey Dijon | 2 tbsp | 50 | 0% | 0% | 0% |
| ★ Italian | 2 tbsp | 35 | 0% | 0% | 0% |
| ★ Raspberry | 2 tbsp | 35 | 0% | 0% | 0% |
| ★ Red Wine | 2 tbsp | 40 | 0% | 0% | 0% |
| ★ White Wine | 2 tbsp | 40 | 0% | 0% | 0% |
| ☻ NEWMAN'S OWN Olive Oil & Vinegar | 2 tbsp | 150 | 25% | 13% | 0% |

| FOOD | Serving Size | Calories | Tot Fat | Sat Fat | Chol |
|---|---|---|---|---|---|
| SEVEN SEAS Dressings—KRAFT | | | | | |
| ★ *Free* Red Wine Vinegar, Fat Free | 2 tbsp | 15 | 0% | 0% | 0% |
| ❖ Red Wine Vinegar & Oil | 2 tbsp | 110 | 17% | 9% | 0% |
| ❖ Red Wine Vinegar & Oil, Reduced Calorie | 2 tbsp | 60 | 8% | 4% | 0% |
| ❖ WISH-BONE Olive Oil Vinaigrette —LIPTON | 2 tbsp | 60 | 7% | 4% | 0% |

### Other Dressings
### Brand Name Foods

| FOOD | Serving Size | Calories | Tot Fat | Sat Fat | Chol |
|---|---|---|---|---|---|
| ★ ESTEE Creamy Garlic | 2 tbsp | 10 | 0% | 0% | 0% |
| ★ FEATHERWEIGHT Creamy Dijon | 2 tbsp | 15 | 1% | 0% | 0% |
| GOOD SEASONS Mixes (prep as dir)—KRAFT | | | | | |
| Ⓐ Mexican Spice | 2 tbsp | 140 | 24% | 13% | 0% |
| Ⓐ Oriental Sesame | 2 tbsp | 150 | 24% | 13% | 0% |
| HIDDEN VALLEY RANCH (Bottled) | | | | | |
| Ⓐ Bacon | 2 tbsp | 150 | 23% | 15% | 3% |
| Ⓐ Fiesta Ranch | 2 tbsp | 140 | 22% | 10% | 3% |
| Ⓐ Original | 2 tbsp | 140 | 22% | 10% | 3% |
| ★ Original, Fat Free | 2 tbsp | 45 | 0% | 0% | 0% |
| ❖ Light Original Ranch, Reduced Calorie | 2 tbsp | 80 | 11% | 5% | 0% |
| KRAFT | | | | | |
| Ⓐ Bacon & Tomato | 2 tbsp | 140 | 22% | 13% | 1% |
| ❖ Creamy Garlic | 2 tbsp | 110 | 16% | 9% | 0% |
| ★ *Free Catalina*, Fat Free | 2 tbsp | 45 | 0% | 0% | 0% |
| ❖ *Herb* Creamy Cucumber Dill | 2 tbsp | 120 | 18% | 10% | 0% |
| ❖ Russian | 2 tbsp | 130 | 15% | 8% | 0% |
| ❖ *Salsa* Ranch | 2 tbsp | 130 | 20% | 10% | 3% |
| ❖ *Salsa* Zesty Garden | 2 tbsp | 70 | 9% | 5% | 0% |
| Ⓐ Sour Cream & Onion Ranch | 2 tbsp | 170 | 28% | 15% | 3% |
| KRAFT *Deliciously Right* Reduced Calorie | | | | | |
| ❖ Bacon and Tomato | 2 tbsp | 60 | 8% | 5% | 1% |
| ❖ *Catalina* French | 2 tbsp | 80 | 7% | 3% | 0% |
| ❖ Cucumber Ranch | 2 tbsp | 60 | 8% | 5% | 0% |
| MARIE'S Dressing & Dip— CAMPBELL'S | | | | | |
| ❖ Poppyseed | 2 tbsp | 150 | 18% | 8% | 3% |
| Ⓐ Sour Cream & Dill | 2 tbsp | 190 | 31% | 15% | 5% |

★ Foods with this symbol have less than or equal to 5% *Daily Value* for <u>all</u> three nutrients (5% Rule).

❖ Foods with this symbol have <u>at least one</u> of the three nutrients greater than 5% *Daily Value* but less than or equal to 20% *Daily Value*.

Ⓐ Foods with this symbol have <u>at least one</u> of the three nutrients greater than 20% *Daily Value* (20% Rule).

| FOOD | Serving Size | Calories | Tot Fat | Sat Fat | Chol |
|------|------|------|------|------|------|
| ❖ MIRACLE WHIP Salad Dressing | | | | | |
| —KRAFT | 1 tbsp | 70 | 11% | 5% | 2% |
| ★ SALAD CELEBRATIONS Russian | | | | | |
| —WEIGHT WATCHERS | 2 tbsp | 45 | 2% | 0% | 3% |
| SEVEN SEAS—KRAFT | | | | | |
| ❖ Green Goddess | 2 tbsp | 120 | 20% | 10% | 0% |
| Ⓐ *Viva* Russian | 2 tbsp | 150 | 25% | 13% | 0% |
| WISH-BONE—LIPTON | | | | | |
| ❖ Creamy Roasted Garlic | 2 tbsp | 140 | 20% | 9% | 0% |
| ❖ Russian | 2 tbsp | 110 | 9% | 4% | 0% |
| ★ Creamy Roasted Garlic, Fat Free | 2 tbsp | 40 | 0% | 0% | 0% |

TOPPERS

**Brand Name Foods**

| FOOD | Serving Size | Calories | Tot Fat | Sat Fat | Chol |
|------|------|------|------|------|------|
| ★ ARNOLD/BROWNBERRY | | | | | |
| Croutons: All flavors—CPC | 2 tbsp | 30 | 2% | 0% | 0% |
| ★ BETTY CROCKER *Bac\*Os* Chips | | | | | |
| or Bits—GENERAL MILLS | 1 tbsp | 30 | 2% | 0% | 0% |
| HORMEL Bacon | | | | | |
| ★ Bacon Bits | 1 tsp | 30 | 2% | 5% | 2% |
| ★ Bacon Pieces | 1 tsp | 25 | 2% | 3% | 3% |
| McCORMICK/SCHILLING Salad Toppins | | | | | |
| ★ Garden Vegetable | 1 tbsp | 30 | 1% | 0% | 0% |
| ★ Oriental | 1 1/3 tbsp | 40 | 3% | 0% | 0% |
| ★ Regular | 1 tbsp | 30 | 1% | 0% | 0% |
| ★ McCORMICK/SCHILLING Salad Toppins: Bac 'n Pieces: Chips or Bits | 1 tbsp | 30 | 1% | 0% | 0% |
| ★ OSCAR MAYER Real Bacon Bits | 1 tbsp | 25 | 2% | 3% | 2% |
| PEPPERIDGE FARM *Salad Toppers* | | | | | |
| —CAMPBELL'S | | | | | |
| ★ Bacon Cheddar | 1 tbsp | 35 | 3% | 0% | 0% |
| ★ Caesar Salad Bar Mix | 1 tbsp | 35 | 3% | 0% | 0% |
| ★ Cinnamon Raisin | 1 tbsp | 35 | 3% | 0% | 0% |
| ★ Garlic Italian | 1 tbsp | 35 | 2% | 0% | 0% |
| PEPPERIDGE FARM Croutons | | | | | |
| —CAMPBELL'S | | | | | |
| ★ Caesar Homestyle | 6 croutons | 35 | 2% | 0% | 0% |
| ★ Cheddar & Romano Cheese | 9 croutons | 30 | 2% | 0% | 0% |
| ★ Cheese & Garlic | 9 croutons | 35 | 2% | 0% | 0% |
| ★ Cracked Pepper & Parmesan | 6 croutons | 35 | 2% | 0% | 0% |
| ★ Olive Oil & Garlic Homestyle | 6 croutons | 30 | 2% | 0% | 0% |
| ★ Onion & Garlic | 9 croutons | 30 | 2% | 0% | 0% |
| ★ Ranch | 9 croutons | 35 | 2% | 0% | 1% |
| ★ Seasoned | 9 croutons | 35 | 2% | 0% | 0% |

| FOOD | Serving Size | Calories | Tot Fat | Sat Fat | Chol |
|------|-------------|----------|---------|---------|------|
| ★ Sourdough Cheese Homestyle | 6 croutons | 30 | 2% | 0% | 0% |
| ★ Zesty Italian Homestyle | 9 croutons | 35 | 2% | 0% | 1% |

# Sandwiches, Spreads, and Luncheon Meats

## LUNCHEON MEATS

### Beef

### Generic Foods

| | | | | | |
|------|-------------|----------|---------|---------|------|
| ❖ Roast Beef | ~ 2 slcs | 60 | 3% | 5% | 8% |

### Brand Name Foods

| | | | | | |
|------|-------------|----------|---------|---------|------|
| ❖ BREAD READY Roast Beef— HORMEL FOODS | 2 oz | 60 | 3% | 5% | 8% |
| ❖ HEALTHY CHOICE Deli-Thin Sliced Roast Beef (chopped and formed)—CONAGRA | 6 slcs | 60 | 2% | 3% | 8% |
| HILLSHIRE FARM *Deli Select* | | | | | |
| ❖ Oven Roasted Cured Beef | 6 slcs | 50 | 1% | 0% | 6% |
| ❖ Roast Beef | 6 slcs | 50 | 1% | 0% | 6% |
| ★ Smoked Beef | 6 slcs | 60 | 1% | 0% | 5% |
| ❖ LIGHT & LEAN 97 Deli Roast Beef—HORMEL FOODS | 2 oz | 60 | 3% | 5% | 8% |
| ❖ OSCAR MAYER *Deli Thin* Roast Beef | 4 slcs | 60 | 2% | 3% | 8% |

### Bologna

### Generic Foods

| | | | | | |
|------|-------------|----------|---------|---------|------|
| Ⓐ Beef Bologna | 2 oz (~ 2 slcs) | 170 | 24% | 33% | 10% |
| Ⓐ Beef/Pork Bologna | 2 oz (~ 2 slcs) | 170 | 24% | 29% | 10% |
| ❖ Turkey Bologna | 2 oz | 110 | 13% | 14% | 18% |

### Brand Name Foods

| | | | | | |
|------|-------------|----------|---------|---------|------|
| HEALTHY CHOICE Cold Cuts— CONAGRA | | | | | |
| ★ Beef Bologna | 1 slc | 35 | 2% | 0% | 3% |
| ★ Bologna w/Turkey, Pork & Beef | 1 slc | 30 | 2% | 0% | 5% |
| ❖ Deli-Thin Sliced Bologna w/ Turkey, Pork, & Beef | 4 slcs | 60 | 2% | 3% | 10% |

★ Foods with this symbol have less than or equal to 5% *Daily Value* for <u>all</u> three nutrients (5% Rule).

❖ Foods with this symbol have <u>at least one</u> of the three nutrients greater than 5% *Daily Value* but less than or equal to 20% *Daily Value*.

Ⓐ Foods with this symbol have <u>at least one</u> of the three nutrients greater than 20% *Daily Value* (20% Rule).

| FOOD | Serving Size | Calories | Tot Fat | Sat Fat | Chol |
|---|---|---|---|---|---|
| ❖ HILLSHIRE FARM *Deli Select* Light Bologna | 6 slcs | 80 | 8% | 12% | 6% |
| ❖ JENNIE-O *Extra Lean* Turkey Bologna | 1 slc | 35 | 2% | 0% | 8% |
| ❖ LOUIS RICH Turkey Bologna— OSCAR MAYER | 1 slc | 50 | 6% | 5% | 7% |
| ❖ MR. TURKEY Turkey Bologna | 2 oz | 120 | 17% | 14% | 13% |
| OSCAR MAYER Bologna | | | | | |
| ❖ Beef | 1 slc | 90 | 12% | 20% | 5% |
| ❖ Beef Light | 1 slc | 60 | 6% | 8% | 3% |
| Ⓐ Garlic (made w/Pork, Chicken, and Beef) | 1 slc | 130 | 18% | 23% | 10% |
| ❖ Light (made w/Pork, Chicken, and Beef) | 1 slc | 50 | 6% | 8% | 5% |
| ❖ Made w/Pork, Chicken, and Beef | 1 slc | 90 | 12% | 15% | 7% |
| ★ Made w/Turkey, Beef, and Pork, Fat Free | 2 slcs | 35 | 0% | 0% | 5% |

### *Chicken*

### Generic Foods

| | | | | | |
|---|---|---|---|---|---|
| ★ Chicken Breast | 1 slc | 30 | 2% | 0% | 5% |

### Brand Name Foods

| | | | | | |
|---|---|---|---|---|---|
| HEALTHY CHOICE Cold Cuts— CONAGRA | | | | | |
| ★ Oven Roasted Chicken Breast | 1 slc | 35 | 2% | 3% | 5% |
| ★ Smoked Chicken Breast | 1 slc | 35 | 2% | 0% | 5% |
| HEALTHY CHOICE Deli-Thin Sliced—CONAGRA | | | | | |
| ❖ Oven Roasted Chicken Breast | 6 slcs | 50 | 0% | 0% | 8% |
| ❖ Smoked Chicken Breast | 6 slcs | 60 | 2% | 3% | 8% |
| ★ HILLSHIRE FARM *Deli Select* Smoked Chicken Breast | 6 slcs | 50 | 0% | 0% | 2% |
| LOUIS RICH Chicken—OSCAR MAYER | | | | | |
| ★ Deluxe Oven Roasted Chicken Breast | 1 slc | 30 | 2% | 0% | 5% |
| ★ Hickory Smoked Chicken Breast | 1 slc | 30 | 2% | 0% | 5% |
| ★ Oven Roasted White Chicken | 1 slc | 40 | 4% | 3% | 5% |
| ❖ LOUIS RICH *Deli-Thin* Chicken Breast, Oven Roasted—OSCAR MAYER | 4 slcs | 60 | 2% | 3% | 8% |
| ❖ MR. TURKEY Smoked Chicken Deli Slices | 2 oz | 60 | 2% | 2% | 10% |
| OSCAR MAYER | | | | | |
| ❖ *Deli Thin* Chicken Breast, Honey Glazed | 4 slcs | 60 | 2% | 0% | 8% |

| FOOD | Serving Size | Calories | Tot Fat | Sat Fat | Chol |
|---|---|---|---|---|---|
| ❖ Oven Roasted Chicken Breast, Fat Free | 4 slcs | 45 | 0% | 0% | 8% |
| TYSON Chicken Breast Lunch Meat, Fat Free | | | | | |
| ❖ Hickory Smoked | 3 slcs | 50 | 0% | 0% | 8% |
| ❖ Honey Flavored | 3 slcs | 50 | 0% | 0% | 8% |
| ❖ Mesquite Flavored | 3 slcs | 50 | 0% | 0% | 8% |
| ❖ Oven Roasted | 3 slcs | 50 | 0% | 0% | 8% |
| ❖ Peppered | 3 slcs | 50 | 0% | 0% | 8% |
| ❖ TYSON White Meat Chicken Roll | 2 oz | 90 | 9% | 10% | 8% |

### Corned Beef
**Generic Foods**

| | | | | | |
|---|---|---|---|---|---|
| ❖ Corned Beef | 1 slc | 40 | 2% | 3% | 7% |

**Brand Name Foods**

| | | | | | |
|---|---|---|---|---|---|
| ❖ HEALTHY CHOICE Deli-Thin Sliced Corned Beef (chopped & formed)—CONAGRA | 6 slcs | 60 | 2% | 3% | 8% |
| ★ HILLSHIRE FARM *Deli Select* Corned Beef | 6 slcs | 60 | 1% | 0% | 5% |
| ❖ LIGHT & LEAN 97 Deli Corned Beef—HORMEL FOODS | 2 oz | 40 | 2% | 3% | 7% |

### Ham
**Generic Foods**

| | | | | | |
|---|---|---|---|---|---|
| ❖ Ham (boiled) | 2 slcs | 100 | 9% | 9% | 10% |

**Brand Name Foods**

| | | | | | |
|---|---|---|---|---|---|
| ❖ BLACK LABEL Chopped Ham —HORMEL FOODS | 2 oz | 140 | 17% | 20% | 10% |
| ❖ BREAD READY Ham—HORMEL FOODS | 2 oz | 70 | 5% | 5% | 10% |
| HEALTHY CHOICE Cold Cuts— CONAGRA | | | | | |
| ❖ Baked Cooked Ham | 3 slcs | 70 | 3% | 3% | 10% |
| ★ Honey Ham | 1 slc | 30 | 2% | 3% | 5% |
| ❖ Smoked Ham | 3 slcs | 70 | 3% | 3% | 10% |
| ❖ Turkey Ham (cured turkey thigh) | 1 slc | 30 | 2% | 3% | 7% |
| HEALTHY CHOICE Deli-Thin Sliced—CONAGRA | | | | | |
| ❖ Baked Cooked Ham | 6 slcs | 60 | 2% | 3% | 10% |

★ Foods with this symbol have less than or equal to 5% *Daily Value* for <u>all</u> three nutrients (5% Rule).

❖ Foods with this symbol have <u>at least one</u> of the three nutrients greater than 5% *Daily Value* but less than or equal to 20% *Daily Value.*

Ⓐ Foods with this symbol have <u>at least one</u> of the three nutrients greater than 20% *Daily Value* (20% Rule).

| FOOD | Serving Size | Calories | Tot Fat | Sat Fat | Chol |
|---|---|---|---|---|---|
| ❖ Honey Ham | 6 slcs | 60 | 2% | 3% | 10% |
| ❖ Smoked Ham | 6 slcs | 60 | 2% | 3% | 8% |
| ❖ Turkey Ham (cured turkey thigh) | 6 slcs | 60 | 2% | 3% | 13% |
| HILLSHIRE FARM *Deli Select* | | | | | |
| ❖ Baked Ham | 6 slcs | 60 | 2% | 3% | 6% |
| ❖ Brown Sugar Baked Ham | 6 slcs | 60 | 2% | 3% | 7% |
| ❖ Cajun Style Ham | 6 slcs | 60 | 2% | 3% | 8% |
| ❖ Honey Ham | 6 slcs | 60 | 2% | 0% | 6% |
| ❖ Lower Sodium Ham | 6 slcs | 60 | 2% | 3% | 6% |
| ❖ Smoked Ham | 6 slcs | 60 | 3% | 0% | 7% |
| ❖ Turkey Ham | 6 slcs | 50 | 1% | 0% | 7% |
| ❖ HORMEL Deli Cooked Ham | 1 oz | 29 | 2% | 8% | 4% |
| ❖ JENNIE-O *Extra Lean* Turkey Ham | 1 slc | 35 | 2% | 0% | 7% |
| LIGHT & LEAN 97—HORMEL FOODS | | | | | |
| ★ *Cuts* Ham | 16 pieces | 35 | 2% | 3% | 5% |
| ❖ Deli Ham | 2 oz | 50 | 3% | 5% | 8% |
| ★ Sliced Ham | 1 slc | 25 | 2% | 3% | 5% |
| LOUIS RICH *Carving Board* Ham —OSCAR MAYER | | | | | |
| ❖ Ham, Smoked | 2 slcs | 50 | 2% | 3% | 8% |
| ❖ Honey Glazed: Thin Carved | 6 slcs | 70 | 3% | 5% | 12% |
| ❖ Honey Glazed: Traditional Carved | 2 slcs | 50 | 2% | 3% | 8% |
| LOUIS RICH Ham—OSCAR MAYER | | | | | |
| ❖ Chopped Turkey Ham | 1 slc | 45 | 4% | 5% | 7% |
| ❖ *Deli Thin* Turkey Ham | 4 slcs | 60 | 2% | 3% | 12% |
| ❖ Honey Cured Turkey Ham | 3 slcs | 70 | 3% | 3% | 15% |
| ❖ Turkey Ham | 1 slc | 35 | 2% | 0% | 7% |
| MR. TURKEY Turkey Ham | | | | | |
| ❖ Chub: Honey or Smoked | 2 oz | 70 | 4% | 5% | 11% |
| ❖ Lunchmeat | 2 oz | 70 | 4% | 5% | 14% |
| OSCAR MAYER Ham | | | | | |
| ❖ Baked | 3 slcs | 60 | 2% | 3% | 10% |
| ❖ Boiled | 3 slcs | 60 | 4% | 5% | 10% |
| ★ Chopped | 1 slc | 45 | 5% | 5% | 5% |
| ❖ Honey | 3 slcs | 70 | 4% | 5% | 10% |
| ❖ Lower Sodium | 3 slcs | 70 | 4% | 5% | 10% |
| ❖ Smoked, Cooked | 3 slcs | 60 | 4% | 5% | 10% |
| OSCAR MAYER *Deli Thin* Ham | | | | | |
| ❖ Boiled | 4 slcs | 50 | 3% | 3% | 8% |
| ❖ Honey | 4 slcs | 60 | 3% | 3% | 8% |
| ❖ Smoked | 4 slcs | 50 | 3% | 3% | 8% |
| OSCAR MAYER *Healthy Favorites* Ham | | | | | |
| ❖ Baked | 4 slcs | 50 | 2% | 0% | 8% |
| ❖ Honey | 4 slcs | 50 | 2% | 3% | 8% |
| ❖ Smoked | 4 slcs | 50 | 2% | 3% | 8% |

| FOOD | Serving Size | Calories | Tot Fat | Sat Fat | Chol |
|------|--------------|----------|---------|---------|------|
| ***Pastrami*** | | | | | |
| **Generic Foods** | | | | | |
| ⊛ Pastrami | 2 oz | 190 | 25% | 29% | 17% |
| **Brand Name Foods** | | | | | |
| ❖ HILLSHIRE FARM *Deli Select* Pastrami | 6 slcs | 60 | 1% | 0% | 6% |
| ❖ LIGHT & LEAN 97 Deli Pastrami —HORMEL FOODS | 2 oz | 50 | 2% | 0% | 7% |
| ❖ LOUIS RICH Turkey Pastrami— OSCAR MAYER | 2 slcs | 45 | 2% | 0% | 10% |
| ❖ MR. TURKEY Turkey Pastrami Deli Slices | 2 oz | 70 | 4% | 4% | 12% |
| ***Salami*** | | | | | |
| **Generic Foods** | | | | | |
| ⊛ Beef Salami | 2 oz (~ 2 slcs) | 180 | 25% | 36% | 11% |
| ⊛ Hard/Dry Salami (pork) | 2 oz | 220 | 29% | 33% | 14% |
| ❖ Pork Salami | 2 oz (~ 2 slcs) | 130 | 16% | 17% | 11% |
| ❖ Turkey Salami | 2 slcs | 110 | 12% | 11% | 15% |
| **Brand Name Foods** | | | | | |
| ⊛ BREAD READY Genoa Salami— HORMEL FOODS | 1 oz | 120 | 17% | 25% | 12% |
| ⊛ HOMELAND Hard Salami— HORMEL FOODS | 1 oz | 110 | 15% | 23% | 12% |
| ❖ HORMEL Italian Dry Salami | 1 oz | 120 | 15% | 20% | 10% |
| ❖ JENNIE-O *Extra Lean* Turkey Salami | 1 slc | 35 | 2% | 0% | 8% |
| LOUIS RICH Salami—OSCAR MAYER | | | | | |
| ❖   Turkey Cotto Salami | 1 slc | 40 | 4% | 5% | 8% |
| ❖   Turkey Salami | 1 slc | 45 | 4% | 5% | 7% |
| ❖ MR. TURKEY Salami Lunchmeat | 2 oz | 90 | 9% | 9% | 10% |
| OSCAR MAYER Salami | | | | | |
| ⊛   Beef Machiach Brand | 2 slcs | 120 | 15% | 25% | 10% |
| ❖   Cotto, Beef | 2 slcs | 90 | 11% | 15% | 12% |
| ❖   Cotto made w/Beef, Pork, and Chicken | 2 slcs | 110 | 14% | 20% | 12% |
| ❖   *Deli Thin* Hard Salami | 4 slcs | 130 | 17% | 20% | 10% |
| ❖   For Beer | 2 slcs | 110 | 14% | 15% | 10% |
| ❖   Genoa | 3 slcs | 100 | 14% | 15% | 8% |
| ❖   Hard | 3 slcs | 100 | 14% | 15% | 8% |

★ Foods with this symbol have less than or equal to 5% *Daily Value* for <u>all</u> three nutrients (5% Rule).
❖ Foods with this symbol have <u>at least one</u> of the three nutrients greater than 5% *Daily Value* but less than or equal to 20% *Daily Value*.
⊛ Foods with this symbol have <u>at least one</u> of the three nutrients greater than 20% *Daily Value* (20% Rule).

| FOOD | Serving Size | Calories | Tot Fat | Sat Fat | Chol |
|------|--------------|----------|---------|---------|------|
| ❖ SAN REMO BRAND Genoa Salami—HORMEL FOODS | 1 oz | 120 | 14% | 20% | 10% |
| ⊘ SANDWICH MAKER Genoa Salami—HORMEL FOODS | 1 oz | 120 | 17% | 25% | 12% |
| ⊘ SANDWICH MAKER Hard Salami—HORMEL FOODS | 1 oz | 110 | 15% | 23% | 12% |

**Turkey**

**Generic Foods**

| | | | | | |
|------|--------------|----------|---------|---------|------|
| ★ Turkey | 1 slc | 40 | 2% | 1% | 5% |

**Brand Name Foods**

| | | | | | |
|------|--------------|----------|---------|---------|------|
| ❖ BREAD READY Turkey: Plain or Smoked—HORMEL FOODS | 2 oz | 50 | 1% | 0% | 10% |
| HEALTHY CHOICE Cold Cuts —CONAGRA | | | | | |
| ★ Honey Roasted or Smoked Turkey | 1 slc | 35 | 2% | 0% | 5% |
| ★ Oven Roasted Turkey Breast | 1 slc | 35 | 2% | 0% | 5% |
| ★ Smoked Turkey Breast | 1 slc | 30 | 2% | 0% | 3% |
| HEALTHY CHOICE Deli-Thin Sliced—CONAGRA | | | | | |
| ❖ Honey Roasted or Smoked Turkey Breast | 6 slcs | 70 | 2% | 3% | 8% |
| ❖ Oven Roasted Turkey Breast | 6 slcs | 60 | 2% | 3% | 7% |
| ❖ Peppered Turkey Breast | 6 slcs | 60 | 2% | 3% | 8% |
| ❖ Smoked Turkey Breast | 6 slcs | 60 | 2% | 3% | 8% |
| HILLSHIRE FARM *Deli Select* | | | | | |
| ★ Honey Roasted Turkey Breast | 6 slcs | 50 | 0% | 0% | 3% |
| ❖ Oven Roasted Turkey Breast | 6 slcs | 50 | 0% | 0% | 6% |
| ❖ Smoked Turkey Breast | 6 slcs | 60 | 1% | 0% | 9% |
| ❖ HORMEL Deli Premium Skinless Turkey Breast | 2 oz | 50 | 1% | 0% | 7% |
| JENNIE-O *Extra Lean* Turkey Breast (sliced) | | | | | |
| ❖ Oven Roasted | 2 slcs | 45 | 0% | 0% | 6% |
| ★ Smoked (95% fat free) | 1 slc | 35 | 2% | 0% | 4% |
| ❖ Smoked (99% fat free) | 2 slcs | 40 | 0% | 0% | 6% |
| ❖ JENNIE-O Natural Choice Premium Turkey Breast (sliced) | 1 slc | 90 | 1% | 0% | 14% |
| LIGHT & LEAN 97—HORMEL FOODS | | | | | |
| ★ *Cuts* Turkey: Regular or Smoked | 16 pcs | 30 | 1% | 0% | 5% |
| ❖ Deli Turkey Breast: Regular or Honey | 2 oz | 50 | 1% | 0% | 7% |
| ★ Turkey Breast | 1 slc | 30 | 1% | 0% | 3% |

| FOOD | Serving Size | Calories | Tot Fat | Sat Fat | Chol |
|---|---|---|---|---|---|
| **LOUIS RICH** *Carving Board*— OSCAR MAYER | | | | | |
| ❖ Turkey Breast Oven Roasted: Traditional Carved | 2 slcs | 40 | 1% | 0% | 7% |
| ❖ Turkey Breast Oven Roasted: Thin Carved | 6 slcs | 60 | 1% | 0% | 8% |
| ❖ Turkey Breast Smoked | 2 slcs | 40 | 1% | 0% | 7% |
| **LOUIS RICH** Cold Cuts: Turkey Breast—OSCAR MAYER | | | | | |
| ★ Hickory Smoked | 1 slc | 25 | 1% | 0% | 3% |
| ★ Honey Roasted | 1 slc | 30 | 2% | 0% | 3% |
| ★ Oven Roasted | 1 slc | 30 | 1% | 0% | 3% |
| ★ Smoked White | 1 slc | 30 | 2% | 0% | 5% |
| ❖ Smoked | 4 slcs | 50 | 2% | 0% | 7% |
| **LOUIS RICH** Fat Free Turkey Breast—OSCAR MAYER | | | | | |
| ★ *Deli-Thin* Oven Roasted | 4 slcs | 40 | 0% | 0% | 5% |
| ★ Hickory Smoked | 1 slc | 25 | 0% | 0% | 3% |
| ★ Oven Roasted | 1 slc | 25 | 0% | 0% | 3% |
| ❖ **LOUIS RICH** *Deli-Thin* Turkey Breast, Oven Roasted—OSCAR MAYER | 4 slcs | 50 | 2% | 0% | 7% |
| ❖ **MR. TURKEY** Turkey Breast Lunchmeat: Regular or Smoked | 2 oz | 60 | 2% | 1% | 6% |
| **OSCAR MAYER** *Deli Thin* Turkey Breast | | | | | |
| ❖ Breast & White Turkey Roasted | 4 slcs | 50 | 2% | 0% | 7% |
| ❖ Roasted | 4 slcs | 50 | 2% | 0% | 7% |
| ❖ Smoked, Honey Roasted | 4 slcs | 60 | 2% | 0% | 7% |
| **OSCAR MAYER** Fat Free Turkey Breast | | | | | |
| ★ Oven Roasted | 4 slcs | 40 | 0% | 0% | 5% |
| ★ Smoked | 4 slcs | 40 | 0% | 0% | 5% |
| **OSCAR MAYER** Oven Roasted Turkey | | | | | |
| ★ Breast | 1 slc | 25 | 1% | 0% | 3% |
| ★ White | 1 slc | 30 | 2% | 0% | 3% |

### *Other Luncheon Meats*
### Generic Foods

| FOOD | Serving Size | Calories | Tot Fat | Sat Fat | Chol |
|---|---|---|---|---|---|
| ⦿ Liverwurst | 2 oz | 180 | 24% | 29% | 29% |
| ⦿ Mortadella (beef & pork) | 2 oz | 170 | 21% | 26% | 10% |

★ Foods with this symbol have less than or equal to 5% *Daily Value* for <u>all</u> three nutrients (5% Rule).
❖ Foods with this symbol have <u>at least one</u> of the three nutrients greater than 5% *Daily Value* but less than or equal to 20% *Daily Value.*
⦿ Foods with this symbol have <u>at least one</u> of the three nutrients greater than 20% *Daily Value* (20% Rule).

| FOOD | Serving Size | Calories | Tot Fat | Sat Fat | Chol |
|---|---|---|---|---|---|
| ⊛ Pimiento Loaf (pork) | 2 oz | 140 | 18% | 21% | 6% |
| ⊛ Thuringer (pork) | 2 oz | 180 | 25% | 33% | 10% |

**Brand Name Foods**

| FOOD | Serving Size | Calories | Tot Fat | Sat Fat | Chol |
|---|---|---|---|---|---|
| ⊛ BREAD READY Pepperoni— | | | | | |
|    HORMEL FOODS | 1 oz | 140 | 20% | 30% | 12% |
| ❖ DI LUSSO Genoa—HORMEL FOODS | 1 oz | 120 | 14% | 20% | 10% |
| ⊛ LEONI BRAND Pepperoni— | | | | | |
|    HORMEL FOODS | 1 oz | 140 | 20% | 30% | 12% |
| ❖ LIGHT & LEAN 97 Deli Cotto | | | | | |
|    Loaf—HORMEL FOODS | 2 oz | 50 | 2% | 3% | 7% |
|    OSCAR MAYER | | | | | |
| ❖   Ham & Cheese Loaf | 1 slc | 70 | 8% | 13% | 7% |
| ❖   Head Cheese | 1 slc | 50 | 6% | 8% | 8% |
| ★   Honey Loaf | 1 slc | 35 | 2% | 0% | 5% |
| ⊛   Liver Cheese, Pork Fat Wrapped | 1 slc | 120 | 15% | 20% | 27% |
| ❖   New England Brand Sausage | 2 slcs | 60 | 4% | 5% | 8% |
| ❖   Old Fashioned Loaf | 1 slc | 60 | 8% | 8% | 5% |
| ❖   Olive Loaf | 1 slc | 70 | 8% | 8% | 7% |
| ⊛   Pepperoni | 15 slcs | 140 | 20% | 25% | 8% |
| ❖   Pickle & Pimiento Loaf | 1 slc | 70 | 9% | 10% | 7% |
| ❖   Spiced Luncheon Loaf | 1 slc | 70 | 8% | 8% | 7% |
|    OSCAR MAYER Thuringer Cervelat | | | | | |
|    Summer Sausage | | | | | |
| ⊛   Beef | 2 slcs | 140 | 18% | 25% | 12% |
| ⊛   Pork | 2 slcs | 140 | 20% | 25% | 13% |
| ⊛ ROSA GRANDE Pepperoni— | | | | | |
|    HORMEL FOODS | 1 oz | 140 | 20% | 30% | 12% |

## MAYONNAISE

**Brand Name Foods**

| FOOD | Serving Size | Calories | Tot Fat | Sat Fat | Chol |
|---|---|---|---|---|---|
|    BEST FOODS Mayonnaises—CPC | | | | | |
| ❖   Light Reduced Calorie Dressing | 1 tbsp | 50 | 8% | 5% | 2% |
| ❖   Real | 1 tbsp | 100 | 17% | 10% | 2% |
| ★   Reduced Fat Cholesterol Free | | | | | |
|    Dressing | 1 tbsp | 40 | 5% | 5% | 0% |
| ❖   Sandwich Spread | 1 tbsp | 50 | 8% | 5% | 0% |
| ❖ FEATHERWEIGHT Soyamaise | | | | | |
|    Mayonnaise | 1 tbsp | 100 | 17% | 10% | 2% |
|    HAIN Mayonnaises | | | | | |
| ❖   Canola Mayonnaise | 1 tbsp | 110 | 18% | 4% | 1% |
| ❖   Safflower Mayonnaise | 1 tbsp | 110 | 18% | 6% | 2% |
| ❖ HEART BEAT Low Calorie | | | | | |
|    Mayonnaise—NUCOA | 1 tbsp | 40 | 6% | 5% | 0% |
|    HELLMAN'S Mayonnaises—CPC | | | | | |
| ❖   Light Reduced Calorie Dressing | 1 tbsp | 50 | 8% | 5% | 2% |
| ❖   Real | 1 tbsp | 100 | 17% | 10% | 2% |

| FOOD | Serving Size | Calories | Tot Fat | Sat Fat | Chol |
|------|------|------|------|------|------|
| ★ Reduced Fat Cholesterol Free Dressing | 1 tbsp | 40 | 5% | 5% | 0% |
| ❖ Sandwich Spread | 1 tbsp | 50 | 8% | 5% | 0% |
| HOLLYWOOD Mayonnaises— | | | | | |
| HAIN PURE FOODS | | | | | |
| ❖ Canola Mayonnaise | 1 tbsp | 110 | 18% | 4% | 1% |
| ❖ Safflower Mayonnaise | 1 tbsp | 110 | 18% | 6% | 2% |
| KRAFT Mayonnaises | | | | | |
| ❖ Real | 1 tbsp | 100 | 17% | 10% | 3% |
| ★ *Free* Dressing, Fat Free | 1 tbsp | 10 | 0% | 0% | 0% |
| ❖ *Light* Dressing | 1 tbsp | 50 | 8% | 5% | 0% |
| ❖ SAFFOLA Mayonnaise | 1 tbsp | 100 | 17% | 8% | 3% |
| WEIGHT WATCHERS Mayonnaises | | | | | |
| ★ Fat Free Dressing | 1 tbsp | 10 | 0% | 0% | 0% |
| ★ Fat Free Whipped Dressing | 1 tbsp | 15 | 0% | 0% | 0% |
| ★ Light | 1 tbsp | 25 | 3% | 0% | 2% |
| ★ Light (Low Sodium) | 1 tbsp | 25 | 3% | 5% | 2% |

### SANDWICH SPREADS

**Brand Name Foods**

| FOOD | Serving Size | Calories | Tot Fat | Sat Fat | Chol |
|------|------|------|------|------|------|
| ★ BEST FOODS *Dijonnaise* | 1 tsp | 10 | 1% | 0% | 0% |
| ❖ KRAFT Sandwich Spread & Burger Sauce | 1 tbsp | 50 | 8% | 3% | 2% |
| MIRACLE WHIP Dressing—KRAFT | | | | | |
| ★ *Free* Nonfat | 1 tbsp | 15 | 0% | 0% | 0% |
| ★ *Light* | 1 tbsp | 40 | 5% | 0% | 0% |
| HORMEL Spreads | | | | | |
| ❖ Deviled Ham | 4 tbsp | 150 | 18% | 20% | 13% |
| Ⓐ Liverwurst Spread | 4 tbsp | 130 | 15% | 18% | 23% |
| ❖ Potted Meat | 4 tbsp | 100 | 11% | 15% | 17% |
| LIBBY'S *Spreadables*—NESTLÉ | | | | | |
| ❖ Chicken | 1/3 cup | 140 | 14% | 9% | 8% |
| ❖ Ham | 1/3 cup | 110 | 7% | 5% | 7% |
| ❖ Tuna | 1/3 cup | 130 | 12% | 6% | 5% |
| ❖ Turkey | 1/3 cup | 150 | 15% | 9% | 8% |
| ❖ LOMA LINDA Sandwich Spread —WORTHINGTON FOODS | 1/4 cup | 80 | 7% | 5% | 0% |
| OSCAR MAYER Spreads | | | | | |
| Ⓐ Braunschweiger (Liver Sausage) | 2 oz | 190 | 26% | 30% | 30% |
| ❖ Sandwich Spread | 2 oz | 130 | 15% | 20% | 8% |
| UNDERWOOD Meat Spreads—PET | | | | | |
| ❖ Chunky Chicken | 1/4 cup | 120 | 13% | 12% | 13% |
| Ⓐ Deviled Ham | 1/4 cup | 160 | 21% | 24% | 15% |

★ Foods with this symbol have less than or equal to 5% *Daily Value* for all three nutrients (5% Rule).
❖ Foods with this symbol have at least one of the three nutrients greater than 5% *Daily Value* but less than or equal to 20% *Daily Value*.
Ⓐ Foods with this symbol have at least one of the three nutrients greater than 20% *Daily Value* (20% Rule).

| FOOD | Serving Size | Calories | Tot Fat | Sat Fat | Chol |
|------|------|------|------|------|------|
| ☻ Honey Ham | 1/4 cup | 180 | 24% | 28% | 15% |
| ☻ Liverwurst | 1/4 cup | 160 | 22% | 25% | 22% |
| ☻ Roast Beef | 1/4 cup | 130 | 17% | 22% | 15% |
| ☻ Sells Liver Pate | 1/4 cup | 160 | 22% | 25% | 22% |

**% DAILY VALUE**

## SANDWICHES

**Generic Foods**

| FOOD | Serving Size | Calories | Tot Fat | Sat Fat | Chol |
|------|------|------|------|------|------|
| ☻ Bacon, Lettuce, and Tomato Sandwich | 1 sandwich | 280 | 24% | 31% | 15% |
| ☻ Cheeseburger | 1 sandwich | 610 | 51% | 71% | 32% |
| ☻ Cheeseburger w/Bacon and Condiments | 1 sandwich | 610 | 57% | 81% | 37% |
| ☻ Ham and Cheese Sandwich | 1 sandwich | 350 | 24% | 32% | 19% |
| ☻ Hamburger w/Cheese | 1 sandwich | 320 | 23% | 32% | 17% |
| ☻ Hamburger w/Cheese, Bacon, and Condiments | 1 sandwich | 610 | 57% | 81% | 37% |
| ☻ Hamburger w/Cheese (large) | 1 sandwich | 610 | 51% | 71% | 32% |
| ☻ Hamburger w/Condiments (large) | 1 sandwich | 510 | 42% | 52% | 29% |
| ☻ Hamburger (large) | 1 sandwich | 430 | 35% | 42% | 24% |
| ☻ Hot Dog | 1 sandwich | 240 | 22% | 26% | 15% |
| ☻ Roast Beef Sandwich (plain) | 1 sandwich | 350 | 21% | 18% | 17% |
| ☻ Roast Beef Submarine Sandwich | 1 sandwich | 410 | 20% | 35% | 24% |
| ☻ Roast Beef w/Cheese Sandwich | 1 sandwich | 480 | 28% | 45% | 26% |
| ☻ Steak Sandwich | 1 sandwich | 460 | 22% | 19% | 24% |
| ☻ Submarine Sandwich w/Cold Cuts | 1 sandwich | 460 | 29% | 34% | 12% |
| ❖ Tuna Salad Sandwich | 1/2 cup | 260 | 16% | 8% | 4% |

**Brand Name Foods**

| FOOD | Serving Size | Calories | Tot Fat | Sat Fat | Chol |
|------|------|------|------|------|------|
| BANQUET Hot Sandwich Toppers —CONAGRA | | | | | |
| ❖ Chicken Ala King | 1 bag | 100 | 6% | 8% | 13% |
| ❖ Creamed Chipped Beef | 1 bag | 100 | 5% | 8% | 8% |
| ❖ Gravy & Sliced Beef | 1 bag | 70 | 3% | 5% | 8% |
| ❖ Gravy & Sliced Turkey | 1 bag | 90 | 6% | 8% | 10% |
| ☻ Salisbury Steak | 1 bag | 220 | 25% | 35% | 8% |
| ❖ Sloppy Joe | 1 bag | 140 | 11% | 15% | 8% |
| FANTASTIC FOODS | | | | | |
| ★ BBQ Nature Burger | 1 patty | 170 | 2% | 0% | 0% |
| ★ Nature Burger | 1 patty | 170 | 5% | 0% | 0% |
| ❖ Tofu Burger | 1 cup | 560 | 18% | 0% | 0% |
| ☻ MRS. PAUL'S Fish Fillet Sandwich w/Cheese—CAMPBELL'S | 1 sandwich | 330 | 23% | 20% | 8% |
| OSCAR MAYER *Lunchables* Lunch Combinations, Deluxe | | | | | |
| ☻ Chicken/Turkey | 1 pkg | 390 | 35% | 60% | 23% |
| ☻ Turkey/Ham | 1 pkg | 370 | 32% | 50% | 22% |

| FOOD | Serving Size | Calories | Tot Fat | Sat Fat | Chol |
|---|---|---|---|---|---|
| OSCAR MAYER *Lunchables* Lunch Combinations, Fun Pack | | | | | |
| ⊛ Bologna/Wild Cherry | 1 pkg | 530 | 43% | 65% | 20% |
| ⊛ Ham/Fruit Punch | 1 pkg | 440 | 31% | 45% | 17% |
| ⊛ Pizza w/Mozzarella/Fruit Punch | 1 pkg | 480 | 26% | 50% | 12% |
| ⊛ Pizza w/Pepperoni/Orange | 1 pkg | 480 | 26% | 40% | 12% |
| ⊛ Turkey/Pacific Cooler | 1 pkg | 450 | 31% | 50% | 17% |
| ⊛ Turkey/Surfer Cooler | 1 pkg | 430 | 23% | 40% | 15% |
| OSCAR MAYER *Lunchables* Lunch Combinations, Low Fat | | | | | |
| ⊛ Ham/Fruit Punch | 1 pkg | 360 | 15% | 23% | 0% |
| ⊛ Ham/Surfer Cooler | 1 pkg | 380 | 15% | 23% | 12% |
| ❖ Turkey/Pacific Cooler | 1 pkg | 360 | 14% | 20% | 10% |
| OSCAR MAYER *Lunchables* Lunch Combinations, Regular | | | | | |
| ⊛ Bologna/American | 1 pkg | 470 | 54% | 80% | 28% |
| ⊛ Ham/Cheddar | 1 pkg | 360 | 32% | 55% | 25% |
| ⊛ Ham/Swiss | 1 pkg | 340 | 31% | 50% | 23% |
| ⊛ Pizza w/Mozzarella/Cheddar | 1 pkg | 330 | 22% | 40% | 12% |
| ⊛ Pizza w/Pepperoni/Mozzarella | 1 pkg | 330 | 23% | 35% | 12% |
| ⊛ Salami/American | 1 pkg | 420 | 45% | 70% | 27% |
| ⊛ Turkey/Cheddar | 1 pkg | 350 | 31% | 55% | 23% |
| ⊛ Turkey/Monterey Jack | 1 pkg | 350 | 32% | 55% | 25% |
| QUICK MEAL Sandwiches— HORMEL FOODS | | | | | |
| ⊛ Bacon/Cheeseburger | 1 sandwich | 440 | 35% | 50% | 30% |
| ⊛ BBQ Beef Sandwich | 1 sandwich | 360 | 25% | 30% | 18% |
| ⊛ BBQ Pork Sandwich | 1 sandwich | 350 | 23% | 30% | 20% |
| ⊛ Beef Burrito | 1 sandwich | 300 | 20% | 30% | 13% |
| ❖ Cheese Burrito | 1 sandwich | 250 | 9% | 10% | 10% |
| ⊛ Cheeseburger | 1 sandwich | 400 | 31% | 45% | 27% |
| ⊛ Cheesey Dog | 1 dog | 310 | 26% | 25% | 15% |
| ❖ Chicken Sandwich | 1 sandwich | 340 | 18% | 15% | 20% |
| ⊛ Chili Cheeseburger | 1 sandwich | 450 | 35% | 50% | 28% |
| ⊛ Chili Dog w/Cheese | 1 dog | 350 | 31% | 35% | 20% |
| ❖ Corn Dog | 1 sandwich | 220 | 17% | 15% | 15% |
| ⊛ Fish Fillet Sandwich | 1 sandwich | 400 | 25% | 20% | 25% |
| ❖ Grilled Chicken Sandwich | 1 sandwich | 300 | 14% | 15% | 20% |
| ⊛ Hamburger | 1 sandwich | 350 | 23% | 30% | 22% |
| ⊛ Jumbo Dog | 1 dog | 350 | 32% | 35% | 18% |
| ⊛ Mini Corn Dog | 1 sandwich | 250 | 23% | 25% | 17% |
| ⊛ Pepperoni Bagel | 1 sandwich | 350 | 23% | 30% | 15% |
| ⊛ Red Chili Burrito | 1 sandwich | 280 | 17% | 23% | 12% |

★ Foods with this symbol have less than or equal to 5% *Daily Value* for <u>all</u> three nutrients (5% Rule).

❖ Foods with this symbol have <u>at least one</u> of the three nutrients greater than 5% *Daily Value* but less than or equal to 20% *Daily Value*.

⊛ Foods with this symbol have <u>at least one</u> of the three nutrients greater than 20% *Daily Value* (20% Rule).

| FOOD | Serving Size | Calories | Tot Fat | Sat Fat | Chol |
|------|-------------|----------|---------|---------|------|
| **SANDWICHES ON-THE-GO!—** | | | | | |
| WEIGHT WATCHERS | | | | | |
| ❖ Chicken, Broccoli & Cheddar Pocket | 1 sandwich | 250 | 9% | 13% | 8% |
| ❖ Deluxe Pizza Pocket | 1 sandwich | 300 | 11% | 13% | 5% |
| ❖ Grilled Chicken | 1 sandwich | 210 | 8% | 10% | 7% |
| ❖ Ham & Cheese Pocket | 1 sandwich | 240 | 11% | 13% | 3% |
| ❖ Hickory Smoked Ham & Cheddar Pretzel | 1 sandwich | 260 | 12% | 15% | 3% |
| ❖ Honey Dijon Turkey Pretzel | 1 sandwich | 230 | 6% | 8% | 8% |
| ❖ Reuben Pocket | 1 sandwich | 250 | 9% | 10% | 7% |
| SARA LEE Croissants | | | | | |
| ❖ Chicken & Broccoli | 1 croissant | 280 | 20% | 18% | 10% |
| Ⓐ Ham & Swiss | 1 croissant | 300 | 25% | 23% | 15% |
| ❖ Original | 1 croissant | 170 | 12% | 15% | 1% |

# Snack Foods

## CHIPS AND PUFFS

### Corn Chips

### Generic Foods

| FOOD | Serving Size | Calories | Tot Fat | Sat Fat | Chol |
|------|-------------|----------|---------|---------|------|
| Corn Chips | | | | | |
| ❖ Barbecue Chips | 1 oz | 150 | 14% | 6% | 0% |
| ❖ Plain Chips | 1 oz | 160 | 14% | 8% | 0% |
| Corn Chip Cones | | | | | |
| Ⓐ Nacho Cheese | 1 oz | 150 | 14% | 38% | 0% |
| Ⓐ Plain | 1 oz | 150 | 12% | 32% | 0% |

### Brand Name Foods

| FOOD | Serving Size | Calories | Tot Fat | Sat Fat | Chol |
|------|-------------|----------|---------|---------|------|
| BARBARA'S BAKERY *Amazing Bakes* | | | | | |
| ★ Blue Corn | 24 chips | 100 | 2% | 0% | 0% |
| ★ Light Salt | 24 chips | 100 | 2% | 0% | 0% |
| ★ Pesto | 24 chips | 100 | 2% | 0% | 0% |
| ★ Quinoa | 24 chips | 100 | 2% | 0% | 0% |
| ❖ BARBARA'S BAKERY Blue Corn Corn Chips: Regular and No Salt Added | 15 chips | 140 | 11% | 4% | 0% |
| BUGLES—GENERAL MILLS | | | | | |
| ★ Nacho | 1 1/3 cups | 160 | 14% | 35% | 0% |
| Ⓐ Original | 1 1/3 cups | 160 | 14% | 41% | 0% |
| Ⓐ Ranch | 1 1/3 cups | 160 | 14% | 39% | 0% |
| Ⓐ Sour Cream & Onion | 1 1/3 cups | 160 | 14% | 39% | 0% |

| FOOD | Serving Size | Calories | Tot Fat | Sat Fat | Chol |
|---|---|---|---|---|---|
| Crisp Baked BUGLES—GENERAL MILLS | | | | | |
| ★ BBQ | 1 1/2 cups | 130 | 4% | 3% | 0% |
| ★ Cheddar Cheese | 1 1/2 cups | 130 | 5% | 3% | 0% |
| ★ Original | 1 1/2 cups | 130 | 4% | 3% | 0% |
| ❖ FEATHERWEIGHT Corn Chips | 1 oz (3/4 cup) | 150 | 12% | 10% | 0% |
| FRITOS Corn Chips—FRITO-LAY | | | | | |
| ❖ BBQ | 1 oz (~ 32 chips) | 160 | 15% | 8% | 0% |
| ❖ Plain | 1 oz (~ 32 chips) | 160 | 15% | 8% | 0% |

**Potato Chips**

**Generic Foods**

| | | | | | |
|---|---|---|---|---|---|
| ❖ Barbecue Flavor | 1 oz | 140 | 14% | 11% | 0% |
| ❖ Cheese Flavor | 1 oz | 140 | 12% | 12% | 0% |
| ❖ Light Potato Chips | 1 oz | 130 | 9% | 6% | 0% |
| ❖ Plain | 1 oz | 150 | 15% | 16% | 0% |
| ❖ Sour Cream and Chives | 1 oz | 150 | 15% | 13% | 1% |

**Brand Name Foods**

| | | | | | |
|---|---|---|---|---|---|
| BAKED LAY'S—FRITO-LAY | | | | | |
| ★ BBQ | 1 oz (~ 11 chips) | 110 | 2% | 0% | 0% |
| ★ Original | 1 oz (~ 11 chips) | 110 | 2% | 0% | 0% |
| BARBARA'S BAKERY Potato Chips | | | | | |
| ❖ Au Gratin | 1 cup | 150 | 15% | 8% | 0% |
| ❖ Barbeque | 1 1/4 cups | 160 | 15% | 5% | 0% |
| ❖ Regular or No Salt | 1 1/4 cups | 150 | 15% | 5% | 0% |
| ❖ Ripple | 1 1/4 cups | 150 | 15% | 5% | 0% |
| ❖ Sweet Potato | 1 cup | 140 | 12% | 5% | 0% |
| ❖ Yogurt & Green Onion | 1 1/4 cups | 150 | 14% | 5% | 0% |
| CAPE COD Potato Chips—ANHEUSER BUSCH | | | | | |
| ❖ Regular | 1 oz (19 chips) | 150 | 12% | 10% | 0% |
| ❖ Sea Salt & Vinegar | 1 oz (18 chips) | 150 | 12% | 10% | 0% |

★ Foods with this symbol have less than or equal to 5% *Daily Value* for all three nutrients (5% Rule).
❖ Foods with this symbol have at least one of the three nutrients greater than 5% *Daily Value* but less than or equal to 20% *Daily Value*.
Ⓐ Foods with this symbol have at least one of the three nutrients greater than 20% *Daily Value* (20% Rule).

| FOOD | Serving Size | Calories | Tot Fat | Sat Fat | Chol |
|------|------|------|------|------|------|
| **EAGLE Potato Chips**—ANHEUSER BUSCH | | | | | |
| ❖ Hawaiian Kettle, Extra Crunchy | 1 oz (19 chips) | 150 | 12% | 10% | 0% |
| ❖ Idaho Russet, Dark & Crunchy | 1 oz (22 chips) | 140 | 11% | 8% | 0% |
| **EAGLE *Ripples* Potato Chips**—ANHEUSER BUSCH | | | | | |
| ❖ Cheddar & Sour Cream, Crispy Cooked | 1 oz (16 chips) | 160 | 17% | 5% | 0% |
| ❖ Mesquite BBQ | 1 oz (19 chips) | 160 | 15% | 10% | 0% |
| ❖ Natural | 1 oz (17 chips) | 150 | 15% | 13% | 0% |
| ❖ Sea Salt & Vinegar, Crispy Cooked | 1 oz (16 chips) | 150 | 12% | 10% | 0% |
| ❖ Sour Cream & Onion | 1 oz (16 chips) | 160 | 15% | 10% | 1% |
| **EAGLE *Thins* Potato Chips**—ANHEUSER BUSCH | | | | | |
| ❖ Crispy Cooked | 1 oz (19 chips) | 150 | 12% | 10% | 0% |
| ❖ Louisiana Spicy Hot, Crispy Cooked | 1 oz (18 chips) | 150 | 12% | 10% | 0% |
| ❖ Mesquite BBQ | 1 oz (19 chips) | 160 | 15% | 10% | 0% |
| ❖ Sour Cream & Onion | 1 oz (19 chips) | 160 | 15% | 10% | 1% |
| ❖ Spicy Fiesta | 1 oz (19 chips) | 160 | 14% | 13% | 0% |
| ❖ *Thins* | 1 oz (20 chips) | 150 | 15% | 13% | 0% |
| **LAY'S Potato Chips**—FRITO-LAY | | | | | |
| ❖ BBQ | 1 oz (~ 20 chips) | 150 | 16% | 10% | 0% |
| ❖ Plain Potato Chips | 1 oz (~ 20 chips) | 150 | 16% | 14% | 0% |
| ❖ Salt & Vinegar | 1 oz (~ 20 chips) | 150 | 16% | 14% | 0% |
| ❖ Sour Cream & Onion | 1 oz (~ 20 chips) | 150 | 16% | 14% | 0% |
| ❖ Tangy Ranch | 1 oz (~ 20 chips) | 150 | 16% | 14% | 0% |
| **LOUISE'S 70% Less Fat Potato Chips** | | | | | |
| ★ Mesquite BBQ | 1 oz | 110 | 4% | 0% | 0% |
| ★ Original | 1 oz | 110 | 4% | 0% | 0% |

| FOOD | Serving Size | Calories | Tot Fat | Sat Fat | Chol |
|------|--------------|----------|---------|---------|------|
| **LOUISE'S FAT-FREE Potato Chips** | | | | | |
| ★ Maui Onion | 1 oz | 110 | 0% | 0% | 0% |
| ★ Mesquite BBQ | 1 oz | 110 | 0% | 0% | 0% |
| ★ No Salt | 1 oz | 110 | 0% | 0% | 0% |
| ★ Original | 1 oz | 110 | 0% | 0% | 0% |
| ★ Vinegar & Salt | 1 oz | 110 | 0% | 0% | 0% |
| **O'BOISIES Potato Snack Chips—** KEEBLER | | | | | |
| ❖ Artificially Flavored Sour Cream & Onion | 1 oz (~ 15 chips) | 150 | 14% | 10% | 0% |
| ❖ Cheddar Flavor | 1 oz (~ 16 chips) | 150 | 15% | 10% | 0% |
| ❖ Original | 1 oz (~ 16 chips) | 150 | 14% | 10% | 0% |
| **POPSTERS**—AMERICAN GRAINS | | | | | |
| ★ Herb & Garlic | 30 g (~ 30 chips) | 110 | 3% | 0% | 0% |
| ★ Original | 30 g (~ 30 chips) | 110 | 3% | 0% | 0% |
| ★ Salt 'n Vinegar | 30 g (~ 30 chips) | 110 | 3% | 0% | 0% |
| **PRINGLES Potato Crisps**—PROCTER & GAMBLE | | | | | |
| ❖ Cheez Ums | 1 oz (~ 14 crisps) | 150 | 15% | 13% | 0% |
| ❖ Original | 1 oz (~ 14 crisps) | 160 | 16% | 14% | 0% |
| ❖ Ranch Flavor | 1 oz (~ 14 crisps) | 150 | 15% | 13% | 0% |
| ❖ Sour Cream 'n Onion | 1 oz (~ 14 crisps) | 160 | 16% | 14% | 0% |
| **PRINGLES Ridges Potato Crisps—** PROCTER & GAMBLE | | | | | |
| ❖ BBQ Flavor | 1 oz (~ 12 crisps) | 150 | 17% | 14% | 0% |
| ❖ Cheddar 'n Sour Cream | 1 oz (~ 12 crisps) | 150 | 17% | 14% | 0% |
| ❖ Original | 1 oz (~ 12 crisps) | 150 | 17% | 14% | 0% |
| **PRINGLES Right Crisp Potato Crisps**—PROCTER & GAMBLE | | | | | |
| ❖ BBQ Flavor | 1 oz (~ 16 crisps) | 140 | 11% | 10% | 0% |

★ Foods with this symbol have less than or equal to 5% *Daily Value* for <u>all</u> three nutrients (5% Rule).

❖ Foods with this symbol have <u>at least one</u> of the three nutrients greater than 5% *Daily Value* but less than or equal to 20% *Daily Value*.

Ⓐ Foods with this symbol have <u>at least one</u> of the three nutrients greater than 20% *Daily Value* (20% Rule).

| FOOD | Serving Size | Calories | Tot Fat | Sat Fat | Chol |
|---|---|---|---|---|---|
| ❖ Original | 1 oz (~ 16 crisps) | 140 | 11% | 10% | 0% |
| ❖ Sour Cream 'n Onion | 1 oz (~ 16 crisps) | 140 | 11% | 10% | 0% |
| RIPPLIN'S Potato Snack Chips— KEEBLER | | | | | |
| ❖ Barbecue Flavor | 12 chips | 150 | 14% | 10% | 0% |
| ❖ Original Flavor | 13 chips | 160 | 17% | 10% | 0% |
| ❖ Ranch Flavor | 12 chips | 150 | 14% | 10% | 0% |
| RUFFLES Potato Chips—FRITO-LAY | | | | | |
| ❖ Cheddar & Sour Cream | 1 oz (17 chips) | 160 | 16% | 15% | 0% |
| ❖ Mesquite Grill BBQ | 1 oz (17 chips) | 150 | 14% | 15% | 0% |
| ❖ Plain | 1 oz (17 chips) | 160 | 16% | 15% | 0% |
| ❖ Ranch | 1 oz (17 chips) | 150 | 14% | 15% | 0% |
| ❖ Reduced Fat | 1 oz (~ 16 chips) | 130 | 10% | 4% | 0% |
| TATO SKINS Potato Snack Chips —KEEBLER | | | | | |
| ❖ Artificially Flavored Sour Cream 'n Onion | 18 chips | 150 | 15% | 8% | 0% |
| ❖ Baked Potato Flavor | 18 chips | 150 | 12% | 8% | 0% |
| ❖ Cheese 'n Bacon | 18 chips | 150 | 14% | 8% | 0% |
| TATO WILDS Tato Skins—KEEBLER | | | | | |
| ❖ Cheese 'n Bacon | 1 oz (18 chips) | 150 | 14% | 8% | 0% |
| ❖ Original Baked Potato | 1 oz (18 chips) | 150 | 12% | 8% | 0% |
| ❖ Sour Cream & Onion | 1 oz (18 chips) | 150 | 15% | 8% | 0% |
| WAVY LAY'S Potato Chips— FRITO-LAY | | | | | |
| ❖ Au Gratin | 1 oz (~ 20 chips) | 150 | 16% | 14% | 0% |
| ❖ Plain | 1 oz (~ 20 chips) | 150 | 16% | 14% | 0% |
| ❖ Sour Cream & Onion | 1 oz (~ 20 chips) | 150 | 16% | 14% | 0% |

*Puffs*

**Brand Name Foods**

| BARBARA'S BAKERY Cheese Puffs | | | | | |
|---|---|---|---|---|---|
| ❖ Cheese Puff Bakes | 1 1/2 cups (~ 36 puffs) | 160 | 17% | 10% | 0% |
| ❖ Jalapeno | 3/4 cup | 150 | 14% | 8% | 0% |

| FOOD | Serving Size | Calories | Tot Fat | Sat Fat | Chol |
|------|------|------|------|------|------|
| ❖ Original | 3/4 cup | 150 | 15% | 8% | 0% |
| ❖ Amazin' Cajun Cheddar | 1 oz | | | | |
| | (~ 23 pcs) | 150 | 15% | 11% | 0% |
| CHEE-TOS Cheese Flavored Snacks—FRITO-LAY | | | | | |
| ❖ Crunchy | 1 oz | | | | |
| | (~ 21 pcs) | 150 | 14% | 11% | 0% |
| ❖ Puffs | 1 oz | | | | |
| | (~ 29 pcs) | 160 | 16% | 12% | 0% |
| EAGLE *Cheegles*—ANHEUSER BUSCH | | | | | |
| ❖ Cheese Ball | 2 1/2 cups | 160 | 15% | 10% | 0% |
| ❖ Cheese Ball, Reduced Fat | 2 1/2 cups | 150 | 9% | 8% | 0% |
| ❖ Cheese Crunch | 1 cup | 160 | 15% | 10% | 0% |
| ❖ FEATHERWEIGHT Cheese Curls | 1 oz | | | | |
| | (2 cups) | 140 | 11% | 10% | 0% |
| HEALTH VALLEY Fat Free Puffs | | | | | |
| ★ Apple Cinnamon Caramel Corn | 1 cup | 110 | 0% | 0% | 0% |
| ★ Cheese Flavor w/Chili | 1 1/2 cups | 110 | 0% | 0% | 0% |
| ★ Cheese Flavor w/Green Onion | 1 1/2 cups | 110 | 0% | 0% | 0% |
| ★ Original Cheese Flavor | 1 1/2 cups | 110 | 0% | 0% | 0% |
| ★ Original Style Caramel Corn | 1 cup | 110 | 0% | 0% | 0% |
| QRUNCH 'UMS—QUAKER | | | | | |
| ★ Butter Popped Corn | 1 oz | | | | |
| | (46 pcs) | 100 | 0% | 0% | 0% |
| ★ Caramel Corn | 1 oz | | | | |
| | (31 pcs) | 100 | 0% | 0% | 0% |
| ★ Cinnamon Cookie | 1 oz | | | | |
| | (21 pcs) | 100 | 0% | 0% | 0% |
| RICE BITES—AMERICAN GRAINS | | | | | |
| ❖ Butter Popcorn | 30 g | | | | |
| | (~ 50 bites) | 140 | 9% | 5% | 0% |
| ❖ Exotic Pepper Cheese | 30 g | | | | |
| | (~ 50 bites) | 140 | 9% | 5% | 0% |
| ❖ Herb & Garlic | 30 g | | | | |
| | (~ 50 bites) | 140 | 9% | 5% | 0% |
| ❖ White Cheddar | 30 g | | | | |
| | (~ 50 bites) | 140 | 9% | 5% | 0% |
| SMART SNACKERS Curls— WEIGHT WATCHERS | | | | | |
| ★ Barbecue Flavored | 1 bag | 60 | 2% | 0% | 0% |
| ★ Cheese | 1 bag | 70 | 4% | 5% | 0% |
| ★ Pizza Flavored | 1 bag | 60 | 3% | 0% | 0% |
| ★ Ranch Flavored | 1 bag | 60 | 3% | 0% | 0% |

★ Foods with this symbol have less than or equal to 5% *Daily Value* for <u>all</u> three nutrients (5% Rule).
❖ Foods with this symbol have <u>at least one</u> of the three nutrients greater than 5% *Daily Value* but less than or equal to 20% *Daily Value*.
🅐 Foods with this symbol have <u>at least one</u> of the three nutrients greater than 20% *Daily Value* (20% Rule).

| FOOD | Serving Size | Calories | Tot Fat | Sat Fat | Chol |
|------|--------------|----------|---------|---------|------|
| ★ ULTRA SLIM-FAST Cheese Curls | 1 oz (~ 28 curls) | 120 | 5% | 3% | 0% |

### Tortilla Chips
### Generic Foods

| FOOD | Serving Size | Calories | Tot Fat | Sat Fat | Chol |
|------|--------------|----------|---------|---------|------|
| ❖ Nacho Cheese Flavored | 1 oz | 140 | 11% | 7% | 0% |
| ❖ Nacho Cheese Flavored, Light | 1 oz | 130 | 7% | 4% | 0% |
| ❖ Plain | 1 oz | 140 | 11% | 7% | 0% |
| ❖ Ranch Flavor | 1 oz | 140 | 10% | 6% | 0% |
| ❖ Taco Flavor | 1 oz | 140 | 11% | 7% | 0% |

### Brand Name Foods

| FOOD | Serving Size | Calories | Tot Fat | Sat Fat | Chol |
|------|--------------|----------|---------|---------|------|
| BAKED TOSTITOS Tortilla Chips —FRITO-LAY | | | | | |
| ★ Cool Ranch | 1 oz (~ 11 chips) | 120 | 5% | 2% | 0% |
| ★ Regular | 1 oz (~ 13 chips) | 110 | 1% | 0% | 0% |
| ❖ BARBARA'S BAKERY Organic Yellow Corn Tortilla Chips, Regular or No Salt Added | 14 chips | 120 | 9% | 5% | 0% |
| BEARITOS Baked Tortilla Chips (Salted or Unsalted)—LITTLE BEAR ORGANIC FOODS | | | | | |
| ★ Blue | 1 oz (~ 21 chips) | 110 | 2% | 0% | 0% |
| ★ White | 1 oz (~ 21 chips) | 110 | 2% | 0% | 0% |
| ★ Yellow | 1 oz (~ 21 chips) | 110 | 2% | 0% | 0% |
| BEARITOS Tortilla Chips (Salted or Unsalted)—LITTLE BEAR ORGANIC FOODS | 1 oz (~ 15 chips) | 140 | 11% | 5% | 0% |
| ❖ Blue Corn | 1 oz (~ 15 chips) | 140 | 11% | 5% | 0% |
| ❖ Yellow Corn | 1 oz (~ 15 chips) | 140 | 11% | 5% | 0% |
| CHACHO'S Flour Tortilla Chips —KEEBLER | | | | | |
| ❖ Cheesy Quesadilla | 14 chips | 150 | 12% | 8% | 1% |
| ❖ Cinnamon Crispana | 13 chips | 150 | 11% | 5% | 0% |
| ❖ Restaurant Style Original | 15 chips | 150 | 12% | 5% | 0% |
| DORITOS Tortilla Chips—FRITO-LAY | | | | | |
| ❖ Cool Ranch | 1 oz (~ 11 chips) | 140 | 11% | 6% | 0% |

| FOOD | Serving Size | Calories | Tot Fat | Sat Fat | Chol |
|---|---|---|---|---|---|
| ❖ Nacho Cheese | 1 oz (~ 11 chips) | 140 | 11% | 6% | 0% |
| EAGLE *Restaurant Style* Tortilla Chips—ANHEUSER BUSCH | | | | | |
| ❖ Chips | 1 oz (13 chips) | 140 | 9% | 3% | 0% |
| ❖ *El Grande* Rounds | 1 oz (9 chips) | 140 | 9% | 5% | 0% |
| ❖ Nacho Thins | 1 oz (12 chips) | 150 | 11% | 5% | 0% |
| ❖ Ranch Thins | 1 oz (12 chips) | 150 | 11% | 5% | 0% |
| ❖ Rounds | 1 oz (11 chips) | 140 | 9% | 3% | 0% |
| ❖ Strips | 1 oz (13 chips) | 140 | 9% | 3% | 0% |
| ❖ Yellow | 1 oz (13 chips) | 140 | 11% | 5% | 0% |
| GUILTLESS GOURMET *Baked Not Fried Tortilla Chips* | 1 oz (~ 22 chips) | 110 | 1% | 0% | 0% |
| ★ Nacho | 4 oz (~ 22 chips) | 110 | 1% | 0% | 0% |
| ★ Original Style | 2 oz (~ 22 chips) | 110 | 1% | 0% | 0% |
| ★ White Corn | 3 oz (~ 22 chips) | 110 | 1% | 0% | 0% |
| OLD EL PASO Tortilla Chips—PET | | | | | |
| ❖ White Corn | 11 chips | 140 | 12% | 5% | 0% |
| ❖ *Nachips* | 9 chips | 150 | 12% | 7% | 0% |
| ❖ TOSTITOS Restaurant Style Tortilla Chips—FRITO-LAY | 1 oz (~ 6 chips) | 130 | 9% | 5% | 0% |

### Other Chips
### Brand Name Foods

| FOOD | Serving Size | Calories | Tot Fat | Sat Fat | Chol |
|---|---|---|---|---|---|
| ❖ BARBARA'S BAKERY *Ray's* Taro Chips | 1 cup | 120 | 9% | 4% | 0% |
| BARBARA'S BAKERY Pinta Blues | | | | | |
| ❖ Picante | 13 chips | 130 | 11% | 8% | 0% |
| ❖ Regular | 14 chips | 130 | 11% | 8% | 0% |

★ Foods with this symbol have less than or equal to 5% *Daily Value* for all three nutrients (5% Rule).
❖ Foods with this symbol have at least one of the three nutrients greater than 5% *Daily Value* but less than or equal to 20% *Daily Value*.
Ⓐ Foods with this symbol have at least one of the three nutrients greater than 20% *Daily Value* (20% Rule).

| FOOD | Serving Size | Calories | Tot Fat | Sat Fat | Chol |
|------|------|------|------|------|------|
| BARBARA'S BAKERY Pinta Chips | | | | | |
| ❖ Nacho | 12 chips | 130 | 9% | 5% | 0% |
| ❖ Regular | 13 chips | 130 | 9% | 8% | 0% |
| ❖ Salsa | 12 chips | 130 | 9% | 5% | 0% |
| PIZZARIAS Pizza Chips—KEEBLER | | | | | |
| ❖ Cheese Pizza Flavor | 14 chips | 150 | 11% | 8% | 1% |
| ❖ Pizza Supreme Flavor | 14 chips | 150 | 11% | 8% | 0% |
| ❖ Zesty Pepperoni Flavor | 14 chips | 150 | 11% | 8% | 1% |
| SUNCHIPS—FRITO-LAY | | | | | |
| ❖ French Onion Multi-Grain | 1 oz (~ 10 chips) | 140 | 10% | 4% | 0% |
| ❖ Original Multi-Grain | 1 oz (~ 11 chips) | 140 | 9% | 4% | 0% |

## DIPS

### Bean

**Brand Name Foods**

| FOOD | Serving Size | Calories | Tot Fat | Sat Fat | Chol |
|------|------|------|------|------|------|
| BEARITOS Fat Free Bean Dips— LITTLE BEAR ORGANIC FOODS | | | | | |
| ★ Black Bean | 2 tbsp | 25 | 0% | 0% | 0% |
| ★ Vegetarian Bean | 2 tbsp | 25 | 0% | 0% | 0% |
| EAGLE Bean Dips—ANHEUSER BUSCH | | | | | |
| ★ Black Bean | 2 tbsp | 35 | 2% | 0% | 0% |
| ★ Mild Bean | 2 tbsp | 40 | 2% | 0% | 0% |
| ★ FRITO-LAY Bean Dip | 2 tbsp | 40 | 2% | 2% | 0% |
| GUILTLESS GOURMET Spicy Bean Dips | 2 tbsp | 30 | 0% | 0% | 0% |
| ★ BBQ Black Bean | 2 tbsp | 35 | 0% | 0% | 0% |
| ★ BBQ Pinto Bean | 2 tbsp | 40 | 0% | 0% | 0% |
| ★ Black Bean | 2 tbsp | 30 | 0% | 0% | 0% |
| ★ Pinto Bean | 2 tbsp | 35 | 0% | 0% | 0% |
| KNORR Bean Dip Mixes | | | | | |
| ★ Black Bean | 1/16 pkg | 10 | 0% | 0% | 0% |
| ★ Mexican Bean | 1/16 pkg | 10 | 0% | 0% | 0% |
| Ⓐ MARIE'S Fiesta Bean—CAMPBELL'S | 2 tbsp | 140 | 22% | 10% | 3% |
| ★ OLD EL PASO Black Bean | 2 tbsp | 20 | 0% | 0% | 0% |
| ★ TOSTITOS Black Bean—FRITO-LAY | 2 tbsp | 25 | 0% | 0% | 0% |

### Salsa

**Brand Name Foods**

| FOOD | Serving Size | Calories | Tot Fat | Sat Fat | Chol |
|------|------|------|------|------|------|
| BEARITOS Salsas—LITTLE BEAR ORGANIC FOODS | | | | | |
| ★ Mild | 2 tbsp | 10 | 0% | 0% | 0% |
| ★ Spicy | 2 tbsp | 10 | 0% | 0% | 0% |

| FOOD | Serving Size | Calories | Tot Fat | Sat Fat | Chol |
|---|---|---|---|---|---|
| ★ Tomatillo | 2 tbsp | 8 | 0% | 0% | 0% |
| DEL MONTE Salsas | | | | | |
| ★ Mexicana | 2 tbsp | 5 | 0% | 0% | 0% |
| ★ Taquera | 2 tbsp | 5 | 0% | 0% | 0% |
| ★ Verde | 2 tbsp | 10 | 0% | 0% | 0% |
| EAGLE Salsa Dips—ANHEUSER BUSCH | | | | | |
| ★ Medium | 2 tbsp | 10 | 0% | 0% | 0% |
| ★ Medium Cheese | 2 tbsp | 40 | 5% | 5% | 1% |
| ★ Mild | 2 tbsp | 10 | 0% | 0% | 0% |
| ★ FRITO-LAY Chunky Salsa: Mild— FRITO-LAY | 2 tbsp | 15 | 0% | 0% | 0% |
| ★ GUILTLESS GOURMET Salsa, Medium | 2 tbsp | 10 | 0% | 0% | 0% |
| HUNT'S Homestyle Salsa— HUNT WESSON | | | | | |
| ★ Alfresco Salsa: Mild or Medium | 2 tbsp | 10 | 0% | 0% | 0% |
| ★ Salsa: Mild, Medium, or Hot | 2 tbsp | 25 | 0% | 0% | 0% |
| LA VICTORIA Salsa | | | | | |
| ★ Brava | 1 tsp | 0 | 0% | 0% | 0% |
| ★ Green Chili | 2 tbsp | 10 | 0% | 0% | 0% |
| ★ Picante: Mild or Medium | 2 tbsp | 10 | 0% | 0% | 0% |
| ★ Ranchera | 2 tbsp | 10 | 0% | 0% | 0% |
| ★ Red or Green Jalapeno | 2 tbsp | 10 | 0% | 0% | 0% |
| ★ Suprema | 2 tbsp | 5 | 0% | 0% | 0% |
| ★ Suprema Mild | 2 tbsp | 10 | 0% | 0% | 0% |
| ★ Thick & Chunky: Mild, Medium, or Hot | 2 tbsp | 10 | 0% | 0% | 0% |
| ★ Victoria | 2 tbsp | 5 | 0% | 0% | 0% |
| ★ LAS PALMAS Salsa Mexicana: Mild, Medium, or Hot—PET | 2 tbsp | 10 | 0% | 0% | 0% |
| ★ NEWMAN'S OWN *Bandito* Salsa, Mild, Medium, or Hot | 2 tbsp | 10 | 0% | 0% | 0% |
| OLD EL PASO Dips | | | | | |
| ★ Cheese 'n Salsa: Mild or Medium | 2 tbsp | 40 | 5% | 5% | 1% |
| ★ Chunky Salsa: Mild or Medium | 2 tbsp | 15 | 0% | 0% | 0% |
| ★ Jalapeno | 2 tbsp | 30 | 1% | 0% | 1% |
| OLD EL PASO Salsa—PET | | | | | |
| ★ Green Chili: Medium | 2 tbsp | 10 | 0% | 0% | 0% |
| ★ Homestyle: Mild or Medium | 2 tbsp | 5 | 0% | 0% | 0% |
| ★ Picante: Mild, Medium, or Hot | 2 tbsp | 10 | 0% | 0% | 0% |
| ★ Pico de Gallo: Medium or Hot | 2 tbsp | 5 | 0% | 0% | 0% |
| ★ Thick 'n Chunky: Mild, Medium, or Hot | 2 tbsp | 10 | 0% | 0% | 0% |
| ★ Thick 'n Chunky Picante: Mild, Medium, or Hot | 2 tbsp | 10 | 0% | 0% | 0% |

★ Foods with this symbol have less than or equal to 5% *Daily Value* for <u>all</u> three nutrients (5% Rule).

❖ Foods with this symbol have <u>at least one</u> of the three nutrients greater than 5% *Daily Value* but less than or equal to 20% *Daily Value*.

Ⓐ Foods with this symbol have <u>at least one</u> of the three nutrients greater than 20% *Daily Value* (20% Rule).

| FOOD | Serving Size | Calories | Tot Fat | Sat Fat | Chol |
|---|---|---|---|---|---|
| ★    Verde: Medium | 2 tbsp | 10 | 0% | 0% | 0% |
| ★ PACE Thick & Chunky Salsa | 2 tbsp | 10 | 0% | 0% | 0% |
| ★ PROGRESSO Italian Salsa: Mild, Medium, or Hot—PET | 2 tbsp | 10 | 0% | 0% | 0% |
| ROSARITA Salsa—HUNT WESSON | | | | | |
| ★    Extra Chunky: Medium | 2 tbsp | 5 | 0% | 0% | 0% |
| ★    Green Tomatillo: Medium | 2 tbsp | 10 | 0% | 0% | 0% |
| ★    Roasted: Mild | 2 tbsp | 10 | 1% | 0% | 0% |
| ★    Traditional: Mild or Medium | 2 tbsp | 5 | 0% | 0% | 0% |
| ★ S & W Salsa | 1/4 cup | 16 | 0% | 0% | 0% |
| TOSTITOS Salsa—FRITO-LAY | | | | | |
| ★    Con Queso | 2 tbsp | 40 | 3% | 3% | 1% |
| ★    Mild | 2 tbsp | 15 | 0% | 0% | 0% |

### Other Dips

### Generic Foods

| FOOD | Serving Size | Calories | Tot Fat | Sat Fat | Chol |
|---|---|---|---|---|---|
| ★ Hummus | 2 tbsp | 60 | 4% | 2% | 0% |

### Brand Name Foods

| FOOD | Serving Size | Calories | Tot Fat | Sat Fat | Chol |
|---|---|---|---|---|---|
| BREAKSTONE'S Sour Cream Dip —KRAFT | | | | | |
| ❖    Bacon & Onion | 2 tbsp | 60 | 8% | 15% | 7% |
| ❖    Chesapeake Clam | 2 tbsp | 50 | 6% | 13% | 10% |
| ❖    French Onion | 2 tbsp | 50 | 6% | 15% | 7% |
| ❖    Jalapeno Cheddar | 2 tbsp | 60 | 6% | 15% | 5% |
| ❖    Toasted Onion | 2 tbsp | 50 | 6% | 15% | 7% |
| CALAVO Guacamole | | | | | |
| ★    Guacamole, Reduced Fat | 2 tbsp | 35 | 4% | 3% | 0% |
| ❖    Mexican Style | 2 tbsp | 50 | 7% | 5% | 0% |
| ❖    Mild | 2 tbsp | 60 | 8% | 5% | 0% |
| ❖    Original Avocado Dip | 2 tbsp | 50 | 7% | 5% | 0% |
| ❖    Spicy | 2 tbsp | 50 | 7% | 5% | 0% |
| ❖    Western Style | 2 tbsp | 50 | 7% | 5% | 0% |
| ❖    Zesty | 2 tbsp | 60 | 8% | 5% | 0% |
| FRITO-LAY'S Dips | | | | | |
| ❖    French Onion Flavor | 2 tbsp | 60 | 8% | 17% | 5% |
| ❖    Jalapeno & Cheddar Flavor Cheese | 2 tbsp | 50 | 5% | 6% | 2% |
| ★    Mild Cheddar Flavor Cheese | 2 tbsp | 50 | 5% | 2% | 2% |
| ★    Nacho Cheese Flavor Cheese | 2 tbsp | 45 | 4% | 4% | 2% |
| ★ GUILTLESS GOURMET Nacho, Spicy | 2 tbsp | 25 | 0% | 0% | 0% |
| KNORR Dip Mixes—CPC | | | | | |
| ★    Chili Caliente | 1/20 pkg | 5 | 0% | 0% | 0% |
| ★    Cracked Pepper Ranch | 1/20 pkg | 5 | 0% | 0% | 0% |
| ★    Garden Dill | 1/20 pkg | 2 | 0% | 0% | 0% |
| ★    Nacho Cheese | 1/16 pkg | 10 | 0% | 0% | 0% |

| FOOD | Serving Size | Calories | Tot Fat | Sat Fat | Chol |
|---|---|---|---|---|---|
| ★ Onion Chive | 1/20 pkg | 5 | 0% | 0% | 0% |
| KNUDSEN Premium Real Sour Cream Dip—KRAFT | | | | | |
| ❖ Bacon & Onion | 2 tbsp | 60 | 8% | 15% | 7% |
| ❖ French Onion | 2 tbsp | 50 | 6% | 15% | 7% |
| ❖ Nacho Cheese | 2 tbsp | 60 | 6% | 15% | 5% |
| KRAFT Dip | | | | | |
| ❖ Avocado | 2 tbsp | 60 | 6% | 15% | 0% |
| ❖ Bacon & Horseradish | 2 tbsp | 60 | 8% | 15% | 0% |
| ❖ Clam | 2 tbsp | 60 | 6% | 15% | 0% |
| ❖ French Onion | 2 tbsp | 60 | 6% | 15% | 0% |
| ❖ Green Onion | 2 tbsp | 60 | 6% | 15% | 0% |
| ❖ Jalapeno | 2 tbsp | 60 | 6% | 15% | 0% |
| ❖ Ranch | 2 tbsp | 60 | 6% | 15% | 0% |
| KRAFT Premium Dip | | | | | |
| ❖ Bacon & Horseradish | 2 tbsp | 50 | 8% | 15% | 5% |
| ❖ Bacon & Onion | 2 tbsp | 60 | 8% | 15% | 5% |
| ❖ Blue Cheese | 2 tbsp | 45 | 6% | 13% | 3% |
| ❖ Clam | 2 tbsp | 45 | 6% | 13% | 3% |
| ❖ Creamy Cucumber | 2 tbsp | 50 | 6% | 15% | 4% |
| ❖ Creamy Onion | 2 tbsp | 45 | 6% | 13% | 3% |
| ❖ French Onion | 2 tbsp | 50 | 6% | 13% | 3% |
| ❖ Jalapeno Cheese | 2 tbsp | 60 | 8% | 15% | 5% |
| ❖ Nacho Cheese | 2 tbsp | 60 | 8% | 15% | 5% |
| ★ LA VICTORIA Chili Dip | 2 tbsp | 10 | 0% | 0% | 0% |
| MARIE'S Dips—CAMPBELL'S | | | | | |
| Ⓐ Bacon Ranch | 2 tbsp | 150 | 25% | 10% | 5% |
| Ⓐ Homestyle Ranch | 2 tbsp | 150 | 22% | 10% | 5% |
| Ⓐ Parmesan Garlic | 2 tbsp | 140 | 22% | 10% | 3% |
| Ⓐ Spinach | 2 tbsp | 140 | 22% | 10% | 3% |
| Ⓐ Sun Dried Tomato | 2 tbsp | 140 | 22% | 10% | 5% |
| ❖ PRICE'S Fiesta Cheese Dip— FROMAGERIE BEL | 2 tbsp | 80 | 10% | 13% | 5% |

## FRUIT SNACKS

### Generic Foods

| FOOD | Serving Size | Calories | Tot Fat | Sat Fat | Chol |
|---|---|---|---|---|---|
| Ⓐ Banana Chips | 1 oz | 150 | 15% | 41% | 0% |
| ❖ Fruit Leather Bars (1 oz) | 1 bar | 110 | 2% | 6% | 0% |
| ★ Fruit Leather Rollups (1 oz) | 1 rollup | 100 | 1% | 1% | 0% |

★ Foods with this symbol have less than or equal to 5% *Daily Value* for all three nutrients (5% Rule).

❖ Foods with this symbol have at least one of the three nutrients greater than 5% *Daily Value* but less than or equal to 20% *Daily Value*.

Ⓐ Foods with this symbol have at least one of the three nutrients greater than 20% *Daily Value* (20% Rule).

| FOOD | Serving Size | Calories | Tot Fat | Sat Fat | Chol |
|------|------|------|------|------|------|
| **Brand Name Foods** | | | | | |
| BETTY CROCKER Assorted Fruit | | | | | |
| —GENERAL MILLS | | | | | |
| ★ *Bugs Bunny* & Friends | 1 pouch | 90 | 2% | 0% | 0% |
| ★ *Rollerblade* | 1 pouch | 90 | 2% | 0% | 0% |
| ★ *Shark Bites* | 1 pouch | 90 | 2% | 0% | 0% |
| ★ *Tasmanian Devil* | 1 pouch | 90 | 2% | 0% | 0% |
| ★ *X Men* | 1 pouch | 90 | 2% | 0% | 0% |
| BETTY CROCKER Fruit Snacks | | | | | |
| —GENERAL MILLS | | | | | |
| ★ *Fruit by the Foot:* All flavors | 1 roll | 80 | 2% | 3% | 0% |
| ★ *Fruit Roll-Ups* (pouch): All flavors | 1 roll | 50 | 1% | 0% | 0% |
| ★ *Fruit String Thing:* All flavors | 1 pouch | 80 | 1% | 0% | 0% |
| ★ *Gushers:* All flavors | 1 pouch | 90 | 2% | 2% | 0% |
| DEL MONTE Fruit Snacks: Yogurt Covered Raisins | | | | | |
| ❖ Strawberry Flavor | 1 bag (1 oz) | 120 | 5% | 15% | 0% |
| ❖ Vanilla Flavor | 1 bag (1 oz) | 120 | 5% | 15% | 0% |
| ⊛ ESTEE Fruit & Nut Mix | 1/4 cup | 210 | 18% | 35% | 1% |
| NATURE'S CHOICE Real Fruit Leathers—BARBARA'S BAKERY | | | | | |
| ★ Apple | 2 bars | 100 | 0% | 0% | 0% |
| ★ Apricot | 2 bars | 100 | 0% | 0% | 0% |
| ★ Cherry | 2 bars | 100 | 0% | 0% | 0% |
| ★ Grape | 2 bars | 100 | 0% | 0% | 0% |
| ★ Raspberry | 2 bars | 100 | 0% | 0% | 0% |
| ★ SMART SNACKERS Apple Chips —WEIGHT WATCHERS | 1 bag | 70 | 0% | 0% | 0% |
| SMART SNACKERS Fruit Snacks —WEIGHT WATCHERS | | | | | |
| ★ Apple | 1 pouch | 50 | 0% | 0% | 0% |
| ★ Cinnamon | 1 pouch | 50 | 0% | 0% | 0% |
| ★ Peach | 1 pouch | 50 | 0% | 0% | 0% |
| ★ Strawberry | 1 pouch | 50 | 0% | 0% | 0% |

## POPCORN

**Note:** *All values for popped popcorn unless otherwise noted.*

**Generic Foods**

| | | | | | |
|------|------|------|------|------|------|
| ★ Air-Popped | 5 cups | 130 | 0% | 0% | 0% |
| ❖ Caramel Coated | 1 cup | 150 | 7% | 6% | 0% |
| ★ Caramel w/Peanuts | 1 cup | 170 | 5% | 2% | 0% |
| ❖ Cheese Flavored | 3 cups | 170 | 17% | 11% | 1% |
| ★ Popcorn (unpopped) | 1/4 cup | 190 | 4% | 1% | 0% |

| FOOD | Serving Size | Calories | Tot Fat | Sat Fat | Chol |
|------|--------------|----------|---------|---------|------|
| ⍟ Popped in Oil | 3 cups | 120 | 9% | 23% | 0% |
| ★ Sugar Coated | 1 cup | 140 | 2% | 2% | 0% |

### Brand Name Foods

| FOOD | Serving Size | Calories | Tot Fat | Sat Fat | Chol |
|------|--------------|----------|---------|---------|------|
| ACT II *Flavor Lover's* Microwave Popcorn—GOLDEN VALLEY | | | | | |
| ❖ Caramel Glaze (5.1 oz bag) | ~ 1/2 bag | 170 | 11% | 8% | 0% |
| ❖ Cheese (3 oz bag) | ~ 1/2 bag | 180 | 16% | 10% | 0% |
| ❖ Cinnamon Toffee Glaze (5.1 oz bag) | ~ 1/2 bag | 170 | 11% | 8% | 0% |
| ❖ Santa Fe Butter (3 oz bag) | ~ 1/2 bag | 170 | 14% | 10% | 0% |
| ACT II Microwave Popcorn— GOLDEN VALLEY | | | | | |
| ★ 96% Fat Free, Butter (3 oz bag) | ~ 1/2 bag | 130 | 2% | 0% | 0% |
| ❖ Butter (3.5 oz bag) | ~ 1/2 bag | 170 | 17% | 13% | 0% |
| ❖ Butter Lovers (3.5 oz bag) | ~ 1/2 bag | 170 | 17% | 13% | 0% |
| ❖ Light Butter (3 oz bag) | ~ 1/2 bag | 130 | 8% | 5% | 0% |
| ❖ Light Natural (3 oz bag) | ~ 1/2 bag | 130 | 8% | 5% | 0% |
| ❖ Natural (3.5 oz bag) | ~ 1/2 bag | 180 | 19% | 13% | 0% |
| BEARITOS Popcorn—LITTLE BEAR ORGANIC FOODS | | | | | |
| ❖ 50% Less Oil | 3 1/2 cups | 140 | 9% | 3% | 0% |
| ❖ Lite Buttery | 3 1/2 cups | 140 | 9% | 3% | 0% |
| ❖ White Cheddar | 3 1/2 cups | 170 | 17% | 8% | 2% |
| CAPE COD Popcorn—ANHEUSER BUSCH | | | | | |
| ❖ All Natural | 3 1/5 cups | 160 | 14% | 10% | 0% |
| ❖ Old Fashioned Butter | 3 cups | 170 | 15% | 15% | 1% |
| ❖ White Cheddar Cheese | 2 1/3 cups | 170 | 18% | 13% | 3% |
| CRACKER JACK—BORDEN | | | | | |
| ❖ Butter Toffee | 2/3 cup | 130 | 7% | 10% | 2% |
| ★ Butter Toffee, Fat Free | 1 cup | 110 | 0% | 0% | 0% |
| ❖ Butter Toffee Clusters | 1 ounce (~ 1/2 cup) | 130 | 7% | 10% | 2% |
| ★ Original | 2/3 cup | 120 | 4% | 3% | 0% |
| ★ Original, Fat Free | 1 cup | 110 | 0% | 0% | 0% |
| CRUNCH 'N MUNCH—AMERICAN HOME FOODS | | | | | |
| ★ Buttery Almond Flavored Popcorn w/Almonds | 1/2 cup | 130 | 5% | 3% | 1% |
| ❖ Buttery Toffee Popcorn w/ Peanuts | 2/3 cup | 140 | 6% | 4% | 1% |
| ★ Buttery Toffee Popcorn w/ Peanuts, Reduced Fat | 1/2 cup | 140 | 4% | 0% | 1% |

★ Foods with this symbol have less than or equal to 5% *Daily Value* for <u>all</u> three nutrients (5% Rule).

❖ Foods with this symbol have <u>at least one</u> of the three nutrients greater than 5% *Daily Value* but less than or equal to 20% *Daily Value*.

⍟ Foods with this symbol have <u>at least one</u> of the three nutrients greater than 20% *Daily Value* (20% Rule).

| FOOD | Serving Size | Calories | Tot Fat | Sat Fat | Chol |
|------|------|------|------|------|------|
| ❖ Candied Popcorn w/Peanuts | 1/2 cup | 130 | 7% | 2% | 0% |
| ★ Caramel Popcorn w/Peanuts | 2/3 cup | 140 | 5% | 4% | 3% |
| ❖ Fudge Coated Buttery Toffee Popcorn w/Peanuts | 1/3 cup | 130 | 8% | 17% | 1% |
| ❖ Maple Flavored Popcorn w/ Walnut Chunks | 2/3 cup | 140 | 6% | 3% | 1% |
| ★ ESTEE Caramel Popcorn | 1 cup | 120 | 2% | 0% | 0% |
| FEATHERWEIGHT Microwave Lite Popcorn | | | | | |
| ❖ Butter flavor | 1 bag | 210 | 9% | 5% | 0% |
| ★ Natural | 1 bag | 160 | 3% | 0% | 0% |
| JIFFY POP Microwave Premium Popcorn—AMERICAN HOME FOODS | | | | | |
| ❖ Butter Flavor Artificially Flavored | 3 cups | 170 | 15% | 8% | 0% |
| ❖ Light Butter Flavor Artificially Flavored | 3 cups | 120 | 8% | 3% | 0% |
| ❖ Natural Flavor | 3 cups | 170 | 15% | 8% | 0% |
| JIFFY POP Popcorn—AMERICAN HOME FOODS | | | | | |
| ❖ Butter | 3 cups | 140 | 11% | 5% | 0% |
| ❖ Natural Flavors | 3 cups | 140 | 11% | 5% | 0% |
| JOLLY TIME Microwave Popcorn —AMERICAN POPCORN COMPANY | | | | | |
| ❖ Butter Flavored | 4 cups | 140 | 13% | 8% | 0% |
| ❖ Butter Flavored Light | 5 cups | 120 | 8% | 6% | 0% |
| ❖ Natural Flavored Light | 5 cups | 120 | 8% | 5% | 0% |
| ★ LOUISE'S FAT FREE Caramel Popcorn | 1 oz | 100 | 0% | 0% | 0% |
| NEWMAN'S OWN Oldstyle Picture Show Microwave Popcorn | | | | | |
| ❖ Butter | 3 1/2 cups | 170 | 17% | 10% | 0% |
| ★ Light Butter | 3 1/2 cups | 110 | 5% | 5% | 0% |
| ★ Light Natural | 3 1/2 cups | 110 | 5% | 5% | 0% |
| ❖ Natural | 3 1/2 cups | 170 | 17% | 10% | 0% |
| ❖ Natural, No Salt | 3 1/2 cups | 160 | 15% | 10% | 0% |
| ORVILLE REDENBACHER'S Microwave Popping Corn (unpopped)—HUNT WESSON | | | | | |
| ❖ Butter Flavor | 2 tbsp | 170 | 19% | 14% | 0% |
| ❖ Butter Flavor, Light | 2 tbsp | 120 | 9% | 6% | 0% |
| ❖ Butter Flavor, No Salt | 2 tbsp | 180 | 19% | 13% | 0% |
| ❖ Caramel | 2 tbsp | 180 | 15% | 12% | 0% |
| ❖ Cheddar Cheese | 2 tbsp | 150 | 14% | 4% | 0% |
| ❖ Natural Flavor | 2 tbsp | 160 | 17% | 12% | 0% |
| ❖ Natural Flavor, Light | 2 tbsp | 110 | 8% | 5% | 0% |
| ❖ Natural Flavor, No Salt | 2 tbsp | 170 | 18% | 13% | 0% |

| FOOD | Serving Size | Calories | Tot Fat | Sat Fat | Chol |
|---|---|---|---|---|---|
| ★ Smart Pop | 2 tbsp | 100 | 4% | 3% | 0% |
| ORVILLE REDENBACHER'S Gourmet Popping Corn (unpopped)—HUNT WESSON | | | | | |
| ★ Hot Air | 2 tbsp | 90 | 1% | 1% | 0% |
| ★ Original | 2 tbsp | 90 | 2% | 1% | 0% |
| ★ White | 2 tbsp | 90 | 2% | 1% | 0% |
| POP-SECRET *By Request* Popcorn —GENERAL MILLS | | | | | |
| ★ Butter | 6 cups | 120 | 4% | 3% | 0% |
| ★ Natural | 6 cups | 120 | 4% | 3% | 0% |
| POP-SECRET *Pop Chips*—GENERAL MILLS | | | | | |
| ★ Butter | 1 oz (~ 31 chips) | 120 | 5% | 3% | 0% |
| ★ Cheddar Cheese | 1 oz (~ 31 chips) | 120 | 5% | 3% | 0% |
| ★ Original | 1 oz (~ 31 chips) | 120 | 5% | 3% | 0% |
| ★ Sour Cream & Onion | 1 oz (~ 31 chips) | 120 | 5% | 3% | 0% |
| POP-SECRET Light Popcorn— GENERAL MILLS | | | | | |
| ❖ Butter | 6 cups | 130 | 8% | 5% | 0% |
| ❖ *Buttery Burst* | 6 cups | 130 | 8% | 5% | 0% |
| ❖ Natural | 6 cups | 130 | 8% | 5% | 0% |
| POP-SECRET Popcorn—GENERAL MILLS | | | | | |
| ❖ Butter | 4 cups | 150 | 15% | 13% | 0% |
| ❖ *Buttery Burst* | 4 cups | 150 | 15% | 13% | 0% |
| ❖ Cheddar Cheese | 5 cups | 150 | 15% | 12% | 0% |
| ❖ Nacho Cheese | 5 cups | 150 | 15% | 12% | 0% |
| ❖ Natural | 4 cups | 150 | 15% | 13% | 0% |
| REDEN-BUDDERS Popping Corn (unpopped)—HUNT WESSON | | | | | |
| ⊛ Herb & Garlic | 2 tbsp | 180 | 20% | 14% | 0% |
| ⊛ Movie Theater | 2 tbsp | 180 | 20% | 14% | 0% |
| ❖ Movie Theater, Light | 2 tbsp | 110 | 8% | 5% | 0% |
| ⊛ Zesty | 2 tbsp | 180 | 20% | 14% | 0% |
| SMART SNACKERS Popcorn— WEIGHT WATCHERS | | | | | |
| ★ Butter Flavor | 1 bag | 90 | 4% | 0% | 0% |
| ★ Butter Toffee | 1 bag | 110 | 4% | 5% | 0% |
| ★ Caramel | 1 bag | 100 | 2% | 0% | 0% |

★ Foods with this symbol have less than or equal to 5% *Daily Value* for <u>all</u> three nutrients (5% Rule).

❖ Foods with this symbol have <u>at least one</u> of the three nutrients greater than 5% *Daily Value* but less than or equal to 20% *Daily Value.*

⊛ Foods with this symbol have <u>at least one</u> of the three nutrients greater than 20% *Daily Value* (20% Rule).

| FOOD | Serving Size | Calories | Tot Fat | Sat Fat | Chol |
|------|------|------|------|------|------|
| ❖  White Cheddar Cheese | 1 bag | 90 | 6% | 5% | 0% |
| ❖  SMARTFOOD Popcorn—FRITO-LAY | 1 3/4 cups | 160 | 15% | 11% | 2% |
| ULTRA SLIM-FAST Popcorn | | | | | |
| ★  Caramel Popcorn | 1/2 cup | 120 | 2% | 0% | 1% |
| ★  Popcorn w/Butter Flavor | 4 1/3 cups | 130 | 5% | 3% | 0% |

## PRETZELS

**Brand Name Foods**

| FOOD | Serving Size | Calories | Tot Fat | Sat Fat | Chol |
|------|------|------|------|------|------|
| BARBARA'S BAKERY Pretzels | | | | | |
| ★  9-Grain Pretzels | 2 pcs | 100 | 2% | 0% | 0% |
| ★  Bavarian Pretzels: Regular or No Salt Added | 2 pcs | 100 | 2% | 0% | 0% |
| ★  Honeysweet Pretzels | 2 pcs | 100 | 2% | 0% | 0% |
| ★  Mini Pretzels: Regular or No Salt Added | 18 pcs | 100 | 2% | 0% | 0% |
| ★  Sesame Sticks | 35 pcs | 110 | 4% | 0% | 0% |
| BEARITOS Pretzels—LITTLE BEAR ORGANIC FOODS | | | | | |
| ★  Big Twist | 6 pretzels | 120 | 0% | 0% | 0% |
| ★  Thin Sticks | 50 pretzels | 120 | 0% | 0% | 0% |
| ★ CAPE COD No Fat Multi Grain Pretzels—ANHEUSER BUSCH | 30 pretzels | 110 | 0% | 0% | 0% |
| EAGLE Pretzels—ANHEUSER BUSCH | | | | | |
| ★  Mini Bites, Low Fat | 1 oz (3/4 cup) | 110 | 2% | 0% | 0% |
| ★  Pretzel Sticks, Low Fat | 1 oz (46 sticks) | 110 | 2% | 0% | 0% |
| ★  Sourdough Hard Bavarian, No Fat | 1 oz (2 pretzels) | 110 | 0% | 0% | 0% |
| ★  Thin Twists, Low Fat | 1 oz (10 pretzels) | 110 | 2% | 0% | 0% |
| ★  Thin Twist, No Fat | 1 oz (10 pretzels) | 100 | 0% | 0% | 0% |
| ESTEE Pretzels | | | | | |
| ★  Nuggets | 30 nuggets | 120 | 2% | 0% | 0% |
| ★  Ranch Nuggets | 23 nuggets | 130 | 3% | 3% | 0% |
| ★  Unsalted | 23 pretzels | 120 | 2% | 0% | 0% |
| ★  Unsalted Dutch | 2 pretzels | 130 | 2% | 0% | 0% |
| ★ FEATHERWEIGHT Pretzels, unsalted | 23 pretzels | 120 | 2% | 0% | 0% |
| KEEBLER Pretzels | | | | | |
| ★  *Butter Braids* | 22 pretzels | 100 | 2% | 0% | 0% |
| ★  *Butter Knots* | 7 pretzels | 100 | 2% | 0% | 0% |
| ★  *Mini Butter Knots* | 18 pretzels | 100 | 2% | 0% | 0% |
| ★  *Traditional Bavarian* | 3 pretzels | 120 | 3% | 3% | 0% |
| ★  *Traditional Knots* | 7 pretzels | 110 | 2% | 0% | 0% |

| FOOD | Serving Size | Calories | Tot Fat | Sat Fat | Chol |
|---|---|---|---|---|---|
| ★ MANISCHEWITZ Original Bagel Shaped Pretzels | 4 pretzels | 110 | 0% | 0% | 0% |
| MISTER SALTY—NABISCO | | | | | |
| ★ Dutch Pretzels | 2 pretzels | 120 | 2% | 0% | 0% |
| ★ Mini Pretzels | ~ 22 pretzels | 110 | 2% | 0% | 0% |
| ★ Pretzel Sticks, Fat Free | ~ 47 pretzels | 110 | 0% | 0% | 0% |
| ★ Pretzel Twists, Fat Free | ~ 9 pretzels | 110 | 0% | 0% | 0% |
| PEPPERIDGE FARM Snack Sticks —CAMPBELL'S | | | | | |
| ★ Pretzel | 9 sticks | 130 | 5% | 0% | 0% |
| ❖ Pumpernickel | 9 sticks | 150 | 9% | 3% | 0% |
| ❖ Sesame | 9 sticks | 150 | 9% | 3% | 0% |
| ❖ Three Cheese | 9 sticks | 140 | 8% | 10% | 2% |
| ROLD GOLD Pretzels—FRITO-LAY | | | | | |
| ★ Bavarian | 1 oz (~3 pretzels) | 120 | 3% | 2% | 0% |
| ★ Thins, Fat Free | 1 oz (~10 pretzels) | 110 | 0% | 0% | 0% |
| ★ Tiny Twist | 1 oz (~ 15 pretzels) | 110 | 2% | 0% | 0% |
| ★ Twists | 1 oz (~ 10 pretzels) | 111 | 2% | 0% | 0% |
| ★ SMART SNACKERS Oat Bran Pretzel Nuggets—WEIGHT WATCHERS | 1 bag | 170 | 4% | 0% | 0% |

## SNACK MIXES

**Generic Foods**

| | | | | | |
|---|---|---|---|---|---|
| ❖ Trail Mix | 1 oz | 130 | 13% | 8% | 0% |
| ❖ Trail Mix, Tropical | 1 oz | 120 | 7% | 12% | 0% |

**Brand Name Foods**

| | | | | | |
|---|---|---|---|---|---|
| CHEERIOS Snack Mixes—GENERAL MILLS | | | | | |
| ❖ Cheddar Cheese | 3/4 cup | 130 | 8% | 5% | 0% |
| ❖ Original w/Peanuts | 3/4 cup | 140 | 8% | 5% | 0% |
| ❖ Sour Cream & Onion | 3/4 cup | 130 | 8% | 5% | 0% |
| ❖ CHEEZ-IT Party Mix—SUNSHINE BISCUITS | 1/2 cup | 140 | 8% | 5% | 0% |
| COMBOS Snacks—M&M/MARS | | | | | |
| ❖ Cheddar Cheese Pretzel | 1 oz | 130 | 8% | 5% | 0% |
| ❖ Cheddar Cheese Cracker | 1 oz | 140 | 12% | 9% | 1% |
| ❖ Chili Cheese w/Corn Shell | 1 oz | 140 | 10% | 6% | 0% |

★ Foods with this symbol have less than or equal to 5% *Daily Value* for <u>all</u> three nutrients (5% Rule).
❖ Foods with this symbol have <u>at least one</u> of the three nutrients greater than 5% *Daily Value* but less than or equal to 20% *Daily Value*.
Ⓐ Foods with this symbol have <u>at least one</u> of the three nutrients greater than 20% *Daily Value* (20% Rule).

| FOOD | Serving Size | Calories | Tot Fat | Sat Fat | Chol |
|------|--------------|----------|---------|---------|------|
| ❖ Mustard Pretzel | 1 oz | 130 | 7% | 3% | 0% |
| ❖ Nacho Cheese Pretzel | 1 oz | 130 | 7% | 4% | 0% |
| ❖ Nacho Cheese w/Tortilla Shell | 1 oz | 140 | 10% | 5% | 0% |
| ❖ Peanut Butter Cracker | 1 oz | 140 | 12% | 7% | 0% |
| ❖ Pepperoni and Cheese Pizza | 1 oz | 140 | 10% | 6% | 1% |
| ❖ Pizzeria Pretzel | 1 oz | 130 | 7% | 4% | 0% |
| ❖ Tortilla Ranch Flavor | 1 oz | 140 | 11% | 8% | 1% |
| ❖ DEL MONTE Sierra Trail Mix | 1 oz | 120 | 9% | 10% | 0% |
| DOLE Trail Mix | | | | | |
| ★ California Style | 1.2 oz | 130 | 4% | 0% | 0% |
| ❖ Hawaiian Style | 1.2 oz | 150 | 6% | 5% | 0% |
| ❖ EAGLE Snack Mix—ANHEUSER BUSCH | 1/2 cup | 150 | 11% | 5% | 0% |
| FISHER Nuts & Crunches—PROCTER & GAMBLE | | | | | |
| ❖ Golden Crisp | 1/4 cup | 140 | 11% | 7% | 0% |
| ❖ Honey Crunch | 1/4 cup | 140 | 9% | 5% | 0% |
| ❖ FISHER Nuts & Fruits Snack Mix: Pineapple & Banana—PROCTER & GAMBLE | 1/4 cup | 140 | 12% | 10% | 0% |
| ❖ FISHER FAVORITES Tropical Fruit Nut and Fruit Mix and Cashews—PROCTER & GAMBLE | 1 oz | 140 | 12% | 6% | 0% |
| ❖ LITTLE DEBBIE Individual Snacks: *Star Crunch* Snack—MCKEE FOODS | 1 pkg (62 g) | 280 | 18% | 13% | 0% |
| PEPPERIDGE FARM *Snack Mix*— CAMPBELL'S | 1/2 cup | 180 | 14% | 8% | 8% |
| ❖ Extra Nutty | 1/2 cup | 180 | 14% | 8% | 8% |
| ❖ Goldfish | 1/2 cup | 150 | 11% | 5% | 3% |
| ❖ Honey Mustard & Onion | 1/2 cup | 180 | 15% | 8% | 1% |
| ❖ Lightly Seasoned | 1/2 cup | 170 | 12% | 5% | 1% |
| ❖ Original Goldfish | 1/2 cup | 170 | 12% | 8% | 2% |
| ❖ Savory | 1/2 cup | 170 | 12% | 5% | 1% |
| ❖ Seasoned | 1/2 cup | 170 | 12% | 5% | 1% |
| ❖ Smokey Cheddar | 1/2 cup | 180 | 15% | 8% | 1% |
| ❖ Snack Mix w/Goldfish | 1/2 cup | 170 | 12% | 5% | 1% |
| ❖ Spicy | 1/2 cup | 170 | 12% | 5% | 1% |
| ❖ Zesty Cheddar Goldfish | 1/2 cup | 180 | 15% | 8% | 1% |
| PLANTERS—NABISCO | | | | | |
| ❖ *Caribbean Crunch* Snack Mix | 1/4 cup | 170 | 17% | 15% | 0% |
| ❖ Chocolate Crisps | 13 pcs | 140 | 10% | 9% | 0% |
| ⦸ *Heat* Snack Mix | 1/4 cup | 190 | 23% | 8% | 0% |
| ⦸ *Honey Crunchers* | 1/4 cup | 190 | 23% | 8% | 0% |
| ⦸ Peanut Butter Chocolates | 4 pcs | 230 | 22% | 27% | 1% |
| PLANTERS *P.B. Crisps* Bite Size Snacks—NABISCO | | | | | |
| ❖ Strawberry Filling & Peanut Butter Creme | 12 pcs | 140 | 9% | 6% | 0% |
| ❖ Sweet Peanut Butter Creme | 12 pcs | 150 | 12% | 7% | 0% |

| FOOD | Serving Size | Calories | Tot Fat | Sat Fat | Chol |
|------|------|------|------|------|------|
| | | | | | |

## SNACK PACKS

**Brand Name Foods**

HANDI-SNACKS—KRAFT
| | | | | | |
|------|------|------|------|------|------|
| ❖ Cheez'n Breadsticks | 1 unit | 130 | 11% | 20% | 5% |
| ⊛ Cheez'n Crackers | 1 unit | 130 | 12% | 23% | 5% |
| ❖ Cheez'n Pretzels | 1 unit | 110 | 9% | 20% | 5% |
| ❖ Mozzarella String Cheese | 1 stick | 80 | 9% | 20% | 7% |
| ❖ Peanut Butter'n Crackers | 1 unit | 180 | 18% | 15% | 0% |
| ❖ Peanut Butter'n Grahamsticks | 1 unit | 170 | 15% | 13% | 0% |

MOO TOWN SNACKERS—SARGENTO
| | | | | | |
|------|------|------|------|------|------|
| ❖ Cheese & Pretzels | 1 unit | 90 | 5% | 10% | 3% |
| ❖ Cheese & Sticks | 1 unit | 100 | 6% | 13% | 3% |

RED DEVIL SNACKERS—PET
| | | | | | |
|------|------|------|------|------|------|
| ⊛ Chunky Chicken | 1 pkg | 270 | 24% | 18% | 15% |
| ⊛ Deviled Ham | 1 pkg | 310 | 34% | 30% | 16% |
| ⊛ Honey Ham | 1 pkg | 340 | 36% | 36% | 16% |

## OTHER SNACKS

**Generic Foods**

| | | | | | |
|------|------|------|------|------|------|
| ❖ Cornnuts: Plain, Barbecue, or Nacho Cheese | 1 oz | 120 | 6% | 4% | 0% |

**Brand Name Foods**

| | | | | | |
|------|------|------|------|------|------|
| ❖ BAKEN-ETS Fried Pork Skins, Traditional—FRITO-LAY | 9 pcs | 80 | 8% | 9% | 8% |
| ❖ FUNYONS Onion Snacks—FRITO-LAY | 1 oz (~ 13 pcs) | 140 | 10% | 7% | 0% |

TOMBSTONE Beef Jerky—KRAFT
| | | | | | |
|------|------|------|------|------|------|
| ★ Beef Jerky | 1 stick | 35 | 0% | 0% | 5% |
| ⊛ Beef Sticks | 1 stick | 110 | 15% | 23% | 7% |
| ⊛ Snappy Sticks | 1 stick | 110 | 15% | 23% | 7% |

---

★ Foods with this symbol have less than or equal to 5% *Daily Value* for <u>all</u> three nutrients (5% Rule).

❖ Foods with this symbol have <u>at least one</u> of the three nutrients greater than 5% *Daily Value* but less than or equal to 20% *Daily Value*.

⊛ Foods with this symbol have <u>at least one</u> of the three nutrients greater than 20% *Daily Value* (20% Rule).

| FOOD | Serving Size | Calories | Tot Fat | Sat Fat | Chol |
|------|------|------|------|------|------|

# Soups

*Note:* *% Daily Values for condensed soups are for soup before dilution with water or milk.*

### BEAN AND LENTIL SOUPS

**Generic Foods**

| FOOD | Serving Size | Calories | Tot Fat | Sat Fat | Chol |
|------|------|------|------|------|------|
| ❖ Bean w/Bacon | 1 cup | 170 | 9% | 8% | 1% |
| ❖ Beans & Frankfurter | 1 cup | 190 | 11% | 11% | 4% |
| ★ Black Bean | 1 cup | 120 | 2% | 2% | 0% |
| ★ Black Turtle Bean | 1 cup | 220 | 1% | 1% | 0% |
| ❖ Lentil w/Ham | 1 cup | 140 | 4% | 6% | 2% |

**Brand Name Foods**

| FOOD | Serving Size | Calories | Tot Fat | Sat Fat | Chol |
|------|------|------|------|------|------|
| BEARITOS Fat Free Homestyle Naturals—LITTLE BEAR ORGANIC FOODS | | | | | |
| ★ Black Bean | 1 cup | 110 | 0% | 0% | 0% |
| ★ Hearty Tex Mex | 1 cup | 115 | 0% | 0% | 0% |
| ★ Lentil | 1 cup | 100 | 0% | 0% | 0% |
| ★ Mixed Bean | 1 cup | 120 | 0% | 0% | 0% |
| ★ Navy Bean | 1 cup | 100 | 0% | 0% | 0% |
| CAMPBELL'S | | | | | |
| ★ *Chunky* (Ready-to-Serve) Old Fashioned Bean 'n Ham | 1 cup | 190 | 3% | 3% | 5% |
| ❖ *Healthy Request* (Condensed) Bean w/Bacon | 1/2 cup | 180 | 8% | 10% | 2% |
| CAMPBELL'S *Home Cookin'* (Ready-to-Serve) | | | | | |
| ★ Bean & Ham | 1 cup | 180 | 2% | 3% | 2% |
| ★ Hearty Lentil | 1 cup | 150 | 3% | 3% | 0% |
| ❖ CAMPBELL'S Microwave (Ready-to-Serve) Bean w/Bacon 'n Ham | 1 container | 180 | 9% | 10% | 3% |
| FANTASTIC FOODS | | | | | |
| ★ Country Lentil | 1 cup | 170 | 1% | 0% | 0% |
| ★ Couscous w/Lentils | 1 cup | 190 | 1% | 0% | 0% |
| ★ Five Bean | 1 cup | 170 | 1% | 0% | 0% |
| ★ Jumpin' Black Bean | 1 cup | 150 | 1% | 0% | 0% |
| ★ Spanish Rice & Bean | 1 cup | 180 | 2% | 0% | 0% |
| HAIN 99% Fat Free | | | | | |
| ★ Black Bean | 1 cup | 150 | 1% | 0% | 0% |
| ★ Vegetarian Lentil | 1 cup | 130 | 2% | 0% | 0% |
| HEALTH VALLEY Fat Free | | | | | |
| ★ 5 Bean Vegetable | 1 cup | 140 | 0% | 0% | 0% |
| ★ Black Bean & Vegetable | 1 cup | 110 | 0% | 0% | 0% |
| ★ Lentil & Carrots | 1 cup | 90 | 0% | 0% | 0% |
| ★ Lentil w/Couscous | 1/3 cup | 130 | 0% | 0% | 0% |

| FOOD | Serving Size | Calories | Tot Fat | Sat Fat | Chol |
|---|---|---|---|---|---|
| ★ Spicy Black Bean w/Couscous | 1/3 cup | 130 | 0% | 0% | 0% |
| ★ Zesty Black Bean w/Rice | 1/3 cup | 100 | 0% | 0% | 0% |
| HEALTHY CHOICE—CONAGRA | | | | | |
| ★ Bean & Ham | 1 cup | 180 | 5% | 5% | 2% |
| ★ Lentil | 1 cup | 150 | 2% | 3% | 0% |
| KNORR Bean Soup Mixes—CPC | | | | | |
| ★ Black Bean | 1 pkg | 190 | 2% | 0% | 0% |
| ★ Hearty Lentil | 1 pkg | 220 | 1% | 0% | 0% |
| ★ Navy Bean | 1 pkg | 140 | 1% | 0% | 0% |
| ★ MANISCHEWITZ Lima Bean (tube style, prep as dir) | 1 cup | 80 | 0% | 0% | 0% |
| ★ OLD EL PASO Black Bean w/ Bacon—PET | 1 cup | 160 | 2% | 2% | 2% |
| ★ PEPPERIDGE FARM Black Bean w/Sherry—CAMPBELL'S | 2/3 cup | 120 | 4% | 3% | 0% |
| PROGRESSO—PET | | | | | |
| ★ Bean and Ham | 1 cup | 160 | 3% | 3% | 4% |
| ★ *Healthy Classics* Lentil | 1 cup | 130 | 2% | 0% | 0% |
| ★ Hearty Black Bean | 1 cup | 170 | 2% | 0% | 1% |
| ★ Lentil | 1 cup | 140 | 3% | 0% | 0% |
| ❖ Lentil w/Sausage | 1 cup | 170 | 11% | 10% | 5% |
| ❖ Macaroni & Bean | 1 cup | 160 | 6% | 4% | 1% |
| ★ *Pasta Soups* Lentil & Shells | 1 cup | 130 | 2% | 0% | 0% |
| ULTRA SLIM-FAST | | | | | |
| ★ Lentil | 1 can | 230 | 5% | 5% | 2% |
| ★ Spicy Chili Bean | 1 can | 240 | 5% | 5% | 1% |
| ★ Vegetable Bean | 1 can | 240 | 5% | 5% | 2% |

BEEF SOUPS

**Generic Foods**

| | | | | | |
|---|---|---|---|---|---|
| ★ Beef Broth | 1 cup | 20 | 1% | 1% | 0% |
| ❖ Beef Noodle | 1 cup | 80 | 5% | 6% | 2% |
| ❖ Beef Stew | 1 cup | 220 | 8% | 9% | 20% |
| Ⓐ Brunswick Stew | 1 cup | 230 | 10% | 8% | 24% |
| ❖ Chili Beef | 1 cup | 170 | 0% | 17% | 4% |
| ❖ Chunky Beef | 1 cup | 170 | 8% | 13% | 5% |

**Brand Name Foods**

| | | | | | |
|---|---|---|---|---|---|
| CAMPBELL'S *Chunky* (Ready-to-Serve) | | | | | |
| ❖ Beef Pasta | 1 cup | 150 | 5% | 5% | 7% |
| ❖ Beef w/Country Vegetables | 1 cup | 160 | 6% | 5% | 8% |

★ Foods with this symbol have less than or equal to 5% *Daily Value* for all three nutrients (5% Rule).

❖ Foods with this symbol have at least one of the three nutrients greater than 5% *Daily Value* but less than or equal to 20% *Daily Value*.

Ⓐ Foods with this symbol have at least one of the three nutrients greater than 20% *Daily Value* (20% Rule).

| FOOD | Serving Size | Calories | Tot Fat | Sat Fat | Chol |
|------|------|------|------|------|------|
| ❖   Chili Beef w/Beans | 1 cup | 230 | 9% | 8% | 5% |
| ❖   Pepper Steak | 1 cup | 140 | 4% | 5% | 7% |
| ❖   Sirloin Burger w/Vegetables | 1 cup | 190 | 14% | 18% | 7% |
| ❖   Steak 'n Potato | 1 cup | 160 | 6% | 5% | 7% |
| ❖ CAMPBELL'S *Homestyle* Old Fashioned Beef Stew | 1/2 cup | 220 | 11% | 15% | 13% |
| CAMPBELL'S (Condensed) | | | | | |
| ★   Beef Broth | 1/2 cup | 15 | 0% | 0% | 1% |
| ★   Beef Noodle | 1/2 cup | 70 | 4% | 5% | 5% |
| ★   Beef w/Vegetables & Barley | 1/2 cup | 80 | 3% | 5% | 5% |
| ★   Beefy Mushroom | 1/2 cup | 70 | 5% | 5% | 3% |
| ❖   Chili Beef Soup w/Beans | 1/2 cup | 170 | 8% | 13% | 5% |
| ★   Consommé Beef | 1/2 cup | 25 | 0% | 0% | 1% |
| ❖   Noodles & Ground Beef | 1/2 cup | 100 | 6% | 10% | 8% |
| ❖ CAMPBELL'S Low Sodium (Ready-to-Serve) Chunky Vegetable Beef | 1 cup | 130 | 5% | 8% | 17% |
| CAMPBELL'S Microwave (Ready-to-Serve) | | | | | |
| ❖   Chili Beef | 1 container | 180 | 8% | 10% | 3% |
| ❖   Chunky Beef | 1 container | 210 | 8% | 5% | 12% |
| ❖   Chunky Sirloin Burger | 1 container | 210 | 12% | 15% | 5% |
| ★ FEATHERWEIGHT Beef Bouillon | 1 1/2 tsp | 15 | 1% | 0% | 0% |
| ★ HEALTH VALLEY Fat Free Beef Broth | 1 cup | 20 | 0% | 0% | 0% |
| HEALTHY CHOICE—CONAGRA | | | | | |
| ★   Beef & Potato | 1 cup | 120 | 2% | 3% | 2% |
| ★   Chili Beef | 1 cup | 170 | 2% | 3% | 3% |
| ★   Vegetable Beef | 1 cup | 130 | 2% | 0% | 1% |
| KNORR—CPC | | | | | |
| ★   Beef Bouillon | 1/2 cube | 20 | 2% | 2% | 0% |
| ★   Oxtail Soup & Recipe Mix | 1/3 pkg | 60 | 3% | 5% | 1% |
| MANISCHEWITZ | | | | | |
| ★   Beef Broth Consommé | 1/2 cup | 10 | 0% | 0% | 0% |
| ★   Beef Vegetable Soup | 1/2 cup | 80 | 3% | 3% | 2% |
| ★ MRS. GRASS Vegetable Beef Flavored Noodle Soup—BORDEN | 1/4 pkg | 70 | 2% | 0% | 0% |
| ❖ NISSIN *Top Ramen* Spicy Beef Flavor | 1/2 pkg | 200 | 12% | 20% | 0% |
| ❖ OLD EL PASO Hearty Beef—PET | 1 cup | 120 | 4% | 7% | 8% |
| ★ PEPPERIDGE FARM Consommé Madrilene—CAMPBELL'S | 2/3 cup | 50 | 1% | 0% | 0% |
| PROGRESSO—PET | | | | | |
| ❖   Beef Barley | 1 cup | 130 | 6% | 8% | 8% |
| ❖   Beef Noodle | 1 cup | 140 | 5% | 7% | 10% |
| PROGRESSO *Healthy Classics*—PET | | | | | |
| ❖   Beef Barley | 1 cup | 140 | 3% | 4% | 6% |
| ★   Beef Vegetable | 1 cup | 150 | 2% | 3% | 4% |
| PROGRESSO *Pasta Soups*—PET | | | | | |
| ❖   Beef Vegetable & Rotini | 1 cup | 120 | 5% | 7% | 7% |

| FOOD | Serving Size | Calories | Tot Fat | Sat Fat | Chol |
|---|---|---|---|---|---|
| ❖ Meatballs & Pasta Pearls | 1 cup | 140 | 11% | 14% | 4% |
| ★ RECIPE SECRETS Beefy Mushroom —LIPTON | 2 tbsp | 35 | 0% | 0% | 0% |
| SOUP STARTER—BORDEN | | | | | |
| ★ Beef Barley Vegetable | 1/8 pkg | 100 | 1% | 0% | 0% |
| ★ Beef Vegetable | 1/8 pkg | 90 | 1% | 0% | 0% |
| ★ Ground Beef Vegetable | 1/8 pkg | 80 | 1% | 0% | 0% |
| ★ Hearty Beef Stew | 1/7 pkg | 80 | 0% | 0% | 0% |
| STEERO Beef Flavored Bouillon —BORDEN | | | | | |
| ★ Cubes | 1 cube | 5 | 0% | 0% | 0% |
| ★ Instant | 1 tsp | 5 | 0% | 0% | 0% |
| ★ Instant, Low Sodium | 1 tsp | 10 | 0% | 0% | 0% |
| ★ SWANSON Clear Beef Broth— CAMPBELL'S | 1 cup | 20 | 2% | 3% | 0% |
| ★ WEIGHT WATCHERS Instant Beef Broth Mix | 1 pkt | 10 | 0% | 0% | 0% |
| WYLER'S Beef Flavored Bouillon —BORDEN | | | | | |
| ★ Cubes | 1 cube | 5 | 0% | 0% | 0% |
| ★ Instant | 1 tsp | 5 | 0% | 0% | 0% |
| ★ Instant, Low Sodium | 1 tsp | 10 | 0% | 0% | 0% |

### CHEESE SOUPS

**Generic Foods**

| | | | | | |
|---|---|---|---|---|---|
| ⊛ Cheese Soup (prep w/milk) | 1 cup | 230 | 22% | 46% | 16% |

**Brand Name Foods**

| | | | | | |
|---|---|---|---|---|---|
| ⊛ CAMPBELL'S Chunky (Ready-to-Serve) Chicken Broccoli Cheese Soup | 1 cup | 200 | 18% | 25% | 8% |
| CAMPBELL'S (Condensed) | | | | | |
| ❖ Broccoli Cheese | 1/2 cup | 110 | 11% | 15% | 3% |
| ⊛ Cheddar Cheese | 1/2 cup | 150 | 15% | 25% | 7% |
| ❖ Nacho Cheese | 1/2 cup | 140 | 12% | 20% | 5% |

### CHICKEN SOUPS

**Generic Foods**

| | | | | | |
|---|---|---|---|---|---|
| ★ Chicken and Rice | 1 cup | 130 | 1% | 5% | 4% |
| ★ Chicken Broth | 1 cup | 40 | 2% | 2% | 0% |

★ Foods with this symbol have less than or equal to 5% Daily Value for all three nutrients (5% Rule).
❖ Foods with this symbol have at least one of the three nutrients greater than 5% Daily Value but less than or equal to 20% Daily Value.
⊛ Foods with this symbol have at least one of the three nutrients greater than 20% Daily Value (20% Rule).

| FOOD | Serving Size | Calories | Tot Fat | Sat Fat | Chol |
|---|---|---|---|---|---|
| ★ Chicken Noodle | 1 cup | 75 | 4% | 3% | 2% |
| ❖ Chunky Chicken | 1 cup | 180 | 1% | 10% | 10% |

**Brand Name Foods**

CAMPBELL'S *Chunky* (Ready-to-Serve)

| | | | | | |
|---|---|---|---|---|---|
| ☻ Chicken Corn Chowder | 1 cup | 250 | 23% | 35% | 8% |
| ❖ Chicken Mushroom Chowder | 1 cup | 210 | 18% | 20% | 3% |
| ❖ Chicken Noodle w/Mushrooms | 1 cup | 140 | 7% | 8% | 10% |
| ❖ Chicken Nuggets w/Vegetables | 1 cup | 150 | 8% | 8% | 5% |
| ❖ Chicken Rice | 1 cup | 130 | 6% | 8% | 5% |
| ★ Chicken Vegetable | 1 cup | 90 | 2% | 3% | 3% |
| ❖ Classic Chicken Noodle | 1 cup | 130 | 6% | 5% | 7% |
| ❖ Old Fashioned Chicken | 1 cup | 130 | 5% | 8% | 7% |

CAMPBELL'S *Healthy Request* (Condensed)

| | | | | | |
|---|---|---|---|---|---|
| ★ Chicken Noodle | 1/2 cup | 70 | 5% | 5% | 5% |
| ★ Chicken Vegetable | 1/2 cup | 80 | 3% | 3% | 2% |
| ★ Chicken w/Rice | 1/2 cup | 70 | 5% | 5% | 3% |

CAMPBELL'S *Healthy Request* (Ready-to-Serve)

| | | | | | |
|---|---|---|---|---|---|
| ★ Chicken Broth | 1 cup | 20 | 0% | 0% | 0% |
| ★ Chicken Corn Chowder | 1 cup | 140 | 5% | 5% | 5% |
| ❖ Hearty Chicken Noodle | 1 cup | 110 | 5% | 5% | 8% |
| ★ Hearty Chicken Rice | 1 cup | 120 | 5% | 5% | 5% |
| ★ Hearty Chicken Vegetable | 1 cup | 120 | 4% | 5% | 5% |

CAMPBELL'S *Home Cookin'* (Ready-to-Serve)

| | | | | | |
|---|---|---|---|---|---|
| ★ Chicken Noodle | 1 cup | 100 | 5% | 5% | 5% |
| ★ Chicken Rice | 1 cup | 110 | 2% | 3% | 5% |
| ★ Chicken Vegetable | 1 cup | 130 | 5% | 5% | 3% |
| ❖ CAMPBELL'S *Homestyle* Chicken Noodle | 1/2 cup | 70 | 4% | 8% | 7% |

CAMPBELL'S (Condensed)

| | | | | | |
|---|---|---|---|---|---|
| ★ Chicken & Stars | 1/2 cup | 70 | 3% | 3% | 1% |
| ★ Chicken Alphabet w/Vegetables | 1/2 cup | 80 | 3% | 5% | 3% |
| ★ Chicken Broth | 1/2 cup | 30 | 3% | 3% | 1% |
| ❖ Chicken Dumplings | 1/2 cup | 80 | 5% | 5% | 8% |
| ★ Chicken Gumbo | 1/2 cup | 60 | 2% | 3% | 3% |
| Chicken Noodle | 1/2 cup | 70 | 4% | 5% | 5% |
| ★ Chicken Noodle O's | 1/2 cup | 80 | 5% | 5% | 5% |
| ★ Chicken Vegetable | 1/2 cup | 80 | 3% | 3% | 3% |
| ★ Chicken w/Rice | 1/2 cup | 70 | 4% | 5% | 1% |
| ★ Chicken w/Wild Rice | 1/2 cup | 70 | 3% | 3% | 3% |
| ★ Chicken Won Ton | 1/2 cup | 45 | 2% | 0% | 5% |
| ★ Curly Noodle w/Chicken Broth | 1/2 cup | 80 | 4% | 5% | 5% |
| ★ Double Noodle in Chicken Broth | 1/2 cup | 100 | 4% | 5% | 5% |

| FOOD | Serving Size | Calories | Tot Fat | Sat Fat | Chol |
|---|---|---|---|---|---|
| ★ CAMPBELL'S Dry Soup & Recipe Mix: Chicken Noodle | 3 tbsp | 90 | 2% | 3% | 3% |
| CAMPBELL'S Low Sodium (Ready-to-Serve) | | | | | |
| ★   Chicken Broth | 1 cup | 25 | 3% | 5% | 2% |
| ❖   Chicken with Noodles | 1 cup | 170 | 8% | 8% | 17% |
| CAMPBELL'S Microwave (Ready-to-Serve) | | | | | |
| ❖   Chicken Noodle | 1 container | 130 | 6% | 5% | 8% |
| ★   Chicken Rice | 1 container | 120 | 4% | 5% | 3% |
| ❖   Chunky Chicken Noodle | 1 container | 160 | 7% | 10% | 12% |
| ★ FANTASTIC FOODS Chicken Free Noodle | 1 cup | 120 | 1% | 0% | 0% |
| ★ FEATHERWEIGHT Chicken Bouillon | 1 1/2 tsp | 15 | 0% | 0% | 0% |
| HAIN Homestyle | | | | | |
| ★   Chicken Broth | 1 cup | 40 | 4% | 2% | 1% |
| ❖   Chicken Noodle | 1 cup | 110 | 6% | 2% | 7% |
| HEALTH VALLEY Fat Free | | | | | |
| ★   Chicken Broth | 1 cup | 30 | 0% | 0% | 0% |
| ★   Chicken Noodle w/Vegetables | 1/3 cup | 80 | 0% | 0% | 0% |
| HEALTHY CHOICE—CONAGRA | | | | | |
| ★   Chicken Corn Chowder | 1 cup | 150 | 5% | 5% | 3% |
| ★   Chicken Noodle | 1 cup | 140 | 5% | 5% | 3% |
| ★   Chicken w/Pasta | 1 cup | 120 | 4% | 5% | 2% |
| ★   Chicken w/Rice | 1 cup | 110 | 5% | 5% | 2% |
| ❖   Hearty Chicken | 1 cup | 130 | 4% | 5% | 7% |
| KNORR Soup Mixes—CPC | | | | | |
| ★   Chicken Bouillon | 1/2 cube | 20 | 2% | 0% | 0% |
| ★   Chicken Flavor Noodle | 1/3 pkg | 90 | 2% | 2% | 5% |
| ★   Chicken Flavor Vegetable | 1 pkg | 100 | 1% | 1% | 0% |
| MANISCHEWITZ | | | | | |
| ★   Chicken w/Kreplach | 1/2 cup | 35 | 2% | 0% | 0% |
| ❖   Chicken w/Matzo Balls | 1/2 cup | 80 | 6% | 10% | 8% |
| ★   Chicken w/Noodles | 1/2 cup | 35 | 1% | 0% | 0% |
| ★   Chicken w/Rice | 1/2 cup | 45 | 5% | 5% | 0% |
| ★   Chicken w/Vegetables | 1/2 cup | 35 | 1% | 0% | 0% |
| ★   Matzo Ball and Soup Mix | 1/4 cup mix | 120 | 2% | 5% | 0% |
| ❖   Matzo Ball Soup | 1 cup | 110 | 8% | 10% | 12% |
| Ⓐ   Matzo Balls in Broth | 1 cup | 220 | 14% | 15% | 27% |
| MRS. GRASS—BORDEN | | | | | |
| ★   Chicken Flavored w/Rice | 1/4 carton | 80 | 2% | 0% | 0% |
| ★   Homestyle Chickeny Flavored Noodle | 1/4 carton | 70 | 2% | 0% | 5% |

★  Foods with this symbol have less than or equal to 5% *Daily Value* for <u>all</u> three nutrients (5% Rule).

❖  Foods with this symbol have <u>at least one</u> of the three nutrients greater than 5% *Daily Value* but less than or equal to 20% *Daily Value*.

Ⓐ  Foods with this symbol have <u>at least one</u> of the three nutrients greater than 20% *Daily Value* (20% Rule).

| FOOD | Serving Size | Calories | Tot Fat | Sat Fat | Chol |
|---|---|---|---|---|---|
| ❖ Noodle Soup w/Real Chicken Broth | 1/4 carton | 60 | 2% | 2% | 7% |
| NISSIN *Cup Noodles* | | | | | |
| Ⓐ Chicken Flavor | 1 container | 300 | 19% | 32% | 1% |
| Ⓐ Chicken Mushroom Flavor | 1 container | 300 | 20% | 32% | 0% |
| NISSIN *Top Ramen* | | | | | |
| ❖ Chicken Sesame Flavor | 1/2 pkg | 200 | 12% | 20% | 0% |
| ★ Low Fat Chicken Flavor | 1/2 pkg | 150 | 2% | 0% | 0% |
| ❖ NISSIN Twin *Cup Noodles* Chicken Flavor | 1 container | 160 | 11% | 18% | 0% |
| OLD EL PASO—PET | | | | | |
| ★ Chicken Vegetable | 1 cup | 110 | 4% | 4% | 5% |
| ❖ Chicken w/Rice | 1 cup | 90 | 3% | 3% | 6% |
| ❖ Hearty Chicken Noodle | 1 cup | 110 | 5% | 4% | 9% |
| PEPPERIDGE FARM—CAMPBELL'S | | | | | |
| ❖ Chicken Curry | 2/3 cup | 170 | 12% | 18% | 8% |
| ❖ Chicken w/Rice | 2/3 cup | 80 | 5% | 8% | 5% |
| PROGRESSO—PET | | | | | |
| ❖ Chickarina | 1 cup | 120 | 8% | 10% | 6% |
| ❖ Chicken & Wild Rice | 1 cup | 100 | 3% | 3% | 6% |
| ❖ Chicken Barley | 1 cup | 110 | 3% | 3% | 6% |
| ★ Chicken Broth | 1 cup | 20 | 1% | 0% | 2% |
| ❖ Chicken Noodle | 1 cup | 80 | 3% | 3% | 7% |
| ❖ Chicken Rice & Vegetable | 1 cup | 110 | 5% | 5% | 6% |
| ❖ Homestyle Chicken & Vegetable | 1 cup | 100 | 4% | 3% | 6% |
| ★ Tortellini in Chicken Broth | 1 cup | 80 | 3% | 4% | 2% |
| PROGRESSO *Healthy Classics*—PET | | | | | |
| ❖ Chicken Noodle | 1 cup | 80 | 3% | 3% | 6% |
| ★ Chicken Rice w/Vegetables | 1 cup | 90 | 2% | 0% | 4% |
| PROGRESSO *Pasta Soups*—PET | | | | | |
| ★ Chicken Vegetable & Penne | 1 cup | 100 | 4% | 3% | 4% |
| ❖ Hearty Chicken & Rotini | 1 cup | 90 | 3% | 3% | 7% |
| ★ Hearty Penne in Chicken Broth | 1 cup | 70 | 1% | 0% | 2% |
| ❖ Spicy Chicken & Penne | 1 cup | 120 | 6% | 6% | 7% |
| SOUP SECRETS Mixes—LIPTON | | | | | |
| ★ Chicken Noodle | 3 tbsp | 80 | 4% | 4% | 5% |
| ❖ Giggle Noodle w/Chicken Broth | 2 tbsp | 80 | 3% | 4% | 6% |
| ❖ Hearty Chicken Noodle | 1/4 cup | 80 | 2% | 3% | 6% |
| ★ Noodle w/Chicken Broth | 2 tbsp | 60 | 3% | 3% | 5% |
| ★ Ring-O-Noodle w/Chicken Broth | 2 tbsp | 70 | 3% | 3% | 6% |
| SOUP STARTER—BORDEN | | | | | |
| ★ Chicken & Rice | 1/8 pkg | 70 | 1% | 0% | 0% |
| ★ Chicken Noodle | 1/8 pkg | 80 | 1% | 0% | 0% |
| ★ Hearty Chicken Vegetable | 1/7 pkg | 70 | 0% | 0% | 0% |
| STEERO Chicken Flavored Bouillon —BORDEN | | | | | |
| ★ Cubes | 1 cube | 5 | 0% | 0% | 0% |
| ★ Instant | 1 tsp | 5 | 0% | 0% | 0% |
| ★ Instant, Low Sodium | 1 tsp | 10 | 0% | 0% | 0% |

| | | | % DAILY VALUE | | |
|---|---|---|---|---|---|
| **FOOD** | **Serving Size** | **Calories** | **Tot Fat** | **Sat Fat** | **Chol** |
| ★ SWANSON Clear Chicken Broth— | | | | | |
| CAMPBELL'S | 1 cup | 30 | 2% | 3% | 0% |
| WEIGHT WATCHERS | | | | | |
| ★ Chicken & Rice | 1 can | 110 | 2% | 0% | 3% |
| ❖ Chicken Noodle | 1 can | 150 | 3% | 3% | 10% |
| ★ Instant Chicken Broth | 1 pkt | 10 | 0% | 0% | 0% |
| WYLER'S Chicken Flavored Bouillon—BORDEN | | | | | |
| ★ Cubes | 1 cube | 5 | 0% | 0% | 0% |
| ★ Instant | 1 tsp | 5 | 0% | 0% | 0% |
| ★ Instant, Low Sodium | 1 tsp | 10 | 0% | 0% | 0% |

## CLAM CHOWDER

**Generic Foods**

| | | | | | |
|---|---|---|---|---|---|
| ★ Manhattan Clam Chowder (prep w/water) | 1 cup | 80 | 1% | 2% | 1% |
| ❖ New England Clam Chowder (prep w/milk) | 1 cup | 160 | 1% | 15% | 7% |
| ★ New England Clam Chowder (prep w/water) | 1 cup | 100 | 4% | 2% | 2% |

**Brand Name Foods**

| | | | | | |
|---|---|---|---|---|---|
| CAMPBELL'S (Ready-to-Serve) New England Clam Chowder | | | | | |
| ⊛ *Chunky* | 1 cup | 250 | 23% | 30% | 3% |
| ★ *Healthy Request* | 1 cup | 110 | 5% | 5% | 3% |
| ⊛ *Home Cookin'* | 1 cup | 210 | 25% | 25% | 2% |
| CAMPBELL'S (Condensed) | | | | | |
| ★ Manhattan Style Clam Chowder | 1/2 cup | 70 | 3% | 3% | 1% |
| ★ New England Clam Chowder | 1/2 cup | 90 | 4% | 3% | 1% |
| CAMPBELL'S Microwave (Ready-to-Serve) | | | | | |
| ⊛ Chunky New England Clam Chowder | 1 container | 290 | 26% | 40% | 7% |
| ⊛ New England Clam Chowder | 1 container | 200 | 22% | 20% | 5% |
| ❖ GORTON'S (Ready-to-Serve) New England Clam Chowder— | | | | | |
| GENERAL MILLS | 1 cup | 140 | 9% | 8% | 6% |
| ❖ HEALTHY CHOICE New England Clam Chowder—CONAGRA | 1 cup | 130 | 4% | 10% | 1% |
| PEPPERIDGE FARM—CAMPBELL'S | | | | | |
| ★ Manhattan Style Clam Chowder | 2/3 cup | 80 | 3% | 3% | 1% |
| ❖ New England Clam Chowder | 2/3 cup | 160 | 12% | 15% | 7% |

★ Foods with this symbol have less than or equal to 5% *Daily Value* for <u>all</u> three nutrients (5% Rule).
❖ Foods with this symbol have <u>at least one</u> of the three nutrients greater than 5% *Daily Value* but less than or equal to 20% *Daily Value*.
⊛ Foods with this symbol have <u>at least one</u> of the three nutrients greater than 20% *Daily Value* (20% Rule).

| FOOD | Serving Size | Calories | Tot Fat | Sat Fat | Chol |
|------|--------------|----------|---------|---------|------|
| **PROGRESSO—**PET | | | | | |
| ★ *Healthy Classics* New England Clam Chowder | 1 cup | 120 | 3% | 3% | 2% |
| ★ Manhattan Clam Chowder | 1 cup | 110 | 3% | 0% | 3% |
| ❖ New England Clam Chowder | 1 cup | 180 | 15% | 14% | 5% |
| ❖ *Pasta Soups* Clam & Rotini Chowder | 1 cup | 200 | 15% | 11% | 4% |

### CREAM SOUPS

**Generic Foods**

| FOOD | Serving Size | Calories | Tot Fat | Sat Fat | Chol |
|------|--------------|----------|---------|---------|------|
| ❖ Cream of Asparagus | 1 cup | 160 | 8% | 17% | 7% |
| ❖ Cream of Celery | 1 cup | 160 | 10% | 20% | 11% |
| ☻ Cream of Chicken (prep w/milk) | 1 cup | 190 | 2% | 23% | 9% |
| ❖ Cream of Chicken (prep w/water) | 1 cup | 120 | 1% | 10% | 3% |
| ❖ Cream of Mushroom (prep w/water) | 1 cup | 130 | 5% | 12% | 1% |
| ❖ Cream of Potato (prep w/milk) | 1 cup | 150 | 8% | 19% | 7% |

**Brand Name Foods**

| FOOD | Serving Size | Calories | Tot Fat | Sat Fat | Chol |
|------|--------------|----------|---------|---------|------|
| ☻ CAMPBELL'S *Chunky* (Ready-to-Serve) Creamy Chicken w/ Mushroom | 1 cup | 210 | 26% | 40% | 7% |
| CAMPBELL'S *Healthy Request* (Condensed) | | | | | |
| ★ Cream of Broccoli | 1/2 cup | 70 | 3% | 5% | 1% |
| ★ Cream of Celery | 1/2 cup | 70 | 3% | 3% | 1% |
| ★ Cream of Chicken | 1/2 cup | 80 | 4% | 5% | 3% |
| ★ Cream of Mushroom | 1/2 cup | 70 | 5% | 5% | 3% |
| CAMPBELL'S *Home Cookin'* (Ready-to-Serve) | | | | | |
| ☻ Cream of Chicken | 1 cup | 200 | 26% | 30% | 5% |
| ❖ Cream of Mushroom | 1 cup | 170 | 20% | 20% | 5% |
| ★ CAMPBELL'S *Homestyle* Cream of Tomato | 1/2 cup | 110 | 4% | 5% | 2% |
| CAMPBELL'S (Condensed) | | | | | |
| ❖ Cream of Asparagus | 1/2 cup | 110 | 11% | 10% | 1% |
| ❖ Cream of Broccoli | 1/2 cup | 100 | 9% | 13% | 1% |
| ❖ Cream of Celery | 1/2 cup | 110 | 11% | 13% | 1% |
| ❖ Cream of Chicken | 1/2 cup | 130 | 12% | 15% | 3% |
| ❖ Cream of Chicken & Broccoli | 1/2 cup | 120 | 12% | 13% | 5% |
| ❖ Cream of Mushroom | 1/2 cup | 110 | 11% | 13% | 1% |
| ❖ Cream of Potato | 1/2 cup | 100 | 5% | 8% | 3% |
| ❖ Cream of Shrimp | 1/2 cup | 100 | 11% | 10% | 7% |
| ❖ Creamy Chicken Mushroom | 1/2 cup | 130 | 14% | 13% | 5% |
| ❖ Creamy Chicken Noodle | 1/2 cup | 130 | 11% | 10% | 5% |

| FOOD | Serving Size | Calories | Tot Fat | Sat Fat | Chol |
|---|---|---|---|---|---|
| ❖ CAMPBELL'S Low Sodium (Ready-to-Serve) Cream of Mushroom | 1 cup | 120 | 15% | 18% | 2% |
| ❖ KNORR Cream of Spinach Soup & Recipe Mix—CPC | 1/3 pkg | 70 | 4% | 6% | 0% |
| KNORR *Chef's Collection* Soupmixes—CPC | | | | | |
| ★ Cream of Broccoli | 1/2 pkg | 60 | 4% | 5% | 2% |
| ★ Cream of Snow Pea | 1/2 pkg | 70 | 3% | 2% | 0% |
| ★ Cream of Wild Mushroom | 1/2 pkg | 90 | 5% | 3% | 0% |
| PEPPERIDGE FARM—CAMPBELL'S | | | | | |
| ❖ Cream of Broccoli | 2/3 cup | 90 | 7% | 15% | 2% |
| Ⓐ Vichyssoise (Cream of Potato & Onion) | 2/3 cup | 120 | 12% | 23% | 5% |
| PROGRESSO—PET | | | | | |
| ❖ Cream of Chicken | 1 cup | 170 | 15% | 17% | 12% |
| ❖ Cream of Mushroom | 1 cup | 140 | 13% | 18% | 6% |
| Ⓐ Creamy Tortellini | 1 cup | 210 | 23% | 38% | 11% |
| ★ *Healthy Classics* Cream of Broccoli—PET | 1 cup | 90 | 4% | 3% | 2% |

MINESTRONE

**Generic Foods**

| | | | | | |
|---|---|---|---|---|---|
| ❖ Minestrone | 1 cup | 80 | 10% | 3% | 1% |

**Brand Name Foods**

| | | | | | |
|---|---|---|---|---|---|
| ★ BEARITOS Homestyle Fat Free Naturals: Minestrone—LITTLE BEAR ORGANIC FOODS | 1 cup | 70 | 0% | 0% | 0% |
| ❖ CAMPBELL'S *Chunky* (Ready-to-Serve) Minestrone | 1 cup | 140 | 8% | 8% | 2% |
| CAMPBELL'S *Healthy Request* (Condensed) | | | | | |
| ★ Minestrone | 1/2 cup | 90 | 2% | 3% | 0% |
| ★ Hearty Minestrone | 1 cup | 120 | 3% | 3% | 1% |
| CAMPBELL'S *Home Cookin'* (Ready-to-Serve) | | | | | |
| ★ Minestrone | 1 cup | 120 | 3% | 5% | 2% |
| ❖ Tuscany Minestrone | 1 cup | 160 | 11% | 8% | 2% |
| ★ CAMPBELL'S (Condensed) Minestrone | 1/2 cup | 100 | 3% | 3% | 1% |
| ★ HAIN 99% Fat Free Minestrone | 1 cup | 150 | 5% | 2% | 0% |

★ Foods with this symbol have less than or equal to 5% *Daily Value* for <u>all</u> three nutrients (5% Rule).
❖ Foods with this symbol have <u>at least one</u> of the three nutrients greater than 5% *Daily Value* but less than or equal to 20% *Daily Value*.
Ⓐ Foods with this symbol have <u>at least one</u> of the three nutrients greater than 20% *Daily Value* (20% Rule).

| FOOD | Serving Size | Calories | Tot Fat | Sat Fat | Chol |
|------|-----------|----------|---------|---------|------|
| ★ HEALTH VALLEY Fat Free Real Italian Minestrone | 1 cup | 80 | 0% | 0% | 0% |
| ★ HEALTHY CHOICE Minestrone —CONAGRA | 1 cup | 110 | 2% | 0% | 0% |
| MANISCHEWITZ | | | | | |
| ★ Minestrone | 1/2 cup | 90 | 2% | 0% | 0% |
| ★ Minestrone (tube style, prep as dir) | 1 cup | 150 | 0% | 0% | 0% |
| ❖ PEPPERIDGE FARM Minestrone —CAMPBELL'S | 2/3 cup | 100 | 6% | 5% | 1% |
| PROGRESSO—PET | | | | | |
| ❖ Beef Minestrone | 1 cup | 140 | 6% | 8% | 9% |
| ❖ Chicken Minestrone | 1 cup | 120 | 5% | 5% | 7% |
| ★ *Healthy Classics* Minestrone | 1 cup | 120 | 4% | 0% | 0% |
| ★ Minestrone | 1 cup | 130 | 4% | 3% | 0% |
| ★ *Pasta Soups* Hearty Minestrone & Shells | 1 cup | 120 | 2% | 0% | 0% |
| ❖ Zesty Minestrone | 1 cup | 150 | 9% | 11% | 4% |
| ★ ULTRA SLIM-FAST Minestrone | 1 can | 240 | 5% | 5% | 1% |
| ★ WEIGHT WATCHERS Minestrone | 1 can | 130 | 3% | 3% | 2% |

## ONION SOUPS

**Generic Foods**

| FOOD | Serving Size | Calories | Tot Fat | Sat Fat | Chol |
|------|-----------|----------|---------|---------|------|
| ★ Onion Soup | 1 cup | 60 | 2% | 1% | 0% |

**Brand Name Foods**

| FOOD | Serving Size | Calories | Tot Fat | Sat Fat | Chol |
|------|-----------|----------|---------|---------|------|
| ★ CAMPBELL'S (Condensed) French Onion | 1/2 cup | 70 | 4% | 0% | 1% |
| ★ CAMPBELL'S Dry Soup & Recipe Mix: Onion | 2 tbsp | 50 | 2% | 0% | 0% |
| KNORR Soup & Recipe Mixes—CPC | | | | | |
| ★ French Onion Soup & Recipe | 1/3 pkg | 45 | 1% | 2% | 0% |
| ★ Leek Soup & Recipe | 1/3 pkg | 70 | 5% | 4% | 0% |
| ❖ MANISCHEWITZ French Onion | 1 cup | 70 | 6% | 2% | 0% |
| ★ MRS. GRASS Recipe, Soup & Dip Mix: Onion—BORDEN | 1/4 packet | 35 | 1% | 0% | 0% |
| ★ PEPPERIDGE FARM French Onion w/Beef Stock—CAMPBELL'S | 2/3 cup | 50 | 2% | 3% | 1% |
| RECIPE SECRETS Mixes—LIPTON | | | | | |
| ★ Beefy Onion | 1 tbsp | 25 | 1% | 0% | 0% |
| ★ Golden Onion | 2 tbsp | 60 | 2% | 0% | 0% |
| ★ Onion | 1 tbsp | 20 | 0% | 0% | 0% |
| ★ Onion Mushroom | 2 tbsp | 35 | 1% | 0% | 0% |

| FOOD | Serving Size | Calories | Tot Fat | Sat Fat | Chol |
|---|---|---|---|---|---|
| | | | | | |

## PEA SOUPS

### Generic Foods

| FOOD | Serving Size | Calories | Tot Fat | Sat Fat | Chol |
|---|---|---|---|---|---|
| ❖ Green Pea | 1 cup | 200 | 12% | 14% | 3% |
| ❖ Split Pea w/Ham | 1 cup | 190 | 15% | 9% | 3% |

### Brand Name Foods

| FOOD | Serving Size | Calories | Tot Fat | Sat Fat | Chol |
|---|---|---|---|---|---|
| ★ BEARITOS Homestyle Naturals Fat Free: Split Pea—LITTLE BEAR ORGANIC FOODS | 1 cup | 90 | 0% | 0% | 0% |
| CAMPBELL'S | | | | | |
| ❖ Chunky (Ready-to-Serve) Split Pea 'n Ham | 1 cup | 190 | 5% | 5% | 7% |
| ★ Healthy Request (Ready-to-Serve) Split Pea w/Ham | 1 cup | 170 | 4% | 5% | 3% |
| ★ Home Cookin' (Ready-to-Serve) Split Pea w/Ham | 1 cup | 170 | 2% | 3% | 2% |
| ★ CAMPBELL'S (Condensed) | 1/2 cup | 180 | 5% | 5% | 1% |
| ★ Green Pea | 1/2 cup | 180 | 5% | 5% | 1% |
| ❖ Split Pea w/Ham & Bacon | 1/2 cup | 180 | 5% | 10% | 1% |
| CAMPBELL'S Low Sodium (Ready-to-Serve) | | | | | |
| ❖ Green Pea | 1 cup | 160 | 6% | 10% | 2% |
| ❖ Split Pea | 1 cup | 190 | 5% | 10% | 2% |
| ★ FANTASTIC FOODS Split Pea | 1 cup | 130 | 1% | 0% | 0% |
| ★ HAIN 99% Fat Free Vegetarian Split Pea | 1 cup | 150 | 1% | 0% | 0% |
| HEALTH VALLEY Fat Free | | | | | |
| ★ Garden Split Pea w/Carrots | 1/2 cup | 130 | 0% | 0% | 0% |
| ★ Split Pea & Carrots | 1 cup | 110 | 0% | 0% | 0% |
| ★ HEALTHY CHOICE Split Pea w/Ham—CONAGRA | 1 cup | 160 | 3% | 5% | 3% |
| MANISCHEWITZ | | | | | |
| ★ Split Pea & Barley (tube style, prep as dir) | 1 cup | 110 | 0% | 0% | 0% |
| ★ Split Pea (tube style, prep as dir) | 1 cup | 140 | 0% | 0% | 0% |
| ❖ PEPPERIDGE FARM Green Pea w/Ham & Sherry Wine— CAMPBELL'S | 2/3 cup | 210 | 9% | 20% | 3% |
| PROGRESSO—PET | | | | | |
| ★ Green Split Pea | 1 cup | 170 | 5% | 5% | 1% |
| ★ Healthy Classics Split Pea | 1 cup | 180 | 4% | 4% | 2% |
| ❖ Split Pea w/Ham | 1 cup | 160 | 6% | 7% | 4% |
| ★ ULTRA SLIM-FAST Split Pea | 1 can | 230 | 4% | 5% | 2% |

★ Foods with this symbol have less than or equal to 5% *Daily Value* for <u>all</u> three nutrients (5% Rule).

❖ Foods with this symbol have <u>at least one</u> of the three nutrients greater than 5% *Daily Value* but less than or equal to 20% *Daily Value*.

Ⓐ Foods with this symbol have <u>at least one</u> of the three nutrients greater than 20% *Daily Value* (20% Rule).

| FOOD | Serving Size | Calories | Tot Fat | Sat Fat | Chol |
|------|------|------|------|------|------|
| | | | | | |

## TOMATO SOUPS

**Generic Foods**

| FOOD | Serving Size | Calories | Tot Fat | Sat Fat | Chol |
|------|------|------|------|------|------|
| ❖ Tomato | 1 cup | 130 | 9% | 9% | 6% |
| ❖ Tomato Bisque | 1 cup | 160 | 3% | 10% | 4% |
| ★ Tomato Rice (prep w/water) | 1 cup | 120 | 0% | 3% | 1% |
| ★ Tomato Vegetable | 1 cup | 60 | 1% | 2% | 0% |
| ❖ Tomato, Beef, and Noodle | 1 cup | 140 | 3% | 8% | 2% |

**Brand Name Foods**

| FOOD | Serving Size | Calories | Tot Fat | Sat Fat | Chol |
|------|------|------|------|------|------|
| CAMPBELL'S | | | | | |
| ★ _Healthy Request_ (Condensed) Tomato | 1/2 cup | 90 | 3% | 3% | 0% |
| ★ _Healthy Request_ (Ready-to-Serve) Tomato Vegetable | 1 cup | 120 | 3% | 3% | 2% |
| CAMPBELL'S (Condensed) | | | | | |
| ★ Fiesta Tomato | 1/2 cup | 60 | 0% | 0% | 0% |
| ★ Italian Tomato w/Basil & Oregano | 1/2 cup | 100 | 1% | 0% | 0% |
| ★ Old Fashioned Tomato Rice | 1/2 cup | 120 | 3% | 3% | 1% |
| ★ Tomato Soup | 1/2 cup | 100 | 3% | 0% | 0% |
| ❖ CAMPBELL'S Low Sodium (Ready-to-Serve) Tomato | 1 cup | 170 | 9% | 13% | 3% |
| ★ HEALTH VALLEY Fat Free Tomato Vegetable | 1 cup | 80 | 0% | 0% | 0% |
| ★ MANISCHEWITZ Tomato | 1/2 cup | 70 | 2% | 0% | 0% |
| ❖ PEPPERIDGE FARM Bacon, Lettuce & Tomato—CAMPBELL'S | 2/3 cup | 130 | 11% | 10% | 2% |
| PROGRESSO—PET | | | | | |
| ★ _Healthy Classics_ Tomato Garden Vegetable | 1 cup | 100 | 2% | 0% | 0% |
| ❖ Tomato Beef & Rotini | 1 cup | 140 | 7% | 7% | 8% |
| ★ Tomato Soup | 1 cup | 90 | 3% | 0% | 0% |
| PROGRESSO _Pasta Soups_—PET | | | | | |
| ★ Hearty Tomato & Rotini | 1 cup | 90 | 1% | 0% | 2% |
| ❖ Tomato Tortellini | 1 cup | 120 | 8% | 8% | 3% |
| ★ RECIPE SECRETS Mix: Italian Herb w/Tomatoes—LIPTON | 2 tbsp | 40 | 1% | 0% | 0% |

## TURKEY SOUPS

**Generic Foods**

| FOOD | Serving Size | Calories | Tot Fat | Sat Fat | Chol |
|------|------|------|------|------|------|
| ❖ Chunky Turkey | 1 cup | 140 | 0% | 6% | 3% |
| ★ Turkey Noodle | 1 cup | 70 | 0% | 3% | 2% |
| ⏀ Turkey Vegetable | 1 cup | 70 | 38% | 4% | 1% |

| FOOD | Serving Size | Calories | Tot Fat | Sat Fat | Chol |
|---|---|---|---|---|---|
| **Brand Name Foods** | | | | | |
| ★ CAMPBELL'S *Healthy Request* (Ready-to-Serve) Turkey Vegetable w/Wild Rice | 1 cup | 120 | 4% | 5% | 5% |
| CAMPBELL'S (Condensed) | | | | | |
| ★   Turkey Noodle | 1/2 cup | 80 | 4% | 5% | 5% |
| ★   Turkey Vegetable | 1/2 cup | 80 | 4% | 5% | 3% |
| ★ CAMPBELL'S Low Sodium (Ready-to-Serve) Turkey Noodle | 1 cup | 60 | 4% | 5% | 3% |
| ★ HEALTHY CHOICE Turkey w/ White & Wild Rice—CONAGRA | 1 cup | 90 | 4% | 5% | 0% |
| ❖ PEPPERIDGE FARM Hunters w/ Turkey, Beef & Burgundy— CAMPBELL'S | 2/3 cup | 130 | 9% | 5% | 5% |

### VEGETABLE SOUPS

| FOOD | Serving Size | Calories | Tot Fat | Sat Fat | Chol |
|---|---|---|---|---|---|
| **Generic Foods** | | | | | |
| ❖ Corn Chowder | 1 cup | 150 | 5% | 0% | 9% |
| ★ Vegetable Beef Soup | 1 cup | 80 | 1% | 4% | 2% |
| **Brand Name Foods** | | | | | |
| ★ BEARITOS Homestyle Fat Free Naturals: Southwest Vegetable —LITTLE BEAR ORGANIC FOODS | 1 cup | 70 | 0% | 0% | 0% |
| CAMPBELL'S *Chunky* (Ready-to-Serve) | | | | | |
| ❖   Mediterranean Vegetable | 1 cup | 140 | 7% | 8% | 2% |
| ⊛   Old Fashioned Potato Ham Chowder | 1 cup | 220 | 22% | 40% | 7% |
| ❖   Old Fashioned Vegetable | 1 cup | 150 | 8% | 8% | 5% |
| ★   Vegetable | 1 cup | 130 | 5% | 5% | 0% |
| CAMPBELL'S *Healthy Request* (Condensed) | | | | | |
| ★   Hearty Vegetable | 1/2 cup | 90 | 2% | 3% | 2% |
| ★   Vegetable | 1/2 cup | 90 | 3% | 3% | 0% |
| ★   Vegetable Beef | 1/2 cup | 80 | 3% | 5% | 2% |
| CAMPBELL'S *Healthy Request* (Ready-to-Serve) | | | | | |
| ★   Hearty Vegetable | 1 cup | 100 | 2% | 0% | 0% |
| ❖   Hearty Vegetable Beef | 1 cup | 140 | 4% | 5% | 7% |
| ★   Southwest Style Vegetable | 1 cup | 150 | 2% | 3% | 0% |

★  Foods with this symbol have less than or equal to 5% *Daily Value* for <u>all</u> three nutrients (5% Rule).
❖  Foods with this symbol have <u>at least one</u> of the three nutrients greater than 5% *Daily Value* but less than or equal to 20% *Daily Value*.
⊛  Foods with this symbol have <u>at least one</u> of the three nutrients greater than 20% *Daily Value* (20% Rule).

| FOOD | Serving Size | Calories | Tot Fat | Sat Fat | Chol |
|---|---|---|---|---|---|
| CAMPBELL'S *Home Cookin'* (Ready-to-Serve) | | | | | |
| ★ Country Vegetable | 1 cup | 110 | 2% | 0% | 2% |
| ❖ Italian Vegetable | 1 cup | 100 | 6% | 8% | 2% |
| ★ Southwestern Vegetable | 1 cup | 130 | 4% | 3% | 0% |
| ★ Vegetable Beef | 1 cup | 120 | 3% | 5% | 2% |
| ★ CAMPBELL'S *Homestyle* Vegetable | 1/2 cup | 70 | 3% | 3% | 0% |
| CAMPBELL'S (Condensed) | | | | | |
| ★ Golden Corn | 1/2 cup | 120 | 5% | 5% | 1% |
| ★ Golden Mushroom | 1/2 cup | 80 | 5% | 5% | 1% |
| ★ Hearty Vegetable w/Pasta | 1/2 cup | 90 | 2% | 0% | 0% |
| ★ Old Fashioned Vegetable | 1/2 cup | 70 | 4% | 3% | 1% |
| ★ Vegetable | 1/2 cup | 90 | 2% | 0% | 1% |
| ★ Vegetable Beef | 1/2 cup | 80 | 3% | 5% | 3% |
| ★ Vegetarian Vegetable | 1/2 cup | 70 | 2% | 0% | 0% |
| ★ CAMPBELL'S Dry Soup & Recipe Mix: Vegetable | 2 tbsp | 35 | 0% | 0% | 0% |
| ★ CAMPBELL'S Low Sodium (Ready-to-Serve) Vegetable | 1 cup | 90 | 2% | 3% | 0% |
| CAMPBELL'S Microwave (Ready-to-Serve) | | | | | |
| ★ Vegetable | 1 container | 100 | 3% | 3% | 0% |
| ★ Vegetable Beef | 1 container | 140 | 1% | 0% | 3% |
| FANTASTIC FOODS | | | | | |
| ★ Broccoli & Cheddar | 1 cup | 130 | 3% | 4% | 1% |
| ❖ Corn & Potato Chowder | 1 cup | 140 | 11% | 0% | 0% |
| ❖ Mushroom | 1 cup | 110 | 7% | 0% | 0% |
| ❖ Vegetable Barley | 1 cup | 120 | 6% | 0% | 0% |
| ❖ Vegetable Curry | 1 cup | 120 | 7% | 0% | 0% |
| ❖ Vegetable Miso | 1 cup | 110 | 10% | 0% | 0% |
| ★ Vegetable Tomato | 1 cup | 130 | 4% | 0% | 0% |
| ★ HAIN Fat Free Vegetable Broth | 1 cup | 35 | 0% | 0% | 0% |
| HEALTH VALLEY Fat Free | | | | | |
| ★ 14 Garden Vegetable | 1 cup | 80 | 0% | 0% | 0% |
| ★ Corn Chowder w/Tomatoes | 1/2 cup | 90 | 0% | 0% | 0% |
| ★ Country Corn & Vegetable | 1 cup | 70 | 0% | 0% | 0% |
| ★ Creamy Potato w/Broccoli | 1/3 cup | 70 | 0% | 0% | 0% |
| ★ Super Broccoli Carotene | 1 cup | 70 | 0% | 0% | 0% |
| ★ Vegetable Barley | 1 cup | 90 | 0% | 0% | 0% |
| ★ Vegetable Power Carotene | 1 cup | 70 | 0% | 0% | 0% |
| HEALTHY CHOICE—CONAGRA | | | | | |
| ★ Country Vegetable | 1 cup | 100 | 1% | 0% | 0% |
| ★ Garden Vegetable | 1 cup | 120 | 2% | 0% | 0% |
| ★ Tomato Garden | 1 cup | 110 | 2% | 3% | 0% |
| KNORR Mixes—CPC | | | | | |
| ★ Potato Leek | 1 pkg | 120 | 1% | 1% | 0% |
| ★ Spring Vegetable Soup & Recipe | 1/3 pkg | 25 | 0% | 0% | 0% |

| FOOD | Serving Size | Calories | Tot Fat | Sat Fat | Chol |
|---|---|---|---|---|---|
| ★ Vegetable Soup & Recipe | 1/4 pkg | 30 | 0% | 0% | 0% |
| ★ Vegetarian Vegetable Bouillon | 1/2 cube | 15 | 2% | 0% | 0% |
| MANISCHEWITZ | | | | | |
| ★ Potato (tube style, prep as dir) | 1 cup | 90 | 0% | 0% | 0% |
| ★ Vegetarian Vegetable | 1/2 cup | 70 | 2% | 0% | 0% |
| MRS. GRASS Mixes—BORDEN | | | | | |
| ★ Homestyle Recipe, Soup & Dip: | | | | | |
| Vegetable | 1/4 packet | 35 | 0% | 0% | 0% |
| ★ Onion-Mushroom Recipe Soup | 1/3 pkg | 60 | 2% | 0% | 0% |
| ★ OLD EL PASO Garden Vegetable | | | | | |
| —PET | 1 cup | 110 | 3% | 3% | 1% |
| PEPPERIDGE FARM—CAMPBELL'S | | | | | |
| ❖ Corn Chowder | 2/3 cup | 140 | 12% | 15% | 3% |
| ❖ Shiitake Mushroom | 2/3 cup | 80 | 5% | 10% | 1% |
| ❖ Watercress | 2/3 cup | 80 | 5% | 13% | 1% |
| PROGRESSO *Pasta Soups*—PET | | | | | |
| ★ Broccoli & Shells | 1 cup | 70 | 1% | 0% | 1% |
| ★ Hearty Vegetable & Rotini | 1 cup | 110 | 2% | 0% | 0% |
| PROGRESSO | | | | | |
| ⊛ Corn Chowder | 1 cup | 180 | 15% | 21% | 4% |
| ★ Escarole in Chicken Broth | 1 cup | 25 | 2% | 0% | 1% |
| ★ *Healthy Classics* Vegetable | 1 cup | 80 | 2% | 0% | 2% |
| ★ Vegetable Soup | 1 cup | 90 | 3% | 2% | 1% |
| ★ RECIPE SECRETS Vegetable Soup | | | | | |
| Mix—LIPTON | 2 tbsp | 30 | 0% | 0% | 0% |
| ★ STEERO Instant Vegetable | | | | | |
| Flavored Bouillon—BORDEN | 1 tsp | 5 | 0% | 0% | 0% |
| ★ SWANSON Vegetable Broth— | | | | | |
| CAMPBELL'S | 1 cup | 20 | 2% | 0% | 0% |
| ★ WEIGHT WATCHERS Vegetable | 1 can | 130 | 2% | 0% | 0% |
| ★ WYLER'S Instant Vegetable | | | | | |
| Flavored Bouillon—BORDEN | 1 tsp | 5 | 0% | 0% | 0% |

## OTHER SOUPS

**Generic Foods**

| | | | | | |
|---|---|---|---|---|---|
| ★ Gazpacho | 1 cup | 60 | 4% | 1% | 0% |
| ⊛ Oyster Stew (prep w/milk) | 1 cup | 130 | 3% | 25% | 11% |
| ❖ Oyster Stew (prep w/water) | 1 cup | 60 | 10% | 13% | 5% |
| ❖ Ratatouille | 1 cup | 270 | 18% | 17% | 0% |
| ❖ Vichyssoise | 1 cup | 150 | 14% | 19% | 7% |

★ Foods with this symbol have less than or equal to 5% *Daily Value* for <u>all</u> three nutrients (5% Rule).
❖ Foods with this symbol have <u>at least one</u> of the three nutrients greater than 5% *Daily Value* but less than or equal to 20% *Daily Value*.
⊛ Foods with this symbol have <u>at least one</u> of the three nutrients greater than 20% *Daily Value* (20% Rule).

| FOOD | Serving Size | Calories | Tot Fat | Sat Fat | Chol |
|------|-------------|----------|---------|---------|------|
| **Brand Name Foods** | | | | | |
| CAMPBELL'S (Condensed) | | | | | |
| ❖ Oyster Stew | 1/2 cup | 90 | 9% | 18% | 7% |
| ★ Teddy Bear Pasta Shapes | 1/2 cup | 80 | 3% | 5% | 1% |
| ★ CAMPBELL'S Ramen Noodle Soup | 1/2 pkg | 150 | 2% | 0% | 0% |
| CASBAH | | | | | |
| ❖ Jambalaya | 1 cup | 110 | 10% | 0% | 0% |
| ★ La Fiesta | 1 cup | 150 | 5% | 0% | 0% |
| ★ Pasta Fasul | 1 cup | 140 | 4% | 0% | 0% |
| ❖ Thai Yum | 1 cup | 140 | 11% | 4% | 0% |
| ★ FANTASTIC FOODS Cha Cha Chili | 1 cup | 170 | 2% | 0% | 0% |
| ★ GOLDEN DIPT Lobster Bisque | | | | | |
| Gourmet—MCCORMICK | ~ 3 tbsp mix | 70 | 3% | 5% | 4% |
| HAIN 99% Fat Free | | | | | |
| ★ Mushroom Barley | 1 cup | 80 | 2% | 0% | 1% |
| ★ Wild Rice | 1 cup | 80 | 2% | 0% | 0% |
| HEALTH VALLEY Fat Free | | | | | |
| ★ Italian Plus Carotene | 1 cup | 80 | 0% | 0% | 0% |
| ★ Pasta Italiano | 1/2 cup | 140 | 0% | 0% | 0% |
| KNORR Soup Mixes—CPC | | | | | |
| ❖ Fine Herbs Soup & Recipe Mix | 1/3 pkg | 100 | 7% | 8% | 1% |
| ★ Fish Bouillon | 1/2 cube | 10 | 2% | 0% | 0% |
| ★ Hot & Sour | 1/3 pkg | 50 | 2% | 2% | 0% |
| MANISCHEWITZ | | | | | |
| ★ Barley & Mushroom | 1/2 cup | 100 | 4% | 3% | 0% |
| ★ Noodle (tube style, prep as dir) | 1 cup | 80 | 1% | 0% | 0% |
| NISSIN *Cup Noodles* | | | | | |
| ⊛ Crab Flavor | 1 container | 290 | 19% | 32% | 0% |
| ⊛ Pork Flavor | 1 container | 290 | 18% | 30% | 1% |
| ❖ NISSIN *Top Ramen* Shrimp Flavor | 1/2 pkg | 200 | 12% | 20% | 0% |
| PEPPERIDGE FARM—CAMPBELL'S | | | | | |
| ★ Crab | 2/3 cup | 80 | 3% | 5% | 3% |
| ★ Gazpacho | 2/3 cup | 70 | 3% | 0% | 0% |
| ⊛ Lobster Bisque w/White Wine | 2/3 cup | 160 | 17% | 25% | 13% |
| ⊛ Oyster Stew | 2/3 cup | 160 | 15% | 35% | 10% |
| ★ PROGRESSO *Healthy Classics* | | | | | |
| Garlic & Pasta—PET | 1 cup | 100 | 2% | 0% | 2% |
| RECIPE SECRETS Soup Mixes—LIPTON | | | | | |
| ★ Golden Herb w/Lemon | 2 tbsp | 35 | 1% | 0% | 1% |
| ★ Savory Herb w/Garlic | 1 tbsp | 35 | 1% | 0% | 0% |
| SOUP SECRETS Soup Mixes—LIPTON | | | | | |
| ❖ Extra Noodle | 3 tbsp | 90 | 2% | 3% | 8% |
| ★ Hearty Noodle | 3 tbsp | 70 | 3% | 3% | 3% |

| FOOD | Serving Size | Calories | Tot Fat | Sat Fat | Chol |
|------|-----|----------|---------|---------|------|
| ★ Noodle | 2 tbsp | 60 | 3% | 3% | 5% |
| ★ Ruffle Pasta | 2 tbsp | 60 | 1% | 0% | 0% |

# Vegetables

## BEANS AND LEGUMES

### Generic Foods

| FOOD | Serving Size | Calories | Tot Fat | Sat Fat | Chol |
|------|-----|----------|---------|---------|------|
| ★ Baked Beans | 1/2 cup | 120 | 1% | 1% | 0% |
| ★ Black | 1/2 cup | 110 | 1% | 1% | 0% |
| ★ Cowpeas (Black-eyed Peas) | 1/2 cup | 100 | 1% | 1% | 0% |
| ★ Fava Beans | 1/2 cup | 90 | 1% | 0% | 0% |
| ❖ Frijoles Beans w/Cheese | 1 cup | 230 | 12% | 20% | 12% |
| ★ Garbanzo Beans | 1/2 cup | 80 | 2% | 1% | 0% |
| ★ Great Northern | 1/2 cup | 120 | 1% | 1% | 0% |
| ★ Kidney | 1/2 cup | 110 | 0% | 0% | 0% |
| ★ Lentils | 1/2 cup | 120 | 1% | 0% | 0% |
| ★ Lima | 1/2 cup | 100 | 0% | 0% | 0% |
| ★ Mung | 1/2 cup | 100 | 1% | 1% | 0% |
| ★ Navy | 1/2 cup | 130 | 1% | 1% | 0% |
| ★ Pinto | 1/2 cup | 110 | 1% | 0% | 0% |
| ❖ Pork & Beans | 1 cup | 270 | 6% | 8% | 6% |
| ❖ Pork & Beans in Tomato Sauce | 1 cup | 250 | 4% | 5% | 6% |
| ★ Refried Beans | 1/2 cup | 140 | 2% | 3% | 0% |
| ★ Split Peas | 1/2 cup | 120 | 1% | 0% | 0% |
| ❖ Tofu | 1/3 cup | 90 | 9% | 4% | 0% |

### Brand Name Foods

ARROWHEAD MILLS Beans (uncooked)

| FOOD | Serving Size | Calories | Tot Fat | Sat Fat | Chol |
|------|-----|----------|---------|---------|------|
| ★ Adzukis | 1/4 cup | 160 | 1% | 0% | 0% |
| ★ Garbanzos | 1/4 cup | 170 | 3% | 0% | 0% |
| ★ Kidneys | 1/4 cup | 160 | 1% | 0% | 0% |
| ★ Lentils, all colors | 1/4 cup | 150 | 0% | 0% | 0% |
| ★ Mung | 1/4 cup | 160 | 1% | 0% | 0% |
| ★ Pinto | 1/4 cup | 150 | 1% | 0% | 0% |
| ❖ Soybeans | 1/4 cup | 70 | 12% | 5% | 0% |
| ★ Split Peas | 1/4 cup | 170 | 1% | 0% | 0% |
| B & M Baked Beans—PET | | | | | |
| ★ 99% Fat Free | 1/2 cup | 160 | 1% | 1% | 0% |
| ★ Barbeque | 1/2 cup | 170 | 3% | 4% | 1% |

★ Foods with this symbol have less than or equal to 5% *Daily Value* for all three nutrients (5% Rule).
❖ Foods with this symbol have at least one of the three nutrients greater than 5% *Daily Value* but less than or equal to 20% *Daily Value.*
Ⓐ Foods with this symbol have at least one of the three nutrients greater than 20% *Daily Value* (20% Rule).

| FOOD | Serving Size | Calories | Tot Fat | Sat Fat | Chol |
|------|--------------|----------|---------|---------|------|
| ★ Brick Oven | 1/2 cup | 180 | 3% | 3% | 1% |
| ★ Extra Hearty | 1/2 cup | 190 | 3% | 4% | 1% |
| ★ Red Kidney | 1/2 cup | 170 | 3% | 3% | 1% |
| ★ With Honey | 1/2 cup | 170 | 2% | 0% | 0% |
| ★ Yellow Eye | 1/2 cup | 170 | 3% | 4% | 1% |
| BEARITOS Vegetarian Beans— LITTLE BEAR ORGANIC FOODS | | | | | |
| ★ Baked Beans, Original | 1/2 cup | 130 | 1% | 0% | 0% |
| ★ Baked Black Beans, Traditional | 1/2 cup | 110 | 1% | 0% | 0% |
| ★ Refried Black Beans, Fat Free | 1/2 cup | 80 | 0% | 0% | 0% |
| CAMPBELL'S Beans | | | | | |
| ★ Baked w/Brown Sugar & Bacon Flavor | 1/2 cup | 170 | 5% | 5% | 2% |
| ★ Barbecue w/Tangy Barbecue Flavor | 1/2 cup | 170 | 4% | 3% | 2% |
| ★ Chili in a Zesty Sauce | 1/2 cup | 130 | 5% | 5% | 3% |
| ★ Homestyle | 1/2 cup | 150 | 3% | 3% | 2% |
| ★ New England Style Baked | 1/2 cup | 180 | 5% | 5% | 2% |
| ★ Old Fashioned | 1/2 cup | 180 | 5% | 5% | 2% |
| ★ Old Fashioned Barbecue | 1/2 cup | 170 | 4% | 3% | 2% |
| ★ Old Fashioned Brown Sugar & Bacon Flavor | 1/2 cup | 170 | 5% | 5% | 2% |
| ★ Pork & Beans in Tomato Sauce | 1/2 cup | 130 | 3% | 3% | 2% |
| ★ Vegetarian in Tomato Sauce | 1/2 cup | 130 | 3% | 5% | 0% |
| ❖ DENNISON'S Lima Beans w/Ham in Sauce—AMERICAN HOME FOODS | 1/2 cup | 150 | 5% | 8% | 5% |
| FRIEND'S Baked Beans—PET | | | | | |
| ★ Original | 1/2 cup | 170 | 1% | 0% | 1% |
| ★ Red Kidney | 1/2 cup | 160 | 1% | 0% | 1% |
| GEBHARDT Beans—HUNT WESSON | | | | | |
| ★ Chili | 1/2 cup | 130 | 2% | 2% | 0% |
| ⊛ Chili w/Beans | 1 cup | 320 | 23% | 29% | 10% |
| ★ Pinto | 1/2 cup | 90 | 2% | 0% | 0% |
| GEBHARDT Refried Beans— HUNT WESSON | | | | | |
| ❖ Jalapeno | 1/2 cup | 110 | 5% | 7% | 0% |
| ❖ Traditional | 1/2 cup | 110 | 4% | 7% | 0% |
| ★ Vegetarian | 1/2 cup | 120 | 4% | 2% | 0% |
| GREEN GIANT Canned Dry Beans in Brine—PILLSBURY | | | | | |
| ★ Black Beans | 1/2 cup | 100 | 0% | 0% | 0% |
| ★ Blackeye Peas | 1/2 cup | 90 | 0% | 0% | 0% |
| ★ Butter Beans | 1/2 cup | 90 | 0% | 0% | 0% |
| ★ Garbanzo Beans | 1/2 cup | 110 | 2% | 0% | 0% |
| ★ Great Northern Beans | 1/2 cup | 100 | 1% | 0% | 0% |
| ★ Kidney Beans: Dark or Light Red | 1/2 cup | 110 | 0% | 0% | 0% |
| ★ Pinto Beans | 1/2 cup | 110 | 1% | 0% | 0% |
| ★ Red Beans | 1/2 cup | 100 | 1% | 0% | 0% |

| FOOD | Serving Size | Calories | Tot Fat | Sat Fat | Chol |
|------|------|------|------|------|------|
| ★ Spicy Chili Beans | 1/2 cup | 110 | 2% | 0% | 0% |
| GREEN GIANT Canned Dry Beans in Sauce—PILLSBURY | | | | | |
| ★ Baked Beans | 1/2 cup | 160 | 2% | 5% | 1% |
| ★ Baked Beans w/Onion | 1/2 cup | 150 | 2% | 3% | 0% |
| ★ Barbeque Beans | 1/2 cup | 140 | 1% | 0% | 0% |
| ★ Honey Bacon Flavored Beans | 1/2 cup | 160 | 1% | 0% | 0% |
| ★ Italian Beans | 1/2 cup | 130 | 2% | 0% | 0% |
| ★ Mexican Beans | 1/2 cup | 120 | 2% | 0% | 0% |
| ★ Pork & Beans w/Tomato Sauce | 1/2 cup | 120 | 2% | 0% | 0% |
| HAIN Legumes | | | | | |
| ★ Black Turtle Beans | 1/2 cup | 100 | 2% | 0% | 0% |
| ★ Chick Peas | 1/2 cup | 120 | 4% | 0% | 0% |
| ★ Dark Red Kidney Beans | 1/2 cup | 110 | 0% | 0% | 0% |
| ★ Great Northern Beans | 1/2 cup | 120 | 1% | 0% | 0% |
| ★ Pinto Beans | 1/2 cup | 110 | 2% | 0% | 0% |
| HAIN Refried Beans | | | | | |
| ★ 99% Fat Free Vegetarian Refried Black Beans | 1/2 cup | 110 | 1% | 0% | 0% |
| ★ Fat Free Vegetarian Refried Beans | 1/2 cup | 90 | 0% | 0% | 0% |
| ★ Vegetarian Refried Beans | 1/2 cup | 70 | 2% | 0% | 0% |
| ★ HARVEST FRESH Baby Lima Beans—GREEN GIANT | 1/2 cup | 80 | 0% | 0% | 0% |
| ★ HEALTH VALLEY Fat Free Honey Baked Beans, Regular or No Salt | 1/2 cup | 110 | 0% | 0% | 0% |
| ★ HEARTLAND Baked Beans—PET | 1/2 cup | 150 | 2% | 0% | 1% |
| ★ HEINZ Vegetarian Beans | 1/2 cup | 130 | 1% | 0% | 0% |
| HUNT'S Beans—HUNT WESSON | | | | | |
| ❖ Big John's Beans & Fixin's | 1/2 cup | 130 | 5% | 6% | 1% |
| ★ Chili Beans | 1/2 cup | 90 | 1% | 0% | 0% |
| ★ Kidney Beans | 1/2 cup | 90 | 1% | 0% | 0% |
| ★ Pork & Beans | 1/2 cup | 130 | 2% | 2% | 0% |
| ★ Small Red Beans | 1/2 cup | 90 | 1% | 0% | 0% |
| LAS PALMAS Refried Beans —PET | | | | | |
| ★ Refried Beans, No Fat | 1/2 cup | 110 | 0% | 0% | 0% |
| ★ Refried Beans | 1/2 cup | 110 | 3% | 4% | 0% |
| ★ Refried Black Beans | 1/2 cup | 120 | 3% | 0% | 0% |
| ⊛ LIBBY'S *Diner* Beans w/Franks —NESTLÉ | 1 container | 330 | 25% | 26% | 14% |

★  Foods with this symbol have less than or equal to 5% *Daily Value* for <u>all</u> three nutrients (5% Rule).
❖  Foods with this symbol have <u>at least one</u> of the three nutrients greater than 5% *Daily Value* but less than or equal to 20% *Daily Value*.
⊛  Foods with this symbol have <u>at least one</u> of the three nutrients greater than 20% *Daily Value* (20% Rule).

| | | | | % DAILY VALUE | | |
| FOOD | Serving Size | Calories | Tot Fat | Sat Fat | Chol |
| --- | --- | --- | --- | --- | --- |
| LUCK'S Pork & Beans | | | | | |
| ★ In Tomato Sauce | 1 cup | 240 | 3% | 1% | 0% |
| ❖ Kidney | 1 cup | 240 | 11% | 13% | 5% |
| ❖ Northern | 1 cup | 230 | 8% | 10% | 3% |
| ❖ Pinto | 1 cup | 200 | 6% | 8% | 0% |
| ❖ w/Limas | 1 cup | 240 | 8% | 2% | 0% |
| ★ MORINU Tofu Silken: All varieties | 1/2 cup | 40 | 3% | 1% | 0% |
| ❖ OLD EL PASO Chili w/Beans —PET | 1 cup | 200 | 11% | 8% | 10% |
| OLD EL PASO Beans—PET | | | | | |
| ★ Black | 1/2 cup | 100 | 2% | 0% | 0% |
| ★ Garbanzo | 1/2 cup | 120 | 4% | 0% | 0% |
| ★ Mexe | 1/2 cup | 110 | 1% | 0% | 0% |
| ★ Pinto | 1/2 cup | 110 | 1% | 0% | 0% |
| ★ Refried | 1/2 cup | 110 | 3% | 4% | 1% |
| ★ Refried, Fat Free | 1/2 cup | 110 | 0% | 0% | 0% |
| ❖ Refried Beans & Cheese | 1/2 cup | 130 | 5% | 8% | 1% |
| ★ Refried Black | 1/2 cup | 120 | 3% | 0% | 0% |
| ★ Refried w/Green Chilies | 1/2 cup | 110 | 1% | 0% | 1% |
| Ⓐ Refried w/Sausage | 1/2 cup | 200 | 20% | 25% | 4% |
| ❖ Spicy Refried | 1/2 cup | 140 | 5% | 7% | 1% |
| ★ Vegetarian Refried | 1/2 cup | 100 | 1% | 0% | 0% |
| PROGRESSO Beans—PET | | | | | |
| ★ Black | 1/2 cup | 100 | 2% | 0% | 0% |
| ★ Cannellini | 1/2 cup | 100 | 1% | 0% | 0% |
| ★ Chick Peas | 1/2 cup | 120 | 4% | 0% | 0% |
| ★ Fava | 1/2 cup | 110 | 1% | 0% | 0% |
| ★ Pinto | 1/2 cup | 110 | 2% | 0% | 0% |
| ★ Red Kidney | 1/2 cup | 110 | 1% | 0% | 0% |
| ROSARITA Refried Beans—HUNT WESSON | | | | | |
| ❖ Bacon | 1/2 cup | 120 | 5% | 6% | 0% |
| ❖ Green Chile | 1/2 cup | 110 | 4% | 9% | 0% |
| ★ Black Beans, Low Fat | 1/2 cup | 110 | 1% | 0% | 0% |
| ❖ Nacho Cheese | 1/2 cup | 140 | 5% | 9% | 0% |
| ❖ Onion | 1/2 cup | 110 | 4% | 7% | 0% |
| ❖ Spicy | 1/2 cup | 120 | 4% | 6% | 0% |
| ❖ Traditional | 1/2 cup | 130 | 4% | 6% | 0% |
| ★ Vegetarian | 1/2 cup | 120 | 3% | 2% | 0% |
| ROSARITA Refried Beans, No Fat —HUNT WESSON | | | | | |
| ★ w/Green Chiles & Lime | 1/2 cup | 100 | 0% | 0% | 0% |
| ★ w/Zesty Salsa | 1/2 cup | 100 | 0% | 0% | 0% |
| S & W Baked Beans | | | | | |
| ★ Brick Oven | 1/2 cup | 160 | 1% | 0% | 0% |
| ★ Honey Mustard | 1/2 cup | 130 | 0% | 0% | 0% |
| ★ Maple Sugar | 1/2 cup | 150 | 1% | 0% | 0% |

| FOOD | Serving Size | Calories | Tot Fat | Sat Fat | Chol |
|------|------|------|------|------|------|
| ★ Sweet Bacon | 1/2 cup | 140 | 2% | 3% | 0% |
| ★ Texas Style Barbecue | 1/2 cup | 140 | 2% | 3% | 0% |
| S & W Beans | | | | | |
| ★ Black Beans, Regular or 50% Less Salt | 1/2 cup | 70 | 0% | 0% | 0% |
| ★ Butter Beans | 1/2 cup | 70 | 0% | 0% | 0% |
| ★ Cajun Style Beans | 1/2 cup | 80 | 3% | 0% | 0% |
| ★ Chili Beans | 1/2 cup | 110 | 2% | 0% | 0% |
| ★ Hot Chipotle Chili Beans | 1/2 cup | 90 | 0% | 0% | 0% |
| ★ Pinquitos | 1/2 cup | 80 | 1% | 0% | 0% |
| ★ Small White Beans | 1/2 cup | 80 | 1% | 0% | 0% |
| ❖ Smokey Ranch Beans | 1/2 cup | 110 | 4% | 6% | 0% |
| ★ Texas Style Chili Makin's | 1/2 cup | 80 | 1% | 0% | 0% |
| SUN LUCK Tofu | | | | | |
| ★ Firm | 3 oz | 60 | 5% | 0% | 0% |
| ★ Soft | 3 oz | 45 | 4% | 0% | 0% |
| ★ Traditional | 3 oz | 60 | 4% | 3% | 0% |
| VAN CAMP'S Pork & Beans— STOKELY-VANCAMP | | | | | |
| ★ Fat Free | 1/2 cup | 130 | 0% | 0% | 0% |
| ★ Regular | 1/2 cup | 110 | 2% | 2% | 0% |
| WESTBRAE NATURAL Fat Free Organic Beans | | | | | |
| ★ Black Beans | 1/2 cup | 90 | 0% | 0% | 0% |
| ★ Great Northern Beans | 1/2 cup | 90 | 0% | 0% | 0% |
| ★ Kidney Beans | 1/2 cup | 80 | 0% | 0% | 0% |
| ★ Pinto Beans | 1/2 cup | 90 | 0% | 0% | 0% |
| ★ Red Beans | 1/2 cup | 90 | 0% | 0% | 0% |
| ★ WESTBRAE NATURAL Low Fat Organic Garbanzo Beans | 1/2 cup | 110 | 3% | 0% | 0% |
| WHITE WAVE Tempeh | | | | | |
| ❖ Five Grain | 3 oz | 140 | 6% | 3% | 0% |
| ❖ Original | 3 oz | 150 | 9% | 5% | 0% |
| ★ Sea Vegetable | 3 oz | 120 | 5% | 0% | 0% |
| ❖ Soy Rice | 3 oz | 140 | 8% | 4% | 0% |
| ❖ Soybean | 1/2 cup | 170 | 10% | 5% | 0% |
| ❖ Wild Rice | 3 oz | 140 | 6% | 3% | 0% |
| ❖ WHITE WAVE Reduced Fat Tofu | 1/3 cup | 90 | 6% | 0% | 0% |

## CANNED VEGETABLES

### Generic Foods

| FOOD | Serving Size | Calories | Tot Fat | Sat Fat | Chol |
|------|------|------|------|------|------|
| ★ Bamboo Shoots (drained) | 2/3 cup | 20 | 1% | 0% | 0% |
| ❖ Candied Sweet Potato | 1/2 cup | 150 | 5% | 7% | 0% |

★ Foods with this symbol have less than or equal to 5% *Daily Value* for all three nutrients (5% Rule).

❖ Foods with this symbol have at least one of the three nutrients greater than 5% *Daily Value* but less than or equal to 20% *Daily Value*.

Ⓐ Foods with this symbol have at least one of the three nutrients greater than 20% *Daily Value* (20% Rule).

| FOOD | Serving Size | Calories | Tot Fat | Sat Fat | Chol |
|---|---|---|---|---|---|
| ★ New Potato | 4 potatoes | 80 | 0% | 0% | 0% |
| ★ Pickled Beets | 1/2 cup | 80 | 0% | 0% | 0% |
| ★ Water Chestnuts | 2/3 cup | 50 | 0% | 0% | 0% |

**Brand Name Foods**

CONTADINA Tomatoes—NESTLÉ
| | | | | | |
|---|---|---|---|---|---|
| ★ Crushed Tomatoes | 1/4 cup | 20 | 0% | 0% | 0% |
| ★ Italian Style Pear Tomatoes | 1/2 cup | 25 | 0% | 0% | 0% |
| ★ Italian Style Stewed Tomatoes | 1/2 cup | 40 | 0% | 0% | 0% |
| ★ Mexican Style Stewed Tomatoes | 1/2 cup | 40 | 0% | 0% | 0% |
| ★ Peeled Whole Tomatoes | 1/2 cup | 25 | 0% | 0% | 0% |
| ★ *Recipe Ready* Tomatoes | 1/2 cup | 25 | 0% | 0% | 0% |
| ★ Stewed Tomatoes | 1/2 cup | 40 | 0% | 0% | 0% |

DEL MONTE Corn, Cream Style
| | | | | | |
|---|---|---|---|---|---|
| ★ Golden | 1/2 cup | 90 | 1% | 0% | 0% |
| ★ Golden Supersweet | 1/2 cup | 60 | 1% | 0% | 0% |
| ★ White | 1/2 cup | 100 | 0% | 0% | 0% |

DEL MONTE Corn, Whole Kernel
| | | | | | |
|---|---|---|---|---|---|
| ★ Golden | 1/2 cup | 90 | 2% | 0% | 0% |
| ★ Golden Supersweet | 1/2 cup | 60 | 2% | 0% | 0% |
| ★ White | 1/2 cup | 80 | 0% | 0% | 0% |

DEL MONTE Stewed Tomatoes
| | | | | | |
|---|---|---|---|---|---|
| ★ Cajun Style | 1/2 cup | 35 | 0% | 0% | 0% |
| ★ Chunky Chili | 1/2 cup | 30 | 0% | 0% | 0% |
| ★ Chunky Pasta | 1/2 cup | 45 | 0% | 0% | 0% |
| ★ Chunky Salsa | 1/2 cup | 35 | 0% | 0% | 0% |
| ★ Italian Style | 1/2 cup | 30 | 0% | 0% | 0% |
| ★ Mexican Style | 1/2 cup | 35 | 0% | 0% | 0% |
| ★ Original Style: Regular or No Salt Added | 1/2 cup | 35 | 0% | 0% | 0% |

DEL MONTE Tomatoes
| | | | | | |
|---|---|---|---|---|---|
| ★ Diced or whole | 1/2 cup | 25 | 0% | 0% | 0% |
| ★ Wedges | 1/2 cup | 35 | 0% | 0% | 0% |

DEL MONTE Vegetables
| | | | | | |
|---|---|---|---|---|---|
| ★ Asparagus (tips or spears) | 1/2 cup | 20 | 0% | 0% | 0% |
| ★ Beets, Pickled | 1/2 cup | 80 | 0% | 0% | 0% |
| ★ Beets (sliced or whole) | 1/2 cup | 35 | 0% | 0% | 0% |
| ★ Carrots (sliced) | 1/2 cup | 35 | 0% | 0% | 0% |
| ★ Green Beans (cut, French Style or whole) | 1/2 cup | 20 | 0% | 0% | 0% |
| ★ Italian Beans | 1/2 cup | 30 | 0% | 0% | 0% |
| ★ Mixed Vegetables | 1/2 cup | 40 | 0% | 0% | 0% |
| ★ New Potatoes (sliced) | 2/3 cup | 60 | 0% | 0% | 0% |
| ★ Peas | 1/2 cup | 60 | 0% | 0% | 0% |
| ★ Peas & Carrots | 1/2 cup | 60 | 0% | 0% | 0% |
| ★ Spinach (chopped or whole leaf) | 1/2 cup | 30 | 0% | 0% | 0% |
| ★ Wax Beans | 1/2 cup | 20 | 0% | 0% | 0% |

| FOOD | Serving Size | Calories | Tot Fat | Sat Fat | Chol |
|------|------|------|------|------|------|
| ★ Zucchini w/Italian Style Tomato Sauce | 1/2 cup | 30 | 0% | 0% | 0% |
| HUNT'S Tomatoes—HUNT WESSON | | | | | |
| ★ Angela Mia Crushed | 1/2 cup | 30 | 0% | 0% | 0% |
| ★ Choice Cut Tomatoes | 1/2 cup | 20 | 0% | 0% | 0% |
| ★ Stewed | 1/2 cup | 30 | 0% | 0% | 0% |
| ★ Whole: Regular or No Salt Added | 2 each | 20 | 0% | 0% | 0% |
| LA CHOY Vegetables—HUNT WESSON | | | | | |
| ★ Bamboo Shoots | 2 tbsp | 5 | 0% | 0% | 0% |
| ★ Bean Sprouts | 1 cup | 10 | 0% | 0% | 0% |
| ★ Chinese Mixed Vegetables | 2/3 cup | 10 | 0% | 0% | 0% |
| ★ Chop Suey Vegetables | 1/2 cup | 15 | 0% | 0% | 0% |
| ★ Water Chestnuts (sliced or whole) | 2 tbsp; 2 whole | 10 | 0% | 0% | 0% |
| ★ LIBBY'S Pumpkin—NESTLÉ | 1/2 cup | 60 | 1% | 0% | 0% |
| PROGRESSO—PET | | | | | |
| ★ Artichoke Hearts | 2 pieces | 35 | 0% | 0% | 0% |
| ★ Italian Style Zucchini | 1/2 cup | 40 | 3% | 0% | 0% |
| SUN LUCK Vegetables | | | | | |
| ★ Baby Sweet Corn | 1/4 cup | 5 | 0% | 0% | 0% |
| ★ Bamboo Shoots (sliced, whole or chunks) | 1/4 cup | 5 | 0% | 0% | 0% |
| ★ Stir-Fry Vegetables | 1/4 cup | 20 | 0% | 0% | 0% |
| ★ Straw Mushroom | 1/4 cup | 20 | 0% | 0% | 0% |
| ★ Straw Mushroom, Stir-Fry | 1/4 cup | 20 | 0% | 0% | 0% |
| ★ Water Chestnut (whole or sliced) | 1/4 cup | 15 | 0% | 0% | 0% |

## DRIED VEGETABLES

**Generic Foods**

| FOOD | Serving Size | Calories | Tot Fat | Sat Fat | Chol |
|------|------|------|------|------|------|
| ★ Tomato, Sun Dried | 1/3 cup | 45 | 1% | 0% | 0% |
| ❖ Tomato, Sun Dried (packed in vegetable oil, drained) | 1/3 cup | 80 | 8% | 3% | 0% |

**Brand Name Foods**

| FOOD | Serving Size | Calories | Tot Fat | Sat Fat | Chol |
|------|------|------|------|------|------|
| SUN LUCK | | | | | |
| ★ Dried Seaweed Hoshi Nori | 1 sheet | 10 | 0% | 0% | 0% |
| ★ Forest Mushroom Shiitake | 1/2 cup (dry) | 0 | 0% | 0% | 0% |

★ Foods with this symbol have less than or equal to 5% *Daily Value* for <u>all</u> three nutrients (5% Rule).
❖ Foods with this symbol have <u>at least one</u> of the three nutrients greater than 5% *Daily Value* but less than or equal to 20% *Daily Value*.
Ⓐ Foods with this symbol have <u>at least one</u> of the three nutrients greater than 20% *Daily Value* (20% Rule).

| FOOD | Serving Size | Calories | Tot Fat | Sat Fat | Chol |
|------|--------------|----------|---------|---------|------|

## FRESH VEGETABLES

*Note:* *% Daily Values for raw vegetables unless otherwise noted.*

**Generic Foods**

| FOOD | Serving Size | Calories | Tot Fat | Sat Fat | Chol |
|------|--------------|----------|---------|---------|------|
| ★ Acorn Squash (baked) | 2/3 cup | 80 | 0% | 0% | 0% |
| ★ Artichoke (boiled) | 1 choke | 60 | 0% | 0% | 0% |
| ★ Artichoke Hearts (boiled) | 1/2 cup | 40 | 0% | 0% | 0% |
| ★ Asparagus | 2/3 cup | 20 | 0% | 0% | 0% |
| ❖ Avocado | 1 oz | 50 | 8% | 4% | 0% |
| ★ Bean Sprouts, Mung | 3/4 cup | 25 | 0% | 0% | 0% |
| ❖ Bean Sprouts, Soybeans | 1 1/4 cups | 110 | 9% | 4% | 0% |
| ★ Beets | 1/2 cup | 30 | 0% | 0% | 0% |
| ★ Bell Pepper | 1/2 pepper | 20 | 0% | 0% | 0% |
| ★ Broccoli | 1 cup | 25 | 0% | 0% | 0% |
| ★ Brussels Sprouts | 1/2 cup | 40 | 0% | 0% | 0% |
| ★ Butternut Squash (baked) | 2/3 cup | 60 | 0% | 0% | 0% |
| ★ Cabbage: Green, Red, or Savoy | 1 1/4 cups | 25 | 0% | 0% | 0% |
| ★ Carrots, Baby (2 3/4") | 9 carrots | 35 | 1% | 0% | 0% |
| ★ Carrots, shredded | 1/2 cup | 45 | 0% | 0% | 0% |
| ★ Cauliflower | 1/2 cup | 20 | 0% | 0% | 0% |
| ★ Celery Stalk | 2 stalks | 15 | 0% | 0% | 0% |
| ★ Corn | 1 ear; 1/2 cup | 90 | 1% | 0% | 0% |
| ★ Cucumber, sliced | 3/4 cup | 10 | 0% | 0% | 0% |
| ★ Eggplant | 1 cup | 20 | 0% | 0% | 0% |
| ★ Endive, chopped | 1 3/4 cups | 15 | 0% | 0% | 0% |
| ★ Fennel Bulb | 1 cup | 30 | 0% | 0% | 0% |
| ★ Green Beans | 2/3 cup | 25 | 0% | 0% | 0% |
| ★ Green Onions | 6 onions | 10 | 0% | 0% | 0% |
| ★ Green Peas | 1/2 cup | 60 | 0% | 0% | 0% |
| ★ Hubbard Squash (boiled and mashed) | 2/3 cup | 50 | 1% | 1% | 0% |
| ★ Jerusalem Artichokes | 1/2 cup | 60 | 0% | 0% | 0% |
| ★ Kale | 2/3 cup | 25 | 1% | 0% | 0% |
| ★ Kohlrabi | 2/3 cup | 25 | 0% | 0% | 0% |
| ★ Lentils, sprouted | 1 cup | 80 | 1% | 0% | 0% |
| ★ Lettuce, Butterhead | 6 leaves | 15 | 0% | 0% | 0% |
| ★ Lettuce, Iceberg | 4 leaves; 1 1/2 cups (chopped) | 10 | 0% | 0% | 0% |
| ★ Lettuce, Romaine, shredded | 1 1/2 cups | 15 | 0% | 0% | 0% |
| ★ Mushrooms, chopped | 1 1/4 cups | 20 | 1% | 0% | 0% |
| ★ Okra | 1/2 cup | 25 | 0% | 0% | 0% |
| ★ Onions, chopped | 1/2 cup | 30 | 0% | 0% | 0% |
| ★ Parsley | 1 tbsp | 2 | 1% | 0% | 0% |
| ★ Parsnips | 1/2 cup | 60 | 0% | 0% | 0% |
| ★ Pumpkin (boiled and mashed) | 1/2 cup | 25 | 0% | 1% | 0% |
| ★ Radishes | 7 radishes | 5 | 0% | 0% | 0% |

| FOOD | Serving Size | Calories | Tot Fat | Sat Fat | Chol |
|---|---|---|---|---|---|
| ★ Rutabagas | 2/3 cup | 35 | 0% | 0% | 0% |
| ★ Snow Peas | 1/2 cup | 35 | 0% | 0% | 0% |
| ★ Spinach, chopped | 1 1/2 cups | 20 | 0% | 0% | 0% |
| ★ Swiss Chard | 2 cups | 15 | 0% | 0% | 0% |
| ★ Tomatillo | 3 tomatillos | 30 | 2% | 0% | 0% |
| ★ Tomatoes | 1 tomato | 25 | 1% | 0% | 0% |
| ★ Turnip Greens | 1/2 cup | 15 | 0% | 0% | 0% |
| ★ Turnips | 2/3 cup | 20 | 0% | 0% | 0% |
| ★ Water Chestnuts | 2/3 cup | 90 | 0% | 0% | 0% |
| ★ Yellow Squash | 1/2 cup | 20 | 0% | 0% | 0% |
| ★ Yellow Wax Beans | 2/3 cup | 25 | 0% | 0% | 0% |
| ★ Zucchini, sliced | 1/2 cup | 20 | 0% | 0% | 0% |

**Brand Name Foods**

| | | | | | |
|---|---|---|---|---|---|
| ★ DOLE Almondine Style Green Beans | 3 oz | 40 | 4% | 0% | 0% |
| DOLE Salad Blend Mix | | | | | |
| ★ Classic | 3.5 oz | 25 | 2% | 0% | 0% |
| ★ Coleslaw | 3.5 oz | 30 | 1% | 0% | 0% |
| ★ French | 3.5 oz | 25 | 1% | 0% | 0% |
| ★ Italian | 3.5 oz | 25 | 2% | 0% | 0% |
| DOLE Salad-In-A-Minute | | | | | |
| ⊛ Caesar | 3.5 oz | 170 | 22% | 8% | 2% |
| ❖ Oriental | 3.5 oz | 110 | 11% | 5% | 0% |
| ❖ Spinach | 3.5 oz | 180 | 14% | 8% | 0% |
| DOLE Vegetable Combinations | | | | | |
| ★ California Style | 3 oz | 30 | 2% | 0% | 0% |
| ★ Garden Style | 3 oz | 30 | 1% | 0% | 0% |
| ★ Italian Style | 3 oz | 25 | 1% | 0% | 0% |
| ★ New England Mix | 3 oz | 50 | 1% | 0% | 0% |
| ★ Oriental Style | 3 oz | 30 | 1% | 0% | 0% |

## FROZEN VEGETABLES

**Brand Name Foods**

AMERICAN MIXTURES—GREEN
GIANT

| | | | | | |
|---|---|---|---|---|---|
| ★ California Style | 3/4 cup | 25 | 0% | 0% | 0% |
| ★ Heartland Style | 1 cup | 30 | 0% | 0% | 0% |
| ★ Manhattan Style | 1 cup | 25 | 0% | 0% | 0% |
| ★ New England | 2/3 cup | 70 | 2% | 0% | 0% |
| ★ San Francisco Style | 3/4 cup | 30 | 0% | 0% | 0% |
| ★ Sante Fe | 3/4 cup | 60 | 0% | 0% | 0% |
| ★ Seattle Style | 3/4 cup | 25 | 0% | 0% | 0% |

★ Foods with this symbol have less than or equal to 5% *Daily Value* for <u>all</u> three nutrients (5% Rule).
❖ Foods with this symbol have <u>at least one</u> of the three nutrients greater than 5% *Daily Value* but less than or equal to 20% *Daily Value.*
⊛ Foods with this symbol have <u>at least one</u> of the three nutrients greater than 20% *Daily Value* (20% Rule).

| FOOD | Serving Size | Calories | Tot Fat | Sat Fat | Chol |
|------|--------------|----------|---------|---------|------|
| ★ Western Style | 3/4 cup | 50 | 2% | 0% | 0% |
| HARVEST FRESH—GREEN GIANT | | | | | |
| ★ Asparagus Cuts | 2/3 cup | 25 | 0% | 0% | 0% |
| ★ Baby Cut Carrots | 2/3 cup | 20 | 0% | 0% | 0% |
| ★ Broccoli Spears | 3.5 oz | 25 | 0% | 0% | 0% |
| ★ Broccoli, Cauliflower & Carrots | 1 cup | 30 | 0% | 0% | 0% |
| ★ Cut Broccoli | 2/3 cup | 25 | 0% | 0% | 0% |
| ★ Cut Green Beans | 2/3 cup | 25 | 0% | 0% | 0% |
| ★ Green Beans & Almonds | 2/3 cup | 60 | 5% | 0% | 0% |
| ★ *LaSueur* Baby Early Peas | 2/3 cup | 70 | 0% | 0% | 0% |
| ★ Mixed Vegetables | 2/3 cup | 50 | 0% | 0% | 0% |
| ★ *Niblets* Corn | 2/3 cup | 80 | 1% | 0% | 0% |
| ★ Shoepeg White Corn | 1/2 cup | 70 | 1% | 0% | 0% |
| ★ Spinach | 1/2 cup | 25 | 0% | 0% | 0% |
| ★ Sugar Snap Peas | 2/3 cup | 50 | 0% | 0% | 0% |
| ★ Sweet Peas | 2/3 cup | 60 | 0% | 0% | 0% |
| ★ Sweet Peas & Pearl Onions | 1/2 cup | 50 | 0% | 0% | 0% |
| MRS. PAUL'S—CAMPBELL'S | | | | | |
| ❖ Corn Fritters | 1 fritter | 130 | 11% | 10% | 2% |
| ⓐ Eggplant Parmigiana | 1/2 cup | 220 | 22% | 20% | 3% |
| ❖ Old Fashioned Onion Rings | 7 rings | 230 | 18% | 13% | 0% |
| ORE-IDA—HEINZ | | | | | |
| ★ Chopped Onions | 3/4 cup | 25 | 0% | 0% | 0% |
| ★ Cob Corn | 1 ear | 180 | 4% | 0% | 0% |
| ★ Mini-Gold Cob Corn | 1 ear | 90 | 2% | 0% | 0% |
| ⓐ Onion Ringers | 6 rings | 240 | 22% | 13% | 0% |
| ★ Stew Vegetables | 2/3 cup | 50 | 0% | 0% | 0% |

## FROZEN VEGETABLE SIDE DISHES

**Brand Name Foods**

| FOOD | Serving Size | Calories | Tot Fat | Sat Fat | Chol |
|------|--------------|----------|---------|---------|------|
| BIRDS EYE *International Recipe* Vegetables—DEAN FOODS | | | | | |
| ❖ Austrian Style | 1/2 cup | 110 | 9% | 16% | 6% |
| ⓐ Bavarian Style | 1 cup | 160 | 12% | 22% | 16% |
| ❖ Italian Style | 1 cup | 140 | 14% | 19% | 5% |
| BIRDS EYE *With Butter Sauce*—DEAN FOODS | | | | | |
| ❖ Tender Sweet Corn | 1/2 cup | 110 | 4% | 7% | 2% |
| ❖ Tender Sweet Peas | 1/2 cup | 90 | 3% | 6% | 2% |
| BIRDS EYE *With Cheese Sauce*—DEAN FOODS | | | | | |
| ❖ Broccoli | 1/2 cup | 70 | 5% | 8% | 3% |
| ❖ Broccoli, Cauliflower & Carrots | 1/2 cup | 60 | 4% | 6% | 2% |
| ❖ Cauliflower | 1/2 cup | 60 | 4% | 7% | 2% |
| BIRDS EYE *With Cream Sauce*—DEAN FOODS | | | | | |
| ★ Peas & Potatoes | 1/2 cup | 70 | 3% | 4% | 1% |

| FOOD | Serving Size | Calories | Tot Fat | Sat Fat | Chol |
|------|-------------|----------|---------|---------|------|
| ★ Small Onions | 1/2 cup | 60 | 3% | 5% | 1% |
| BUDGET GOURMET *Side Dishes*— | | | | | |
| ALL AMERICAN GOURMET | | | | | |
| ❖ Mandarin Vegetables | 1 pkg | 180 | 20% | 15% | 3% |
| Ⓐ New England Recipe Vegetables | 1 pkg | 240 | 24% | 33% | 8% |
| Ⓐ Spinach Au Gratin | 1 pkg | 150 | 17% | 33% | 11% |
| Ⓐ Spring Vegetables in Cheese Sauce | 1 pkg | 150 | 15% | 25% | 8% |
| GREEN GIANT Butter Sauce | | | | | |
| Vegetables—PILLSBURY | | | | | |
| ❖ Baby Brussels Sprouts | 2/3 cup | 60 | 2% | 8% | 1% |
| ❖ Baby Lima Beans | 2/3 cup | 120 | 4% | 10% | 1% |
| ★ Broccoli Spears | 4 oz | 50 | 2% | 5% | 1% |
| ❖ Broccoli, Cauliflower, Carrots, | | | | | |
| Corn & Sweet Peas | 3/4 cup | 60 | 3% | 8% | 1% |
| ❖ Broccoli, Pasta, Sweet Peas, Corn | | | | | |
| & Red Peppers | 3/4 cup | 70 | 3% | 8% | 1% |
| ★ Cut Leaf Spinach | 1/2 cup | 40 | 2% | 5% | 1% |
| ❖ *LeSueur* Baby Early Peas | 3/4 cup | 100 | 3% | 8% | 1% |
| ★ Mixed Vegetables | 3/4 cup | 70 | 3% | 5% | 1% |
| ❖ *Niblets* Corn | 2/3 cup | 130 | 5% | 8% | 1% |
| ❖ Shoepeg White Corn | 3/4 cup | 120 | 4% | 8% | 1% |
| ❖ Sweet Peas | 3/4 cup | 100 | 3% | 8% | 1% |
| GREEN GIANT Cheese Flavored | | | | | |
| Sauce Vegetables—PILLSBURY | | | | | |
| ★ Broccoli | 2/3 cup | 70 | 4% | 5% | 1% |
| ❖ Broccoli, Cauliflower, & Carrots | 2/3 cup | 80 | 4% | 8% | 1% |
| ★ Cauliflower | 1/2 cup | 60 | 4% | 3% | 1% |
| GREEN GIANT Cream Sauce | | | | | |
| Vegetables—PILLSBURY | | | | | |
| ★ Cream Style Corn | 1/2 cup | 110 | 2% | 0% | 0% |
| ❖ Creamed Spinach | 1/2 cup | 80 | 5% | 8% | 0% |
| INTERNATIONAL MIXTURES— | | | | | |
| GREEN GIANT | | | | | |
| ❖ English Style Cheddar | 4 oz | 120 | 8% | 10% | 2% |
| ❖ French Style Garlic Dijon | 4 oz | 60 | 5% | 10% | 3% |
| ❖ Italian Style Parmesan | 4 oz | 70 | 4% | 8% | 2% |
| ★ Japanese Style Teriyaki | 4 oz | 50 | 0% | 0% | 0% |
| ❖ Normandy Style Mushroom | 4 oz | 80 | 5% | 10% | 3% |
| ★ Oriental Style Rice | 8 oz | 180 | 1% | 0% | 0% |
| STOUFFER'S Side Dishes—NESTLÉ | | | | | |
| Ⓐ Corn Soufflé | ~ 1/2 cup | 170 | 11% | 8% | 22% |
| ❖ Creamed Spinach | ~ 1/2 cup | 150 | 18% | 20% | 5% |
| ❖ Green Bean Mushroom Casserole | ~ 1/2 cup | 130 | 12% | 10% | 3% |
| Ⓐ Spinach Soufflé | ~ 1/2 cup | 150 | 15% | 10% | 40% |

★ Foods with this symbol have less than or equal to 5% *Daily Value* for all three nutrients (5% Rule).

❖ Foods with this symbol have at least one of the three nutrients greater than 5% *Daily Value* but less than or equal to 20% *Daily Value*.

Ⓐ Foods with this symbol have at least one of the three nutrients greater than 20% *Daily Value* (20% Rule).

| FOOD | Serving Size | Calories | Tot Fat | Sat Fat | Chol |
|---|---|---|---|---|---|
| ❖ Welsh Rarebit | ~ 1/4 cup | 120 | 14% | 20% | 7% |
| TAJ Vegetable Dishes | | | | | |
| ❖ Asparagus & Baby Carrots Curry | 12 oz | 380 | 20% | 5% | 0% |
| ❖ Eggplant Bhartha | 1 pkg | 300 | 15% | 5% | 0% |
| ❖ Mushrooms & Green Peas Curry | 12 oz | 390 | 20% | 5% | 0% |

POTATOES

### Fresh Prepared Potatoes

**Generic Foods**

| FOOD | Serving Size | Calories | Tot Fat | Sat Fat | Chol |
|---|---|---|---|---|---|
| ❖ French Fries | 1 1/4 cups | 200 | 14% | 15% | 0% |
| ★ Mashed Potatoes | 2/3 cup | 120 | 5% | 5% | 1% |
| ★ Potato (baked or boiled w/flesh and skin) | 1/2 potato | 110 | 0% | 0% | 0% |
| Ⓐ Potato au Gratin | 1 cup | 320 | 29% | 58% | 19% |
| ❖ Potato Hash | 1/2 cup | 150 | 15% | 19% | 0% |
| ❖ Potato Hush Puppies | 3 pcs | 220 | 14% | 7% | 10% |
| Ⓐ Potato Pancakes | 2 pancakes | 200 | 17% | 11% | 23% |
| Ⓐ Scalloped Potatoes | 1 cup | 210 | 14% | 28% | 10% |
| ★ Sweet Potato (baked or boiled) | 1 whole | 120 | 0% | 0% | 0% |
| ★ Yams (baked or broiled) | 1 whole | 160 | 0% | 0% | 0% |

### Frozen Potatoes

**Brand Name Foods**

| FOOD | Serving Size | Calories | Tot Fat | Sat Fat | Chol |
|---|---|---|---|---|---|
| ACT II Microwave French Fries (3.1 oz)—GOLDEN VALLEY | | | | | |
| ❖ Original/Regular Flavor | 1 box | 220 | 18% | 13% | 0% |
| ❖ Sour Cream/Chives Flavor | 1 box | 240 | 18% | 13% | 0% |
| ❖ Zesty Flavor | 1 box | 240 | 18% | 13% | 0% |
| Ⓐ BUDGET GOURMET Light & Healthy Entrées Baked Potato w/Broccoli & Cheese—ALL AMERICAN GOURMET | 10.5 oz | 270 | 12% | 25% | 8% |
| BUDGET GOURMET Side Dishes —ALL AMERICAN GOURMET | | | | | |
| Ⓐ Cheddared Potatoes | 5.5 oz | 260 | 26% | 45% | 13% |
| Ⓐ Cheddared Potatoes & Broccoli | 5.25 oz | 170 | 13% | 30% | 9% |
| Ⓐ Three Cheese Potatoes | 6.125 oz | 230 | 19% | 34% | 11% |
| HEALTHY CHOICE Entrées— CONAGRA | | | | | |
| ❖ Cheddar Broccoli Potatoes | 1 meal | 310 | 7% | 10% | 4% |
| ❖ Garden Potato Casserole | 1 meal | 200 | 6% | 6% | 3% |
| LYNDEN FARMS Potatoes—NESTLÉ | | | | | |
| ❖ Crinkle Fries | 3 oz | 120 | 7% | 9% | 1% |
| ❖ French Fries | 3 oz | 120 | 6% | 7% | 1% |
| ❖ Hash Brown Patties | 1 patty | 110 | 13% | 13% | 3% |

| FOOD | Serving Size | Calories | Tot Fat | Sat Fat | Chol |
|------|--------------|----------|---------|---------|------|
| ❖ Hash Brown Potatoes | 2/3 cup | 150 | 10% | 15% | 2% |
| ❖ Shoestring Fries | 3 oz | 140 | 9% | 7% | 1% |
| ❖ Spuds w/Skins | 3 oz | 130 | 7% | 7% | 1% |
| ❖ Steak Fries | 3 oz | 130 | 7% | 12% | 2% |
| ❖ Steakhouse Fries w/Skins | 3 oz | 110 | 5% | 7% | 1% |
| ❖ Tater Rounds | 12 rounds | 160 | 13% | 20% | 3% |
| ❖ Tater Triangles | 3 triangles | 140 | 9% | 14% | 3% |
| ❖ Taters | 9 taters | 150 | 11% | 13% | 2% |
| MRS. PAUL'S Sweet Potatoes— CAMPBELL'S | | | | | |
| ★ Candied Sweet Potatoes | 5 fl oz | 330 | 2% | 3% | 0% |
| ★ Candied Sweet Potatoes 'n Apples | 1 cup | 270 | 0% | 0% | 2% |
| ORE-IDA—HEINZ | | | | | |
| ❖ Bacon Artificial Flavor *Tater Tots* | 3 oz ( 9 tots) | 150 | 10% | 9% | 0% |
| ★ Cheddar Browns | 1 patty | 90 | 4% | 5% | 2% |
| ❖ Cottage Fries | 3 oz (~ 14 fries) | 130 | 6% | 6% | 0% |
| ★ Country Style Dinner Fries | 3 oz (~ 8 fries) | 110 | 5% | 5% | 0% |
| ★ Country Style Hash Browns | 1 cup | 60 | 0% | 0% | 0% |
| ❖ Crispers! | 3 oz (~ 17 fries) | 220 | 19% | 11% | 0% |
| ❖ *Crispy Crowns!* | 3 oz (12 pcs) | 190 | 17% | 10% | 0% |
| ❖ *Crispy Crunchies!* | 3 oz (~ 12 fries) | 160 | 13% | 8% | 0% |
| ❖ *Deep Fries* Crinkle Cuts | 3 oz (~ 18 fries) | 160 | 10% | 6% | 0% |
| ❖ *Deep Fries* French Fries | 3 oz (~ 22 fries) | 160 | 11% | 6% | 0% |
| ❖ *Fast Fries* | 3 oz (~ 23 fries) | 140 | 9% | 10% | 0% |
| ❖ *Fast Fries* Ranch Flavor | 3 oz (~ 22 fries) | 150 | 11% | 6% | 0% |
| ❖ Golden Crinkles | 3 oz (~ 16 fries) | 120 | 6% | 4% | 0% |
| ❖ Golden Fries | 3 oz (~16 fries) | 120 | 6% | 3% | 0% |
| ❖ Golden Patties | 1 patty | 140 | 11% | 6% | 0% |
| ❖ Golden Twirls | 3 oz (~ 28 fries) | 160 | 11% | 6% | 0% |
| ❖ *Hot Tots* | 3 oz ( 9 tots) | 150 | 10% | 6% | 0% |
| ❖ Microwave Crinkle Cuts | 1 pkg | 180 | 12% | 7% | 0% |
| ❖ Microwave Hash Browns | 1 patty | 110 | 9% | 8% | 0% |
| ❖ Microwave *Tater Tots* | 1 pkg | 190 | 15% | 13% | 0% |

★ Foods with this symbol have less than or equal to 5% *Daily Value* for <u>all</u> three nutrients (5% Rule).

❖ Foods with this symbol have <u>at least one</u> of the three nutrients greater than 5% *Daily Value* but less than or equal to 20% *Daily Value*.

Ⓐ Foods with this symbol have <u>at least one</u> of the three nutrients greater than 20% *Daily Value* (20% Rule).

| FOOD | Serving Size | Calories | Tot Fat | Sat Fat | Chol |
|------|--------------|----------|---------|---------|------|
| ❖ *Nacho Crispers!* | 3 oz (~ 10 fries) | 170 | 14% | 14% | 0% |
| ★ Natural Butter Flavor Mashed Potatoes | 1/2 cup | 80 | 3% | 3% | 1% |
| ❖ Onion *Tater Tots* | 3 oz (9 tots) | 150 | 10% | 9% | 0% |
| ❖ Pixie Crinkles | 3 oz (~33 fries) | 140 | 8% | 4% | 0% |
| ★ Potato Wedges w/Skin | 3 oz (~ 9 fries) | 110 | 4% | 4% | 0% |
| ★ Potatoes O'Brien | 3/4 cup | 60 | 0% | 0% | 0% |
| ❖ Shoestrings | 3 oz (~ 8 fries) | 150 | 8% | 5% | 0% |
| ★ Shredded Hash Browns | 1 patty | 70 | 0% | 0% | 0% |
| Ⓐ *Snackin' Fries:* Regular or Extra Zesty | 1 pkg | 340 | 31% | 18% | 0% |
| ★ Southern Style Hash Browns | 3/4 cup | 70 | 0% | 0% | 0% |
| Ⓐ *Tater ABC's* | 3 oz (10 pcs) | 190 | 17% | 22% | 0% |
| ❖ *Tater Tots* | 3 oz ( 9 tots) | 160 | 12% | 7% | 0% |
| ❖ *Texas Crispers!* | 3 oz | 170 | 15% | 13% | 0% |
| ❖ Toaster Hash Browns | 2 patties | 190 | 18% | 10% | 0% |
| ❖ Topped Baked Potato Broccoli & Cheese | 1/2 baker | 150 | 6% | 9% | 3% |
| ❖ Topped Baked Potato Salsa & Cheese | 1/2 baker | 160 | 7% | 8% | 3% |
| ❖ Waffle Fries | 3 oz ( ~15 fries) | 140 | 8% | 7% | 0% |
| ❖ *Zesties!* | 3 oz (~ 12 fries) | 160 | 13% | 8% | 0% |
| ORE-IDA Twice Baked Potato— HEINZ | | | | | |
| ❖ Butter Flavor | 1 baker | 200 | 13% | 14% | 0% |
| ❖ Cheddar Cheese | 1 baker | 190 | 12% | 11% | 0% |
| ❖ Ranch Flavor | 1 baker | 180 | 9% | 9% | 0% |
| ❖ Sour Cream & Chives | 1 baker | 180 | 10% | 9% | 0% |
| STOUFFER'S *Lean Cuisine* Entrées —NESTLÉ | | | | | |
| ❖ Deluxe Cheddar Potato | 1 pkg | 270 | 15% | 18% | 10% |
| ❖ *Lunch Express:* Broccoli & Cheddar Cheese Sauce over Baked Potato | 1 pkg | 250 | 14% | 20% | 8% |
| STOUFFER'S Side Dishes—NESTLÉ | | | | | |
| ❖ Potatoes Au Gratin | ~ 1/2 cup | 130 | 9% | 13% | 5% |
| ❖ Scalloped Potatoes | ~ 1/2 cup | 130 | 9% | 5% | 2% |
| ❖ WEIGHT WATCHERS Baked Potatoes: Broccoli & Cheese | 1 entrée | 230 | 11% | 10% | 3% |

| FOOD | Serving Size | Calories | Tot Fat | Sat Fat | Chol |
|------|------|------|------|------|------|
| *Potato Mixes* | | | | | |
| **Brand Name Foods** | | | | | |
| BETTY CROCKER *Cheddar Classics* Potatoes (prep as dir)—GENERAL MILLS | | | | | |
| ❖ Cheddar & Bacon | 1/2 cup | 160 | 10% | 7% | 1% |
| ❖ Cheddar & Sour Cream | 1/2 cup | 170 | 10% | 8% | 2% |
| ❖ Three Cheese | 1/2 cup | 150 | 9% | 7% | 1% |
| ❖ White Cheddar | 1/2 cup | 150 | 10% | 8% | 1% |
| BETTY CROCKER *Potato Buds* Potato Mixes (prep as dir)— GENERAL MILLS | | | | | |
| ❖ Cheddar Cheese | 2/3 cup | 190 | 15% | 10% | 1% |
| ❖ Original | 2/3 cup | 160 | 12% | 8% | 1% |
| ❖ Sour Cream 'n Chive | 2/3 cup | 190 | 16% | 12% | 2% |
| BETTY CROCKER *Potato Shakers* (prep as dir)—GENERAL MILLS | | | | | |
| ❖ Original | 3/4 cup | 170 | 7% | 3% | 1% |
| ❖ Parmesan | 3/4 cup | 170 | 7% | 4% | 1% |
| ❖ Zesty Cheddar | 3/4 cup | 170 | 8% | 5% | 1% |
| BETTY CROCKER *Potatoes Express* (prep as dir)—GENERAL MILLS | | | | | |
| ❖ Broccoli Au Gratin | 2/3 cup | 130 | 6% | 6% | 1% |
| ❖ Cheddar Cheese | 2/3 cup | 140 | 6% | 6% | 1% |
| ❖ Creamy Scalloped | 2/3 cup | 180 | 12% | 9% | 2% |
| BETTY CROCKER Homestyle Potato (prep as dir)—GENERAL MILLS | | | | | |
| ❖ American Cheese | 1/2 cup | 150 | 10% | 8% | 1% |
| ❖ Broccoli Au Gratin | 1/2 cup | 150 | 10% | 7% | 1% |
| ❖ Cheddar Cheese | 1/2 cup | 160 | 10% | 8% | 1% |
| ❖ Cheesy Scalloped | 1/2 cup | 150 | 10% | 8% | 1% |
| BETTY CROCKER Specialty Potatoes (prep as dir)— GENERAL MILLS | | | | | |
| ❖ Au Gratin (9 oz box) | 1/2 cup | 160 | 9% | 7% | 1% |
| ❖ Cheddar 'n Bacon | 1/2 cup | 160 | 10% | 7% | 2% |
| ❖ Hash Brown | 1/2 cup | 200 | 12% | 7% | 0% |
| ❖ Julienne | 1/2 cup | 140 | 9% | 8% | 2% |
| ❖ Scalloped (8.25 oz box) | 1/2 cup | 160 | 10% | 8% | 1% |
| ❖ Scalloped Potatoes 'n Ham | 1/2 cup | 160 | 10% | 8% | 1% |
| ❖ Smokey Cheddar | 1/2 cup | 150 | 9% | 7% | 1% |
| ❖ Sour Cream 'n Chive | 1/2 cup | 160 | 11% | 9% | 2% |

★ Foods with this symbol have less than or equal to 5% *Daily Value* for all three nutrients (5% Rule).

❖ Foods with this symbol have at least one of the three nutrients greater than 5% *Daily Value* but less than or equal to 20% *Daily Value*.

Ⓐ Foods with this symbol have at least one of the three nutrients greater than 20% *Daily Value* (20% Rule).

| FOOD | Serving Size | Calories | Tot Fat | Sat Fat | Chol |
|---|---|---|---|---|---|
| BETTY CROCKER Twice Baked Potatoes (prep as dir)—GENERAL MILLS | | | | | |
| ❹ Cheddar & Bacon | 2/3 cup | 210 | 17% | 14% | 28% |
| ❹ Mild Cheddar & Onion | 2/3 cup | 210 | 18% | 15% | 28% |
| ❹ Sour Cream & Chive | 2/3 cup | 200 | 17% | 15% | 29% |
| HUNGRY JACK Potatoes (prep as dir)—PILLSBURY | | | | | |
| ❖ Au Gratin | 1/2 cup | 150 | 8% | 16% | 5% |
| ❖ Cheesy Scalloped | 1/2 cup | 150 | 9% | 16% | 4% |
| ★ KNORR Potato Pancake Mix—CPC | 1/4 pkg | 150 | 1% | 0% | 0% |
| MANISCHEWITZ | | | | | |
| ❖ Potato Kugel (prep as dir) | 1/8 cup | 70 | 2% | 6% | 0% |
| ★ Potato Pancakes (prep as dir) | 3 cakes | 80 | 1% | 4% | 0% |
| RECIPE SECRETS For Potatoes—LIPTON | | | | | |
| ❖ California Onion | 1 tbsp | 60 | 8% | 4% | 2% |
| ❖ Classic Garlic Herb | 1 tbsp | 50 | 8% | 4% | 1% |
| ❖ Savory Cheddar | 1 tbsp | 60 | 8% | 5% | 2% |
| SHAKE 'N BAKE PERFECT POTATOES—KRAFT | | | | | |
| ❖ Crispy Cheddar | 1/6 packet | 30 | 3% | 6% | 2% |
| ★ Herb and Garlic | 1/6 packet | 20 | 0% | 0% | 0% |

# Fast Foods

ARBY'S

**Breakfast Items**

| | | | | | |
|---|---|---|---|---|---|
| ❖ Bacon | 1 serv | 90 | 11% | 15% | 5% |
| ❹ Biscuit (Plain) | 1 serv | 280 | 23% | 15% | 0% |
| ❖ Blueberry Muffin | 1 serv | 230 | 14% | 10% | 8% |
| ❖ Cinnamon Nut Danish | 1 serv | 360 | 17% | 5% | 0% |
| ❹ Croissant (Plain) | 1 serv | 220 | 18% | 35% | 8% |
| ❹ Egg Portion (pan fried or grilled) | 1 serv | 95 | 12% | 10% | 60% |
| ❹ French-Toastix (w/o powdered sugar) | 6 pcs | 430 | 32% | 25% | 0% |
| ❖ Ham | 1 serv | 45 | 2% | 3% | 7% |
| ❹ Sausage | 1 serv | 163 | 23% | 30% | 8% |
| ❖ Swiss | 1 serv | 45 | 5% | 10% | 4% |
| ★ Table Syrup | 1 serv | 100 | 0% | 0% | 0% |

**Chicken**

| | | | | | |
|---|---|---|---|---|---|
| ❹ Breaded Chicken Fillet | 1 serv | 536 | 43% | 25% | 15% |
| ❹ Chicken Cordon Bleu | 1 serv | 623 | 51% | 40% | 26% |
| ❹ Chicken Fingers | 2 pcs | 290 | 25% | 10% | 11% |
| ❖ Grilled Chicken BBQ | 1 serv | 388 | 20% | 15% | 14% |

| FOOD | Serving Size | Calories | Tot Fat | Sat Fat | Chol |
|------|------|------|------|------|------|
| ⊛ Grilled Chicken Deluxe | 1 serv | 430 | 31% | 20% | 20% |
| ⊛ Roast Chicken Club | 1 serv | 546 | 48% | 45% | 19% |
| ⊛ Roast Chicken Deluxe | 1 serv | 433 | 34% | 25% | 11% |
| ⊛ Roast Chicken Santa Fe | 1 serv | 436 | 34% | 30% | 18% |

**Desserts**

| FOOD | Serving Size | Calories | Tot Fat | Sat Fat | Chol |
|------|------|------|------|------|------|
| ⊛ Apple Turnover | 1 serv | 330 | 22% | 35% | 0% |
| ⊛ Butterfinger Polar Swirl | 1 serv | 457 | 28% | 40% | 9% |
| ⊛ Cheesecake (Plain) | 1 serv | 320 | 35% | 70% | 32% |
| ⊛ Cherry Turnover | 1 serv | 320 | 20% | 25% | 0% |
| ❖ Chocolate Chip Cookie | 1 serv | 125 | 9% | 10% | 3% |
| ⊛ Heath Polar Swirl | 1 serv | 543 | 34% | 25% | 13% |
| ⊛ Oreo Polar Swirl | 1 serv | 482 | 34% | 50% | 12% |
| ⊛ Peanut Butter Cup Polar Swirl | 1 serv | 517 | 37% | 40% | 11% |
| ⊛ Snickers Polar Swirl | 1 serv | 511 | 29% | 35% | 11% |

**Light Menu**

| FOOD | Serving Size | Calories | Tot Fat | Sat Fat | Chol |
|------|------|------|------|------|------|
| ★ Garden Salad (w/o dressing) | 1 serv | 61 | 1% | 0% | 0% |
| ❖ Roast Beef Deluxe | 1 serv | 296 | 15% | 15% | 14% |
| ❖ Roast Chicken Deluxe | 1 serv | 276 | 9% | 10% | 11% |
| ❖ Roast Chicken Salad | 1 serv | 149 | 3% | 3% | 10% |
| ❖ Roast Turkey Deluxe | 1 serv | 260 | 11% | 10% | 11% |
| ★ Side Salad (w/o dressing) | 1 serv | 23 | 0% | 0% | 0% |

**Other Sandwiches**

| FOOD | Serving Size | Calories | Tot Fat | Sat Fat | Chol |
|------|------|------|------|------|------|
| ⊛ Fish Fillet | 1 serv | 529 | 42% | 35% | 14% |
| ⊛ Ham 'n Cheese | 1 serv | 359 | 22% | 25% | 18% |
| ❖ Ham 'n Cheese Melt | 1 serv | 329 | 20% | 20% | 13% |

**Potatoes**

| FOOD | Serving Size | Calories | Tot Fat | Sat Fat | Chol |
|------|------|------|------|------|------|
| ★ Baked Potato (Plain) | 1 serv | 355 | 0% | 0% | 0% |
| ⊛ Baked Potato w/Margarine & Sour Cream | 1 serv | 578 | 37% | 45% | 8% |
| ⊛ Broccoli 'n Cheddar Baked Potato | 1 serv | 571 | 31% | 25% | 4% |
| ⊛ Cheddar Curly Fries | 1 serv | 333 | 28% | 20% | 1% |
| ⊛ Curly Fries | 1 serv | 300 | 23% | 15% | 0% |
| ⊛ Deluxe Baked Potato | 1 serv | 736 | 55% | 80% | 20% |
| ❖ French Fries | 1 serv | 246 | 20% | 15% | 0% |
| ❖ Potato Cakes | 2 pcs | 204 | 18% | 10% | 0% |

**Roast Beef Sandwiches**

| FOOD | Serving Size | Calories | Tot Fat | Sat Fat | Chol |
|------|------|------|------|------|------|
| ⊛ Arby's Melt w/Cheddar | 1 sandwich | 368 | 28% | 30% | 10% |
| ⊛ Arby-Q | 1 sandwich | 431 | 28% | 30% | 12% |
| ⊛ Bac'n Cheddar Deluxe | 1 sandwich | 539 | 52% | 50% | 15% |

★ Foods with this symbol have less than or equal to 5% *Daily Value* for <u>all</u> three nutrients (5% Rule).

❖ Foods with this symbol have <u>at least one</u> of the three nutrients greater than 5% *Daily Value* but less than or equal to 20% *Daily Value*.

⊛ Foods with this symbol have <u>at least one</u> of the three nutrients greater than 20% *Daily Value* (20% Rule).

| | FOOD | Serving Size | Calories | Tot Fat | Sat Fat | Chol |
|---|---|---|---|---|---|---|
| ⊛ | Beef 'n Cheddar | 1 sandwich | 487 | 43% | 45% | 17% |
| ⊛ | Giant Roast Beef | 1 sandwich | 555 | 43% | 55% | 24% |
| ⊛ | Junior Roast Beef | 1 sandwich | 324 | 22% | 25% | 10% |
| ⊛ | Regular Roast Beef | 1 sandwich | 388 | 29% | 35% | 14% |
| ⊛ | Super Roast Beef | 1 sandwich | 523 | 42% | 45% | 14% |

**Salad Dressings**

| | | | | | | |
|---|---|---|---|---|---|---|
| ⊛ | Blue Cheese Dressing | 1 serv | 290 | 48% | 30% | 17% |
| ⊛ | Buttermilk Ranch Dressing | 1 serv | 350 | 58% | 30% | 2% |
| ⊛ | Honey French Dressing | 1 serv | 280 | 35% | 15% | 0% |
| ❖ | Red Ranch Dressing | 1 serv | 75 | 9% | 5% | 0% |
| ★ | Reduced Calorie Buttermilk Ranch Dressing | 1 serv | 50 | 0% | 0% | 0% |
| ★ | Reduced Calorie Italian Dressing | 1 serv | 20 | 2% | 0% | 0% |
| ⊛ | Thousand Island Dressing | 1 serv | 260 | 40% | 20% | 10% |

**Sauces and Spreads**

| | | | | | | |
|---|---|---|---|---|---|---|
| ★ | Arby's Sauce | 1 serv | 15 | 0% | 0% | 0% |
| ★ | Barbeque Sauce | 1 serv | 30 | 0% | 0% | 0% |
| ★ | Beef Stock Au Jus | 1 serv | 10 | 0% | 0% | 0% |
| ★ | Cheddar Cheese Sauce | 1 serv | 35 | 5% | 5% | 1% |
| ❖ | Horsey Sauce | 1 serv | 60 | 8% | 5% | 2% |
| ★ | Ketchup | 1 serv | 16 | 0% | 0% | 0% |
| ★ | Light Cholesterol Free Mayonnaise | 1 serv | 12 | 2% | 0% | 0% |
| ⊛ | Mayonnaise | 1 serv | 110 | 18% | 35% | 2% |
| ★ | Mustard, German Style | 1 serv | 5 | 0% | 0% | 0% |
| ❖ | Non-Separating Italian Sub Sauce | 1 serv | 70 | 11% | 5% | 0% |
| ❖ | Parmesan Cheese Sauce | 1 serv | 70 | 11% | 5% | 2% |
| ❖ | Reduced Calorie Honey Mayonnaise | 1 serv | 70 | 11% | 5% | 7% |
| ⊛ | Tartar Sauce | 1 serv | 140 | 23% | 10% | 10% |

**Shakes**

| | | | | | | |
|---|---|---|---|---|---|---|
| ❖ | Chocolate Shake | 1 serv | 451 | 18% | 15% | 12% |
| ❖ | Jamocha Shake | 1 serv | 384 | 15% | 15% | 12% |
| ❖ | Vanilla Shake | 1 serv | 360 | 18% | 20% | 12% |

**Soups**

| | | | | | | |
|---|---|---|---|---|---|---|
| ❖ | Boston Clam Chowder (made w/whole milk) | 1 serv | 190 | 14% | 15% | 8% |
| ❖ | Cream of Broccoli (made w/whole milk) | 1 serv | 160 | 12% | 20% | 8% |
| ❖ | Lumberjack Mixed Vegetable | 1 serv | 90 | 6% | 10% | 2% |
| ❖ | Old Fashion Chicken Noodle | 1 serv | 80 | 3% | 0% | 7% |
| ❖ | Potato w/Bacon (made w/whole milk) | 1 serv | 170 | 11% | 15% | 7% |
| ❖ | Timberline Chili | 1 serv | 220 | 15% | 20% | 10% |

% DAILY VALUE

| FOOD | Serving Size | Calories | Tot Fat | Sat Fat | Chol |
|------|--------------|----------|---------|---------|------|
| ⓐ Wisconsin Cheese (made w/ whole milk) | 1 serv | 280 | 28% | 35% | 12% |

**Sub Roll Sandwiches**

| FOOD | Serving Size | Calories | Tot Fat | Sat Fat | Chol |
|------|--------------|----------|---------|---------|------|
| ⓐ French Dip | 1 sandwich | 475 | 34% | 40% | 18% |
| ⓐ Hot Ham 'n Swiss | 1 sandwich | 500 | 35% | 35% | 23% |
| ⓐ Italian Sub | 1 sandwich | 675 | 55% | 65% | 28% |
| ⓐ Philly Beef 'n Swiss | 1 sandwich | 755 | 72% | 75% | 30% |
| ⓐ Roast Beef Sub | 1 sandwich | 700 | 65% | 70% | 28% |
| ⓐ Triple Cheese Melt | 1 sandwich | 720 | 69% | 80% | 30% |
| ⓐ Turkey Sub | 1 sandwich | 550 | 42% | 35% | 22% |

BOSTON MARKET

**Baked Goods**

| FOOD | Serving Size | Calories | Tot Fat | Sat Fat | Chol |
|------|--------------|----------|---------|---------|------|
| ⓐ Brownie | 1 pc | 450 | 42% | 35% | 27% |
| ⓐ Chocolate Chip Cookie | 1 cookie | 340 | 26% | 31% | 8% |
| ❖ Corn Bread | 1 loaf | 200 | 9% | 8% | 8% |
| ❖ Hot Cinnamon Apples | 3/4 cup | 250 | 7% | 2% | 0% |
| ❖ Oatmeal Raisin Cookie | 1 cookie | 320 | 20% | 12% | 8% |

**Cold Side Dishes**

| FOOD | Serving Size | Calories | Tot Fat | Sat Fat | Chol |
|------|--------------|----------|---------|---------|------|
| ⓐ Caesar Side Salad | 4 oz | 210 | 26% | 22% | 7% |
| ⓐ Cole Slaw | 3/4 cup | 280 | 25% | 12% | 8% |
| ❖ Cranberry Relish | 3/4 cup | 370 | 8% | 2% | 0% |
| ★ Fruit Salad (Fall) | 3/4 cup | 70 | 1% | 0% | 0% |
| ❖ Mediterranean Pasta Salad | 3/4 cup | 170 | 15% | 12% | 3% |
| ⓐ Tortellini Salad | 3/4 cup | 380 | 37% | 23% | 30% |

**Entrées**

| FOOD | Serving Size | Calories | Tot Fat | Sat Fat | Chol |
|------|--------------|----------|---------|---------|------|
| ⓐ 1/2 Chicken (w/skin) | 10 oz | 630 | 57% | 50% | 123% |
| ⓐ 1/4 Dark Meat chicken (w/skin) | 5 oz | 330 | 34% | 30% | 60% |
| ⓐ 1/4 Dark Meat Chicken (w/o skin) | ~ 4 oz | 210 | 15% | 12% | 50% |
| ⓐ 1/4 White Meat Chicken (w/skin) | 5 oz | 330 | 26% | 22% | 58% |
| ⓐ 1/4 White Meat Chicken (w/o skin) | ~ 4 oz | 160 | 6% | 5% | 32% |
| ⓐ Chunky Chicken Salad | 3/4 cup | 390 | 46% | 26% | 48% |
| ⓐ Ham | 5 oz | 230 | 15% | 20% | 25% |
| ⓐ Meatloaf | 5 oz | 340 | 28% | 35% | 40% |
| ⓐ Original Chicken Pot Pie | 1 pie | 750 | 52% | 45% | 38% |

★ Foods with this symbol have less than or equal to 5% *Daily Value* for <u>all</u> three nutrients (5% Rule).
❖ Foods with this symbol have <u>at least one</u> of the three nutrients greater than 5% *Daily Value* but less than or equal to 20% *Daily Value*.
ⓐ Foods with this symbol have <u>at least one</u> of the three nutrients greater than 20% *Daily Value* (20% Rule).

| FOOD | Serving Size | Calories | Tot Fat | Sat Fat | Chol |
|---|---|---|---|---|---|
| ⊛ Rotisserie Turkey | 5 oz | 170 | 2% | 3% | 33% |
| ⊛ Vegetable Pot Pie | 1 pie | 350 | 18% | 35% | 12% |

**Hot Side Dishes**

| FOOD | Serving Size | Calories | Tot Fat | Sat Fat | Chol |
|---|---|---|---|---|---|
| ❖ BBQ Baked Beans | 3/4 cup | 330 | 14% | 3% | 3% |
| ❖ Butternut Squash | 3/4 cup | 160 | 9% | 5% | 5% |
| ★ Chicken Gravy | 1 oz | 150 | 2% | 0% | 0% |
| ⊛ Creamed Spinach | 3/4 cup | 300 | 37% | 75% | 25% |
| ⊛ Homestyle Mashed Potatoes & Gravy | 3/4 cup | 200 | 14% | 25% | 8% |
| ❖ Macaroni & Cheese | 3/4 cup | 280 | 15% | 7% | 7% |
| ⊛ Mashed Potatoes | 2/3 cup | 180 | 12% | 25% | 8% |
| ★ New Potatoes | 3/4 cup | 140 | 5% | 2% | 0% |
| ❖ Rice Pilaf | 2/3 cup | 180 | 8% | 5% | 0% |
| ★ Steamed Vegetables | 2/3 cup | 35 | 1% | 0% | 0% |
| ❖ Stuffing | 3/4 cup | 310 | 18% | 0% | 0% |
| ❖ Whole Kernel Corn | 3/4 cup | 190 | 6% | 5% | 0% |
| ❖ Zucchini Marinara | 3/4 cup | 80 | 6% | 2% | 0% |

**Soups, Salads, and Sandwiches**

| FOOD | Serving Size | Calories | Tot Fat | Sat Fat | Chol |
|---|---|---|---|---|---|
| ⊛ Caesar Salad Entrée | 10 oz | 520 | 66% | 60% | 13% |
| ⊛ Caesar Salad w/o Dressing | 8 oz | 240 | 20% | 35% | 8% |
| ⊛ Chicken Breast Sandwich | 1 sandwich | 420 | 8% | 5% | 33% |
| ⊛ Chicken Caesar Salad | 13 oz | 670 | 72% | 63% | 40% |
| ❖ Chicken Soup | 3/4 cup | 80 | 5% | 5% | 8% |
| ⊛ Chunky Chicken Salad Sandwich | 1 sandwich | 640 | 48% | 25% | 48% |

BURGER KING

**Breakfast Dishes**

| FOOD | Serving Size | Calories | Tot Fat | Sat Fat | Chol |
|---|---|---|---|---|---|
| ⊛ CROISSAN'WICH w/Bacon, Egg & Cheese | 1 sandwich | 350 | 37% | 40% | 75% |
| ⊛ CROISSAN'WICH w/Ham, Egg & Cheese | 1 sandwich | 350 | 34% | 35% | 77% |
| ⊛ CROISSAN'WICH w/Sausage, Egg & Cheese | 1 sandwich | 530 | 63% | 70% | 85% |
| ⊛ French Toast Sticks | 1 serving | 500 | 42% | 35% | 0% |
| ❖ Hash Browns | 1 serving | 220 | 18% | 15% | 0% |

**Burgers**

| FOOD | Serving Size | Calories | Tot Fat | Sat Fat | Chol |
|---|---|---|---|---|---|
| ⊛ Cheeseburger | 1 burger | 300 | 22% | 30% | 15% |
| ⊛ Double Cheeseburger | 1 burger | 600 | 55% | 85% | 45% |
| ⊛ Double Cheeseburger w/Bacon | 1 burger | 640 | 60% | 90% | 48% |
| ⊛ Double WHOPPER | 1 burger | 860 | 86% | 95% | 57% |
| ⊛ Double WHOPPER w/Cheese | 1 burger | 950 | 97% | 120% | 65% |
| ❖ Hamburger | 1 burger | 260 | 15% | 20% | 10% |

| FOOD | Serving Size | Calories | Tot Fat | Sat Fat | Chol |
|---|---|---|---|---|---|
| ⊛ WHOPPER | 1 burger | 630 | 60% | 55% | 30% |
| ⊛ WHOPPER JR. | 1 burger | 410 | 37% | 40% | 20% |
| ⊛ WHOPPER JR. w/Cheese | 1 burger | 460 | 43% | 50% | 25% |
| ⊛ WHOPPER w/Cheese | 1 burger | 720 | 71% | 80% | 38% |
| **Condiments** | | | | | |
| ⊛ Mayonnaise | 2 tbsp | 210 | 35% | 15% | 7% |
| ⊛ Tartar Sauce | 2 tbsp | 180 | 29% | 15% | 5% |
| **Dipping Sauces** | | | | | |
| ★ Barbecue | 2 tbsp | 35 | 0% | 0% | 0% |
| ★ Honey | 2 tbsp | 90 | 0% | 0% | 0% |
| ⊛ Ranch | 2 tbsp | 170 | 26% | 15% | 0% |
| ★ Sweet & Sour | 2 tbsp | 45 | 0% | 0% | 0% |
| **Salad Dressings** | | | | | |
| ⊛ Bleu Cheese | 2 tbsp | 160 | 23% | 20% | 10% |
| ❖ French | 2 tbsp | 140 | 15% | 10% | 0% |
| ⊛ Ranch | 2 tbsp | 180 | 29% | 20% | 3% |
| ★ Reduced Calorie Light Italian | 2 tbsp | 15 | 1% | 0% | 0% |
| ❖ Thousand Island | 2 tbsp | 140 | 18% | 15% | 5% |
| **Sandwiches** | | | | | |
| ⊛ BK Big Fish | 1 sandwich | 720 | 66% | 40% | 20% |
| ⊛ BK BROILER Chicken | 1 sandwich | 540 | 45% | 30% | 27% |
| ⊛ Chicken | 1 sandwich | 700 | 66% | 45% | 20% |
| **Shakes** | | | | | |
| ❖ Chocolate Shake (medium) | 1 shake | 310 | 11% | 20% | 7% |
| ❖ Chocolate Shake (medium, syrup added) | 1 shake | 460 | 11% | 20% | 7% |
| ❖ Strawberry Shake (medium, syrup added) | 1 shake | 430 | 11% | 20% | 7% |
| ❖ Vanilla Shake (medium) | 1 shake | 310 | 11% | 20% | 7% |
| **Side Orders** | | | | | |
| ⊛ Broiled Chicken Salad (w/o dressing) | 1 salad | 200 | 15% | 25% | 20% |
| ❖ CHICKEN TENDERS | 6 pcs | 250 | 18% | 15% | 12% |
| ⊛ Dutch Apple Pie | 1 pie | 310 | 23% | 15% | 0% |
| ⊛ French Fries (medium) | 1 serv | 400 | 31% | 25% | 0% |

★  Foods with this symbol have less than or equal to 5% *Daily Value* for <u>all</u> three nutrients (5% Rule).
❖  Foods with this symbol have <u>at least one</u> of the three nutrients greater than 5% *Daily Value* but less than or equal to 20% *Daily Value.*
⊛  Foods with this symbol have <u>at least one</u> of the three nutrients greater than 20% *Daily Value* (20% Rule).

| FOOD | Serving Size | Calories | Tot Fat | Sat Fat | Chol |
|------|------|------|------|------|------|
| ❖ Garden Salad (w/o dressing) | 1 salad | 90 | 8% | 15% | 5% |
| Ⓐ Onion Rings | 1 serv | 310 | 22% | 10% | 0% |
| ❖ Side Salad (w/o dressing) | 1 salad | 50 | 5% | 10% | 2% |

## CHICK-FIL-A

### Sandwiches

| FOOD | Serving Size | Calories | Tot Fat | Sat Fat | Chol |
|------|------|------|------|------|------|
| ❖ Chargrilled Chicken | 1 sandwich | 280 | 5% | 5% | 13% |
| ❖ Chargrilled Chicken (no bun, no pickles) | 1 sandwich | 130 | 5% | 5% | 10% |
| Ⓐ Chargrilled Chicken Club (no dressing) | 1 sandwich | 390 | 18% | 25% | 23% |
| ❖ Chargrilled Chicken Deluxe | 1 sandwich | 290 | 5% | 5% | 13% |
| ❖ CHICK-N-Q | 1 sandwich | 370 | 20% | 15% | 7% |
| ❖ Chicken | 1 sandwich | 290 | 14% | 10% | 17% |
| ❖ Chicken (no bun, no pickles) | 1 sandwich | 160 | 12% | 10% | 15% |
| ❖ Chicken Deluxe | 1 sandwich | 300 | 14% | 10% | 17% |
| ❖ Chicken Salad (on whole wheat) | 1 sandwich | 320 | 8% | 10% | 3% |

### Specialties

| FOOD | Serving Size | Calories | Tot Fat | Sat Fat | Chol |
|------|------|------|------|------|------|
| ❖ CHICK-N-STRIPS | 4 pcs | 230 | 12% | 10% | 7% |
| ★ GRILLED 'N LITES | 2 skewers | 100 | 3% | 0% | 0% |
| ❖ Hearty Breast of Chicken Soup | 1 cup | 215 | 2% | 0% | 15% |
| Ⓐ Nuggets | 8 pcs | 290 | 21% | 15% | 20% |

### Desserts

| FOOD | Serving Size | Calories | Tot Fat | Sat Fat | Chol |
|------|------|------|------|------|------|
| Ⓐ Cheesecake | 1 slc | 270 | 32% | 45% | 3% |
| Ⓐ Cheesecake w/Blueberry Topping | 1 slc | 290 | 35% | 50% | 3% |
| Ⓐ Cheesecake w/Strawberry Topping | 1 slc | 290 | 35% | 50% | 3% |
| Ⓐ Fudge Nut Brownie | 1 pc | 350 | 25% | 15% | 10% |
| ❖ ICEDREAM (small cone) | 1 serv | 140 | 6% | 5% | 13% |
| Ⓐ ICEDREAM (small cup) | 1 serv | 350 | 15% | 15% | 23% |
| Ⓐ Lemon Pie | 1 slc | 280 | 34% | 30% | 2% |

### French Fries

| FOOD | Serving Size | Calories | Tot Fat | Sat Fat | Chol |
|------|------|------|------|------|------|
| ❖ WAFFLE POTATO FRIES (small) | 1 serv | 290 | 15% | 20% | 2% |

### Salads

| FOOD | Serving Size | Calories | Tot Fat | Sat Fat | Chol |
|------|------|------|------|------|------|
| ★ Carrot & Raisin Salad (small) | 1 serv | 150 | 3% | 0% | 2% |
| ❖ Chargrilled Chicken Garden Salad | 1 serv | 170 | 5% | 5% | 8% |
| ❖ Chicken Salad Plate | 1 serv | 290 | 8% | 0% | 12% |
| ❖ CHICKEN-N-STRIPS Salad | 1 serv | 290 | 14% | 10% | 7% |
| ❖ Cole Slaw (small) | 1 serv | 130 | 9% | 5% | 5% |
| ★ Tossed Salad | 1 serv | 70 | 0% | 0% | 0% |

| FOOD | Serving Size | Calories | Tot Fat | Sat Fat | Chol |
|------|------|------|------|------|------|

## DAIRY QUEEN

### Desserts

| FOOD | Serving Size | Calories | Tot Fat | Sat Fat | Chol |
|------|------|------|------|------|------|
| ☻ Banana Split | 1 serv | 510 | 17% | 40% | 10% |
| ☻ BUSTER BAR | 1 bar | 450 | 45% | 45% | 5% |
| ☻ Chocolate Cone, Large | 1 cone | 350 | 17% | 40% | 10% |
| ☻ Chocolate Cone, Regular | 1 cone | 230 | 11% | 25% | 7% |
| ☻ Chocolate Dipped Cone, Regular | 1 cone | 330 | 25% | 40% | 7% |
| ☻ Chocolate Sundae, Regular | 1 serv | 300 | 11% | 25% | 7% |
| ☻ DILLY BAR | 1 bar | 210 | 20% | 30% | 3% |
| ☻ DQ Frozen Cake Slice | 1 slice | 380 | 28% | 40% | 7% |
| ❖ DQ Sandwich | 1 sandwich | 140 | 6% | 10% | 2% |
| ☻ HEATH BLIZZARD, Regular | 1 serv | 820 | 55% | 85% | 20% |
| ☻ HEATH BLIZZARD, Small | 1 serv | 560 | 35% | 55% | 13% |
| ☻ HEATH BREEZE, Regular | 1 serv | 680 | 32% | 30% | 5% |
| ❖ HEATH BREEZE, Small | 1 serv | 450 | 18% | 15% | 3% |
| ☻ Hot Fudge Brownie *Delight* | 1 serv | 710 | 45% | 70% | 12% |
| ★ McMISTY, Regular | 1 serv | 250 | 0% | 0% | 0% |
| ☻ NUTTY DOUBLE FUDGE | 1 serv | 580 | 34% | 50% | 12% |
| ☻ PEANUT BUSTER Parfait | 1 serv | 710 | 49% | 50% | 10% |
| ☻ QC Chocolate BIG SCOOP | 1 cone | 310 | 22% | 50% | 12% |
| ☻ QC Vanilla BIG SCOOP | 1 cone | 300 | 22% | 45% | 12% |
| ☻ Strawberry BLIZZARD, Regular | 1 serv | 740 | 25% | 55% | 17% |
| ☻ Strawberry BLIZZARD, Small | 1 serv | 500 | 18% | 40% | 12% |
| ★ Strawberry BREEZE, Regular | 1 serv | 590 | 2% | 3% | 2% |
| ★ Strawberry BREEZE, Small | 1 serv | 400 | 1% | 3% | 2% |
| ☻ STRAWBERRY WAFFLE CONE SUNDAE | 1 cone | 350 | 18% | 25% | 7% |
| ☻ Vanilla Cone, Large | 1 cone | 340 | 15% | 35% | 10% |
| ☻ Vanilla Cone, Regular | 1 cone | 230 | 11% | 25% | 7% |
| ❖ Vanilla Cone, Small | 1 cone | 140 | 6% | 15% | 5% |
| ★ Yogurt Cone, Large | 1 cone | 260 | 1% | 3% | 2% |
| ★ Yogurt Cone, Regular | 1 cone | 180 | 1% | 3% | 1% |
| ★ Yogurt Cup, Large | 1 serv | 230 | 1% | 3% | 1% |
| ★ Yogurt Cup, Regular | 1 serv | 170 | 1% | 3% | 1% |
| ★ Yogurt Strawberry Sundae, Regular | 1 serv | 200 | 1% | 3% | 1% |

### French Fries

| FOOD | Serving Size | Calories | Tot Fat | Sat Fat | Chol |
|------|------|------|------|------|------|
| ☻ Large | 1 serv | 390 | 28% | 20% | 0% |
| ☻ Regular | 1 serv | 300 | 22% | 15% | 0% |
| ❖ Regular Onion Rings | 1 serv | 240 | 18% | 15% | 0% |
| ❖ Small | 1 serv | 210 | 15% | 10% | 0% |

★ Foods with this symbol have less than or equal to 5% *Daily Value* for <u>all</u> three nutrients (5% Rule).
❖ Foods with this symbol have <u>at least one</u> of the three nutrients greater than 5% *Daily Value* but less than or equal to 20% *Daily Value*.
☻ Foods with this symbol have <u>at least one</u> of the three nutrients greater than 20% *Daily Value* (20% Rule).

| FOOD | Serving Size | Calories | Tot Fat | Sat Fat | Chol |
|------|--------------|----------|---------|---------|------|
| **Hamburgers** | | | | | |
| ⊛ Double Hamburger | 1 burger | 460 | 38% | 60% | 32% |
| ⊛ Double Hamburger w/Cheese | 1 burger | 570 | 52% | 90% | 40% |
| ⊛ DQ Homestyle Ultimate Burger | 1 burger | 700 | 72% | 105% | 47% |
| ⊛ Single Hamburger | 1 burger | 310 | 20% | 30% | 15% |
| ⊛ Single Hamburger w/Cheese | 1 burger | 365 | 28% | 45% | 20% |
| **Salads and Dressings** | | | | | |
| ⊛ Garden Salad (w/o dressing) | 1 salad | 200 | 20% | 35% | 62% |
| ❖ Reduced Calorie French Dressing | 2 tbsp | 90 | 8% | 5% | 0% |
| ★ Side Salad (w/o dressing) | 1 salad | 25 | 0% | 0% | 0% |
| ⊛ Thousand Island Dressing | 2 tbsp | 225 | 32% | 15% | 8% |
| **Sandwiches** | | | | | |
| ⊛ 1/4 Pound SUPER DOG | 1 sandwich | 590 | 58% | 80% | 20% |
| ❖ BBQ Beef | 1 sandwich | 225 | 6% | 5% | 7% |
| ⊛ Breaded Chicken Fillet | 1 sandwich | 430 | 31% | 20% | 18% |
| ⊛ Breaded Chicken Fillet w/Cheese | 1 sandwich | 480 | 38% | 35% | 23% |
| ⊛ Fish Fillet | 1 sandwich | 370 | 25% | 15% | 15% |
| ⊛ Fish Fillet w/Cheese | 1 sandwich | 450 | 32% | 30% | 20% |
| ❖ Grilled Chicken Fillet | 1 sandwich | 300 | 12% | 10% | 17% |
| ⊛ Hot Dog | 1 sandwich | 280 | 25% | 30% | 8% |
| ⊛ Hot Dog w/Cheese | 1 sandwich | 330 | 32% | 45% | 12% |
| ⊛ Hot Dog w/Chili | 1 sandwich | 320 | 29% | 35% | 10% |
| **Shakes** | | | | | |
| ⊛ Chocolate Shake, Regular | 1 shake | 540 | 22% | 40% | 15% |
| ⊛ Vanilla Malt, Regular | 1 shake | 610 | 22% | 40% | 15% |
| ⊛ Vanilla Shake, Large | 1 shake | 600 | 25% | 50% | 17% |
| ⊛ Vanilla Shake, Regular | 1 shake | 520 | 22% | 40% | 15% |

## DOMINO'S PIZZA

| FOOD | Serving Size | Calories | Tot Fat | Sat Fat | Chol |
|------|--------------|----------|---------|---------|------|
| **12" Deep Dish Pizza** (8 slices per pizza) | | | | | |
| ⊛ Cheese | 2 slcs | 560 | 37% | 45% | 11% |
| ⊛ Ham | 2 slcs | 580 | 38% | 47% | 13% |
| ⊛ Italian Sausage & Mushroom | 2 slcs | 620 | 43% | 54% | 14% |
| ⊛ Pepperoni | 2 slcs | 620 | 45% | 56% | 15% |
| ⊛ Veggie | 2 slcs | 580 | 38% | 46% | 11% |
| ⊛ X-tra Cheese & Pepperoni | 2 slcs | 670 | 51% | 67% | 18% |
| **12" Hand-Tossed Pizza** (8 slices per pizza) | | | | | |
| ⊛ Cheese | 2 slcs | 340 | 15% | 22% | 6% |

| FOOD | Serving Size | Calories | Tot Fat | Sat Fat | Chol |
|------|------|------|------|------|------|
| ⊛ Ham | 2 slcs | 360 | 16% | 23% | 88% |
| ⊛ Italian Sausage & Mushroom | 2 slcs | 400 | 21% | 31% | 10% |
| ⊛ Pepperoni | 2 slcs | 410 | 23% | 33% | 11% |
| ⊛ Veggie | 2 slcs | 360 | 16% | 23% | 6% |
| ⊛ X-tra Cheese & Pepperoni | 2 slcs | 460 | 29% | 43% | 14% |

**12" Thin Crust Pizza**

| | | | | | |
|------|------|------|------|------|------|
| ⊛ Cheese | 1/3 pizza | 360 | 24% | 32% | 9% |
| ⊛ Ham | 1/3 pizza | 390 | 25% | 33% | 12% |
| ⊛ Italian Sausage & Mushroom | 1/3 pizza | 440 | 33% | 43% | 14% |
| ⊛ Pepperoni | 1/3 pizza | 450 | 35% | 46% | 14% |
| ⊛ Veggie | 1/3 pizza | 390 | 26% | 33% | 9% |
| ⊛ X-tra Cheese & Pepperoni | 1/3 pizza | 510 | 43% | 60% | 19% |

HARDEE'S

**Breakfast Dishes**

| | | | | | |
|------|------|------|------|------|------|
| ⊛ Bacon & Egg Biscuit | 1 serv | 490 | 42% | 45% | 52% |
| ⊛ Bacon, Egg & Cheese Biscuit | 1 serv | 530 | 48% | 55% | 52% |
| ⊛ BIG COUNTRY BREAKFAST w/Bacon | 1 serv | 740 | 66% | 65% | 102% |
| ⊛ BIG COUNTRY BREAKFAST w/Sausage | 1 serv | 930 | 94% | 95% | 113% |
| ⊛ BISCUIT 'N GRAVY | 1 serv | 510 | 43% | 45% | 5% |
| ⊛ CINNAMON 'N RAISIN Biscuit | 1 serv | 370 | 28% | 25% | 0% |
| ⊛ Country Ham Biscuit | 1 serv | 430 | 34% | 30% | 8% |
| ⊛ FRISCO Breakfast Sandwich w/Ham | 1 serv | 450 | 34% | 40% | 58% |
| ⊛ Ham Biscuit | 1 serv | 400 | 31% | 25% | 5% |
| ⊛ Ham, Egg & Cheese Biscuit | 1 serv | 500 | 42% | 50% | 57% |
| ⊛ Regular Hash Rounds | 1 serv | 230 | 22% | 15% | 0% |
| ⊛ RISE 'N SHINE Biscuit | 1 serv | 390 | 32% | 30% | 0% |
| ⊛ Sausage & Egg Biscuit | 1 serv | 560 | 54% | 55% | 57% |
| ⊛ Sausage Biscuit | 1 serv | 510 | 48% | 50% | 8% |
| ★ Three Pancakes | 1 serv | 280 | 3% | 5% | 5% |
| ⊛ Three Pancakes w/1 Sausage Patty | 1 serv | 430 | 25% | 30% | 13% |
| ❖ Three Pancakes w/2 Bacon Strips | 1 serv | 350 | 14% | 15% | 8% |
| ⊛ Ultimate Omelet Biscuit | 1 serv | 530 | 46% | 55% | 58% |

**Desserts**

| | | | | | |
|------|------|------|------|------|------|
| ❖ BIG COOKIE | 1 cookie | 280 | 18% | 20% | 5% |
| ★ COOL TWIST Cone: Chocolate | 1 cone | 180 | 3% | 5% | 5% |
| ★ COOL TWIST Cone: Vanilla | 1 cone | 170 | 3% | 5% | 3% |

★   Foods with this symbol have less than or equal to 5% *Daily Value* for <u>all</u> three nutrients (5% Rule).
❖   Foods with this symbol have <u>at least one</u> of the three nutrients greater than 5% *Daily Value* but less than or equal to 20% *Daily Value*.
⊛   Foods with this symbol have <u>at least one</u> of the three nutrients greater than 20% *Daily Value* (20% Rule).

| FOOD | Serving Size | Calories | Tot Fat | Sat Fat | Chol |
|------|-------------|----------|---------|---------|------|
| ★ COOL TWIST Cone: Vanilla/ Chocolate | 1 cone | 180 | 3% | 5% | 3% |
| ❖ COOL TWIST Sundae: Hot Fudge | 1 sundae | 290 | 9% | 15% | 7% |
| ★ COOL TWIST Sundae: Strawberry | 1 sundae | 210 | 3% | 5% | 3% |

**Entrees**

| FOOD | Serving Size | Calories | Tot Fat | Sat Fat | Chol |
|------|-------------|----------|---------|---------|------|
| ⊛ Chicken Thigh | 1 serv | 330 | 23% | 20% | 20% |
| ⊛ Chicken Breast | 1 serv | 370 | 23% | 20% | 25% |
| ❖ Chicken Leg | 1 serv | 170 | 11% | 10% | 15% |
| ❖ Chicken Wing | 1 serv | 200 | 12% | 10% | 10% |

**French Fries**

| FOOD | Serving Size | Calories | Tot Fat | Sat Fat | Chol |
|------|-------------|----------|---------|---------|------|
| ❖ Small | 1 serv | 240 | 15% | 15% | 0% |
| ⊛ Medium | 1 serv | 350 | 23% | 20% | 0% |
| ⊛ Large | 1 serv | 430 | 28% | 25% | 0% |

**Salads**

| FOOD | Serving Size | Calories | Tot Fat | Sat Fat | Chol |
|------|-------------|----------|---------|---------|------|
| ★ Fat Free French Dressing | 2 tbsp | 70 | 0% | 0% | 0% |
| ⊛ Garden Salad | 1 salad | 210 | 20% | 45% | 13% |
| ❖ Grilled Chicken Salad | 1 salad | 150 | 5% | 5% | 20% |
| ⊛ Ranch Dressing | 2 tbsp | 290 | 45% | 20% | 8% |
| ★ Side Salad (w/o dressing) | 1 salad | 25 | 1% | 2% | 0% |
| ⊛ Thousand Island Dressing | 2 tbsp | 250 | 35% | 15% | 12% |

**Sandwiches**

| FOOD | Serving Size | Calories | Tot Fat | Sat Fat | Chol |
|------|-------------|----------|---------|---------|------|
| ⊛ Bacon Cheeseburger | 1 burger | 600 | 55% | 75% | 17% |
| ⊛ BIG DELUXE Burger | 1 burger | 530 | 46% | 65% | 13% |
| ⊛ Cheeseburger | 1 burger | 300 | 20% | 35% | 8% |
| ⊛ Chicken Fillet | 1 sandwich | 470 | 26% | 15% | 17% |
| ⊛ FISHERMAN'S FILLET | 1 sandwich | 500 | 34% | 30% | 20% |
| ⊛ FRISCO Burger | 1 burger | 760 | 77% | 90% | 23% |
| ❖ Hamburger | 1 burger | 260 | 14% | 20% | 7% |
| ⊛ Hot Ham 'N Cheese | 1 sandwich | 350 | 20% | 30% | 17% |
| ⊛ Marinated Chicken Grill | 1 sandwich | 340 | 15% | 10% | 22% |
| ⊛ MUSHROOM 'N' SWISS Burger | 1 burger | 520 | 42% | 65% | 15% |
| ⊛ Quarter Pound Cheeseburger | 1 burger | 490 | 38% | 60% | 12% |
| ⊛ Regular Roast Beef | 1 sandwich | 270 | 17% | 25% | 8% |

**Shakes**

| FOOD | Serving Size | Calories | Tot Fat | Sat Fat | Chol |
|------|-------------|----------|---------|---------|------|
| ❖ Chocolate | 1 shake | 370 | 8% | 15% | 10% |
| ❖ Peach | 1 shake | 390 | 6% | 15% | 8% |
| ❖ Strawberry | 1 shake | 420 | 6% | 15% | 7% |
| ❖ Vanilla | 1 shake | 350 | 8% | 15% | 7% |

| FOOD | Serving Size | Calories | Tot Fat | Sat Fat | Chol |
|---|---|---|---|---|---|

**Side Dishes**

| | FOOD | Serving Size | Calories | Tot Fat | Sat Fat | Chol |
|---|---|---|---|---|---|---|
| Ⓐ | Cole Slaw | 1/2 cup | 240 | 31% | 15% | 3% |
| ★ | Gravy | 1.5 oz | 20 | 1% | 2% | 0% |
| ★ | Mashed Potatoes | 1/2 cup | 70 | 1% | 2% | 0% |

Jᴀᴄᴋ ɪɴ ᴛʜᴇ Bᴏx

**Breakfast Dishes**

| | FOOD | Serving Size | Calories | Tot Fat | Sat Fat | Chol |
|---|---|---|---|---|---|---|
| Ⓐ | BREAKFAST JACK | 1 serv | 300 | 18% | 25% | 62% |
| ★ | COUNTRY CROCK SPREAD | 1 tsp | 25 | 5% | 0% | 0% |
| ★ | Grape Jelly | 1 tsp | 40 | 0% | 0% | 0% |
| ❖ | Hash Browns | 1 serv | 160 | 17% | 13% | 0% |
| Ⓐ | Pancake Platter | 1 serv | 610 | 34% | 45% | 33% |
| ★ | Pancake Syrup | 1/4 cup | 120 | 0% | 0% | 0% |
| Ⓐ | Sausage Crescent | 1 serv | 580 | 66% | 64% | 62% |
| Ⓐ | Scrambled Egg Platter | 1 serv | 560 | 49% | 45% | 127% |
| Ⓐ | Scrambled Egg Pocket | 1 serv | 430 | 32% | 40% | 118% |
| Ⓐ | Sourdough Breakfast Sandwich | 1 sandwich | 380 | 31% | 35% | 78% |
| Ⓐ | Supreme Crescent | 1 serv | 530 | 51% | 50% | 70% |
| Ⓐ | Ultimate Breakfast Sandwich | 1 sandwich | 620 | 54% | 55% | 152% |

**Finger Foods**

| | FOOD | Serving Size | Calories | Tot Fat | Sat Fat | Chol |
|---|---|---|---|---|---|---|
| ★ | Barbecue Sauce | 2 tbsp | 45 | 0% | 0% | 0% |
| Ⓐ | Buttermilk House Sauce | 2 tbsp | 130 | 20% | 25% | 3% |
| ❖ | Chicken Strips (breaded) | 4 pcs | 290 | 20% | 15% | 17% |
| Ⓐ | Chicken Strips (breaded) | 6 pcs | 450 | 31% | 25% | 27% |
| Ⓐ | Chicken Taquitos | 5 pcs | 350 | 23% | 15% | 13% |
| Ⓐ | Chicken Taquitos | 8 pcs | 560 | 39% | 25% | 22% |
| Ⓐ | Egg Rolls | 3 pcs | 440 | 37% | 35% | 10% |
| Ⓐ | Egg Rolls | 5 pcs | 750 | 63% | 60% | 17% |
| ★ | Hot Sauce | 1 tsp | 5 | 0% | 0% | 0% |
| ★ | Sweet & Sour Sauce | 2 tbsp | 40 | 0% | 0% | 0% |

**Hamburgers**

| | FOOD | Serving Size | Calories | Tot Fat | Sat Fat | Chol |
|---|---|---|---|---|---|---|
| Ⓐ | 1/4 lb. Burger | 1 burger | 510 | 42% | 50% | 22% |
| Ⓐ | Bacon Bacon Cheeseburger | 1 burger | 710 | 69% | 75% | 37% |
| Ⓐ | Cheeseburger | 1 burger | 330 | 23% | 30% | 12% |
| Ⓐ | Double Cheeseburger | 1 burger | 450 | 37% | 60% | 25% |
| Ⓐ | Grilled Sourdough Burger | 1 burger | 670 | 66% | 80% | 37% |
| ❖ | Hamburger | 1 burger | 280 | 17% | 20% | 8% |
| Ⓐ | JUMBO JACK | 1 burger | 560 | 49% | 50% | 22% |
| Ⓐ | JUMBO JACK w/Cheese | 1 burger | 610 | 55% | 60% | 27% |

★   Foods with this symbol have less than or equal to 5% *Daily Value* for <u>all</u> three nutrients (5% Rule).
❖   Foods with this symbol have <u>at least one</u> of the three nutrients greater than 5% *Daily Value* but less than or equal to 20% *Daily Value*.
Ⓐ   Foods with this symbol have <u>at least one</u> of the three nutrients greater than 20% *Daily Value* (20% Rule).

| FOOD | Serving Size | Calories | Tot Fat | Sat Fat | Chol |
|---|---|---|---|---|---|
| ✬ The Colossus Burger | 1 burger | 940 | 92% | 125% | 55% |
| ✬ Ultimate Cheeseburger | 1 burger | 830 | 88% | 130% | 43% |

**Mexican Food**

| | | | | | |
|---|---|---|---|---|---|
| ❖ Guacamole | 2 tbsp | 50 | 6% | 3% | 0% |
| ★ Salsa | 2 tbsp | 10 | 0% | 0% | 0% |
| ✬ Super Taco | 1 taco | 280 | 26% | 30% | 10% |
| ❖ Taco | 1 taco | 190 | 17% | 20% | 7% |

**Salad Dressings**

| | | | | | |
|---|---|---|---|---|---|
| ✬ Bleu Cheese Dressing | 4 tbsp | 210 | 28% | 16% | 5% |
| ✬ Buttermilk House Dressing | 4 tbsp | 290 | 45% | 54% | 7% |
| ★ Low Calorie Italian | 4 tbsp | 25 | 2% | 0% | 0% |
| ✬ Thousand Island | 4 tbsp | 250 | 38% | 20% | 7% |

**Salads**

| | | | | | |
|---|---|---|---|---|---|
| ✬ Garden Chicken | 1 salad | 200 | 14% | 20% | 22% |
| ❖ Side | 1 salad | 70 | 6% | 13% | 3% |

**Sandwiches**

| | | | | | |
|---|---|---|---|---|---|
| ✬ Chicken | 1 sandwich | 400 | 28% | 20% | 15% |
| ✬ Chicken Caesar | 1 sandwich | 520 | 40% | 30% | 18% |
| ❖ Chicken Fajita Pita | 1 sandwich | 290 | 12% | 15% | 12% |
| ✬ Chicken Supreme | 1 sandwich | 620 | 55% | 55% | 25% |
| ✬ Country Fried Steak | 1 sandwich | 450 | 38% | 35% | 12% |
| ✬ Fish Supreme | 1 sandwich | 590 | 49% | 40% | 20% |
| ✬ Grilled Chicken Fillet | 1 sandwich | 430 | 29% | 25% | 22% |
| ✬ Monterey Roast Beef | 1 sandwich | 540 | 46% | 45% | 25% |
| ✬ Smoked Chicken Cheddar & Bacon | 1 sandwich | 540 | 46% | 55% | 27% |
| ✬ Sourdough Ranch Chicken | 1 sandwich | 490 | 32% | 30% | 22% |
| ✬ Spicy Crispy Chicken | 1 sandwich | 560 | 42% | 25% | 17% |

**Shakes**

| | | | | | |
|---|---|---|---|---|---|
| ❖ Chocolate Milk Shake (regular) | 1 shake | 390 | 9% | 18% | 8% |
| ❖ Strawberry Milk Shake (regular) | 1 shake | 330 | 11% | 20% | 10% |
| ❖ Vanilla Milk Shake (regular) | 1 shake | 350 | 11% | 20% | 10% |

**Sides and Desserts**

| | | | | | |
|---|---|---|---|---|---|
| ✬ Cheesecake | 1 serv | 310 | 28% | 25% | 22% |
| ✬ Chocolate Chip Cookie Dough Cheesecake | 1 serv | 360 | 28% | 40% | 15% |
| ✬ Cinnamon Churritos | 1 serv | 330 | 32% | 25% | 7% |
| ✬ Hot Apple Turnover | 1 turnover | 350 | 29% | 20% | 0% |
| ✬ Jumbo Fries | 1 serv | 400 | 29% | 25% | 0% |
| ✬ Onion Rings | 1 serv | 380 | 35% | 30% | 0% |
| ✬ Regular French Fries | 1 serv | 350 | 26% | 20% | 0% |

| FOOD | Serving Size | Calories | Tot Fat | Sat Fat | Chol |
|---|---|---|---|---|---|
| ❧ Seasoned Curly Fries | 1 serv | 360 | 31% | 25% | 0% |
| ❖ Small French Fries | 1 serv | 220 | 17% | 13% | 0% |
| ❧ Super Scoop French Fries | 1 serv | 590 | 45% | 35% | 0% |
| **Teriyaki Bowls** | | | | | |
| ❖ Beef Teriyaki | 1 bowl | 640 | 5% | 5% | 8% |
| ❖ Chicken Teriyaki | 1 bowl | 580 | 2% | 2% | 10% |

## KFC

| FOOD | Serving Size | Calories | Tot Fat | Sat Fat | Chol |
|---|---|---|---|---|---|
| **Breads** | | | | | |
| ❖ Biscuit | 1 biscuit | 220 | 18% | 15% | 1% |
| ★ Breadstick | 1 breadstick | 110 | 5% | 0% | 0% |
| ❖ Cornbread | 1 cornbread | 230 | 20% | 11% | 14% |
| ★ Sourdough Roll | 1 roll | 130 | 3% | 1% | 0% |
| **COLONEL'S Rotisserie Gold Chicken** | | | | | |
| ❧ Dark Quarter (skin removed by customer) | 4.1 oz | 220 | 19% | 18% | 43% |
| ❧ Dark Quarter (w/skin) | 5.1 oz | 330 | 36% | 33% | 54% |
| ❧ White Quarter (skin & wing removed by customer) | 4.1 oz | 200 | 9% | 9% | 32% |
| ❧ White Quarter (w/skin & wing) | 6.2 oz | 340 | 29% | 27% | 52% |
| **EXTRA TASTY CRISPY Chicken** | | | | | |
| ❧ Center Breast | 4.1 oz | 330 | 29% | 20% | 25% |
| ❧ Drumstick | 2.3 oz | 190 | 19% | 15% | 22% |
| ❧ Side Breast | 4.1 oz | 400 | 42% | 30% | 25% |
| ❧ Thigh | 3.8 oz | 380 | 45% | 35% | 30% |
| ❧ Whole Wing | 2.1 oz | 240 | 26% | 20% | 22% |
| **Hot & Spicy Chicken** | | | | | |
| ❧ Center Breast | 4.4 oz | 360 | 34% | 25% | 27% |
| ❖ Drumstick | 2.4 oz | 180 | 19% | 15% | 18% |
| ❧ Side Breast | 4.2 oz | 400 | 43% | 30% | 35% |
| ❧ Thigh | 4.2 oz | 370 | 42% | 30% | 33% |
| ❧ Whole Wing | 2.1 oz | 220 | 25% | 20% | 22% |
| **ORIGINAL RECIPE Chicken** | | | | | |
| ❧ Center Breast | 3.6 oz | 260 | 22% | 20% | 31% |
| ❧ Drumstick | 2.0 oz | 150 | 14% | 10% | 25% |
| ❧ Side Breast | 2.9 oz | 250 | 23% | 20% | 26% |

★ Foods with this symbol have less than or equal to 5% *Daily Value* for all three nutrients (5% Rule).
❖ Foods with this symbol have at least one of the three nutrients greater than 5% *Daily Value* but less than or equal to 20% *Daily Value*.
❧ Foods with this symbol have at least one of the three nutrients greater than 20% *Daily Value* (20% Rule).

| FOOD | Serving Size | Calories | Tot Fat | Sat Fat | Chol |
|---|---|---|---|---|---|
| ⊛ Thigh | 3.4 oz | 290 | 32% | 25% | 37% |
| ❖ Whole Wing | 1.9 oz | 170 | 17% | 15% | 20% |
| **Potatoes and Rice** | | | | | |
| ❖ Crispy Fries | 1 serv | 210 | 17% | 16% | 1% |
| ★ Garden Rice | 1 serv | 80 | 1% | 0% | 0% |
| ★ Mashed Potatoes w/Gravy | 1 serv | 70 | 2% | 5% | 1% |
| ❖ Potato Wedges | 1 serv | 190 | 14% | 14% | 1% |
| **Salads** | | | | | |
| ❖ Cole Slaw | 1 serv | 110 | 9% | 5% | 2% |
| ★ Garden Salad | 1 serv | 15 | 0% | 0% | 0% |
| ❖ Italian Dressing | 2 tbsp | 15 | 1% | 0% | 0% |
| ⊛ Macaroni Salad | 1 serv | 250 | 27% | 13% | 4% |
| ❖ Pasta Salad | 1 serv | 140 | 12% | 7% | 0% |
| ❖ Potato Salad | 1 serv | 180 | 17% | 8% | 4% |
| ⊛ Ranch Dressing | 2 tbsp | 170 | 28% | 13% | 3% |
| **Snackables** | | | | | |
| ❖ CHICKEN LITTLES Sandwich | 1 sandwich | 170 | 15% | 10% | 6% |
| ⊛ COLONEL'S Chicken Sandwich | 1 sandwich | 480 | 42% | 30% | 16% |
| ⊛ HOT WINGS Pieces | 6 pcs | 470 | 51% | 40% | 50% |
| ⊛ KENTUCKY NUGGETS | 6 pcs | 280 | 28% | 20% | 22% |
| **Specials** | | | | | |
| ❖ Macaroni & Cheese | 1 serv | 160 | 13% | 13% | 5% |
| ★ MEAN GREENS | 1 serv | 50 | 3% | 4% | 2% |
| ★ Red Beans & Rice | 1 serv | 110 | 4% | 4% | 1% |
| **Vegetables** | | | | | |
| ★ BBQ Baked Beans | 1 serv | 130 | 3% | 3% | 1% |
| ❖ Corn on the Cob | 1 cob | 220 | 18% | 9% | 0% |
| ★ Green Beans | 1 serv | 35 | 2% | 2% | 1% |
| ❖ Vegetable Medley Salad | 1 serv | 130 | 7% | 3% | 0% |

## LITTLE CAESARS

| FOOD | Serving Size | Calories | Tot Fat | Sat Fat | Chol |
|---|---|---|---|---|---|
| **Dessert** | | | | | |
| ⊛ Chocolate Ravioli | 1 serv | 140 | 14% | 27% | 1% |
| **Entrées** | | | | | |
| ⊛ Lasagna | 1 serv | 720 | 56% | 93% | 33% |
| ❖ Spaghetti | 1 serv | 260 | 9% | 9% | 3% |
| ❖ Spaghetti, Little Bucket | 1 serv | 530 | 19% | 17% | 5% |
| ❖ Veal Parmesan | 1 serv | 260 | 9% | 9% | 3% |

| FOOD | Serving Size | Calories | Tot Fat | Sat Fat | Chol |
|------|-----|----------|---------|---------|------|

**Pizzas**

| | | | | | | |
|---|---|---|---|---|---|---|
| ❖ | Crazy Bread | 1 slc | 110 | 5% | 3% | 0% |
| ★ | Crazy Sauce | 1 serv | 70 | 1% | 0% | 0% |
| Ⓐ | Slice Slice | 1 serv | 800 | 52% | 81% | 21% |

**Pizzas with Cheese**

| | | | | | | |
|---|---|---|---|---|---|---|
| Ⓐ | Small Round (6 slcs) | 2 slcs | 390 | 20% | 34% | 11% |
| Ⓐ | Medium Round (8 slcs) | 2 slcs | 400 | 21% | 35% | 11% |
| Ⓐ | Large Round (10 slcs) | 2 slcs | 420 | 24% | 40% | 13% |
| Ⓐ | Small PAN PAN (6 slcs) | 2 slcs | 370 | 20% | 33% | 11% |
| Ⓐ | Medium PAN PAN (9 slcs) | 2 slcs | 360 | 19% | 31% | 10% |
| Ⓐ | Large PAN PAN (12 slcs) | 2 slcs | 370 | 20% | 33% | 11% |

**Pizzas with Pepperoni**

| | | | | | | |
|---|---|---|---|---|---|---|
| Ⓐ | Small Round (6 slcs) | 2 slcs | 420 | 26% | 40% | 11% |
| Ⓐ | Medium Round (8 slcs) | 2 slcs | 440 | 27% | 41% | 11% |
| Ⓐ | Large Round (10 slcs) | 2 slcs | 470 | 30% | 47% | 13% |
| Ⓐ | Small PAN PAN (6 slcs) | 2 slcs | 410 | 25% | 39% | 11% |
| Ⓐ | Medium PAN PAN (9 slcs) | 2 slcs | 400 | 24% | 37% | 10% |
| Ⓐ | Large PAN PAN (12 slcs) | 2 slcs | 410 | 25% | 39% | 11% |
| Ⓐ | Baby PAN! PAN! | 1 pizza | 620 | 37% | 61% | 16% |

**Salads**

| | | | | | | |
|---|---|---|---|---|---|---|
| ❖ | Antipasto | 1 serv | 180 | 18% | 9% | 6% |
| ❖ | Caesar | 1 serv | 140 | 8% | 15% | 4% |
| ❖ | Greek | 1 serv | 170 | 15% | 0% | 12% |
| ★ | Tossed | 1 serv | 120 | 5% | 2% | 0% |

**Sandwiches**

| | | | | | | |
|---|---|---|---|---|---|---|
| Ⓐ | Big Veal Deal | 1 sandwich | 530 | 40% | 29% | 19% |
| Ⓐ | Chicken | 1 sandwich | 530 | 38% | 21% | 24% |
| Ⓐ | Ham & Cheese | 1 sandwich | 670 | 57% | 19% | 14% |
| Ⓐ | Italian | 1 sandwich | 720 | 66% | 37% | 18% |
| Ⓐ | Tuna | 1 sandwich | 730 | 59% | 27% | 21% |
| Ⓐ | Turkey | 1 sandwich | 560 | 35% | 18% | 15% |
| Ⓐ | Vegetarian | 1 sandwich | 870 | 82% | 51% | 29% |

### LONG JOHN SILVER'S

**À la Carte**

| | | | | | | |
|---|---|---|---|---|---|---|
| ❖ | Batter-Dipped Fish | 1 pc | 180 | 17% | 14% | 10% |
| ★ | Batter-Dipped Shrimp | 1 pc | 30 | 3% | 3% | 3% |

★ Foods with this symbol have less than or equal to 5% *Daily Value* for <u>all</u> three nutrients (5% Rule).

❖ Foods with this symbol have <u>at least one</u> of the three nutrients greater than 5% *Daily Value* but less than or equal to 20% *Daily Value*.

Ⓐ Foods with this symbol have <u>at least one</u> of the three nutrients greater than 20% *Daily Value* (20% Rule).

| FOOD | Serving Size | Calories | Tot Fat | Sat Fat | Chol |
|------|------|------|------|------|------|
| ❖ CHICKEN PLANK | 1 pc | 120 | 9% | 8% | 5% |
| ❖ Cole Slaw (drained on fork) | ~ 1/2 cup | 140 | 9% | 5% | 5% |
| ❖ Corn Cobbette | 1 pc | 140 | 12% | 0% | 0% |
| ❖ Crispy Fish | 1 serv | 150 | 12% | 11% | 7% |
| ⓐ Fries | 1 serv (3 oz) | 250 | 23% | 13% | 0% |
| ★ Green Beans | 1/2 cup | 20 | 1% | 1% | 0% |
| ★ Hushpuppy | 1 pc | 70 | 3% | 2% | 2% |
| ❖ Rice | 1/2 cup | 190 | 6% | 5% | 0% |
| ★ Roll | 1 roll | 110 | 1% | 1% | 0% |
| ❖ Seafood Chowder w/Cod | ~ 1 cup | 140 | 9% | 9% | 7% |
| ❖ Seafood Gumbo w/Cod | ~ 1 cup | 120 | 12% | 11% | 8% |

**Baked À la Carte**

| | | | | | |
|------|------|------|------|------|------|
| ❖ Chicken, Light Herb | 1 serv | 120 | 6% | 6% | 20% |
| ⓐ Fish w/Lemon Crumb | 3 pcs | 150 | 2% | 3% | 37% |

**Baked Entrées**

| | | | | | |
|------|------|------|------|------|------|
| ⓐ Chicken w/rice, green beans, slaw, roll w/o margarine | 1 serv | 590 | 23% | 17% | 25% |
| ⓐ Fish w/Lemon Crumb w/rice, green beans, slaw, roll w/o margarine | 3 pcs | 610 | 20% | 11% | 42% |
| ⓐ Light Portion Fish w/Lemon Crumb w/rice, side salad w/o dressing | 2 pcs | 330 | 8% | 5% | 25% |

**Chicken Entrées**

| | | | | | |
|------|------|------|------|------|------|
| ⓐ CHICKEN PLANKS w/fries | 2 pcs | 490 | 40% | 29% | 10% |
| ⓐ CHICKEN PLANKS w/fries, slaw & 2 hushpuppies | 3 pcs | 890 | 68% | 48% | 18% |

**Combos**

| | | | | | |
|------|------|------|------|------|------|
| ⓐ 1 Fish, 1 Chicken w/fries | 1 serv | 550 | 49% | 34% | 15% |
| ⓐ 1 Fish, 2 Chickens w/fries, slaw & 2 hushpuppies | 1 serv | 950 | 75% | 53% | 25% |
| ⓐ 2 Fish, 4 Shrimp, 3 oz Clams w/fries, slaw & 2 hushpuppies | 1 serv | 1240 | 108% | 76% | 47% |
| ⓐ 2 Fish, 5 Shrimp, 1 Chicken w/ fries, slaw & 2 hushpuppies | 1 serv | 1160 | 100% | 71% | 45% |
| ⓐ 2 Fish, 8 Shrimp w/fries, slaw & 2 hushpuppies | 1 serv | 1140 | 100% | 71% | 48% |

**Condiments**

| | | | | | |
|------|------|------|------|------|------|
| ★ Creamy Italian Dressing | 1 pkt | 30 | 5% | 0% | 0% |
| ★ Honey Mustard Sauce | 1 pkt | 20 | 1% | 1% | 0% |
| ⓐ Ranch Dressing | 1 pkt | 180 | 29% | 18% | 1% |
| ⓐ Sea Salad Dressing | 1 pkt | 140 | 23% | 30% | 1% |

| FOOD | Serving Size | Calories | Tot Fat | Sat Fat | Chol |
|---|---|---|---|---|---|
| ★  Seafood Sauce | 1 pkt | 14 | 1% | 1% | 0% |
| ★  Sweet & Sour Sauce | 1 pkt | 20 | 1% | 1% | 0% |
| ❖  Tartar Sauce | 1 pkt | 50 | 8% | 5% | 0% |
| **Desserts** | | | | | |
| Ⓐ  Apple Pie | 1 serv | 320 | 20% | 23% | 1% |
| Ⓐ  Cherry Pie | 1 serv | 360 | 20% | 22% | 2% |
| Ⓐ  Chocolate Chip Cookie | 1 serv | 230 | 14% | 29% | 3% |
| ❖  Lemon Pie | 1 serv | 340 | 14% | 15% | 15% |
| ❖  Oatmeal Raisin Cookie | 1 serv | 160 | 15% | 10% | 5% |
| Ⓐ  Pineapple Cream Cheese Cake | 1 serv | 310 | 28% | 45% | 3% |
| Ⓐ  Walnut Brownie | 1 serv | 440 | 34% | 27% | 7% |
| **Finger Foods** | | | | | |
| ❖  Batter-Dipped Fish | 1 pc | 180 | 17% | 14% | 10% |
| ❖  CHICKEN PLANKS | 2 pcs | 240 | 18% | 16% | 10% |
| **Fish Entrées** | | | | | |
| Ⓐ  Crispy Fish w/fries, slaw & 2 hushpuppies | 3 pcs fish | 980 | 77% | 57% | 23% |
| Ⓐ  Fish & Fries | 2 pcs | 610 | 57% | 40% | 20% |
| Ⓐ  Fish & More w/fries, slaw & 2 hushpuppies | 2 pcs fish | 890 | 74% | 51% | 25% |
| **Salads** | | | | | |
| ❖  Ocean Chef Salad w/ 1 hushpuppy | 1 serv | 110 | 2% | 2% | 13% |
| Ⓐ  Seafood Salad w/1 hushpuppy | 1 serv | 380 | 48% | 26% | 18% |
| ★  Side Salad w/o dressing | 1 serv | 25 | 1% | 0% | 0% |
| **Sandwiches** | | | | | |
| ❖  Batter-Dipped Chicken w/o sandwich sauce | 1 sandwich | 280 | 12% | 11% | 5% |
| ❖  Batter-Dipped Fish w/o sandwich sauce | 1 sandwich | 340 | 20% | 16% | 10% |
| **Seafood Entrées** | | | | | |
| Ⓐ  Clams w/fries, slaw & 2 hushpuppies | 6 oz | 990 | 80% | 55% | 25% |
| Ⓐ  Shrimp w/fries, slaw & 2 hushpuppies | 10 pcs | 840 | 72% | 49% | 33% |

★  Foods with this symbol have less than or equal to 5% *Daily Value* for <u>all</u> three nutrients (5% Rule).
❖  Foods with this symbol have <u>at least one</u> of the three nutrients greater than 5% *Daily Value* but less than or equal to 20% *Daily Value*.
Ⓐ  Foods with this symbol have <u>at least one</u> of the three nutrients greater than 20% *Daily Value* (20% Rule).

| FOOD | Serving Size | Calories | Tot Fat | Sat Fat | Chol |
|------|------|------|------|------|------|
| **McDonald's** | | | | | |
| **Breakfast** | | | | | |
| ☯ Bacon, Egg & Cheese Biscuit | 1 biscuit | 440 | 40% | 40% | 80% |
| ❖ Biscuit | 1 biscuit | 260 | 20% | 15% | 0% |
| ☯ Breakfast Burrito | 1 burrito | 280 | 26% | 20% | 45% |
| ★ CHEERIOS | 1 serv | 80 | 2% | 0% | 0% |
| ☯ Egg McMUFFIN | 1 muffin | 280 | 17% | 20% | 78% |
| ❖ English Muffin | 1 muffin | 170 | 6% | 5% | 0% |
| ❖ Hash Browns | 1 serv | 130 | 11% | 5% | 0% |
| ☯ Hotcakes  (Plain) | 1 serv | 245 | 22% | 5% | 3% |
| ❖ Hotcakes (Margarine and Syrup) | 1 serv | 435 | 18% | 10% | 3% |
| ☯ Sausage | 1 serv | 160 | 23% | 25% | 15% |
| ☯ Sausage Biscuit | 1 biscuit | 420 | 43% | 40% | 15% |
| ☯ Sausage Biscuit w/Egg | 1 biscuit | 505 | 51% | 50% | 87% |
| ☯ Sausage McMUFFIN | 1 muffin | 345 | 31% | 35% | 20% |
| ☯ Sausage McMUFFIN w/Egg | 1 muffin | 430 | 38% | 40% | 90% |
| ☯ Scrambled Eggs (2 eggs) | 1 serv | 140 | 15% | 15% | 142% |
| ★ WHEATIES | 1 serv | 90 | 2% | 0% | 0% |
| **Chicken McNUGGETS and Sauces** | | | | | |
| ★ Barbeque Sauce | 1 serv | 50 | 1% | 0% | 0% |
| ☯ Chicken McNUGGETS | 6 pcs | 270 | 23% | 18% | 18% |
| ★ Honey | 1 serv | 45 | 0% | 0% | 0% |
| ★ Hot Mustard Sauce | 1 serv | 70 | 5% | 3% | 2% |
| ★ Sweet 'N Sour Sauce | 1 serv | 60 | 0% | 0% | 0% |
| **Desserts** | | | | | |
| ☯ Baked Apple Pie | 1 pie | 280 | 23% | 10% | 0% |
| ☯ Chocolaty Chip Cookies | 1 serv | 330 | 23% | 20% | 2% |
| ❖ Hot Caramel Lowfat Frozen Yogurt Sundae | 1 sundae | 270 | 5% | 8% | 5% |
| ❖ Hot Fudge Lowfat Frozen Yogurt Sundae | 1 sundae | 240 | 5% | 10% | 2% |
| ❖ McDONALDLAND Cookies | 1 serv | 290 | 14% | 5% | 0% |
| ★ Strawberry Lowfat Frozen Yogurt Sundae | 1 sundae | 210 | 2% | 3% | 2% |
| ★ Vanilla Lowfat Frozen Yogurt Cone | 1 cone | 110 | 2% | 3% | 2% |
| **French Fries** | | | | | |
| ☯ Large | 1 serv | 400 | 34% | 25% | 0% |
| ☯ Medium | 1 serv | 320 | 26% | 18% | 0% |
| ❖ Small | 1  serv | 220 | 18% | 13% | 0% |
| **Muffins/Danish** | | | | | |
| ❖ Apple Bran Muffin | 1 muffin | 180 | 0% | 10% | 0% |

| FOOD | Serving Size | Calories | Tot Fat | Sat Fat | Chol |
|------|------|------|------|------|------|
| ⓐ Apple Danish | 1 danish | 360 | 25% | 25% | 13% |
| ⓐ Cheese Danish | 1 danish | 400 | 34% | 40% | 23% |
| ⓐ Cinnamon Raisin Danish | 1 danish | 430 | 34% | 35% | 17% |
| ⓐ Raspberry Danish | 1 danish | 390 | 25% | 25% | 15% |

**Salads and Dressings**

| | | | | | |
|------|------|------|------|------|------|
| ⓐ Chef Salad | 1 salad | 170 | 14% | 20% | 37% |
| ⓐ Chunky Chicken Salad | 1 salad | 150 | 6% | 5% | 27% |
| ⓐ Garden Salad | 1 salad | 50 | 3% | 3% | 22% |
| ❖ Side Salad | 1 salad | 30 | 2% | 3% | 10% |
| ★ Croutons | 1 serv | 50 | 3% | 3% | 0% |
| ★ Bacon Bits | 1 serv | 15 | 2% | 3% | 0% |
| ⓐ 1000 Island Dressing | 1 pkt | 225 | 23% | 25% | 13% |
| ⓐ Bleu Cheese Dressing | 1 pkt | 250 | 31% | 25% | 12% |
| ★ Lite Vinaigrette Dressing | 1 pkt | 50 | 3% | 3% | 0% |
| ⓐ Ranch Dressing | 1 pkt | 220 | 31% | 20% | 7% |
| ❖ Red French Reduced Calorie Dressing | 1 pkt | 160 | 12% | 5% | 0% |

**Sandwiches**

| | | | | | |
|------|------|------|------|------|------|
| ⓐ BIG MAC | 1 burger | 500 | 40% | 45% | 33% |
| ⓐ Cheeseburger | 1 burger | 305 | 20% | 25% | 17% |
| ❖ Chicken Fajita | 1 sandwich | 190 | 12% | 10% | 12% |
| ⓐ FILET-O-FISH | 1 sandwich | 370 | 28% | 20% | 17% |
| ❖ Hamburger | 1 burger | 255 | 14% | 15% | 12% |
| ⓐ McCHICKEN | 1 sandwich | 470 | 38% | 25% | 20% |
| ⓐ McGrilled Chicken | 1 sandwich | 400 | 18% | 20% | 27% |
| ❖ McLEAN DELUXE | 1 burger | 320 | 15% | 20% | 20% |
| ⓐ McLEAN DELUXE w/Cheese | 1 burger | 370 | 22% | 25% | 25% |
| ⓐ QUARTER POUNDER | 1 burger | 410 | 31% | 40% | 28% |
| ⓐ QUARTER POUNDER w/Cheese | 1 burger | 510 | 45% | 55% | 38% |

**Shakes**

| | | | | | |
|------|------|------|------|------|------|
| ❖ Chocolate Shake | 1 shake | 350 | 9% | 20% | 8% |
| ❖ Strawberry Shake | 1 shake | 340 | 8% | 15% | 8% |
| ❖ Vanilla Shake | 1 shake | 310 | 8% | 15% | 8% |

## PIZZA HUT

**BIGFOOT Pizzas**

| | | | | | |
|------|------|------|------|------|------|
| ⓐ Cheese | 2 slcs | 270 | 18% | 30% | 11% |
| ⓐ Pepperoni | 2 slcs | 410 | 22% | 30% | 13% |

★ Foods with this symbol have less than or equal to 5% *Daily Value* for <u>all</u> three nutrients (5% Rule).
❖ Foods with this symbol have <u>at least one</u> of the three nutrients greater than 5% *Daily Value* but less than or equal to 20% *Daily Value*.
ⓐ Foods with this symbol have <u>at least one</u> of the three nutrients greater than 20% *Daily Value* (20% Rule).

| FOOD | Serving Size | Calories | Tot Fat | Sat Fat | Chol |
|------|--------------|----------|---------|---------|------|
| ⊛ Pepperoni, Mushroom, and Italian Sausage | 2 slcs | 430 | 25% | 40% | 14% |

**Hand Tossed Pizzas (Medium)**

| FOOD | Serving Size | Calories | Tot Fat | Sat Fat | Chol |
|------|--------------|----------|---------|---------|------|
| ❖ Beef | 1 slc | 260 | 14% | 20% | 9% |
| ❖ Cheese | 1 slc | 240 | 11% | 20% | 8% |
| ❖ Ham | 1 slc | 210 | 8% | 15% | 7% |
| ⊛ Italian Sausage | 1 slc | 270 | 17% | 25% | 10% |
| ⊛ MEAT LOVER'S | 1 slc | 310 | 17% | 30% | 13% |
| ❖ Pepperoni | 1 slc | 240 | 12% | 20% | 8% |
| ⊛ PEPPERONI LOVER'S | 1 slc | 310 | 22% | 30% | 13% |
| ⊛ Pork Topping | 1 slc | 270 | 15% | 25% | 9% |
| ⊛ Super Supreme | 1 slc | 300 | 20% | 25% | 11% |
| ⊛ Supreme | 1 slc | 280 | 18% | 25% | 10% |
| ❖ VEGGIE LOVER'S | 1 slc | 220 | 9% | 15% | 6% |

**Pan Pizzas (Medium)**

| FOOD | Serving Size | Calories | Tot Fat | Sat Fat | Chol |
|------|--------------|----------|---------|---------|------|
| ⊛ Beef | 1 slc | 290 | 20% | 25% | 9% |
| ⊛ Cheese | 1 slc | 260 | 17% | 25% | 8% |
| ❖ Ham | 1 slc | 240 | 14% | 15% | 7% |
| ⊛ Italian Sausage | 1 slc | 290 | 23% | 25% | 10% |
| ⊛ MEAT LOVER'S | 1 slc | 340 | 28% | 35% | 13% |
| ❖ Pepperoni | 1 slc | 270 | 18% | 20% | 8% |
| ⊛ PEPPERONI LOVER'S | 1 slc | 330 | 26% | 35% | 13% |
| ⊛ Pork Topping | 1 slc | 290 | 22% | 25% | 9% |
| ⊛ Super Supreme | 1 slc | 320 | 26% | 30% | 11% |
| ⊛ Supreme | 1 slc | 310 | 23% | 30% | 10% |
| ❖ VEGGIE LOVER'S | 1 slc | 240 | 15% | 15% | 6% |

**PERSONAL PAN PIZZA**

| FOOD | Serving Size | Calories | Tot Fat | Sat Fat | Chol |
|------|--------------|----------|---------|---------|------|
| ⊛ Pepperoni Supreme | Whole pizza | 640 | 43% | 50% | 18% |
| ⊛ Supreme | Whole pizza | 720 | 52% | 60% | 22% |

**THIN 'N CRISPY Pizzas (Medium)**

| FOOD | Serving Size | Calories | Tot Fat | Sat Fat | Chol |
|------|--------------|----------|---------|---------|------|
| ⊛ Beef | 1 slc | 230 | 17% | 25% | 9% |
| ⊛ Cheese | 2 slcs | 410 | 25% | 40% | 17% |
| ⊛ Ham | 2 slcs | 370 | 22% | 30% | 15% |
| ⊛ Italian Sausage | 2 slcs | 470 | 37% | 50% | 21% |
| ⊛ MEAT LOVER'S | 1 slc | 230 | 20% | 30% | 13% |
| ⊛ Pepperoni | 2 slcs | 430 | 31% | 40% | 17% |
| ⊛ PEPPERONI LOVER'S | 1 slc | 290 | 25% | 35% | 14% |
| ⊛ Pork Topping | 1 slc | 240 | 18% | 25% | 9% |
| ⊛ Super Supreme | 1 slc | 270 | 22% | 30% | 12% |
| ⊛ Supreme | 1 slc | 260 | 20% | 25% | 10% |
| ❖ VEGGIE LOVER'S | 1 slc | 190 | 11% | 15% | 6% |

| FOOD | Serving Size | Calories | Tot Fat | Sat Fat | Chol |
|------|-------------|----------|---------|---------|------|

## TACO BELL

### Border Lights

Tacos

| | | | | | | |
|---|---|---|---|---|---|---|
| ❖ | LIGHT Taco | 1 serv | 140 | 8% | 8% | 7% |
| ❖ | LIGHT Taco Supreme | 1 serv | 160 | 8% | 8% | 7% |
| ❖ | LIGHT Soft Taco | 1 serv | 180 | 8% | 12% | 8% |
| ❖ | LIGHT Soft Taco Supreme | 1 serv | 200 | 8% | 12% | 8% |
| ❖ | LIGHT Chicken Soft Taco | 1 serv | 180 | 8% | 5% | 10% |

Burritos

| | | | | | | |
|---|---|---|---|---|---|---|
| ❖ | LIGHT Bean Burrito | 1 serv | 330 | 9% | 10% | 2% |
| ❖ | LIGHT Chicken Burrito | 1 serv | 290 | 9% | 8% | 10% |
| ❖ | LIGHT Burrito Supreme | 1 serv | 350 | 12% | 15% | 8% |
| ❖ | LIGHT 7-Layer Burrito | 1 serv | 440 | 14% | 10% | 2% |
| Ⓐ | LIGHT Chicken Burrito Supreme | 1 serv | 410 | 15% | 10% | 22% |

Salad

| | | | | | | |
|---|---|---|---|---|---|---|
| Ⓐ | LIGHT Taco Salad w/chips | 1 serv | 680 | 38% | 40% | 17% |
| Ⓐ | LIGHT Taco Salad without chips | 1 serv | 330 | 14% | 22% | 17% |

### Burritos

| | | | | | | |
|---|---|---|---|---|---|---|
| Ⓐ | 7 Layer Burrito | 1 serv | 485 | 32% | 40% | 9% |
| ❖ | Bean Burrito | 1 serv | 391 | 18% | 20% | 2% |
| Ⓐ | Beef Burrito | 1 serv | 432 | 29% | 40% | 19% |
| Ⓐ | Big Beef BURRITO SUPREME | 1 serv | 525 | 38% | 55% | 24% |
| Ⓐ | BURRITO SUPREME | 1 serv | 443 | 29% | 45% | 16% |
| Ⓐ | Chicken Burrito | 1 serv | 345 | 20% | 25% | 19% |
| Ⓐ | Chicken BURRITO SUPREME | 1 serv | 520 | 35% | 45% | 42% |
| Ⓐ | Chili Cheese Burrito | 1 serv | 391 | 28% | 45% | 16% |
| Ⓐ | Combo Burrito | 1 serv | 412 | 25% | 30% | 11% |
| Ⓐ | Steak BURRITO SUPREME | 1 serv | 500 | 35% | 55% | 25% |

### Side Orders and Condiments

| | | | | | | |
|---|---|---|---|---|---|---|
| ★ | Green Sauce | 1 serv | 4 | 0% | 0% | 0% |
| ★ | Guacamole | 1 serv | 36 | 5% | 5% | 0% |
| ★ | Hot Taco Sauce | 1 serv | 2 | 0% | 0% | 0% |
| ★ | Mild Taco Sauce | 1 serv | 0 | 0% | 0% | 0% |
| ❖ | Nacho Cheese Sauce | 1 serv | 51 | 6% | 10% | 1% |
| ★ | Picante Sauce | 1 serv | 3 | 0% | 0% | 0% |
| ★ | Pico de Gallo | 1 serv | 6 | 0% | 0% | 0% |
| Ⓐ | Ranch Dressing | 1 serv | 136 | 22% | 15% | 7% |
| ★ | Red Sauce | 1 serv | 10 | 0% | 0% | 0% |
| ★ | Salsa | 1 serv | 27 | 0% | 0% | 0% |
| ★ | Seasoned Rice | 1 serv | 110 | 5% | 5% | 2% |

★   Foods with this symbol have less than or equal to 5% *Daily Value* for <u>all</u> three nutrients (5% Rule).
❖   Foods with this symbol have <u>at least one</u> of the three nutrients greater than 5% *Daily Value* but less than or equal to 20% *Daily Value*.
Ⓐ   Foods with this symbol have <u>at least one</u> of the three nutrients greater than 20% *Daily Value* (20% Rule).

| FOOD | Serving Size | Calories | Tot Fat | Sat Fat | Chol |
|------|--------------|----------|---------|---------|------|
| ❖ Sour Cream | 1 serv | 44 | 6% | 15% | 5% |

**Specialty Items**

| FOOD | Serving Size | Calories | Tot Fat | Sat Fat | Chol |
|------|--------------|----------|---------|---------|------|
| Ⓐ Beef MEXMELT | 1 serv | 262 | 22% | 35% | 13% |
| ❖ Cinnamon Twists | 1 serv | 139 | 9% | 0% | 0% |
| Ⓐ Mexican Pizza | 1 serv | 574 | 58% | 60% | 17% |
| Ⓐ Nachos | 1 serv | 345 | 28% | 30% | 3% |
| Ⓐ Nachos BELLGRANDE | 1 serv | 633 | 52% | 60% | 16% |
| Ⓐ Nachos Supreme | 1 serv | 364 | 28% | 25% | 6% |
| ❖ Pintos 'N Cheese | 1 serv | 190 | 14% | 20% | 5% |
| Ⓐ Taco Salad | 1 serv | 838 | 85% | 80% | 26% |

**Tacos and Tostadas**

| FOOD | Serving Size | Calories | Tot Fat | Sat Fat | Chol |
|------|--------------|----------|---------|---------|------|
| ❖ Chicken Soft Taco | 1 serv | 223 | 15% | 20% | 19% |
| Ⓐ Soft Taco | 1 serv | 223 | 17% | 25% | 11% |
| Ⓐ SOFT TACO SUPREME | 1 serv | 268 | 23% | 40% | 16% |
| ❖ Steak Soft Taco | 1 serv | 27 | 14% | 20% | 10% |
| Ⓐ Taco | 1 serv | 180 | 17% | 25% | 11% |
| Ⓐ TACO SUPREME | 1 serv | 225 | 23% | 35% | 16% |
| ❖ Tostada | 1 serv | 242 | 17% | 20% | 5% |

## TACO JOHN'S

**Burritos**

| FOOD | Serving Size | Calories | Tot Fat | Sat Fat | Chol |
|------|--------------|----------|---------|---------|------|
| ❖ Bean | 1 burrito | 340 | 17% | 15% | 5% |
| Ⓐ Beef | 1 burrito | 420 | 29% | 32% | 14% |
| Ⓐ Combination | 1 burrito | 380 | 21% | 28% | 10% |
| Ⓐ Super | 1 burrito | 420 | 29% | 33% | 12% |

**Desserts**

| FOOD | Serving Size | Calories | Tot Fat | Sat Fat | Chol |
|------|--------------|----------|---------|---------|------|
| ★ Apple Flauta | 1 serv | 80 | 2% | 1% | 0% |
| ❖ Cherry Flauta | 1 serv | 140 | 5% | 4% | 0% |
| Ⓐ Choco Taco | 1 taco | 320 | 26% | 55% | 7% |
| ❖ Churro | 1 serv | 150 | 12% | 9% | 1% |
| ❖ Cream Cheese Flauta | 1 serv | 180 | 12% | 15% | 3% |

**Fajitas**

| FOOD | Serving Size | Calories | Tot Fat | Sat Fat | Chol |
|------|--------------|----------|---------|---------|------|
| Ⓐ Chicken Fajita Burrito | 1 serv | 360 | 18% | 25% | 16% |
| Ⓐ Chicken Fajita Salad (no dressing) | 1 serv | 560 | 53% | 48% | 18% |
| ❖ Chicken Fajita Softshell | 1 serv | 220 | 13% | 15% | 11% |

**Kid's Meals**

| FOOD | Serving Size | Calories | Tot Fat | Sat Fat | Chol |
|------|--------------|----------|---------|---------|------|
| Ⓐ w/Crispy Taco | 1 serv | 580 | 51% | 48% | 10% |
| Ⓐ w/Softshell Taco | 1 serv | 620 | 50% | 49% | 11% |
| Ⓐ w/Taco Burger | 1 serv | 670 | 52% | 51% | 12% |

| FOOD | Serving Size | Calories | Tot Fat | Sat Fat | Chol |
|------|--------------|----------|---------|---------|------|
| **Platters** | | | | | |
| ⓐ Chimichanga Platter | 1 platter | 920 | 54% | 68% | 17% |
| ⓐ Double Enchilada | 1 platter | 900 | 56% | 65% | 24% |
| ⓐ Sampler | 1 platter | 1280 | 78% | 93% | 32% |
| ⓐ Smothered Burrito | 1 platter | 970 | 58% | 73% | 20% |
| **Side Orders and Extras** | | | | | |
| ❖ Beans ("Refried") | 1 serv | 300 | 12% | 8% | 3% |
| ⓐ Chili (Texas Style w/2 Saltine Crackers) | 1 serv | 300 | 22% | 33% | 16% |
| ⓐ Mexican Rice | 1 cup | 570 | 27% | 24% | 0% |
| ⓐ Nachos | 1 serv | 290 | 26% | 19% | 2% |
| ⓐ POTATO OLES w/Nacho Cheese | 1 serv | 520 | 52% | 43% | 2% |
| ❖ Salad Dressing: House | 2 tbsp | 110 | 18% | 9% | 0% |
| **Special Features** | | | | | |
| ⓐ MEXI ROLLS w/Guacamole | 1 serv | 840 | 70% | 59% | 15% |
| ⓐ MEXI ROLLS w/Nacho Cheese | 1 serv | 810 | 66% | 53% | 15% |
| ⓐ MEXI ROLLS w/Salsa | 1 serv | 750 | 57% | 53% | 15% |
| ⓐ MEXI ROLLS w/Sour Cream | 1 serv | 850 | 72% | 53% | 15% |
| ⓐ Mexican Pizza | 1 serv | 640 | 55% | 68% | 18% |
| ⓐ SIERRA CHICKEN FILLET SANDWICH | 1 sandwich | 500 | 32% | 28% | 14% |
| ⓐ Super Nachos | 1 serv | 850 | 77% | 77% | 17% |
| ⓐ Taco Salad (no dressing) | 1 salad | 470 | 47% | 42% | 7% |
| **Tacos** | | | | | |
| ❖ Crispy | 1 serv | 180 | 16% | 19% | 7% |
| ⓐ Softshell | 1 serv | 280 | 17% | 21% | 7% |
| ⓐ TACO BRAVO | 1 serv | 330 | 21% | 22% | 8% |
| ⓐ Taco Burger | 1 serv | 280 | 17% | 22% | 9% |

WENDY'S

| FOOD | Serving Size | Calories | Tot Fat | Sat Fat | Chol |
|------|--------------|----------|---------|---------|------|
| **Baked Potato** | | | | | |
| ⓐ Bacon & Cheese | 1 each | 530 | 28% | 20% | 7% |
| ⓐ Broccoli & Cheese | 1 each | 460 | 22% | 13% | 0% |
| ⓐ Cheese | 1 each | 560 | 35% | 40% | 10% |
| ⓐ Chili & Cheese | 1 each | 610 | 37% | 45% | 15% |
| ★ Plain | 10 oz | 310 | 0% | 0% | 0% |
| ❖ Sour Cream & Chives | 1 each | 380 | 9% | 20% | 5% |
| ❖ Sour Cream | 1 pkt | 60 | 9% | 20% | 3% |

★ Foods with this symbol have less than or equal to 5% *Daily Value* for <u>all</u> three nutrients (5% Rule).
❖ Foods with this symbol have <u>at least one</u> of the three nutrients greater than 5% *Daily Value* but less than or equal to 20% *Daily Value.*
ⓐ Foods with this symbol have <u>at least one</u> of the three nutrients greater than 20% *Daily Value* (20% Rule).

| FOOD | Serving Size | Calories | Tot Fat | Sat Fat | Chol |
|------|--------------|----------|---------|---------|------|
| ❖ Whipped Margarine | 1 pkt | 60 | 8% | 5% | 0% |
| **Chicken Nuggets** | | | | | |
| ★ Barbeque Sauce | 1 pkt | 50 | 0% | 0% | 0% |
| ★ Honey | 1 pkt | 45 | 0% | 0% | 0% |
| ❋ Nuggets | 6 pcs | 280 | 31% | 25% | 17% |
| ★ Sweet & Sour Sauce | 1 pkt | 45 | 0% | 0% | 0% |
| ★ Sweet Mustard Sauce | 1 pkt | 50 | 2% | 0% | 0% |
| **Chili** | | | | | |
| ❖ Cheddar Cheese, shredded | 2 tbsp | 70 | 9% | 15% | 5% |
| ❖ Large | 12 oz | 290 | 14% | 20% | 20% |
| ★ Saltine Crackers | 2 crackers | 25 | 1% | 0% | 0% |
| ❖ Small | 8 oz | 190 | 9% | 13% | 13% |
| **Desserts** | | | | | |
| ❋ Chocolate Chip Cookie | 1 cookie | 270 | 17% | 40% | 5% |
| ❋ Frosty Dairy Dessert, small | 12 oz | 340 | 15% | 25% | 13% |
| ❋ Frosty Dairy Dessert, medium | 16 oz | 460 | 20% | 35% | 18% |
| ❋ Frosty Dairy Dessert, large | 20 oz | 570 | 26% | 45% | 23% |
| **French Fries** | | | | | |
| ❖ Small | 1 serv | 240 | 18% | 13% | 0% |
| ❋ Medium | 1 serv | 340 | 26% | 20% | 0% |
| ❋ Biggie | 1 serv | 420 | 31% | 20% | 0% |
| **Fresh Salads to Go (without Dressing)** | | | | | |
| ❖ Caesar Side Salad | 1 each | 110 | 8% | 10% | 5% |
| ❖ Deluxe Garden Salad | 1 each | 110 | 9% | 5% | 0% |
| ❖ Grilled Chicken Salad | 1 each | 200 | 12% | 8% | 17% |
| ★ Side Salad | 1 each | 60 | 5% | 3% | 0% |
| ★ Soft Breadstick | 1 stick | 130 | 5% | 3% | 2% |
| ❋ Taco Salad | 1 each | 580 | 46% | 55% | 25% |
| **GARDEN SPOT Salad Bar** | | | | | |
| ★ Applesauce | 2 tbsp | 30 | 0% | 0% | 0% |
| ★ Bacon Bits | 2 tbsp | 40 | 2% | 3% | 2% |
| ★ Broccoli | 1/4 cup | 0 | 0% | 0% | 0% |
| ★ Cantaloupe, sliced | 1 pc | 15 | 0% | 0% | 0% |
| ★ Carrots | 1/4 cup | 5 | 0% | 0% | 0% |
| ★ Cauliflower | 2 tbsp | 0 | 0% | 0% | 0% |
| ❖ Cheddar Chips | 2 tbsp | 70 | 6% | 5% | 0% |
| ❖ Cheese (imitation), shredded | 2 tbsp | 50 | 6% | 5% | 0% |
| ❖ Chicken Salad | 2 tbsp | 70 | 8% | 5% | 0% |
| ★ Chives | 1 tbsp | 0 | 0% | 0% | 0% |
| ★ Chow Mein Noodles | 1/4 cup | 35 | 3% | 0% | 0% |
| ★ Cole Slaw | 2 tbsp | 45 | 5% | 0% | 2% |

| FOOD | Serving Size | Calories | Tot Fat | Sat Fat | Chol |
|---|---|---|---|---|---|
| ★ Cottage Cheese | 2 tbsp | 30 | 2% | 5% | 2% |
| ★ Croutons | 2 tbsp | 30 | 2% | 0% | 0% |
| ★ Cucumbers | 2 slc | 0 | 0% | 0% | 0% |
| ⊛ Eggs, hard cooked | 2 tbsp | 40 | 5% | 5% | 37% |
| ★ Green Peas | 2 tbsp | 15 | 0% | 0% | 0% |
| ★ Green Peppers | 2 pcs | 0 | 0% | 0% | 0% |
| ★ Honeydew Melon, sliced | 1 pc | 20 | 0% | 0% | 0% |
| ★ Jalapeno Peppers | 1 tbsp | 0 | 0% | 0% | 0% |
| ★ Lettuce (Iceberg/Romaine) | 1 cup | 10 | 0% | 0% | 0% |
| ★ Mushrooms | 1/2 cup | 0 | 0% | 0% | 0% |
| ★ Olives, Black | 2 tbsp | 15 | 2% | 0% | 0% |
| ★ Orange, sectioned | 1 pc | 10 | 0% | 0% | 0% |
| ★ Pasta Salad | 2 tbsp | 25 | 0% | 0% | 0% |
| ★ Peaches, sliced | 1 pc | 15 | 0% | 0% | 0% |
| ★ Pepperoni, sliced | 6 slcs | 30 | 5% | 5% | 2% |
| ★ Pineapple, chunked | 4 pcs | 20 | 0% | 0% | 0% |
| ❖ Potato Salad | 2 tbsp | 80 | 11% | 13% | 2% |
| ★ Pudding, Chocolate | 1/4 cup | 70 | 5% | 3% | 0% |
| ★ Pudding, Vanilla | 1/4 cup | 70 | 5% | 3% | 0% |
| ★ Red Onions | 3 rings | 0 | 0% | 0% | 0% |
| ❖ Seafood Salad | 1/4 cup | 70 | 6% | 3% | 0% |
| ★ Sesame Breadstick | 1 stick | 15 | 0% | 0% | 0% |
| ★ Strawberries | 1 each | 10 | 0% | 0% | 0% |
| ★ Strawberry Banana Dessert | 1/4 cup | 30 | 0% | 0% | 0% |
| ❖ Sunflower Seeds and Raisins | 2 tbsp | 80 | 8% | 3% | 0% |
| ★ Tomato, wedged | 1 pc | 5 | 0% | 0% | 0% |
| ❖ Turkey Ham, diced | 2 tbsp | 50 | 6% | 5% | 8% |
| ★ Watermelon, wedged | 1 pc | 20 | 0% | 0% | 0% |

## Hamburgers

| | | | | | |
|---|---|---|---|---|---|
| ⊛ Big Bacon Classic | 1 each | 640 | 55% | 65% | 37% |
| ⊛ Cheeseburger Kids' Meal | 1 each | 310 | 20% | 25% | 15% |
| ❖ Hamburger, Kids' Meal | 1 each | 270 | 14% | 15% | 12% |
| ⊛ Jr. Bacon Cheeseburger | 1 each | 440 | 38% | 40% | 22% |
| ⊛ Jr. Cheeseburger | 1 each | 320 | 20% | 25% | 15% |
| ⊛ Jr. Cheeseburger Deluxe | 1 each | 390 | 31% | 35% | 17% |
| ❖ Jr. Hamburger | 1 each | 270 | 14% | 15% | 12% |
| ⊛ Plain Single | 1 each | 350 | 23% | 30% | 23% |
| ⊛ Single w/Everything | 1 each | 440 | 35% | 35% | 25% |

## Salad Dressings

| | | | | | |
|---|---|---|---|---|---|
| ⊛ Blue Cheese | 2 tbsp | 180 | 29% | 15% | 5% |
| ❖ Celery Seed | 2 tbsp | 100 | 11% | 5% | 3% |
| ❖ French | 2 tbsp | 120 | 17% | 8% | 0% |

★ Foods with this symbol have less than or equal to 5% *Daily Value* for <u>all</u> three nutrients (5% Rule).

❖ Foods with this symbol have <u>at least one</u> of the three nutrients greater than 5% *Daily Value* but less than or equal to 20% *Daily Value*.

⊛ Foods with this symbol have <u>at least one</u> of the three nutrients greater than 20% *Daily Value* (20% Rule).

| | FOOD | Serving Size | Calories | Tot Fat | Sat Fat | Chol |
|---|---|---|---|---|---|---|
| ★ | French, Fat Free | 2 tbsp | 35 | 0% | 0% | 0% |
| ❖ | French, Sweet Red | 2 tbsp | 130 | 15% | 8% | 0% |
| ❖ | HIDDEN VALLEY Ranch | 2 tbsp | 90 | 15% | 8% | 3% |
| ❖ | HIDDEN VALLEY Ranch, Reduced Fat, Reduced Calorie | 2 tbsp | 60 | 8% | 5% | 3% |
| Ⓐ | Italian Caesar | 2 tbsp | 150 | 25% | 13% | 5% |
| ❖ | Italian, Golden | 2 tbsp | 90 | 11% | 5% | 0% |
| ★ | Italian, Reduced Fat, Reduced Calorie | 2 tbsp | 40 | 5% | 3% | 0% |
| Ⓐ | Salad Oil | 1 tbsp | 130 | 22% | 10% | 0% |
| ❖ | Thousand Island | 2 tbsp | 130 | 20% | 10% | 3% |
| ★ | Wine Vinegar | 1 tbsp | 0 | 0% | 0% | 0% |

**Sandwich Components**

| | FOOD | Serving Size | Calories | Tot Fat | Sat Fat | Chol |
|---|---|---|---|---|---|---|
| Ⓐ | 1/4 lb. Hamburger Patty | 1 each | 190 | 18% | 25% | 23% |
| ❖ | American Cheese, Jr. | 1 slc | 45 | 6% | 13% | 3% |
| ❖ | American Cheese | 1 slc | 70 | 9% | 20% | 5% |
| ★ | Bacon | 1 slc | 30 | 4% | 5% | 2% |
| ❖ | Breaded Chicken Fillet | 1 pc | 220 | 15% | 10% | 18% |
| ❖ | Grilled Chicken Fillet | 1 pc | 100 | 4% | 3% | 17% |
| ❖ | Jr. Hamburger Patty | 1 each | 90 | 9% | 13% | 12% |
| ★ | Kaiser Bun | 1 bun | 190 | 5% | 3% | 0% |
| ★ | Ketchup | 1 tsp | 10 | 0% | 0% | 0% |
| ★ | Lettuce | 1 leaf | 0 | 0% | 0% | 0% |
| ❖ | Mayonnaise | 1 1/2 tsp | 70 | 11% | 5% | 2% |
| ★ | Mustard | 1/2 tsp | 0 | 0% | 0% | 0% |
| ★ | Onion | 4 rings | 0 | 0% | 0% | 0% |
| ★ | Pickles | 4 slcs | 0 | 0% | 0% | 0% |
| ★ | Reduced Calorie Honey Mustard | 1 tsp | 25 | 2% | 0% | 0% |
| ★ | Sandwich Bun | 1 bun | 160 | 4% | 3% | 0% |
| ★ | Tomatoes | 1 slc | 5 | 0% | 0% | 0% |

**Sandwiches**

| | FOOD | Serving Size | Calories | Tot Fat | Sat Fat | Chol |
|---|---|---|---|---|---|---|
| Ⓐ | Breaded Chicken Sandwich | 1 each | 450 | 31% | 20% | 20% |
| Ⓐ | Chicken Club Sandwich | 1 each | 520 | 38% | 30% | 25% |
| ❖ | Grilled Chicken Sandwich | 1 each | 290 | 11% | 8% | 18% |

**Superbar** (where Available)

| | FOOD | Serving Size | Calories | Tot Fat | Sat Fat | Chol |
|---|---|---|---|---|---|---|
| ★ | Alfredo Sauce | 1/4 cup | 30 | 2% | 0% | 0% |
| ★ | Cheese Sauce | 1/4 cup | 25 | 2% | 0% | 0% |
| ❖ | Macaroni & Cheese | 1/2 cup | 130 | 9% | 13% | 2% |
| ❖ | Parmesan Cheese, grated | 2 tbsp | 70 | 8% | 15% | 5% |
| ★ | Picante Sauce | 2 tbsp | 10 | 0% | 0% | 0% |
| ★ | Refried Beans | 1/4 cup | 80 | 5% | 5% | 0% |
| ★ | Rice, Spanish | 1/4 cup | 60 | 2% | 0% | 0% |
| ★ | Rotini | 1/2 cup | 90 | 3% | 0% | 0% |
| Ⓐ | Sour Topping | 2 tbsp | 60 | 8% | 25% | 0% |

| | FOOD | Serving Size | Calories | Tot Fat | Sat Fat | Chol |
|---|---|---|---|---|---|---|
| ★ | Spaghetti Meat Sauce | 1/4 cup | 45 | 2% | 3% | 2% |
| ★ | Spaghetti Sauce | 1/4 cup | 30 | 0% | 0% | 0% |
| ❖ | Taco Chips | 8 chips | 120 | 11% | 5% | 0% |
| ❖ | Taco Meat | 2 tbsp | 80 | 6% | 5% | 5% |
| ★ | Taco Sauce | 2 tbsp | 10 | 0% | 0% | 0% |
| ❖ | Taco Shells | 1 shell | 60 | 6% | 3% | 0% |
| ★ | Tortilla, Flour | 1 tortilla | 110 | 4% | 3% | 0% |

★ Foods with this symbol have less than or equal to 5% *Daily Value* for <u>all</u> three nutrients (5% Rule).

❖ Foods with this symbol have <u>at least one</u> of the three nutrients greater than 5% *Daily Value* but less than or equal to 20% *Daily Value*.

Ⓐ Foods with this symbol have <u>at least one</u> of the three nutrients greater than 20% *Daily Value* (20% Rule).

# Resources

*American Institute for Cancer Research Newsletter*, Winter 1994, Issue 46:5.

Browne, Mona Boyd, RD. *Label Facts for Healthful Eating: Educator's Resource Guide*. National Food Processors Association in cooperation with FDA and FSIS. 1993.

Code of Federal Register. *Food & Drug Administration, HHS*. Part 101—Food Labeling. 1994.

Code of Federal Register. *Food Safety and Inspection Service (Meat, Poultry), USDA*. Part 317.300 to 317.400—Nutrition Labeling. 1994.

Department of Health and Human Services, Public Health Service, Food and Drug Administration, *Nutrition Labeling and Education Act of 1990: Student Manual*. Revised: May 1993.

Hildwine, Regina. "The Challenges of Nutrition Facts: The Food Industry Implement Mandatory Nutrition Labeling." *Nutrition Today*. Sep/Oct 1993: 26–29.

*How Much Sugar Is Added to Your Food?* The University of Georgia Cooperative Extension Service. December, 1993.

"The New Food Label, HFL-40." *FDA Backgrounder: Current & Useful Information from the Food & Drug Administration, BG94-2*. April 1994.

*The New Food Label*. North Dakota State University Extension Service & USDA. FN-524. June 1993.

*New Rules on Calling Foods "Healthy" Issued for All Food Products*. Food and Drug Administration, HHS.

Porter, Donna. "Food Labeling Reform: The Journey from Science to Policy." *Nutrition Today*. Sep/Oct 1993: 7–12.

Schor, Danielle, and Charles Edwards. "USDA's Role: Nutrition Labeling of Meat and Poultry Products." *Nutrition Today*. Sep/Oct 1993: 21-25.

"The Sugar Sleuth: What's Behind the Sugar Listing on the New Food Labels." *Dannon Dialogue*. Vol. 2, Issue 3, Summer 1993.

*Understanding Food Labels* (brochure). The American Dietetic Association. 1993.

*Using The Food Label* (booklet). National Food Processors Association, in cooperation with FDA and FSIS. 1993.

Wilkening, Virginia. "FDA's Regulations to Implement the NLEA." *Nutrition Today*. Sep/Oct 1993: 13–20.

# Acknowledgments

The author wishes to thank the following food manufacturers for providing product information (valid as of spring 1995) that appears in this book. Their names may be shortened in the food section due to space limitations.

Alpine Lace Brands, Inc.
American Home Foods, Inc.
Archway Cookies, Inc.
Arrowhead Mills
Barbara's Bakery, Inc.
Beatrice Cheese, Inc.
Ben & Jerry's
Blue Diamond Growers
Borden, Inc.
Bumble Bee Seafoods Inc.
Cadbury Beverages, Inc.
Calavo Foods, Inc.
Campbell Soup Company
Campbell Taggart, Inc.
Clorox Company (The)
Coca-Cola Foods
ConAgra Frozen Foods
Continental Mills, Inc.
CPC International Inc.
Dannon Company, Inc. (The)
Dean Foods Vegetable Company
Del Monte Foods
Dole Food Company
Dreyer's Grand Ice Cream
Eagle Snacks, Inc. (Anheuser Busch Company)
Estee Corporation (The)
Frito-Lay
Fromageries Bel, Inc.
General Mills, Inc.
Ghirardelli Chocolate Company

Golden Valley Microwave Foods, Inc. (A ConAgra Company)
Good Humor-Breyers Ice Cream
Guiltless Gourmet
H.J. Heinz Company
Hain Pure Foods
Health Valley Foods
Hershey Foods
Hillshire Farm & Kahn's
Hormel Foods Corporation
Hunt Wesson Foods
Imagine Foods
J.R. Knudsen
Jennie-O Foods, Inc.
Kashi Company
Keebler Company
Kellogg's
Kikkoman International Inc.
Kraft General Foods
La Victoria Foods, Inc.
Land O'Lakes, Inc.
Lawry's Foods, Inc.
Little Bear Organic Foods
Louise's, Inc.
M&M/Mars (Division of Mars, Inc.)
Malt-O-Meal Company
Mama Tish's
Manischewitz
McCormick & Company, Inc.
McKee Foods Corporation
Mother's Cake & Cookie Company

Nabisco Foods Group
Nestlé USA, Inc.
Newman's Own Inc.
Nissin Foods (USA) Company, Inc.
Ocean Spray Cranberries, Inc.
Oscar Mayer Foods Corporation
Pace Foods
Pepsi-Cola Company
Pet Inc.
Pillsbury Company (The)
Planters LifeSavers Company
Procter & Gamble Company (The)
Quaker Oats Company (The)
Reckitt & Colman
S & W Fine Foods
Saffola Quality Foods
Sara Lee Bakery
Sargento of Wisconsin
Slim-Fast Foods Company

Smucker's
Stagg Foods, Inc.
Stella D'Oro
Stonyfield Farm
Sun Luck
Sunshine Biscuits, Inc.
Taj Gourmet Foods
Thomas J. Lipton Company
Tofutti Brands, Inc.
Tootsie Roll Industries, Inc.
Tyson Foods, Inc.
Uncle Ben's, Inc.
Weight Watcher's International, Inc.
Westbrae Natural Foods
Worthington Foods, Inc.

*Other Sources:*
  $N^2$ Computing, *Nutritionist IV*
  Independent market research

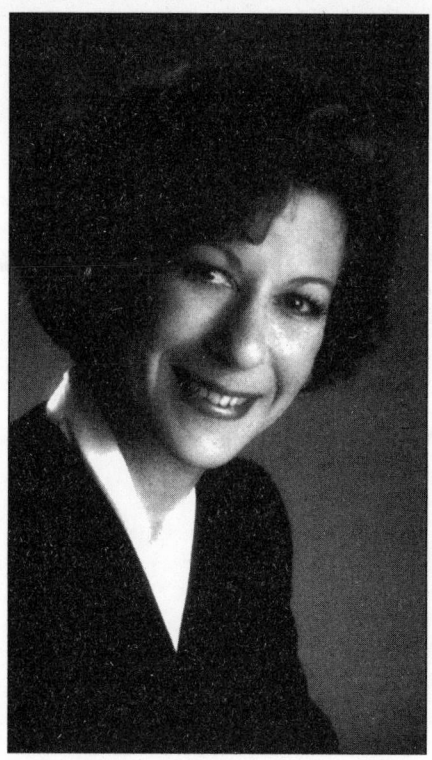

Roberta Schwartz Wennik, M.S., R.D., is the author of *Drawing the Line on Fat and Cholesterol,* a patented "connect-the-dots" approach to learning to eat less fat and cholesterol. A newspaper columnist and freelance author, her articles have appeared in such magazines as *Mature Outlook, Fit,* and *Health and Fitness.* As a nutrition educator, speaker, and writer, she has helped many achieve a healthier lifestyle. She lives and runs her consulting business, HealthPro, in Edmonds, Washington.